Textbook of Clinical Echocardiography

TEXTBOOK OF CLINICAL ECHOCARDIOGRAPHY

CATHERINE M. OTTO, MD

Professor of Medicine

Director, Training Program in Cardiovascular Disease

University of Washington School of Medicine

Associate Director, Echocardiography Laboratory

Co-Director, Adult Congenital Heart Disease Clinic

University of Washington Medical Center

Seattle, Washington

THIRD EDITION

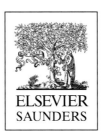

ELSEVIER
SAUNDERS

ELSEVIER
SAUNDERS
An Imprint of Elsevier

The Curtis Center
170 S Independence Mall W 300E
Philadelphia, Pennsylvania 19106

TEXTBOOK OF CLINICAL ECHOCARDIOGRAPHY
Third Edition

NOTICE

Medicine is an ever-changing field. Standard safety precautions must be followed, but as new research and clinical experience broaden our knowledge, changes in treatment and drug therapy may become necessary or appropriate. Readers are advised to check the most current product information provided by the manufacturer of each drug to be administered to verify the recommended dose, the method and duration of administration, and contraindications. It is the responsibility of the licensed prescriber, relying on experience and knowledge of the patient, to determine dosages and the best treatment for each individual patient. Neither the publisher nor the author assumes any liability for any injury and/or damage to persons or property arising from this publication.

The Publisher

Library of Congress Cataloging-in-Publication Data

Otto, Catherine M.
    Textbook of clinical echocardiography / Catherine M. Otto.—3rd ed.
        p. ; cm.
    Includes index.
    ISBN-13: 978–0–7216–0789–4   ISBN-10: 0–7216–0789–6
    1. Echocardiography. I. Title.
    [DNLM: 1. Echocardiography. 2. Hearth Diseases—ultrasonography. WG 141.5.E2 O91t 2004]
  RC683.5.U5O87 2004
  616.1′207547—dc22   2004046758

Acquisitions Editor: Anne Lenehan
Developmental Editor: Vera Ginsburgs
Production Services Manager: Joan Sinclair
Project Manager: Cecelia Bayruns

ISBN-13: 978–0–7216–0789–4
ISBN-10: 0–7216–0789–6

Printed in China

Last digit is the print number: 9 8 7 6 5 4

PREFACE
The Third Edition

Echocardiography is an integral part of clinical cardiology with important applications in the initial diagnosis, clinical management, and decision making for patients with a wide range of cardiovascular diseases. In addition to examinations performed in the echocardiography laboratory, echocardiographic techniques now are used in a variety of other clinical settings, including the coronary care unit, intensive care unit, operating room, emergency department, catheterization laboratory, and electrophysiology laboratory, both for diagnosis and for monitoring the effects of therapeutic interventions. There continues to be expansion of echocardiographic applications given the detailed and precise anatomic and physiologic information that can be obtained with this technique at relatively low cost and with minimal risk to the patient.

This textbook on general clinical echocardiography is intended to be read by individuals new to echocardiography and by those interested in updating their knowledge in this area. The text is aimed primarily at cardiology fellows on their basic echocardiography rotation but also will be of value to residents and fellows in general internal medicine, radiology, anesthesiology, and emergency medicine, as well as to cardiac sonographer students. For physicians in practice, this textbook provides a concise and practical update. A more advanced discussion of the impact of echocardiographic data in clinical medicine is available in a second book, *The Practice of Clinical Echocardiography* (CM Otto [ed], 2002), also published by Elsevier.

Introductory chapters include practical ultrasound physics, normal tomographic transthoracic and transesophageal views, flow patterns, and indications for echocardiography. A new chapter provides an introduction to other echocardiography modalities. Some of these specialized modalities are practiced by most echocardiographers and are integrated into subsequent chapters (e.g., stress, contrast, handheld echocardiography). Other echocardiographic modalities are still in development, such as three-dimensional echocar-

diography, or are utilized by cardiologists with subspecialization in interventional procedures, such as intracardiac and intravascular ultrasound. Physicians and sonographers using these advanced techniques will need to refer to the suggested readings for more information.

The remainder of the book is organized by disease category (e.g., cardiomyopathy or valvular stenosis), emphasizing a clinical (rather than a technical) approach to echocardiographic diagnosis. In each chapter, basic principles for echocardiographic evaluation of that disease category are reviewed, the echocardiographic approach and differential diagnosis are discussed in detail, limitations and technical considerations are emphasized, and alternate diagnostic approaches are delineated. Schematic diagrams are used to illustrate basic concepts; echocardiographic images and Doppler data show typical and unusual findings in patients with each disease process. Transthoracic and transesophageal images are used throughout the text, reflecting their use in clinical practice. Tables are used frequently to summarize studies validating quantitative echocardiographic methods.

At the end of each chapter a selected list of annotated references is included. These references are suggestions for the individual who is interested in reading more about a particular subject. Additional relevant articles can be found in the suggested readings or in *The Practice of Clinical Echocardiography*. An on-line medical reference database is the best place to obtain more recent publications and to obtain a comprehensive list of all journal articles on a specific topic.

In the third edition, the text of all the chapters has been revised to reflect recent advances in the field, the suggested readings have been updated, and the majority of the figures have been replaced with recent examples that more clearly illustrate the disease process. The schematic drawings have been redrawn in color and a core set of tomographic sections has been converted to full-color anatomic illustrations to improve the understanding of three-dimensional anatomic relationships in cardiac imaging. Key points now are highlighted as bulleted lists throughout the text. The chapters on diastolic function and valvular regurgitation have undergone extensive revision so that readers familiar with previous editions may want to re-read these chapters.

A special feature of the third edition that grew out of my experience teaching fellows and sonographers is a new section at the end of each chapter: The Echo Exam. This section serves as a summary of the important concepts in each chapter and provides examples of the quantitative calculations used in the day-to-day clinical practice of echocardiography. The information in The Echo Exam is arranged as lists, tables, and figures for clarity. My hope is that The Echo Exam will also serve as a quick reference guide when a review is needed and in daily practice in the echocardiography laboratory.

It should be emphasized that this textbook is only a starting point or frame of reference for learning echocardiography. Appropriate training in echocardiography includes competency in the acquisition and interpretation of echocardiographic and Doppler data in real time. Additional training is needed for performance of stress and transesophageal examinations. Further, echocardiography continues to evolve so that as new techniques, such as three-dimensional echocardiography, become practical and widely available, practitioners will need to update their knowledge. Obviously, a textbook cannot replace the experience gained in performing studies on patients with a range of disease processes, and still photographs do not replace the need for acquisition and review of real-time data. Clearly defined guidelines for training in echocardiography have been published, as referenced in Chapter 5, that provide a framework for determining clinical competency in this technique. Although this textbook is not a substitute for appropriate training and experience, I hope it will enhance the learning experience of those new to the field and provide a review for those with prior training and experience.

CATHERINE M. OTTO, MD

ACKNOWLEDGMENTS

The cardiac sonographers at the University of Washington provided invaluable input into the third edition of the *Textbook of Clinical Echocardiography* in our many sessions discussing details of image acquisition and the optimal echocardiography examination. Their skill in obtaining superb images provides the basis of many of the figures in this book. My thanks to Caryn L. D'Jang, Rachel R. Elizalde, Michelle C. Fujioka, Carolyn J. Gardner, Jessica Lane, Scott G. Simicich, Rebecca G. Schwaegler, Ren Singh, David Stolte, Erin Trent, and Todd R. Zwink.

Special thanks go to my colleagues at the University of Washington who shared their expertise and generously provided illustrations for this edition. J. David Godwin provided the chest radiographs, aortogram, computed tomography scans, and magnetic resonance images; Douglas K. Stewart provided the coronary angiograms, ventriculograms, and intravascular ultrasound images; both Steven L. Goldberg and Robert W. Rho introduced me to intravascular ultrasound and provided images; James H. Caldwell contributed examples of radionuclide studies; Dennis D. Reichenbach photographed the stenotic prosthetic valve; and Florence H. Sheehan thoughtfully prepared new three-dimensional echocardiographic examples for this book. Thanks also are extended to those individuals who kindly gave permission for reproduction of previously published figures.

The input of the University of Washington Cardiology Fellows was key in preparing this new edition. In particular, Kelley R. Branch deserves special thanks for assisting me with image acquisition. Starr Kaplan is to be commended for her skills as a medical illustrator and for providing such clear and detailed anatomic drawings. My thanks to Anne Lenehan at Elsevier for being such a supportive editor. Finally, a great deal of appreciation is due to Sharon A. Kemp, my assistant, and, of course, innumerable thanks are due to my family for their constant encouragement, patience, and support.

CONTENTS

GLOSSARY

Abbreviations Used in Figures, Tables, and Equations

2D = two-dimensional

3D = three-dimensional

A-long = apical long-axis

A-mode = amplitude mode (amplitude versus depth)

A = late (atrial) diastolic velocity peak or area (depends on context)

A2C = apical two-chamber

A4C = apical four-chamber

AcT = acceleration time

a_{dur} = duration of pulmonary venous atrial reversal velocity

A_{dur} = duration of atrial filling velocity

AF = atrial fibrillation

A_m = myocardial tissue late diastolic velocity

AMVL = anterior mitral valve leaflet

ant = anterior

Ao = aortic or aorta

AR = aortic regurgitation

AS = aortic stenosis

ASD = atrial septal defect

ASH = asymmetrical septal hypertrophy

ATVL = anterior tricuspid valve leaflet

AV = atrioventricular

AVA = aortic valve area

AVR = aortic valve replacement

BAV = balloon aortic valvuloplasty

BP = blood pressure

BSA = body surface area

C-TGA = congenitally corrected transposition of the great arteries

C = chordae

c = propagation velocity of sound in tissue

CAD = coronary artery disease

cath = cardiac catheterization

CBV = catheter balloon valvuloplasty

cm = centimeters

C_m = specific heat of tissue

cm/s = centimeters per second

CO = cardiac output

Cont eq = continuity equation valve area

cos = cosine

CS = coronary sinus

CSA = cross-sectional area

CT = computed tomography

CW = continuous wave

Cx = circumflex coronary artery

D = diameter

DA = descending aorta

dB = decibels

dP/dt = rate of change in pressure over time

DT = deceleration time

dT/dt = rate of increase in temperature

$dyne \cdot s \cdot cm^{-5}$ = units of resistance

E = early diastolic peak velocity

ECG = electrocardiogram

echo = echocardiography

ED = end-diastole

EDD = end-diastolic dimension

EDV = end-diastolic volume

EF = ejection fraction

E_m = myocardial tissue early diastolic velocity

endo = endocardium

epi = epicardium

EPSS = E-point septal separation

ES = end-systole

ESD = end-systolic dimension

ESPVR = end-systolic pressure-volume relationship

ESV = end-systolic volume

ETT = exercise treadmill test

Δf = frequency shift

f = frequency

FL = false lumen

F_n = near field

FN = false negative

F_o = resonance frequency

FP = false positive

F_s = scattered frequency

FSV = forward stroke volume

F_t = transmitted frequency

fx = function

HCM = hypertrophic cardiomyopathy

HOCM = hypertrophic obstructive cardiomyopathy

HPRF = high pulse repetition frequency

HR = heart rate

HV = hepatic vein

I = intensity of ultrasound exposure
IAS = interatrial septum
ID = indicator dilution
inf = inferior
IV = intravenous
IVC = inferior vena cava
IVCT = isovolumic contraction time
IVRT = isovolumic relaxation time
kHz = kilohertz
L = length
LA = left atrium
LAA = left atrial appendage
LAD = left anterior descending coronary artery
LAE = left atrial enlargement
lat = lateral
LCC = left coronary cusp
LLAT = left lateral
LMCA = left main coronary artery
LPA = left pulmonary artery
LSPV = left superior pulmonary vein
LV = left ventricle
LVE = left ventricular extension branch or left
    ventricular enlargement (depends on context)
LV-EDP = left ventricular end-diastolic pressure
LVH = left ventricular hypertrophy
LVI = left ventricular inflow
LVID = left ventricular internal dimension
LVO = left ventricular outflow
LVOT = left ventricular outflow tract
M = myxoma
M-mode = motion display (depth versus time)
MAC = mitral annular calcification
MB = moderator band
MI = myocardial infarction
MR = mitral regurgitation
MRI = magnetic resonance imaging
MS = mitral stenosis
MV = mitral valve
MVA = mitral valve area
MVL = mitral valve leaflet
MVR = mitral valve replacement
n = number of subjects
NBTE = nonbacterial thrombotic endocarditis
NCC = noncoronary cusp
ΔP = pressure gradient
P = pressure
PA = pulmonary artery
pAn = pseudoaneurysm
PAP = pulmonary artery pressure
PD = pulsed Doppler
PDA = patent ductus arteriosus or posterior
    descending artery (depends on context)
PE = pericardial effusion
PEP = preejection period
PET = positron-emission tomography
PISA = proximal isovelocity surface area
PLAX = parasternal long-axis
PM = papillary muscle

PMVL = posterior mitral valve leaflet
PR = pulmonic regurgitation
PRF = pulse repetition frequency
PRFR = peak rapid filling rate
PS = pulmonic stenosis
PSAX = parasternal short-axis
PTCA = percutaneous transluminal coronary
    angioplasty
PV = pulmonary vein
PV_a = pulmonary venous atrial reversal velocity
PV_D = pulmonary venous peak diastolic velocity
PV_S = pulmonary venous peak systolic velocity
PVC = premature ventricular contraction
PWT = posterior wall thickness
Q = volume flow rate
Q_p = pulmonic volume flow rate
Q_s = systemic volume flow rate
r = ventricular radius or correlation coefficient
    (depends on context)
RA = right atrium
RAE = right atrial enlargement
RAM = random access memory
RAO = right anterior oblique
RAP = right atrial pressure
RCA = right coronary artery
RCC = right coronary cusp
Re = Reynolds number
RF = regurgitant fraction
RJ = regurgitant jet
R_o = radius of microbubble
ROA = regurgitant orifice area
RPA = right pulmonary artery
RSPV = right superior pulmonary vein
RSV = regurgitant stroke volume
RV = right ventricle
RVE = right ventricular enlargement
RVH = right ventricular hypertrophy
RVI = right ventricular inflow
RVO = right ventricular outflow
RVOT = right ventricular outflow tract
SAM = systolic anterior motion
SC = subcostal
SEE = standard error of the estimate
SPPA = spatial peak pulse average
SPTA = spatial peak temporal average
SSN = suprasternal notch
ST = septal thickness
STJ = sinotubular junction
STVL = septal tricuspid valve leaflet
SV = stroke volume or sample volume (depends
    on context)
SVC = superior vena cava
SWMA = segmental wall motion abnormality
$T_{1/2}$ = pressure half-time
T = thrombus
TD = thermodilution
TEE = transesophageal echocardiography
TGA = transposition of the great arteries

TGC = time gain compensation
TL = true lumen
TN = true negatives
TOF = tetralogy of Fallot
TP = true positives
TPV = time to peak velocity
TR = tricuspid regurgitation
TS = tricuspid stenosis
TSV = total stroke volume
TTE = transthoracic echocardiography

TV = tricuspid valve
v = velocity
V = volume or velocity (depends on context)
VAS = ventriculo-atrial septum
Veg = vegetation
V_{max} = maximum velocity
VSD = ventricular septal defect
VTI = velocity-time integral
WPW = Wolff-Parkinson-White syndrome
Z = acoustic impedance

Symbol	Greek Name	Used for
α	alpha	frequency
γ	gamma	viscosity
Δ	delta	difference
θ	theta	angle
λ	lambda	wavelength
μ	mu	micro-
π	pi	mathematical constant (approx. 3.14)
ρ	rho	tissue density
σ	sigma	wall stress
τ	tau	time constant of ventricular relaxation

UNITS OF MEASURE

Variable	Unit	Definition
Amplitude	dB	Decibels = a logarithmic scale describing the amplitude ("loudness") of the sound wave
Angle	Degrees	Degree = $(\pi/180)$rad. Example: intercept angle
Area	cm^2	Square centimeters. A two-dimensional measurement (e.g., end-systolic area) or a calculated value (e.g., continuity equation valve area)
Frequency (f)	Hz	Hertz (cycles per second)
	kHz	Kilohertz = 1000 Hz
	MHz	Megahertz = 1,000,000 Hz
Length	cm	Centimeter (1/100 m)
	mm	Millimeter (1/1000 m or 1/10 cm)
Mass	g	Grams. Example: LV mass
Pressure	mm Hg	Millimeters of mercury, 1 mm Hg = 1333.2 dyne/cm^2, where dyne measures force in cm · g · s^{-2}
Resistance	dyne · s · cm^{-5}	Measure of vascular resistance
Time	S	Second
	ms	Millisecond (1/1000 s)
	μs	Microsecond
Ultrasound intensity	W/cm^2	Where watt (W) = joule per second and joule = m^2 · kg · s^{-2} (unit of energy)
	mW/cm^2	
Velocity (v)	m/s	Meters per second
	cm/s	Centimeters per second
Velocity-time integral (VTI)	cm	Integral of the Doppler velocity curve (cm/s) over time(s), in units of cm
Volume	cm^3	Cubic centimeters
	mL	Milliliter, 1 mL = 1 cm^3
	L	Liter = 1000 mL
Volume flow rate (Q)		Rate of volume flow across a valve or in cardiac output
	L/min	L/min = liters per minute
	mL/s	mL/s = milliliters per second
Wall stress	dyne/cm^2	Units of meridional or circumferential wall stress
	kdyn/cm^2	Kilodynes per cm^2
	kPa	Kilopascals where 1 kPa = 10 kdyn/cm^2

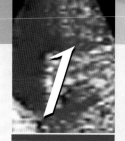

PRINCIPLES OF ECHOCARDIOGRAPHIC IMAGE ACQUISITION AND DOPPLER ANALYSIS

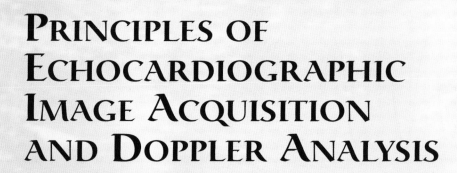

An understanding of the basic principles of ultrasound imaging and Doppler echocardiography is essential both during data acquisition and for correct interpretation of the ultrasound information. Although, at times, current instruments provide instantaneous images so clear and detailed that it seems as if we can "see" the heart and blood flow directly, in actuality, we always are looking at images and flow data generated by complex analyses of ultrasound waves reflected and backscattered from the patient's body. Knowledge of the strengths of this technique and, more importantly, its limitations is critical for correct clinical diagnosis and patient treatment. On one hand, echocardiography can be used for decision making with a high degree of accuracy in a variety of clinical settings. On the other hand, if an ultrasound artifact is mistaken for an anatomic abnormality, a patient might undergo needless, expensive, and potentially risky diagnostic tests or therapeutic interventions.

In this chapter, a brief (and necessarily simplified) overview of the basic principles of cardiac ultrasound imaging and flow analysis is presented.

The reader is referred to the Suggested Reading at the end of the chapter for more information on these subjects. Because the details of image processing, artifact formation, and Doppler physics become more meaningful with experience, some readers may choose to return to this chapter after reading other sections of this book and after participating in some echocardiographic examinations.

BASIC PRINCIPLES OF ULTRASOUND

Ultrasound Waves

Sound waves are mechanical vibrations that induce alternate refractions and compressions of any physical medium through which they pass. Like other waves, sound waves are described in terms of (Fig. 1–1)

- frequency–cycles per second, or hertz (Hz),
- wavelength–millimeters (mm),
- amplitude–decibels (dB),
- velocity of propagation.

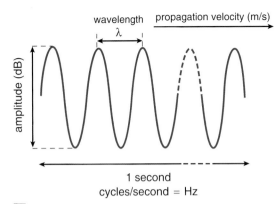

FIGURE 1–1. Schematic diagram of an ultrasound wave.

The velocity of propagation depends on each carrying medium and is approximately 1540 m/s in blood.

Humans can hear sound waves with frequencies between 20 Hz and 20 kHz; frequencies higher than this range are termed *ultrasound*. Diagnostic medical ultrasound typically uses transducers with a frequency between 1 million and 20 million Hz or 1 and 20 MHz.

Wavelength (λ) times frequency (f) equals the propagation velocity c:

$$c = \lambda f \qquad (1\text{–}1)$$

Because the propagation velocity in the heart is constant at 1540 m/sec, the wavelength for any transducer frequency can be calculated as

$$\lambda \,(\text{mm}) = 1.54 / f \,(\text{MHz}) \qquad (1\text{–}2)$$

as shown in Figure 1–2. Wavelength is important in diagnostic applications for at least two reasons:

■ Image resolution is no greater than 1 to 2 wavelengths (typically about 1 mm).
■ The depth of penetration of the ultrasound wave into the body is directly related to wavelength—shorter wavelengths penetrate a shorter distance than longer wavelengths.

Thus, there is an obvious tradeoff between image resolution (shorter wavelength or higher frequency preferable) and depth penetration (longer wavelength or lower frequency preferable).

The *amplitude* (e.g., "loudness") of an ultrasound wave is described in terms of decibels. Decibels (dB) are logarithmic units based on a ratio of the measured value V of acoustic pressure to a reference value R such that

$$\text{dB} = 20 \log(V/R) \qquad (1\text{–}3)$$

Thus a ratio of 10,000 to 1 is

$$20 \times \log(10,000) = 20 \times 4 = 80 \,\text{dB}$$

a ratio of 1000 to 1 is

$$20 \times \log(1000) = 20 \times 3 = 60 \,\text{dB}$$

a ratio of 100 to 1 is

$$20 \times \log(100) = 20 \times 2 = 40 \,\text{dB}$$

and a ratio of 2 to 1 is

$$20 \times \log(2) = 20 \times 0.3 = 6 \,\text{dB}$$

A simple rule to remember is that a 6-dB change represents a doubling or halving of the

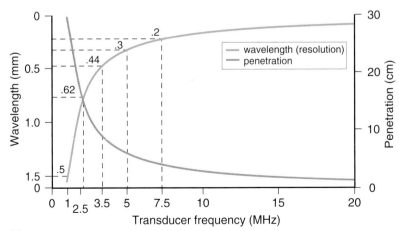

FIGURE 1–2. Graph of transducer frequency (*horizontal axis*) versus wavelength and penetration of the ultrasound signal in soft tissue. Wavelength has been plotted inversely to show that resolution increases with increasing transducer frequency while penetration decreases. The specific wavelengths for transducer frequencies of 1, 2.5, 3.5, 5, and 7.5 MHz are shown.

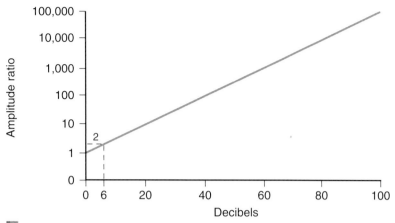

FIGURE 1–3. Graph of the decibel scale (*horizontal axis*) showing the logarithmic relationship with the amplitude ratio (*vertical axis*). Note that a doubling or halving of the amplitude ratio corresponds to a 6-dB change.

signal amplitude (Fig. 1–3). The advantages of the decibel scale are that a very large range can be compressed into a smaller number of values and that low-amplitude (weak) signals can be displayed alongside very high-amplitude (strong) signals.

Interaction of Ultrasound Waves with Tissues

The interaction of ultrasound waves with the organs and tissues of the body can be described in terms of (Fig. 1–4):

- reflection,
- scattering,
- refraction, and
- attenuation.

Reflection

The basis of ultrasound imaging is *reflection* of the transmitted ultrasound signal from internal structures. Ultrasound is reflected at tissue boundaries and interfaces, with the amount of ultrasound reflected dependent on the relative change in acoustic impedance between the two tissues. Acoustic impedance Z depends on tissue density (p) and on the propagation velocity in that tissue (c):

$$Z = pc \qquad (1\text{–}4)$$

Differences in acoustic impedance largely relate to differences in tissue density, but the velocity of propagation can differ as well (e.g., bone has a propagation velocity about twice as fast as blood). Smooth tissue boundaries with a lateral dimension greater than the wavelength of the ultrasound beam act as specular, or "mirror-like," reflectors. The amount of ultrasound reflected is constant for

a given interface, although the amount received back at the transducer varies with angle because (like light reflected from a mirror) the angle of incidence and reflection is equal. Optimal return of reflected ultrasound occurs at a perpendicular angle (90°). Remembering this fact is crucial for obtaining diagnostic ultrasound images. It also accounts for ultrasound "dropout" in a two-dimensional (2D) image when too little or no reflected ultrasound reaches the transducer due to a parallel alignment between the ultrasound beam and tissue interface.

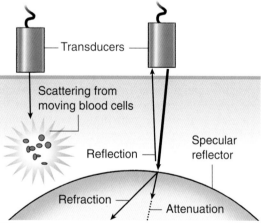

FIGURE 1–4. Diagram of the interaction between ultrasound and body tissues. Doppler analysis is based on the scattering of ultrasound in all directions from moving blood cells with a resulting change in frequency of the ultrasound received at the transducer. 2D imaging is based on reflection of ultrasound from tissue interfaces (specular reflectors). Attenuation limits the depth of ultrasound penetration. Refraction, a change in direction of the ultrasound wave, results in imaging artifacts.

Scattering

Small structures (<1 wavelength in lateral dimension) result in *scattering* of the ultrasound signal instead of reflection. Unlike a reflected beam, scattered ultrasound energy may be radiated in all directions. Only a small amount of the scattered signal reaches the receiving transducer, and the amplitude of a scattered signal is 100 to 1000 times (40–60 dB) less than the amplitude of the returned signal from a specular reflector. Scattering of ultrasound from moving blood cells is the basis of Doppler echocardiography. While some argue that the size of a single red blood cell (7–10 μm) is so much smaller (20 times) than the wavelength of ultrasound (0.2–1 mm) that it is unlikely to be an effective scatterer, most investigators consider that detectable scattering occurs due to thousands of blood cells being present in the sound beam. However, the evidence suggests that variation in hematocrit over the clinical range has little effect on the Doppler signal as used in clinical applications.

Refraction

Ultrasound waves can be *refracted*–deflected from a straight path–as they pass through a medium with a different acoustic impedance. Refraction of an ultrasound beam is analogous to refraction of light waves as they pass through a curved glass lens (e.g., prescription eyeglasses). Refraction allows enhanced image quality by using acoustic "lenses" to focus the ultrasound beam. However, refraction also occurs in unplanned ways during image formation, resulting in ultrasound artifacts, most notably the "double-image" artifact.

Attenuation

As ultrasound penetrates into the body, signal strength is progressively *attenuated* due to absorption of the ultrasound energy by conversion to heat, as well as by reflection and scattering. Overall attenuation is frequency dependent such that lower ultrasound frequencies penetrate deeper into the body than higher frequencies. The depth of penetration for adequate imaging tends to be limited to approximately 200 wavelengths. This translates roughly into a penetration depth of 30 cm for a 1-MHz transducer, 6 cm for a 5-MHz transducer, and 1.5 cm for a 20-MHz transducer, although diagnostic images at depths greater than these postulated limits can be obtained with state-of-the-art equipment.

Clinically, attenuation, as much as resolution, dictates the need for a particular transducer frequency in a specific clinical setting. For example, visualization of distal structures from the apical approach in a large adult patient often requires a low-frequency transducer. From a transesophageal approach, the same structures can be imaged (at better resolution) with a higher-frequency transducer.

Attenuation also depends on acoustic impedance and on the mismatch in impedance between adjacent structures. This factor is important in transducer design so that the signal is not attenuated significantly before it leaves the transducer. It also is important during the examination. Because air has a very high acoustic impedance, any air between the transducer and the cardiac structures of interest results in substantial signal attenuation. This is avoided on transthoracic examinations by use of a water-soluble gel to form an airless contact between the transducer and the skin and on transesophageal examination by maintaining close contact between the transducer and the esophageal wall. The air-filled lungs are avoided by careful patient positioning and the use of acoustic "windows" that allow access of the ultrasound beam to the cardiac structures without intervening lung tissue. Other intrathoracic air (e.g., pneumomediastinum, residual air after cardiac surgery) results in poor ultrasound tissue penetration due to attenuation, resulting in suboptimal image quality.

TRANSDUCERS

Piezoelectric Crystal

Ultrasound transducers use a piezoelectric crystal both to generate and to receive ultrasound waves (Fig. 1–5). A piezoelectric crystal is a material (such as quartz or a titanate ceramic) with the property that applied electric current results in alignment of polarized particles perpendicular to the face of the crystal with consequent expansion of crystal size. When an alternating electric current is applied, the crystal alternately compresses and expands, generating an ultrasound wave. The frequency that a transducer emits depends on the nature and thickness of the piezoelectric material.

Conversely, when an ultrasound wave strikes the piezoelectric crystal, an electric current is generated. Thus, the crystal can serve both as a "receiver" and as a "transmitter." The ultrasound transducer transmits a brief burst of ultrasound and then switches to the "receive mode" to await the reflected ultrasound signals from the intracardiac acoustic interfaces. This cycle is repeated temporally and spatially to generate ultrasound images. Image formation is based on the *time delay* between ultrasound transmission and return of

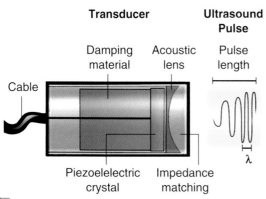

FIGURE 1-5. Schematic diagram of an ultrasound transducer. The piezoelectric crystal both produces and receives ultrasound signals, with the electric input/output transmitted to the instrument via the cable. Damping material allows a short pulse length (improved resolution). The shape of the piezoelectric crystal, an acoustic lens, or electronic focusing (with a phased-array transducer) are used to modify the beam geometry. The material of the transducer surface provides impedance matching with the skin. The ultrasound pulse length for 2D imaging is short (1–6 ms), typically consisting of two wavelengths (l). "Ring down"—the decrease in frequency and amplitude in the pulse—depends on damping and determines bandwidth (the range of frequencies in the signal).

the reflected signal. Deeper structures have a longer time of flight than shallower structures, with the exact depth calculated based on the speed of sound in blood and the interval between the transmitted burst of ultrasound and return of the reflected signal.

The burst, or pulse, of ultrasound generated by the piezoelectric crystal is very brief, typically 1 to 6 ms, because a short pulse length results in improved axial (along the length of the beam) resolution. Damping material is used to control the ring-down time of the crystal and, hence, the pulse length. Pulse length also is determined by frequency, because a shorter time is needed for the same number of cycles at higher frequencies.

The range of frequencies contained in the pulse is described as its *frequency bandwidth*. A wider bandwidth allows better axial resolution due to the ability of the system to produce a narrow pulse. Transducer bandwidth also affects the range of frequencies that can be detected by the system with a wider bandwidth allowing better resolution of structures distant from the transducer. The stated frequency of a transducer represents the center frequency of the pulse.

Types of Transducers

The simplest type of ultrasound transducer is based on a single piezoelectric crystal (Table 1–1).

Alternate pulsed transmission and reception periods allow repeated sampling along a single line, with the sampling rate limited only by the time delay needed for return of the reflected ultrasound wave from the depth of interest. Single nonmoving crystal transducers are used for A-mode (amplitude versus depth) or M-mode (depth versus time) cardiac recordings when a high sampling rate is desirable.

Formation of a tomographic cardiac ultrasound image is based on mechanical or electronic sweeping of the ultrasound beam across the plane of interest. This type of tomographic imaging—*sector scanning*—is used for cardiac applications, rather than a linear array of parallel ultrasound beams, to allow a faster frame rate (to show cardiac motion) and because the smaller transducer size (aperture or "footprint") fits into the narrow acoustic windows used in echocardiography. Mechanical sector scanners actually move the crystal in the transducer in either a rotational or a "wobble" fashion. Mechanical transducers have the advantage of a high signal-to-noise ratio but the disadvantages of limited Doppler capabilities and potential mechanical malfunction and now are rarely used for cardiac applications. A phased-array sector scanner consists of a series of ultrasound crystals arranged so that the beam can be electronically "steered" using combinations of the available elements. There are no moving parts prone to malfunction, and all Doppler modalities can be performed. The phased-array transducer currently is the most common type of transducer used for echocardiography.

TABLE 1–1
Ultrasound Transducers

Piezoelectric Crystal Arrangements

Single (or double) crystal
Mechanical
Phased-array
Annular array

Types

Transthoracic
Transesophageal
Intravascular

Characteristics

Frequency
Focal depth
Bandwidth
Aperture ("footprint")
Power output

Continuous-wave Doppler examinations use two crystals of a phased-array transducer or two separate crystals in a dedicated nonimaging transducer, with one crystal continuously transmitting and the other continuously receiving the ultrasound waves.

Beam Shape and Focusing

Beam shape and size vary predictably with distance from the transducer. However, the three-dimensional (3D) shape of the ultrasound beam generated by a transducer is complex (Fig. 1–6) and depends on several factors, some of which can be manipulated in the design of the transducer and some of which are inherent to ultrasound physics. For an unfocused beam, the initial segment of the beam is columnar in shape (near field F_n) with a length dependent on the diameter D of the transducer face and wavelength λ:

$$F_n = D^2/4\lambda \qquad (1\text{-}5)$$

For a 3.5-MHz transducer with a 5-mm diameter aperture, this corresponds to a columnar length of 1.4 cm. Beyond this region, the ultrasound beam diverges (far field), with the angle of divergence θ determined as

$$\sin\theta = 1.22\lambda/D \qquad (1\text{-}6)$$

This equation indicates a divergence angle of 6° beyond the near field, resulting in an ultrasound beam width of approximately 4.4 cm at a depth of 20 cm for this 3.5-MHz transducer. With a 10-mm diameter aperture, F_n would be 5.7 cm

and beam width at 20 cm would be approximately 2.5 cm (Fig. 1–7).

The shape and focal depth (narrowest point) of the primary beam can be altered by making the surface of the piezoelectric crystal concave or by addition of an acoustic lens. This allows generation of a beam with optimal characteristics at the depth of most cardiac structures, but again, divergence of the beam beyond the focal zone occurs. Some transducers allow manipulation of the focal zone during the examination. Even with focusing, the ultrasound beam generated by each transducer has a lateral (azimuthal) and an elevational dimension that depends on the transducer aperture, frequency, and focusing. Beam geometry for phased-array transducers also depends on the size, spacing, and arrangement of the piezoelectric crystals in the array.

In addition to the main ultrasound beam, dispersion of ultrasound energy laterally from a single-crystal transducer results in formation of side lobes at an angle u from the central beam where $\sin\theta = m\lambda/D$, and m is an integer describing sequential side lobes (i.e., 1, 2, 3, and so on) (Fig. 1–8). Reflected or backscattered signals from these side lobes may be received by the transducer, resulting in image or flow artifacts. With phased-array transducers, additional accessory beams termed *grating lobes* also occur as a result of constructive interference of ultrasound wave fronts (Fig. 1–9). Both the side lobes and the grating lobes affect the lateral (azimuthal) resolution of the transducer.

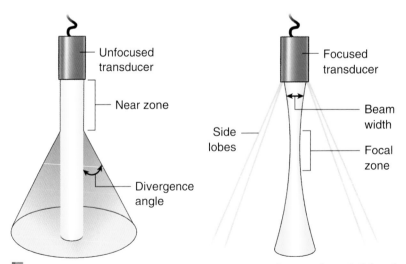

FIGURE 1–6. Schematic diagram of beam geometry for an unfocused (*left*) and focused (*right*) transducer. The length of the near zone and the divergence angle in the far field depend on transducer frequency and aperture. The focal zone of a focused transducer can be adjusted, but beam width still depends on depth. Side lobes (and grating lobes with phased-array transducers) occur with both focused and unfocused transducers and, like the central beam, are three-dimensional.

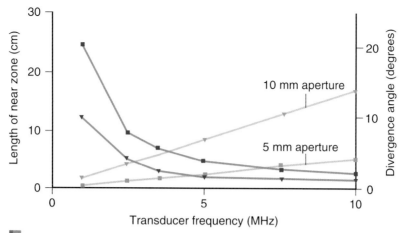

FIGURE 1–7. Graph of transducer frequency (*horizontal axis*) versus length of the near zone (*yellow lines*) and divergence angle (*blue lines*) for an unfocused 5- (*squares*) and 10-mm (*triangles*) diameter aperture transducer. Equations (1.5) and (1.6) were used to generate these curves.

FIGURE 1–8. *Top:* Diagram showing the positions at which side lobes will form. Side lobes occur at the points where the distances traversed by the ultrasound pulse from each edge of the crystal face differ by exactly one wavelength. Note that the distance from the left edge of the crystal point at point P_1 to the position of side lobe 1 is exactly one wavelength longer than the distance from point P_2 at the extreme right edge of the crystal to the position of side lobe 1. *Bottom:* The beam intensity plot formed by sweeping along an arc at focal length F. (From Geiser EA: Chapter 25. In: Skorton DJ, Schelbert AR, Wolf GL, Brundage BH (eds): Marcus Cardiac Imaging, 2nd ed. Philadelphia: WB Saunders, 1996, p 280. Used with permission.)

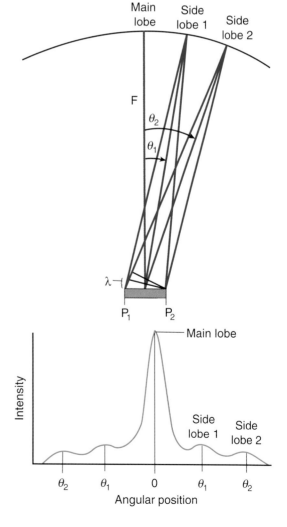

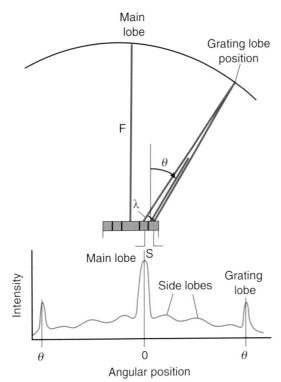

FIGURE 1-9. *Top:* Diagram showing the position of grating lobes in phased-array transducers. The position of grating lobes is determined by the spacing between the centers of independent crystal elements in the transducer. At any point where the path length between the two crystal elements differs by one wavelength, a grating lobe is formed. The grating lobe is formed at an angle u that depends on the wavelength l of the crystals and spacing S between the crystal elements. *Bottom:* The beam intensity plot formed at focal length F. (From Geiser EA: Chapter 25. In: Skorton DJ, Schelbert AR, Wolf GL, Brundage BH (eds): Marcus Cardiac Imaging, 2nd ed. Philadelphia: WB Saunders, 1996, p 283. Used with permission.)

Resolution

Image resolution occurs for each of three dimensions (Table 1-2): (1) *axial resolution,* that is, along the length of the ultrasound beam; (2) *lateral* or *azimuthal resolution,* that is, the resolution side to side across the 2D image; and (3) *elevational resolution,* that is, the thickness of the tomographic "slice."

Of these three resolutions, axial resolution is most precise, so quantitative measurements are made most reliably using data derived from a perpendicular alignment between the ultrasound beam and the structure of interest (Fig. 1-10). Axial resolution depends on the transducer frequency, bandwidth, and pulse length. Because the smallest resolvable distance between two specular reflectors with conventional ultra-

TABLE 1-2
Determinants of Resolution in 2D Imaging
Axial Resolution
Transducer frequency
Transducer bandwidth
Pulse length
Lateral (Azimuthal) Resolution
Transducer frequency
Beam width (focusing) at each depth*
Aperture (width) of transducer
Bandwidth
Side and grating lobe levels
Elevational Resolution
Transducer frequency
Beam width in elevational plane

*Most important.

sound is 1 wavelength, higher-frequency (shorter-wavelength) transducers have greater axial resolution. A wider bandwidth also improves resolution by allowing a shorter pulse, thus avoiding overlap between the reflected ultrasound signals from two adjacent reflectors.

Lateral resolution varies with the depth of the specular reflector from the transducer, being most dependent on beam width at each depth. With a

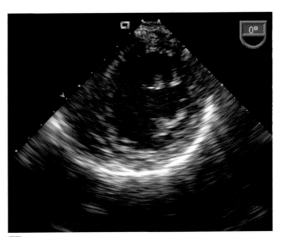

FIGURE 1-10. Two-dimensional echocardiographic view of the left ventricle from a transesophageal approach at end-diastole. Even with excellent image quality, as in this example, the effect of beam width can be appreciated by comparing the length of reflections from the endocardium near the transducer and more distal reflectors (point 2). Note the relative "dropout" of the epicardium and endocardium when parallel to the ultrasound beam.

narrow beam width in the focal region, lateral resolution may approach axial resolution, and a point target will appear as a point on the 2D image. At greater depths, beam width diverges so a point target results in a reflected signal as wide as the beam width. The lack of lateral resolution at greater depths accounts for the "blurring" of the image in the far field. If the 2D image is examined carefully, progressive widening of the echo signals from similar targets along the ultrasound beam can be appreciated. Erroneous interpretations occur when the effects of beam width are not recognized. For example, beam width artifact from a strong specular reflector in the tomographic plane may appear as a linear abnormal structure. Other factors that affect lateral resolution are transducer frequency, aperture, bandwidth, and side and grating lobe levels.

Resolution in the elevational plane is more difficult to recognize on the 2D image but is equally important in the echocardiographic examination. The thickness of the tomographic plane is variable over the 2D image, depending on transducer design and focusing, both of which affect beam width in the elevational plane at each depth. In general, cardiac ultrasound images have a "thickness" of approximately 3 to 10 mm depending on depth and the specific transducer used. The tomographic image generated by the instrument, in effect, includes reflected and backscattered signals from this entire thickness. Strong reflectors adjacent to the image plane may appear to be "in" the image plane due to elevational beam width. Even more distant strong reflectors may appear superimposed on the tomographic plane due to side lobes in the elevational plane. Examples include a calcified aortic valve appearing as a "mass" in the left atrium on apical views or a linear echo in the aortic lumen from an adjacent calcified atheroma appearing as a possible dissection flap.

These principles of ultrasound imaging also apply to 3D echocardiography as discussed in Chapter 4.

ULTRASOUND INSTRUMENTS AND IMAGING MODALITIES

A-Mode/M-Mode

Historically, cardiac ultrasound began with a single-crystal transducer display of the amplitude (*A*) of reflected ultrasound versus depth on an oscilloscope screen. An A-mode display may still be shown on the 2D image screen to aid the examiner in optimal adjustment of the instrument controls. Repeated pulse transmission and receive cycles allow rapid updating of the amplitude

versus depth information so that rapidly moving structures, such as the aortic or mitral valve leaflets, can be identified by their characteristic timing and pattern of motion (Fig. 1–11).

With the time dimension shown explicitly on the horizontal axis and each amplitude signal along the length of the ultrasound beam converted to a corresponding gray-scale level, a *motion (M) mode display* is produced. M-mode recordings originally were made by rolling light-sensitive paper under the brightness versus depth display. Now the M-mode data can be recorded on paper or shown on the video monitor either "scrolling" or "sweeping" across the screen at 50 to 100 mm/s. While a single-crystal transducer had to be aligned based on the M-mode output alone, 2D imaging allows guidance of the M-mode beam to ensure an appropriate angle between the M line and the structures of interest.

Because only a single "line of sight" is included in an A-mode or M-mode tracing, the repetition frequency of the pulse transmission and receive phase of the transducer (the pulse repetition frequency) is limited only by the time needed for the ultrasound beam to travel to the maximum depth of interest and back to the transducer. Even a depth of 20 cm requires only 0.26 ms (given a speed of propagation of 1540 m/s), allowing a pulse frequency up to 3850 times per second. In actual practice, sampling rates of about 1800 times per second are used. This extremely high sampling rate is valuable for accurate evaluation of rapid normal intracardiac motion such as valve

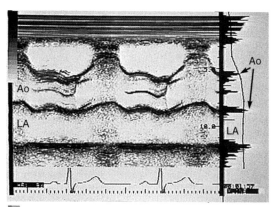

FIGURE 1–11. An A-mode (along right edge) and M-mode recording of aortic root (Ao), left atrium (LA), and aortic valve motion. On the A-mode recording, the anterior and posterior aortic root (with valve closure in the center) and posterior left atrial wall are clearly identified. The rapid sampling rate of M-mode recording allows visualization of aortic valve motion. The line representing the time gain compensation curve is shown at the right of the image, superimposed on the A-mode signal.

opening and closing. It also allows detection of high-frequency fluttering of the anterior mitral leaflet in patients with aortic regurgitation and the rapid oscillating motion of valvular vegetations. In addition, continuously moving structures, such as the ventricular endocardium, may be identified more accurately when motion versus time, as well as depth, is displayed clearly on the M-mode recording.

Two-dimensional Echocardiography

Image Production

A 2D echocardiographic image is generated from the data obtained by mechanically or electronically "sweeping" the ultrasound beam across the tomographic plane. Because a finite time is needed for each scan line of data (depending on the depth of interest), the time needed to acquire all the data for one image frame is directly related to the number of scan lines. Thus, there is a tradeoff between scan line density and image frame rate– the number of images per second. For cardiac applications, a high frame rate ($\geq$30 frames per second) is desirable for accurate display of cardiac motion. This frame rate allows 33 ms per frame or 128 scan lines per 2D image at a displayed depth of 20 cm.

The reflected ultrasound signals for each scan line are received by the piezoelectric crystal and a small electric signal generated with (1) an amplitude proportional to incident angle and acoustic impedance, and (2) timing proportional to distance from the transducer. This signal undergoes complex manipulation to form the final image displayed on the monitor. Typical processing includes signal amplification, time-gain compensation, filtering (to reduce noise), compression, and rectification. Envelope detection generates a bright spot for each signal along the scan line, which then undergoes analog-to-digital scan conversion, since the original polar coordinate data must be fit to a rectangular matrix with appropriate interpolation for missing matrix elements. This image is subject to further "postprocessing" to enhance the visual appreciation of tomographic anatomy and is displayed in "real time" (nearly simultaneous with data acquisition) on the monitor screen.

While standard ultrasound imaging is based on reflection of the fundamental transmitted frequency from tissue interfaces, *tissue harmonic imaging* instead is based on the harmonic frequency energy generated as the ultrasound signal propagates through the tissues. These harmonic frequencies result from the nonlinear effects of the interaction of ultrasound with tissue and have two

properties key to generation of harmonic images. First, the strength of the harmonic signal increases with depth of propagation. Second, stronger fundamental frequencies produce stronger harmonics. Thus harmonic imaging reduces near-field and side lobe artifacts and improves endocardial definition, particularly in patients with poor fundamental frequency images (Fig. 1–12). Because valves and other planar objects may appear thicker than normal with harmonic imaging, most examiners use both standard and harmonic imaging as needed throughout the examination.

Instrument Settings

Many of the elements in the process of image formation are features of a particular instrument that cannot be modified by the operator. Other elements can be manipulated as data are acquired ("preprocessing") or as stored data are reviewed ("postprocessing"). Incorporation of a continuous-loop digital memory to store a series (16–128) of polar images in random access memory facilitates the evaluation of the effect of postprocessing options on the displayed image.

Standard imaging controls available in most ultrasound systems include:

■ *Power output*: This control adjusts the total ultrasound energy delivered by the transducer in the transmitted bursts, thus resulting in higher-amplitude reflected signals (see "Bioeffects and Safety").

■ *Gain*: In contrast to power output, the gain control adjusts the displayed amplitude of the received signals, similar to the volume control in an audio system.

■ *Time-gain compensation* (TGC): The TGC panel allows differential adjustment of gain along the length of the ultrasound beam. Near-field gain can be set lower (because reflected signals are stronger) with a gradually increased gain over the midfield ("ramp" or "slope") and a higher gain in the far field (since reflected signals are weaker). A TGC curve is shown at the right side of Figure 1–11. On some instruments, near-field and far-field gains beyond the range of the TGC are adjusted separately.

■ *Depth*: The displayed depth affects the pulse repetition frequency and frame rate of the image, as well as allowing maximal display of the area of interest on the screen. Standard depth settings show the entire plane (from the transducer down), while "resolution" or "magnification" modes focus on a specific depth range of interest.

■ *Gray scale/dynamic range*: The number of levels of gray in the image, or *dynamic range,* can be

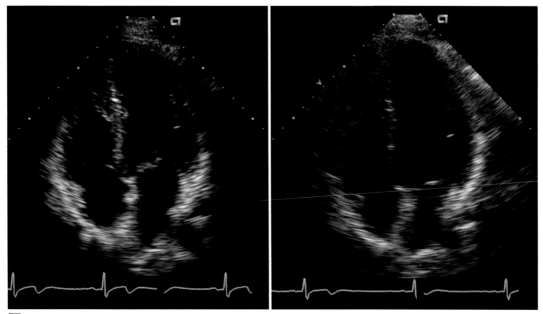

■ FIGURE 1–12. Images obtained in an apical four-chamber view with tissue harmonic imaging (*left*) show improved endocardial definition and reduced near-field artifact compared to standard fundamental frequency images (*right*).

adjusted to provide an image with marked contrast between light and dark areas or a gradation of gray levels between the lightest and darkest areas. A variation of standard gray scale is to use a color intensity for each amplitude value.

Other typical instrument controls include preprocessing and postprocessing settings that change the appearance of the displayed image. Note that image quality and resolution depend on scan-line density (as well as the factors listed in Table 1–2). Scan-line density (or frame rate or both) can be increased by using a lower depth setting or by narrowing the sector to less than the standard 60° wide image.

Imaging Artifacts

Imaging artifacts include (1) extraneous ultrasound signals that result in the appearance of "structures" that are not actually present (at least at that location), (2) failure to visualize structures that are present, and (3) an image of a structure that differs in size and/or shape from its actual appearance. Obviously, recognition of image artifacts is important for both the individual performing the study and the individual interpreting the echocardiographic data (Table 1–3).

The most common image "artifact" is *suboptimal image quality* due to poor ultrasound tissue penetration related to the patient's body habitus

with interposition of high-impedance tissues (e.g., adipose tissue, lung, or bone) between the transducer and cardiac structures. While, strictly speaking, poor image quality is not an "artifact," a low signal-to-noise ratio makes accurate diagnosis difficult and precludes quantitative measurements. In many patients with suboptimal ultrasound penetration, image quality often is improved by use of tissue harmonic imaging. In some cases, transesophageal imaging may be needed to make an accurate diagnosis.

Acoustic shadowing (Fig. 1–13) occurs when a structure with a marked difference in acoustic impedance (e.g., prosthetic valve, calcium) blocks transmission of the ultrasound wave beyond that point. The image appears devoid of reflected signals distal to this structure, because no signal penetrates beyond the shadowing structure. The shape of the shadow (like a light shadow) follows the ultrasound path, so that a small structure near the transducer casts a large shadow. When shadowing occurs, an alternate acoustic window is needed for evaluation of the area of interest. In some cases, a different transthoracic view will suffice. In other cases (e.g., prosthetic mitral valve), transesophageal imaging may be necessary.

Reverberations (Figs. 1–14 and 1–15) are multiple linear high-amplitude echo signals originating from two strong specular reflectors and resulting in a back-and-forth reflection of the ultrasound

TABLE 1–3

Ultrasound Imaging Artifacts

Artifact	Mechanism	Example(s)
Suboptimal image quality	Poor ultrasound tissue penetration	Body habitus (obesity, lung disease) Postcardiac surgery
Acoustic shadowing	Reflection of all the ultrasound signal by a strong specular reflector	Prosthetic valve Calcification
Reverberations	Reverberation between two strong parallel reflectors	Prosthetic valve
Beam width	Superimposition of structures within the beam profile (including side lobes) into a single tomographic image	Aortic valve "in" left atrium Atheroma "in" aortic lumen
Lateral resolution	Displayed width of a point target varies with depth	Excessive width of calcified mass or prosthetic valve
Refraction	Deviation of ultrasound signal from a straight path along the scan line	Double aortic valve or left ventricular image in short-axis view
Range ambiguity	Echo from previous pulse reaches transducer on next cycle	Second, deeper, heart image
Electronic processing	Instrument-specific	Variable

signal before it returns to the transducer. On the image, reverberations appear as relatively parallel, irregular, dense lines extending from the structure into the far field. Like acoustic shadowing, prominent reverberations limit evaluation of structures in the far field. In less dramatic cases,

reverberations may appear to represent abnormal structures. For example, in the parasternal long-axis view, a linear echo in the aortic root may originate as a reverberation from anterior structures (e.g., ribs) rather than representing a dissection flap.

The term *beam width artifact* is applied to two separate sources of image artifacts. First, remember that all the structures within the 3D volume

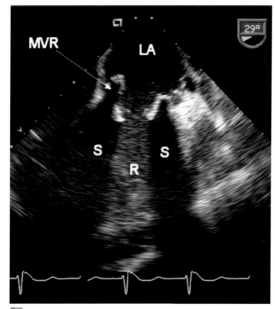

■ FIGURE 1–13. Example of acoustic shadowing and reverberations. Transesophageal view of the left atrium (LA) and left ventricle shows shadowing (S) by the sewing ring of a tissue mitral valve with reverberations (R) from the valve further obscuring the left ventricle.

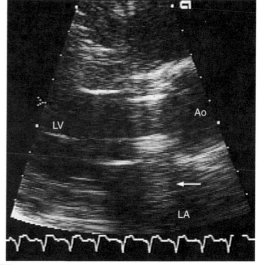

■ FIGURE 1–14. An example of reverberations on transthoracic imaging. Parasternal long-axis view of a mechanical aortic valve prosthesis with reverberations (*arrow*) obscuring the left atrium.

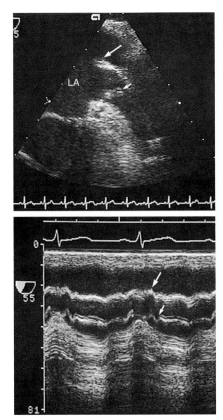

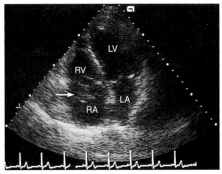

FIGURE 1-16. Example of beam width artifact. Apparent "mass" in the right atrium (*arrow*) in the apical four-chamber view is beam width artifact from a calcified aortic valve.

FIGURE 1-15. Reverberation artifact on transesophageal echocardiography (*top*) with the reverberation from the prominent ridge between the left atrial appendage (*large arrow*) mimicking the appearance of a mass in the left atrial appendage (*small arrow*). M-mode (*bottom*) shows the artifact motion (*small arrow*) parallels that of the atrial ridge (*large arrow*). With a slight change in transducer position, this artifact was no longer seen.

reflected signal. For example, the struts on a prosthetic valve can appear much longer than their actual dimension due to poor lateral resolution. Sometimes, beam width artifacts can be mistaken for abnormal structures such as a valvular vegetation, an intracardiac mass, or an aortic dissection flap.

The appearance of a side-by-side double image results from ultrasound *refraction* as it passes through a tissue proximal to the structure of interest. This artifact often is seen in parasternal short-axis views of the aortic valve or left ventricle, where a second valve or left ventricle is "seen" medial to and partly overlapping the actual valve or left ventricle (Fig. 1–17). The explanation for this appearance is that the transmitted ultrasound beam is deviated from a straight path (the scan line) by refraction as it passes through a tissue

of the ultrasound beam are displayed in a single tomographic plane. In the focal zone of the beam, the 3D volume is quite small and the tomographic "slice" is narrow. In the far zone, however, strong reflectors at the edge of a larger beam will be superimposed on structures in the central zone of the beam although signal intensity falls off at the edges of the beam. In addition, strong reflectors in side lobes of the beam will be displayed in the tomographic section corresponding to the main beam. This type of beam width artifact can result in an image "showing" a calcified aortic valve in the middle of the atrium in an apical four-chamber view (Fig. 1–16).

The second type of beam width artifact is a consequence of varying lateral resolution at different imaging depths. A point target appears as a line whose length depends on the beam characteristics at that depth and the amplitude of the

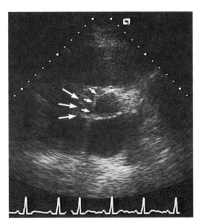

FIGURE 1-17. Example of refraction. An overlapping double image of the aortic valve is seen in a parasternal short-axis view due to refraction of the ultrasound beam by intervening tissues. The actual (*short arrows*) and duplicate aortic valves (*long arrows*) are indicated.

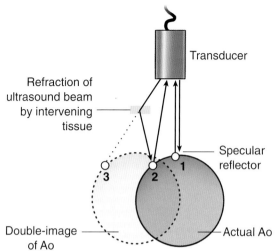

FIGURE 1–18. Schematic diagram showing the mechanism of a double-image artifact on 2D echocardiography. An ultrasound pulse reflected from point 1 of the left ventricular endocardium returns to the transducer and is shown appropriately as a bright spot in the correct position on the 2D image. Later in the scan, an ultrasound pulse is refracted by an intervening tissue so that the beam is reflected back to the transducer from point 2. However, this reflected signal is shown along the transmission scan line (point 3) because this is the presumed origin of the reflected signal. Ao, aorta in cross-section.

near the transducer. When this refracted beam is reflected by the endocardium back to the transducer, the reflected signal is assumed to have originated from the scan line of the transmitted pulse (Fig. 1–18) and thus is displayed on the image in the wrong location.

Range ambiguity occurs when echo signals from an earlier pulse cycle reach the transducer on the next "listen cycle" for that scan line, resulting in deep structures appearing closer to the transducer than their actual location. The appearance of an anatomically unexpected echo within a cardiac chamber often is due to range ambiguity, as can be demonstrated by the disappearance or a change in position of this artifact when the depth setting (and pulse-repetition frequency) is changed. Another type of range ambiguity is the appearance of an apparent second heart, deeper than the actual heart–a double image on the vertical axis. This type of range ambiguity results from echoes being re-reflected by a structure close to the transducer (such as a rib), being re-reflected by the cardiac structures and thus received at the transducer at a time *twice* normal. This artifact can be eliminated (or obscured) by decreasing the depth setting or adjusting the transducer position to a better acoustic window.

Electronic processing artifacts can be difficult to identify and vary from instrument to instrument. In addition, types of artifacts other than those listed have been described.

Doppler Echocardiography

Doppler Equation

Doppler echocardiography is based on the change in frequency of the backscattered signal from small moving structures (red blood cells) intercepted by the ultrasound beam. A visual analogy is that Doppler scattering from blood is similar to scattering of light in fog, while imaging is similar to reflections from a mirror. A stationary target, if much smaller than the wavelength, will scatter ultrasound in all directions, with the frequency of the scattered signal being the same as the transmitted frequency when observed from any direction. A moving target, however, will backscatter ultrasound to the transducer so that the frequency observed when the target is moving *toward* the transducer is higher and the frequency observed when the target is moving *away* from the transducer is lower than the original transmitted frequency (Fig. 1–19). This Doppler effect is known to all of us from audio examples of the change in sound of a car horn, siren, or train whistle as it moves toward (higher pitch) and then away (lower pitch) from the observer.

The difference in frequency between the transmitted frequency (F_T) and the scattered signal received back at the transducer (F_S) is the Doppler shift:

$$\text{Doppler shift} = (F_S - F_T) \qquad (1\text{–}7)$$

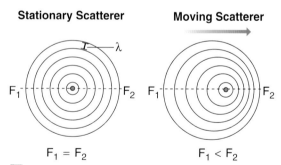

FIGURE 1–19. The Doppler effect. A stationary scatterer (*left*) scatters ultrasound symmetrically in all directions with a wavelength identical to the transmitted wavelength and with the same frequency in all directions (no Doppler shift). A moving scatterer (*right*) also scatters ultrasound symmetrically in all directions. However, the frequency will be higher when the scatterer is moving toward the transducer (F_2) than when it is moving away from the transducer (F_1) due to the movement of the scatterer resulting in waves closer together in advance of and further apart behind the moving object.

Doppler shifts are in the audible range (0–20 kHz) for intracardiac velocities using diagnostic ultrasound transducer frequencies. The relationship between the Doppler shift and blood flow velocity (V, in m/s) is expressed in the Doppler equation:

$$V = \frac{c(F_S - F_T)}{2F_T(\cos\theta)} \qquad (1-8)$$

where c is the speed of sound in blood (1540 m/s), θ is the intercept angle between the ultrasound beam and the direction of blood flow, and 2 is a factor to correct for the transit time both *to* and *from* the scattering source (Fig. 1–20).

Note that intercept angle is critically important in calculation of blood flow velocity. The cosine of an angle of 0° or 180° (parallel toward or away from the transducer) is 1, allowing this term to be ignored when the ultrasound beam is aligned parallel to the direction of blood flow. In contrast, the cosine of 90° is *zero,* indicating that no Doppler shift will be recorded if the ultrasound beam is perpendicular to blood flow.

In cardiac Doppler applications, the ultrasound beam is aligned as parallel with the direction of blood flow as possible so that the cos θ can be assumed to be 1. Because the direction of intracardiac blood flow can be difficult to ascertain and is not predictable from the 2D image, especially with abnormal flow patterns, attempts to "correct" for intercept angle may result in significant errors in velocity calculations. Furthermore, even when blood flow direction is apparent in a 2D plane, direction in the elevational plane remains unknown. Deviation from a parallel intercept angle up to 20° results in only a 6% error in blood velocity calculation. However, a 60° intercept angle results in a 50% underestimation of flow velocity. The importance of intercept angle is particularly underlined in the setting of abnormal blood flow with high-velocity jets, such as in valvular stenosis. Note that although angle correction for the presumed direction of blood flow is used in some peripheral vascular applications, this approach is not acceptable for cardiac applications due to the likelihood that the "correction" will be erroneous.

Spectral Analysis and Doppler Instrument Controls

When the backscattered signal is received at the transducer, the difference between the transmitted and backscattered signal is determined by "comparing" the two waveforms. This is a complex process, because multiple frequencies are present in the backscattered signal. Typically, the frequency content of the signal is analyzed by a process known as a *fast Fourier transform* (FFT) that derives the component frequencies of a complex signal. Alternate methods of frequency analysis also may be used, such as the analog Chirp-Z method.

The display generated by this frequency analysis is termed *spectral analysis* (Fig. 1–21). By convention, this display shows time on the horizontal axis, the zero baseline in the center, and frequency shifts toward the transducer above and frequency shifts away from the transducer below the baseline. Because multiple frequencies exist at any time point, each frequency signal is displayed as a pixel on the vertical axis, with the gray (or color) scale indicating the amplitude (or loudness) and the position on the vertical axis indicating the blood flow velocity (or frequency shift) component. Thus at each time point the spectral display shows

■ blood flow direction,
■ velocity (or frequency shift), and
■ signal amplitude.

Each of these components is displayed at 4-ms intervals (or 250 times per second) simultaneous with data acquisition.

Pulsed and continuous-wave Doppler instrument controls typically include

■ power output–the electrical energy transmitted to the transducer,
■ receiver gain–the degree of amplification of returning signals,
■ "wall" or high-pass filters–elimination of low-frequency Doppler shifts due to motion of myocardium and valves (allowing only the higher frequencies to pass the filter),

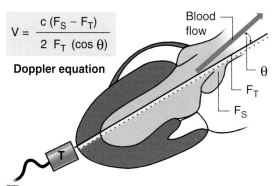

$$V = \frac{c(F_S - F_T)}{2\,F_T\,(\cos\theta)}$$

Doppler equation

■ FIGURE 1–20. The Doppler equation. The velocity V of blood flow can be calculated from the speed of sound in blood c, transducer frequency F_T, backscattered frequency F_S and the cosine of the angle θ between the ultrasound beam and direction of blood flow.

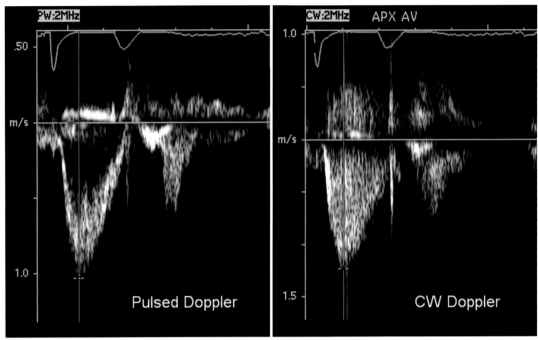

■ **FIGURE 1–21.** Examples of pulsed (*left*) and continuous wave (CW, *right*) spectral Doppler displays. Left ventricular outflow recorded from an apical approach is shown in the standard format. The baseline has been moved from the middle of the vertical axis to display the antegrade flow signal. Velocities toward the transducer are shown above and velocities away from the transducer below the baseline. The velocity range is determined by the Nyquist limit ($\frac{1}{2}$ PRF) with pulsed Doppler echo. Velocities are shown in shades of gray corresponding to the amplitude (decibels) of the signal. Note the "envelope" of flow with pulsed Doppler because flow is sampled at a specific intracardiac location with relatively uniform blood flow velocities. With continuous wave Doppler the curve is "filled in" due to multiple blood flow velocities along the entire length of the ultrasound beam.

■ baseline shift—moves the zero line toward the top or bottom of the display,

■ velocity range—expands or compresses the scale (within the limits for each Doppler modality, as discussed subsequently),

■ postprocessing options—these often include "reject," "compression," and "dynamic range" (i.e., number of shades of gray).

In addition, pulsed Doppler controls include

■ sample volume depth,
■ sample volume length, and
■ the number of sample volumes (high pulse repetition frequency Doppler echo).

The Doppler modality may be integrated with 2D imaging for each of the three major Doppler modalities: continuous-wave, pulsed, and color Doppler flow imaging. However, while color Doppler flow imaging is nearly always conjoined with 2D imaging, pulsed Doppler signal quality is optimized when the 2D image is "frozen," and continuous-wave Doppler is optimized using a dedicated, small-footprint transducer with no 2D imaging.

Continuous-Wave Doppler Ultrasound

Continuous-wave Doppler uses two ultrasound crystals—one continuously transmits and one continuously receives the ultrasound signal. The major advantage of this Doppler modality is that very high–frequency shifts (velocities) can be measured accurately because sampling is continuous. The potential disadvantage of continuous-wave Doppler is that signals from the entire length of the ultrasound beam are recorded simultaneously. However, even with overlap of flow data, a given signal often is characteristic in timing, shape, and direction, allowing correct identification of the origin of the signal. In some cases, other methods (2D echo, color, pulsed Doppler) must be used to determine the depth of origin of the Doppler signal.

Continuous-wave Doppler optimally is performed with a dedicated, nonimaging transducer with two crystals. This type of transducer has a high signal-to-noise ratio and a small footprint, allowing it to fit into small acoustic windows (e.g., between ribs) and to be angled to obtain a parallel intercept angle between the ultrasound beam and the direction of blood flow. Use of a simultaneous imaging transducer may be helpful in some cases but signal quality may be poorer, angulation is more difficult, and the 2D image may distract the operator from optimizing the *flow* signal instead of the anatomic image (which may not coincide).

Careful technique yields a Doppler spectral signal that has a smooth contour with a well-defined edge and maximum velocity, as well as with clearly defined onset and end of flow. The audible signal is tonal and smooth. A continuous-wave Doppler velocity curve is "filled in" because lower-velocity signals proximal and distal to the point of maximum velocity also are recorded. Note that while the maximum frequency shift depends on the intercept angle between the Doppler beam and the flow of interest, amplitude (gray-scale intensity), shape, and audible quality are less dependent on intercept angle. Thus, a "good quality" Doppler signal may be recorded at a nonparallel intercept angle, resulting in underestimation of flow velocity. The empirical method to ensure a parallel intercept angle is to examine the flow of interest from multiple windows with transducer angulation both in the plane of view and in the elevational plane to discover the highest-frequency shift. The highest value found is then assumed to represent a parallel intercept angle.

Pulsed Doppler Ultrasound

Pulsed Doppler echocardiography allows sampling of blood flow velocities from a specific intracardiac depth. A pulse of ultrasound is transmitted, and then, after an interval determined by the depth of interest, the transducer briefly "samples" the backscattered signals. This transducer cycle of transmit-wait-receive is repeated at an interval termed the *pulse repetition frequency* (PRF) (Fig. 1–22). Because the "wait" interval is determined by the depth of interest—the time it takes ultrasound to travel to and from this depth—each transducer cycle is longer for increasing depths. Thus, the PRF also is depth dependent, being high at shallow depths and low for more distant sites.

The depth of interest in pulsed Doppler echo is called the *sample volume* because signals from a small volume of blood are sampled, with the width and height of this volume dependent on beam geometry. The length of the sample volume can be varied by adjusting the length of the transducer "receive" interval. Typically, a sample volume length of 3 mm is used to balance range resolution and signal quality, but a longer (5–

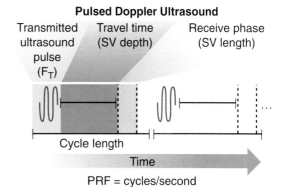

Pulsed Doppler Ultrasound

■ **FIGURE 1–22.** With pulsed Doppler ultrasound, the transducer goes through a repetitive cycle of transmission of an ultrasound pulse at the transducer frequency (F_t), a waiting period determined by the time needed for the signal to travel to and from the depth of interest, and a receive phase when the backscattered signals are sampled. The travel-time duration determines sample volume depth. The duration of the receive phase determines sample volume.

10 mm) or shorter (1–2 mm) sample volume may be useful in specific cases.

Because pulsed Doppler echo repeatedly samples the returning signal, there is a maximum limit to the frequency shift (or velocity) that can be measured unambiguously. A waveform must be sampled at least twice in each cycle for accurate determination of wavelength. A visual analogy is a motion picture film of a moving wagon wheel. If the frame rate is at least twice as fast as the rotation of the wheel, the forward rotation of the wheel is "seen." If the frame rate and rotation speed are the same, the wheel will appear to stay still. Even slower frame rates result in the appearance of the wheel going backward (Fig. 1–23). This phenomenon of ambiguity in the speed and/or direction of the sampled signal is

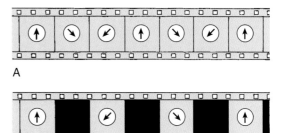

■ **FIGURE 1–23.** Visual analogy for aliasing. The filmstrip in (*A*) shows a wheel rotating clockwise. If the frame rate of the film (or sampling rate) is halved as in (*B*), the wheel will appear to move counterclockwise when the film is played. (From Otto CM, Pearlman AS: Echocardiography 2:141, 1985. Used with permission.)

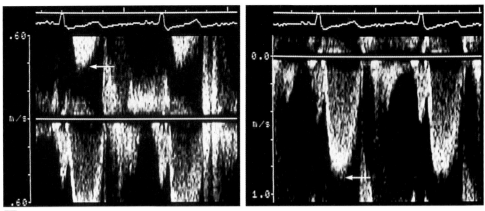

■ **FIGURE 1–24.** The velocity of left ventricular (LV) outflow recorded from an apical approach exceeds the Nyquist limit so that aliasing occurs (*left*) with the appearance of the peak of the outflow curve in the reverse channel (*arrow*). This degree of aliasing can be resolved by shifting the baseline (*right*), in effect an electronic "cut and paste" of the spectral display.

known as *signal aliasing*. For the frequency of an ultrasound waveform to be correctly identified, it must be sampled at least twice per wavelength. Thus, the maximum detectable frequency shift (the *Nyquist limit*) is one half the PRF.

If the velocity of interest exceeds the Nyquist limit by a small degree, signal aliasing is seen with the signal cut off at the edge of the display and the "top" of the waveform appearing in the reverse channel (Fig. 1–24). In these cases, baseline shift (in effect an electronic "cut and paste") restores the expected velocity curve and allows calculation of maximum velocity. When velocities further exceed the Nyquist limit, repeat "wrap-around" of the signal occurs first into the reverse channel, then back to the forward channel, and so on. Occasionally, the shape of the waveform can be discerned (Fig. 1–25), but more often only an undifferentiated band of velocity signals can be

appreciated (Fig. 1–26). Note that nonlaminar disturbed flow and aliased laminar high-velocity flow will appear (and sound) similar on spectral analysis. Methods that can be used to resolve aliasing include

- using continuous-wave Doppler ultrasound,
- increasing the PRF to the maximum for that depth,
- increasing the number of sample volumes (high-PRF Doppler),
- using a lower-frequency transducer, or
- shifting the baseline.

Continuous-wave Doppler is the most reliable approach to resolving aliasing for very high velocities. The other approaches are useful when the aliased velocity exceeds the Nyquist limit by a modest degree (e.g., less than or equal to twice the Nyquist limit).

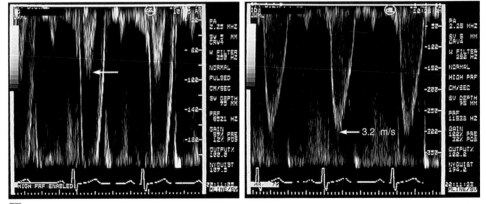

■ **FIGURE 1–25.** In this case, left ventricular (LV) outflow velocity exceeds 2 × the Nyquist limit so that aliasing persists even after baseline shift (*left*). The "wrapped around" peak velocity is clearly seen (*arrow*). With high-PRF Doppler, the maximum velocity is resolved in this patient with a subaortic membrane (*right*).

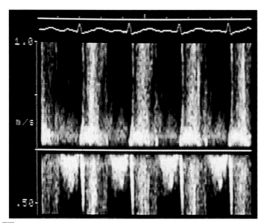

FIGURE 1–26. Severe aliasing results in a band of frequency shifts due to multiple "wraparounds" of the velocity signal. The maximum velocity cannot be reliably identified unless continuous-wave Doppler ultrasound is used.

High-PRF Doppler is the deliberate use of range ambiguity to increase the maximum velocity that can be measured with pulsed Doppler echo (Fig. 1–27). When the transducer sends out a pulse, backscattered signals from the entire length of the ultrasound beam return to the transducer. Range resolution is achieved by sampling only those signals in the short interval corresponding to the depth of interest. However, signals from exactly twice as far away as the sample volume will reach the transducer during the "receive" phase of the next cycle. Thus signals from "harmonics" at 2X 3X, 4X, and so on the

sample volume depth, have the potential of being analyzed. Usually signal strength is low and there are few moving scatterers at these depths, so that this range ambiguity can be ignored. If, instead, the sample volume is placed purposely at one half the depth of interest, backscattered signals from this sample volume (SV_1) and a second sample volume (SV_2) twice as far away (i.e., the depth of interest) will return to the transducer during the "receive" phase (albeit one cycle later). This recording of the signal of interest at a higher PRF allows measurement of higher velocities without signal aliasing. An even higher PRF can be achieved by using additional (three or four) proximal sample volumes. Of course, the limitation of this approach is range ambiguity. The spectral analysis now includes signals from each of the sample volume depths. As with continuous-wave Doppler, the origin of the signal of interest must be determined based on ancillary data.

Color Flow Imaging

Doppler color flow imaging is based on the principles of pulsed Doppler echocardiography. However, rather than one sample volume depth along the ultrasound beam, multiple sample volumes (or multigates) are evaluated along each sampling line (Fig. 1–28). By combining data from adjacent lines, a 2D image of intracardiac flow is generated.

Along each scan line, a pulse of ultrasound is transmitted, and then the backscattered signals are

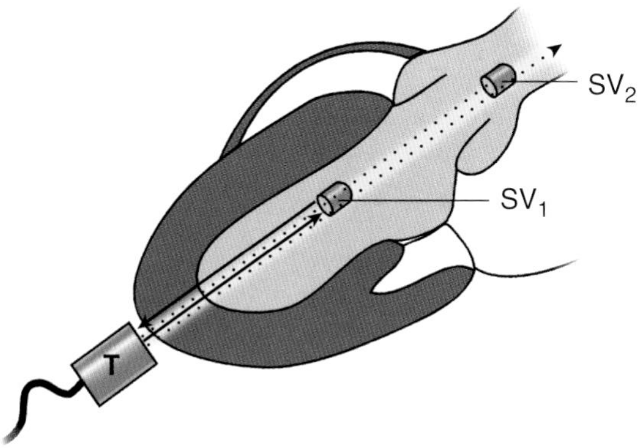

FIGURE 1–27. High-pulse-repetition frequency (PRF) Doppler ultrasound. High-PRF Doppler is based on the concept that with a given sample volume depth (SV_1), some ultrasound will penetrate beyond that depth. Backscattered signals from exactly twice the set depth (SV_2) will return to the transducer (T) during the receive phase of the next cycle. Thus, signals from both sample volume depths are recorded simultaneously.

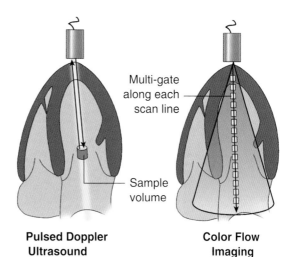

Pulsed Doppler Ultrasound **Color Flow Imaging**

FIGURE 1–28. With pulsed Doppler, the sample volume depth is determined by the time needed for ultrasound to travel to and from the depth of interest (*left*). With color flow imaging, multiple sample volume "gates" along each scan line are interrogated, with this process repeated for scan lines across the 2D image (*right*).

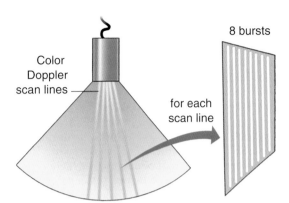

FIGURE 1–29. Along each color Doppler scan line, several (typically eight) bursts of ultrasound are transmitted and received to allow adequate velocity resolution.

TABLE 1–4
Determinants of Color Frame Rate

Depth of sector (pulse-repetition frequency)
Sector width (number of scan lines)
Density of scan lines (number of scan lines)
Number of ultrasound bursts along each sector line
  (burst length)

received from each "gate" or sample volume along that scan line. To calculate accurate velocity data, several bursts along each scan line are used—typically eight—which is known as the *burst length* (Fig. 1–29). The PRF, as for conventional pulsed Doppler, is determined by the maximum depth of the Doppler signals.

Because multiple signals are analyzed along each scan line, an audible output is not helpful and, since only a brief sample of the backscattered signal is available for analysis, an accurate spectral analysis is not possible. Instead, signals from the eight sampling lines at each position are analyzed to obtain mean velocity estimates for each sample volume along the scan line. Velocities are displayed using a color scale showing flow toward the transducer in red and flow away from the

transducer in blue, with the shade of color indicating velocity up to the Nyquist limit. The option of displaying "variance" allows an additional color (usually green) to be added to indicate that the mean velocity for each of the eight bursts had excessive variability. Variance can be seen with nonlaminar disturbed flow or with laminar aliased high-velocity flow.

This process is repeated for each adjacent scan line across the image plane. Because each of these processes takes a finite time depending on the speed of sound in tissue, the rapidity with which this image can be updated (the frame rate) depends on a combination of these factors (Table 1–4). During the examination, these variables may be adjusted to optimize frame rate or velocity resolution, as dictated by the specific clinical situation (Fig. 1–30).

In addition to depth and sector scan width, color flow instrument settings typically include low-pass filter settings, gain, and power output. Most instruments provide several choices of the color "map" used to display velocity information. Velocity alone, velocity plus variance, or a power-mode display can be used. As for conventional

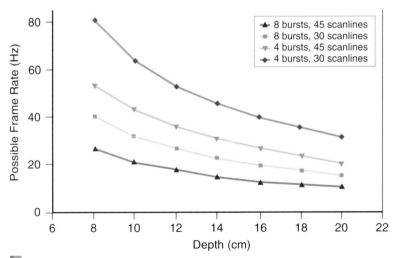

FIGURE 1–30. Graph of the maximum possible color Doppler frame rate (*y* axis) versus depth (*x* axis) for 8 or 4 bursts per scan line and 30 or 45 scan lines per frame. Note that at a depth of 16 cm, a frame rate 20 or greater can be achieved only by decreasing the burst length to 4 or narrowing the sector to 30 scan lines.

TABLE 1–5

Spectral Doppler Echo Artifacts

Artifact	Result
Nonparallel intercept angle	Underestimation of velocity
Aliasing	Inability to measure maximum velocity
Range ambiguity	Doppler signals from more than one depth along the ultrasound beam are recorded
Beam width	Overlap of Doppler signals from adjacent flows
Mirror image	Spectral display shows unidirectional flow both above and below the baseline
Electronic interference	Bandlike interference signal obscures Doppler flow
Transit-time effect	Change in the velocity of the ultrasound wave as it passes through a moving media results in slight overestimation of Doppler shifts

pulsed Doppler, the zero baseline can be shifted and the PRF adjusted to vary the velocity range.

Doppler Artifacts

SPECTRAL DOPPLER (CONTINUOUS WAVE AND PULSED). Many Doppler artifacts are related to ultrasound physics and beam geometry, analogous to those seen with 2D imaging. Others are specific to Doppler echocardiography (Table 1–5).

Clinically, the most important potential artifact is *velocity underestimation* due to a nonparallel intercept angle between the ultrasound beam and the direction of blood flow (Fig. 1–31). Velocity underestimation can occur with either pulsed or continuous-wave Doppler techniques and is of most concern when measuring high-velocity jets due to valve stenosis, regurgitation, or other

intracardiac abnormalities. Attention to technical details with interrogation of the flow signal from multiple acoustic windows and careful angulation is needed to avoid velocity underestimation.

With pulsed Doppler echo, *signal aliasing* limits the maximum measurable velocity. If the examiner recognizes that aliasing has occurred, appropriate steps can be taken to resolve the velocity data if needed. Again the examiner needs to recognize that aliasing can be due to nonlaminar disturbed flow, as well as to high-velocity laminar flow.

Range ambiguity is inherent to continuous-wave Doppler but can occur with pulsed Doppler as well. With a sample volume positioned close to the transducer, strong signals from twice (or three times) the depth of the sample volume will be

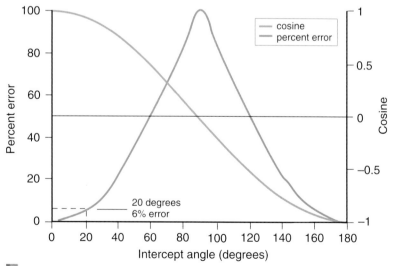

■ **FIGURE 1–31.** The importance of a parallel intercept angle between the ultrasound beam and direction of blood flow is shown. The cosine function versus intercept angle (*horizontal axis*) varies from 1 at a parallel angle (0° and 180°) to 0 at a perpendicular angle (90°). The percentage error if cos is assumed to be 1 in the Doppler equation but, in fact, the intercept angle is *not* parallel; it varies from only 6% at a 20° angle to 50% at a 60° angle and 100% for perpendicular flows. At a perpendicular (90°) intercept angle, no blood flow velocities are recorded.

received in the next "receive" phase and may be misinterpreted as originating from the set sample volume depth. For example, in an apical four-chamber view, placement of a sample volume in the left ventricular apex at half the distance to the mitral annulus results in a spectral display showing the inflow signal across the mitral valve from the "second" sample volume depth. This phenomenon of range ambiguity is used constructively in the high-PRF Doppler mode.

Beam width (and side or grating lobes) affects the Doppler signal, as occurs with 2D imaging, resulting in superimposition of spatially adjacent flow signals on the spectral display. For example, left ventricular outflow and inflow may be seen on the same recording, especially with continuous-wave Doppler. Similarly, the left ventricular inflow signal may be seen superimposed on the aortic regurgitant jet (Fig. 1–32).

A mirror-image artifact is common with spectral analysis, appearing as a symmetric signal of somewhat less intensity than the actual flow signal in the opposite direction flow channel (Fig. 1–33). Mirroring often can be reduced or eliminated by decreasing the power output or gain of the instrument. Interrogation of a flow signal from a near-perpendicular angle can result in flow signals on both sides of the baseline that must be distinguished from artifact.

Electronic interference appears as a band of signals across the spectral display that may obscure the flow signals. These artifacts are due to inadequate shielding of other electric instruments in the examination environment and are particularly common during studies in the intensive care unit or operating room.

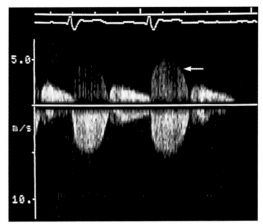

■ **FIGURE 1–33.** A mirror-image Doppler artifact with apparent weaker flow signals in the reverse channel (*arrow*).

The *transit time effect* is the change in propagation speed that occurs as an ultrasound wave passes through a moving medium, such as blood. This phenomenon is separate from the Doppler effect (which affects the backscattered signal) and is the basis of volume flow measurement with a transit-time flow probe. On the spectral display, the transit-time effect may result in a slight broadening of the velocity range at a given time point ("blurring" on the vertical axis), which potentially can result in slight overestimation of velocity. Some investigators argue that this should not happen, since the ultrasound signal passes through the moving blood in both directions—out (adding) and back (subtracting). In either case, this effect is insignificant clinically.

COLOR DOPPLER FLOW IMAGING. Color flow artifacts again relate to the physics of 2D and Doppler flow image generation (Table 1–6). *Shadowing* may be prominent distal to strong reflectors with absence of both 2D and flow data within the acoustic shadow.

Ghosting is the appearance of brief (usually one or two frames) large color patterns that overlay anatomic structures and do not correspond to underlying flow patterns. This artifact is caused by strong moving reflectors (such as prosthetic valve disks). Typically, this artifact is a uniform red or blue color, but it may be coded with a variance scale depending on the instrument. It is inconsistent from beat to beat.

Color Doppler gain settings have a dramatic effect on the color flow image. Extensive gain settings result in a uniform speckled pattern across the 2D image plane due to random *background noise*. Conversely, too low a gain setting results in a smaller displayed flow area than is actually present, an effect colloquially known as "dial-a-

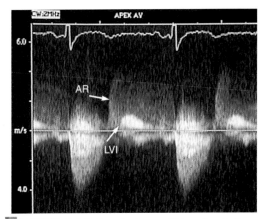

■ **FIGURE 1–32.** Doppler beam width artifact is demonstrated by the simultaneous display of superimposed aortic regurgitation (AR) and left ventricular (LV) inflow curves.

TABLE 1–6

Color Doppler Artifacts

Artifact	Appearance
Shadowing	Absence of flow signal distal to strong reflector
Ghosting	Brief flashes of color that overlay anatomic structures and do not correlate with flow patterns
Background noise	Speckled color pattern over 2D sector due to excessive gain
Underestimation of flow signal	Loss of true flow signals due to inadequate gain
Intercept angle	Change in color (or absence at 90°) due to the angle between the flowstream and ultrasound beam across the image plane
Aliasing	"Wraparound" of color display results in a "variance" display even for laminar flow.
Electronic interference	Linear or complex color patterns across the 2D image

jet." Most experienced echocardiographers recommend setting the gain level just below the level of random background noise to optimize the flow signal.

As for any Doppler technique, the *intercept angle* between the ultrasound beam and direction of blood flow *for each scan line* affects the color display in terms of both direction and velocity. Thus a uniform flow velocity traversing the image plane may appear red (toward the transducer) at one side of the sector and blue (away from the transducer) at the other edge of the sector, with a black area in the center where the flow direction is perpendicular to the ultrasound beam (Fig. 1–34).

Flow velocities that exceed the Nyquist limit at any given depth result in *signal aliasing*. Aliasing on color flow results in "wraparound" of the velocity signal, similar to that seen on a spectral display, so that an aliased velocity toward the transducer (should be red) will appear to be traveling away from the transducer (displayed in blue). Aliasing on color flow images is very common; for example, the left ventricular inflow stream appears red and then blue (due to aliasing) in the apical view (Fig. 1–35). Color aliasing can be used to advantage to quantitate flow based on the proximal isovelocity surface area method described in Chapter 12. In some cases, aliasing results in a variance display (due to an apparent range of velocities at that site), emphasizing that a variance display does not always indicate disturbed flow.

Electronic interference on color flow displays is instrument dependent. As with other electric interference artifacts, it is most likely to occur in settings where numerous other instruments or devices are in use (e.g., operating room, intensive-care unit). Sometimes it appears as a linear multicolored band on the image along a few scan lines; sometimes more complex patterns are seen. Caution is needed in that sometimes electronic interference results in suppression of the color

flow signal. This artifact can be recognized by the absence of normal antegrade flow patterns.

RECORDING DEVICES

There are several reasons to record the echocardiographic examination, including

■ later review and/or quantitation;
■ documentation;

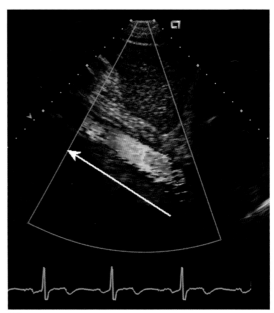

■ **FIGURE 1–34.** Color flow in the proximal abdominal aorta showing the importance of intercept angle on the color display. Although flow in systole goes from right to left across the image plane as shown by the arrow, flow on the right side of the image appears blue (because flow is directed toward the transducer but exceeds the Nyquist limit and thus has aliased to blue) and flow on the left side of the image appears red (because a larger intercept angle results in underestimation of velocity, which now is below the Nyquist limit).

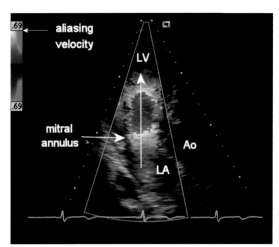

■ **FIGURE 1–35.** A normal left ventricular (LV) inflow signal (*top*) shows aliasing from red to blue at the mitral annulus level, because the velocity exceeds the Nyquist limit of 69 cm/s.

- communication with the patient, referring physician, and other consultants;
- comparison with any future studies in that patient; and
- clinical research.

Because the entire examination may be quite lengthy, depending on the specific findings in each patient, only selected segments of the examination are recorded.

Recordings on paper can be made of M-mode, spectral Doppler, or single 2D or color flow images using a variety of page-printing devices. These recordings are of limited utility for 2D and color flow because only a single frame of information is displayed.

Video recordings are a useful method for recording data with the advantage that a large number of sequential frames can be recorded and replayed in "real time" at low cost. On videotape, the frame rate is 30 frames per second, with each frame consisting of two interlaced "fields" of information. One disadvantage of videotape is that when the tape is stopped, only one field is displayed, resulting in degradation of image quality. Other limitations of videotape are the frame rate (which is less than the achievable 2D frame rate with some ultrasound systems), image degradation in the digital-to-analog recording mode, the storage space required, and the difficulty of rapid access to different data on the same videotape. Recording video data on optical discs may obviate some of these limitations.

Most laboratories now use digital recording and storage of echocardiographic data with the advantages of high image quality, rapid access to the data in any order, and the ability to manipulate the data in terms of image processing (such as contrast) and display formats (such as a cine-loop side-by-side display). The major limitation of digital storage is the immense amount of data contained in an echocardiographic examination (10 minutes of videotape at 30 frames per second = 18,000 image frames), which requires a combination of careful editing of the recorded data, large data storage systems, and compression of the image data (without loss of image quality). These problems have largely been resolved with current computers. Another advantage of digital storage is that selected images and cine-loops are accessible to referring physicians using the medical center's information system.

EXAMINATION TECHNIQUE

The echocardiographic examination is performed by the physician or by a trained cardiac sonographer under the supervision of a qualified physician. Guidelines and recommendations for education and training in echocardiography for both sonographers and physicians have been published, as referenced in Chapter 5.

At the time of a transthoracic echocardiographic examination, the patient is positioned comfortably for each view in either a left lateral decubitus or supine position. Electrocardiographic electrodes are attached for display of a single lead (usually lead II) on the instrument display to aid in timing cardiac events. Specially designed echocardiographic examination stretchers provide apical cutouts for optimal transducer positioning at the apex. The transducer is applied to the chest and upper abdomen using a water-soluble gel to obtain good contact without intervening air. The time needed to perform an echocardiographic examination depends on the specific clinical situation—from a few minutes in a critically ill patient to document cardiac tamponade to more than 1 hour to quantitate multiple lesions in a patient with complex valvular or congenital heart disease.

An echocardiographic examination is a technically demanding procedure, and most examiners find a significant learning curve in their ability to obtain diagnostic data. The specific examination approaches are detailed in Chapter 2 (for transthoracic) and Chapter 3 (for transesophageal) for normal anatomy and flow patterns and throughout this book for specific disease states. The examination also includes appropriate use of the echocardiographic data in patient treatment, as discussed in Chapter 5 and throughout the text.

BIOEFFECTS AND SAFETY

The use of ultrasound for diagnostic cardiac imaging has no known adverse biologic effects. However, ultrasound waves do have the potential to cause significant bioeffects depending on the intensity of exposure. Thus, the physician and cardiac sonographer must be aware of potential bioeffects in assessing the overall safety of the procedure.

Bioeffects

Ultrasound bioeffects can be divided into three basic categories:

- Thermal effects
- Cavitation
- Other (such as torque forces and microstreaming)

Thermal effects predominate with diagnostic ultrasound examinations. As the ultrasound wave passes through a tissue, heating occurs due to absorption of the mechanical energy of the sound wave. The rate of increase in temperature dT/dt depends on the absorption coefficient of the tissue for a given frequency a, the density r, and specific heat C_m of the tissue and the intensity I of ultrasound exposure:

$$dT/dt = 2\alpha I/\rho C_m \qquad (1\text{--}9)$$

Increases in temperature due to ultrasound exposure are offset by heat loss due to blood flow through the tissue (convective loss) and heat diffusion. More dense tissues (such as bone) heat more rapidly than less dense tissues (such as fat). However, the actual elevation in temperature for a specific tissue is difficult to predict both because of the complexity of the entire biologic system and because it is difficult to assess accurately the intensity of exposure. In addition, the actual degree of tissue heating depends on transducer frequency, focus, power output, depth, perfusion, and tissue density.

Cavitation is the creation or vibration of small gas-filled bodies by the ultrasound beam. Cavitation tends to occur only with higher-intensity exposures. Microbubbles resonate (expand and decrease in size) depending on their dimension in relation to the sound wave with a resonance frequency F_0 defined by the radius of the microbubble (R_0 in microns):

$$F_0 = 3260/R_0 \qquad (1\text{--}10)$$

Microbubbles also can be created by ultrasound by expansion of small cavitation nuclei. Cavitation has not been shown to occur with ultrasound exposure due to diagnostic ultrasound systems. However, this effect may be more important when gas-filled bodies are introduced into the ultrasound field, such as with the use of contrast echocardiography.

Other ultrasound bioeffects occur only with much higher exposures than occur with diagnostic ultrasound. These effects include microstreaming, torque forces, and other complex biologic effects.

Safety

The intensity I of ultrasound exposure can be expressed in several ways. The most commonly used unit of measure of intensity is power per area, where power is energy over a specific interval:

$$I = \text{power}/\text{area} = \text{watt}/\text{cm}^2 \qquad (1\text{--}11)$$

The maximum overall intensity is then described as the highest exposure within the beam (spatial peak) averaged over the period of exposure (temporal average) and is known as the *spatial peak temporal average* (SPTA) *intensity*. Another common measure is the *spatial peak pulse average*, defined as the average pulse intensity at the spatial location where the pulse intensity is maximum. The US Food and Drug Administration provides two maximum allowed limits for I_{SPTA} for cardiac applications: a regulated application-specific limit of $430\,\text{mW/cm}^2$, and an output display standard of $720\,\text{mW/cm}^2$, which allows the echocardiographer to balance the potential risks of ultrasound exposure with the benefit of the diagnostic test.

A major limitation of measuring the intensity of ultrasound exposure is that while measuring the *output* of the transducer is straightforward (e.g., in a water bath), estimating the actual tissue *exposure* is more difficult due to attenuation and other interactions with the tissue. Furthermore, tissue exposure is limited only to transmission periods and the time the ultrasound beam dwells at a specific point, both of which are considerably shorter than the total examination time. Other indices that incorporate these factors have been developed to better define the exposure levels with diagnostic ultrasound. These measures include the thermal index (TI) and the mechanical index (MI).

The soft tissue TI is based on the ratio of transmitted acoustic power to the power needed to increase tissue temperature by 1°C:

$$\text{TI} = W_p/W_{\text{deg}}$$

where W_p is a power parameter calculated from output power and acoustic attenuation and W_{deg}

is the estimated power needed to increase the tissue temperature by 1°C. There are different thermal indexes for bone and cranial bone, which are less relevant for cardiac ultrasound. The MI describes the nonthermal effects of ultrasound (cavitation and other effects) as the ratio of peak rarefactional pressure and the square root of transducer frequency, with the specific definition

$$\text{MI} = [\rho_{r.3}/(f_c^{1/2})]/C_{MI}$$

where C_{MI} equals $1\,\text{Mpa}\,\text{MHz}^{-1/2}$, $\rho_{r.3}$ is the attenuated peak-rarefactional pressure in Mpa, and f_c is the center frequency of the transducer in MHz.

An MI or TI less than 1 is generally considered safe, with higher numbers indicating a higher probability of a biologic effect. These indexes are displayed only on instruments capable of exceeding a MI or TI of 1. With a higher index, the benefit of the diagnostic examination must be balanced against the benefits of the diagnostic examination. The TI is most important with Doppler and color flow imaging whereas the MI is most important with 2D imaging.

While any biologic effect is likely to be small, a prudent approach is to

■ perform echocardiography only when indicated clinically (see Chapter 5), as part of an approved research protocol, or in appropriate teaching settings;
■ know the power output and exposure intensity of different modalities (imaging and Doppler) of each instrument;
■ limit the power output and exposure time as much as possible within the constraints of acquiring the necessary information;
■ keep up to date on any new scientific findings or data relating to possible adverse effects.

SUGGESTED READING

1. Kremkau FW: Diagnostic Ultrasound: Principles and Instruments, 6th ed. Philadelphia: WB Saunders, 2002.
   Basic textbook with chapters on ultrasound, transducers, imaging instruments, Doppler effect, spectral instrumentation, color-Doppler instrumentation, artifacts, and safety. Each chapter has a review section with multiple-choice questions. A comprehensive examination (with answers) is included.

2. Geiser EA: Echocardiography: physics and instrumentation. In: Skorton DJ, Schelbert HR, Wolf GL, Brundage BH (eds): Marcus Cardiac Imaging: A Companion to Braunwald's Heart Disease, 2nd ed. Philadelphia: WB Saunders, 1996, pp 273–291.
   Advanced chapter on echocardiographic instrumentation with excellent diagrams.

3. Martin RW: Interaction of ultrasound with tissue, approaches to tissue characterization, and measurement accuracy. In: Otto CM (ed): The Practice of Clinical Echocardiography, 2nd ed. Philadelphia: WB Saunders, 2002, pp 183–201.
   Detailed discussion of beam patterns, ultrasound properties of tissue, scattering and measurement error. An excellent overview for the clinician. 87 references.

4. Zagzebski JA: Essentials of Ultrasound Physics. St Louis: Mosby, 1996.
   Review of ultrasound physics for the beginning student. Concise text with clear schematic illustrations and tables. Topics covered include physics of diagnostic ultrasound, image storage and display, Doppler instrumentation, and bioeffects. Questions for review included with each chapter. Additional suggested readings.

5. Powis RL, Schwartz RA: Practical Doppler Ultrasound for the Clinician. Baltimore: Williams & Williams, 1991.
   Detailed but understandable book describing Doppler ultrasound techniques. An introduction to basic ultrasound principles and basic fluid dynamics also is provided.

6. Thomas JD, Rubin DN: Tissue harmonic imaging: why does it work? J Am Soc Echocardiog 11:803–808, 1998.
   Discussion with clear illustrations of the physical basis of tissue harmonic imaging. Contrast harmonic imaging is based on generation of harmonic frequencies by vibrating microbubbles. Tissue harmonics are generated by the nonlinear effects of ultrasound wave propagation through tissue. Instrumentation factors critical to generation of tissue harmonic images include a wide dynamic range, a narrow transmit spectrum, and a sharp receiver filter.

7. Hatle L, Angelsen B: Doppler Ultrasound in Cardiology: Physical Principles and Clinical Applications, 2nd ed. Philadelphia: Lea & Febiger, 1985.
   Excellent and detailed presentation on the Doppler effect, the physics of blood flow, Doppler instrumentation, and clinical applications of Doppler.

8. Harris RA, Follett DH, Halliwell M, Wells PNT: Ultimate limits in ultrasonic imaging resolution. Ultrasound Med Biol 17:547–558, 1991.
   Detailed review on ultrasound image resolution for readers interested in the technical details of this problem; 61 references.

9. Skorton DJ, Collins SM, Greenleaf JF, Meltzer RS, et al: Ultrasound bioeffects and regulatory issues: an introduction for the echocardiographer. J Am Soc Echocardiogr 1:240–251, 1988.
   Excellent review of bioeffects and safety prepared by the ASE Committee on Physics and Instrumentation.

10. Meltzer RS: Food and Drug Administration ultrasound device regulation: the output display standard, the "mechanical index" and ultrasound safety. J Am Soc Echocardiogr 9:216–220, 1996.
    Brief review of ultrasound bioeffects and cavitation-related bioeffects with a discussion of the potential impact, advantages, and disadvantages of regulation of ultrasound instrument output.

11. Fowlkes JB, Holland CK: Mechanical bioeffects from diagnostic ultrasound: AIUM consensus statements. J Ultrasound Med 19:69–72, 2000.
    Section 1: Conclusions and recommendations, pp 73–76.
    Section 2: Definitions and description of nonthermal mechanisms, pp 77–84.
    Section 3: Selected biological properties of tissues: potential determinants of susceptibility to ultrasound-induced bioeffects, pp 85–96.
    Section 4: Bioeffects in tissues with gas bodies, pp 97–108.

Section 5: Nonthermal bioeffects in the absence of well-defined gas bodies, pp 109–119.

Section 6: Mechanical bioeffects in the presence of gas-carrier ultrasound contrast agents, pp 120–142.

Section 7: Discussion of the mechanical index and other exposure parameters, pp 143–148.

Section 8: Clinical relevance, references, pp 149–168.

AIUM Consensus Development Conferences on ultrasound safety and bioeffects. Detailed document with 8 sections as listed.

12. Frizzell LA: Conclusions regarding biological effects of ultrasound for diagnostically relevant exposures. J Ultrasound Med 13:69–72, 1994.

Summary of AIUM conference held in 1992 on the Bioeffects and Safety of Diagnostic Ultrasound including definitions of the Mechanical Index (MI) and Tissue Thermal Index (TTI). Updated clinical statements are available at the AIUM web site (http://www.aium.org).

13. Miller DL: Update on safety of diagnostic ultrasonography. J Clin Ultrasound 19:531–540, 1991.

Readable review of ultrasound bioeffects; 39 references.

14. AMA Council on Scientific Affairs: Medical diagnostic ultrasound instrumentation and clinical interpretation: report of the Ultrasonography Task Force. JAMA 265:1155–1159, 1991.

AMA Council on Scientific Affairs' report on diagnostic ultrasound. Review of basic principles of ultrasound with emphasis on ultrasound artifacts.

15. Barnett SB, Kossoff G, Edwards MJ: Is diagnostic ultrasound safe? Current international consensus on the thermal mechanism. Med J Aust 160:33–37, 1994.

Review of the thermal effects of diagnostic ultrasound that concludes that there is no evidence of adverse effects for exposures resulting in temperatures less than 38.5°C.

16. Henderson J, Willson K, Jago JR, Whittinhgam TA: A survey of the acoustic outputs of diagnostic ultrasound equipment in current clinical use. Ultrasound in Med Biol 21:699–705, 1995.

Detailed report on the maximum acoustic power generated by 45 probes from 17 scanners using different imaging and Doppler modalities.

17. Abbott JG: Rationale and derivation of the MI and TI: a review. Ultrasound Med Biol 3:341–441, 1999.

Summary of the measurements, calculations and clinical implications of the mechanical index (MI) and thermal index (TI) for use in the output display standard (ODS) on ultrasound instruments.

18. Barnett SB, Haar GR, Ziskin MC, Rott HD, Duck FA, Maeda K: International recommendations and guidelines for the safe use of diagnostic ultrasound in medicine. Ultrasound Med Biol 26:355–366, 2000.

Review article based on symposium sponsored by the World Federation for Ultrasound in Medicine and Biology (WFUMB) comparing national and international recommendations on the safe use of diagnostic ultrasound. Includes summary of US Food and Drug Administration (FDA) regulation by application specific limits on acoustic power and the newer approach of user responsibility for appropriate use based on real time display of safety indices.

The Echo Exam *Basic Principles*

Sound Waves

f = frequency
λ = wavelength
c = velocity of propagation
$c = \lambda f$

Ultrasound-Tissue Interaction

Reflection	Imaging
Scattering	Doppler
Refraction	Beam focusing
	Artifacts
Attenuation	Penetration

Resolution

Axial	Transducer frequency
	Bandwidth
	Pulse length
Lateral	Depth
Elevational	Depth

Frame Rate

Depth
Sector width

Imaging Instrument Settings

Transducer frequency
Power output
Gain
Time gain compensation (TCG)
Depth
Dynamic range
Sector width

Doppler Modalities

Pulsed	Spectral display
	Anatomic location
	Signal aliasing
CW	Spectral display
	High velocity flow
	Range ambiguity
Color	Visual 2D display
	Quantitation problematic

Doppler Equation

$$v = \frac{c(\Delta F)}{2F_T(\cos\theta)}$$

c = speed of sound in blood (1540 m/s)
θ is the intercept angle with flow
F_T = transducer frequency
ΔF = Doppler frequency shift

Spectral Doppler Instrument Settings

Power output
Receiver gain
Wall (high-pass) filters
Baseline shift
Velocity range
Post-processing
Sample volume depth (pulsed)
Sample volume length (pulsed)
Number of sample volumes (HPRF)

Ultrasound Safety

Bioeffects	Thermal
	Cavitation
	Other

Perform echos appropriately
Know power output and exposure intensities
Limit power output and exposure as possible

Optimization of Doppler Recordings

Modality	Data Optimization	Common Artifacts
Pulsed	2D guided with "frozen" image Parallel to flow Small sample volume Velocity scale at Nyquist limit Adjust baseline for aliasing Use low wall filters Adjust gain and dynamic range	Nonparallel angle with underestimation of velocity Signal aliasing. Nyquist limit = 1/2 pulse repetition frequency (PRF) Signal strength/noise
Continuous wave	Dedicated nonimaging transducer Parallel to flow Adjust velocity scale so flow fits and fills the displayed range Use high wall filters Adjust gain and dynamic range	Nonparallel angle with underestimation of velocity Range ambiguity Beam width Transit time effect
Color flow	Use minimal depth and sector width for flow of interest (best frame rate) Adjust gain just below random noise Color scale at Nyquist limit	Shadowing Ghosting Electronic interference

Principles of Doppler Quantitation

Method	Assumptions/Characteristics	Examples of Clinical Applications
Volume flow $SV = CSA \times VTI$	• Laminar flow • Flat flow profile • Cross-sectional area (CSA) and velocity time integral (VTI) measured at same site	• Cardiac output • Continuity equation for valve area • Regurgitant volume calculations • Intracardiac shunts, pulmonary-to-systemic flow ratio
Velocity-pressure relationship $\Delta P = 4v^2$	• Flow-limiting orifice • CW Doppler signal recorded parallel to flow	• Stenotic valve gradients • Calculation of pulmonary pressures • Left ventricular dP/dt
Spatial flow patterns	• Proximal flow convergence region • Narrow flow stream in orifice (vena contracta) • Downstream flow disturbance	• Detection of valve regurgitation and intracardiac shunts • Level of obstruction • Quantitation of regurgitant severity

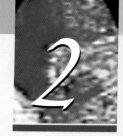

TRANSTHORACIC VIEWS, NORMAL ANATOMY, AND FLOW PATTERNS

BASIC IMAGING PRINCIPLES

Tomographic Imaging

Echocardiography provides tomographic images of cardiac structures and blood flow, analogous to a thin "slice" through the heart. In contrast, angiographic techniques provide silhouette-type images; that is, structures at different distances from the imaging device are superimposed onto a single two-dimensional (2D) image. Each approach has specific advantages and disadvantages (Table 2–1). For example, a silhouette technique allows definition of the entire length of a coronary artery in a single image even though the vessel transverses numerous tomographic planes. Conversely, a single-plane right anterior oblique angiogram of the left ventricle allows assessment of regional wall motion only for those segments that form the edge of the silhouette. The lateral wall is superimposed on the opacified chamber and cannot be evaluated.

TABLE 2–1		
Tomographic versus Silhouette Imaging		
	Tomographic	**Silhouette**
Advantages	Detailed anatomic information in a single image plane	Imaging of an entire 3D structure (such as a coronary artery)
Disadvantages	Cardiac motion	Superimposition of structures
	Need to integrate data from multiple planes	

Tomographic images provide detailed anatomic data in a given image plane. However, complete evaluation of the cardiac chambers and valves requires integration of information from multiple tomographic images. Small structures that transverse numerous tomographic planes (such as the coronary arteries) are difficult to evaluate fully. Another potential problem with tomographic imaging is movement of the heart with respiration and during the cardiac cycle. Respiratory variation in cardiac location is recognized easily by its timing, but movement of the heart during the cardiac cycle is a problem because it may not be obvious on the 2D image. Cardiac motion relative to surrounding structures is described in three dimensions as

- translation (movement of the heart as a whole in the chest),
- rotation (circular motion around the long axis of the left ventricle),
- torsion (unequal rotational motion at the apex versus the base of the left ventricle).

Even if the 2D image plane is fixed in position, the location of underlying structures may vary between systole and diastole. For example, in the apical four-chamber view, adjacent segments (which may be supplied by different coronary arteries) of the left ventricle may be seen in systole versus diastole.

Nomenclature of Standard Views

Each tomographic image is defined by its acoustic *window* (the position of the transducer) and *view* (the image plane) (Table 2–2). The standard three orthogonal echocardiographic image planes are determined by the axis of the heart itself (with the left ventricle as the major point of reference) rather than by skeletal or external body landmarks (Fig. 2–1). The reference points on the heart are the apex, defined as the tip of the left ventricle, and the base, defined as the valve annulus region. The three standard image planes then are:

- *Long-axis plane*: Parallel to the long axis of the left ventricle, defined as an imaginary line drawn through the left ventricular apex and the center of the left ventricular base, with the image plane intersecting the center of the aortic valve
- *Short-axis plane*: Perpendicular to the long-axis of the ventricle, resulting in circular cross-sectional views of the left ventricle
- *Four-chamber plane* (also called the horizontal long axis plane): Perpendicular to both long- and short-axis views, resulting in an image plane from the apex to the base intersecting the right and left ventricles and atria

This standard terminology also applies to other cardiac tomographic imaging techniques and to visualization of cardiac anatomy with three-dimensional (3D) echocardiography.

Acoustic windows are transducer positions that allow ultrasound access to the cardiac structures. The bony thoracic cage and adjacent air-filled lung limit the possible acoustic windows, making patient positioning and sonographer experience critical factors in obtaining diagnostic images. Transthoracic images typically are obtained from parasternal, apical, subcostal, and suprasternal

TABLE 2–2		
Transthoracic Echo Image Orientation Nomenclature		

Window (Transducer Location)

Parasternal
Apical
Subcostal
Suprasternal

Image Planes

Long-axis
Short-axis
Four-chamber

Reference Points

Apex
Base
Lateral
Medial

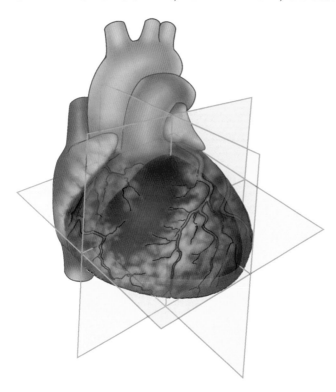

■ **FIGURE 2–1.** The three basic image planes used in transthoracic echocardiography. The long-axis view extends from the left ventricular apex through the aortic valve plane. The short-axis view is perpendicular to the long-axis view resulting in a circular view of the left ventricle. The four-chamber view is perpendicular to both the long- and short-axis views and includes the left ventricular apex, right ventricle, and left and right atria.

notch acoustic windows. The transducer motions used to obtain the desired view are described as follows (Fig. 2–2):

■ *Move* the transducer to a different position on the chest
■ *Tilt or point* the transducer tip with a rocking motion to image different structures in the same tomographic plane
■ *Angle* the transducer from side to side to obtain different tomographic planes somewhat parallel to the original image plane
■ *Rotate* the image plane at a single position to obtain intersecting tomographic planes

Image Orientation

Most laboratories follow the American Society of Echocardiography (ASE) guidelines for image orientation in adults, although many pediatric cardiologists use alternate formats. The recommended orientation is with the transducer position (narrowest portion of the sector scan) at the top of the screen so that structures nearer to the transducer are at the top and structures farther from the transducer are at the bottom of the image. This orientation aids in prompt recognition of ultrasound artifacts, shadowing, and reverberations, because the display of the origin of the ultrasound signal is the same for all acoustic windows and image planes.

The lateral (in short-axis views) and superior (in long-axis views) cardiac structures are displayed on the right side of the screen, which is similar to the format used for other tomographic imaging techniques. Short-axis views can be thought of as the observer looking from the apex toward the cardiac base; long-axis views, as the observer looking from the left toward the right side of the heart. The four-chamber (horizontal long-axis) plane is displayed with lateral structures on the right side of the screen and medial structures on the left side (as for the short-axis view).

Technical Quality

Image quality depends on the degree of ultrasound tissue penetration, as well as on the instrument used, transducer frequency, instrument settings, and the sonographer's skill. Acoustic access to the cardiac structures is determined by body habitus, specifically how the heart is positioned in the chest relative to the lungs and chest wall. Conditions that increase the separation between the transducer and the cardiac structures (e.g., adipose tissue), decrease ultrasound penetration (e.g., scar tissue), or interpose air-containing tissues between the transducer and the heart (e.g., chronic lung disease, recent cardiac surgery) lead to poor image quality. Transesophageal images tend to show better structure

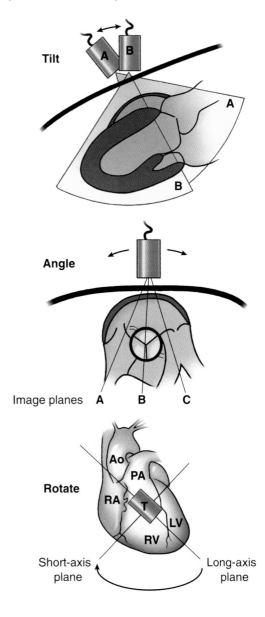

FIGURE 2–2. Transducer motion at a given acoustic window using the example of a left parasternal transducer position. *Tilt*: The transducer is "rocked" to provide images (*A* or *B*) in the same tomographic plane. *Angle*: Different image planes (perpendicular to the plane of the figure at lines *A, B,* and *C*) are obtained by angulation of the transducer. *Rotation*: The transducer is "twisted" with a circular motion to provide a different image plane while maintaining the same orientation between the transducer itself and the chest wall.

definition because of greater ultrasound penetration given the shorter distance between the transducer and the cardiac structures, the use of a higher-frequency transducer, and the absence of interposed lung. On transthoracic studies, optimal patient positioning for each acoustic window brings the cardiac structures against the chest wall. In addition, respiratory variation can be used to the sonographer's advantage by having the patient suspend respiration briefly in whatever phase of the respiratory cycle yields the best image quality. Unfortunately, even with careful attention to examination technique, echocardiographic images remain suboptimal in some patients.

Echocardiographic Image Interpretation

The physician uses the tomographic 2D echocardiographic images to build a mental 3D reconstruction of the cardiac chambers and valves, or uses a 3D echocardiographic data set to examine anatomy in specific image planes (see Chapter 4). To do this, an understanding of image planes and orientation and the technical aspects of image acquisition (e.g., in recognizing artifacts) is needed along with a detailed knowledge of cardiac anatomy. A list of anatomic terminology is shown in Table 2–3. Recording images as the tomographic plane is moved between standard

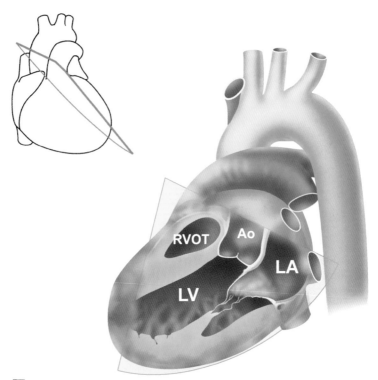

FIGURE 2–3. Parasternal long axis view. The line drawing shows the position of the image plane on an anterior view of the heart. The 3D heart is rotated to the left to show anatomic details of the image plane. In diastole, the long axis view shows the aortic root (Ao) anterior to the left atrium (LA) and the basal segments of the left ventricle (LV) and mitral valve. The aortic root typically is seen beyond the level of the sinotubular junction. The aortic valve is closed with the right coronary and noncoronary cusps visualized. The anterior and posterior leaflets of the open mitral valve are seen. The segments of the left ventricle imaged are the basal and mid-ventricular segments of the anterior septum and posterior wall. The medial papillary muscle has been shown for reference, although slight medial angulation is needed to visualize this structure in the long-axis view. The right ventricular outflow tract (RVOT) is anterior, while the coronary sinus in the atrioventricular groove.

image planes is important for this analysis and ensures that abnormalities that lie outside or between our arbitrary "standard" views are not missed. In complex cases, the physician may need to perform part of the study to appreciate the 3D relationship of the different image planes. Information obtained from anatomic 2D imaging then is integrated with physiologic Doppler data and clinical information in the final echocardiographic interpretation.

TRANSTHORACIC TOMOGRAPHIC VIEWS

The normal anatomy as seen on echocardiography is described below for each tomographic view. The best views for specific cardiac structures are indicated in Table 2–4, expected changes with

aging are shown in Table 2–5, and normal dimensions are shown in Table 2–6.

Parasternal Window

Long-Axis Views

With the patient in a left lateral decubitus position and the transducer in the left third or fourth intercostal space, adjacent to the sternum, a long-axis view of the heart is obtained that bisects the long axis of both aortic and mitral valves (Figs. 2–3 and 2–4). The patient's position may need adjustment between a steep left lateral and nearly supine position based on the images obtained in each subject. The *aortic root,* sinuses of Valsalva, sinotubular junction, and proximal 3 to 4 cm of the ascending aorta are seen in long axis. Further segments of the ascending aorta may be demonstrated by

TABLE 2-3	
Terminology for Normal Echocardiographic Anatomy	
Aortic root	Sinuses of Valsalva Sinotubular junction Coronary ostia
Aortic valve	Right, left, and noncoronary cusps Nodules of Arantius Lambl's excrescence
Mitral valve	Anterior and posterior leaflets Chordae (primary, secondary, tertiary; basal and marginal) Commissures (medial and lateral)
Left ventricle	Wall segments (see Chapter 8) Septum, free wall Base, apex Medial and lateral papillary muscles
Right ventricle	Inflow segment Moderator band Outflow tract (conus) Supraventricular crest Anterior, posterior, and conus papillary muscles
Tricuspid value	Anterior, septal, and posterior leaflets Chordae Commissures
Right atrium	Right atrial appendage SVC, IVC junctions Valve of IVC (Chiari network) Crista terminalis Fossa ovalis Patent foramen ovale
Left atrium	Left atrial appendage Superior and inferior left pulmonary veins Superior and inferior right pulmonary veins Ridge at junction of left atrial appendage and left superior pulmonary vein
Pericardium	Oblique sinus Transverse sinus

SVC, Superior vena cava; IVC, inferior vena cava.

TABLE 2-4	
Transthoracic Echo: Views for Specific Cardiac Structures	
Anatomic Structures	**Best Views**
Aortic valve	Parasternal long-axis (PLAX) Parasternal short-axis (PSAX) Apical long-axis Anteriorly angulated apical 4-chamber
Mitral valve (MV)	PLAX PSAX-mitral valve level Apical 4-chamber Apical long-axis
Pulmonic valve	PSAX (aortic valve level) RV outflow Subcostal short-axis (aortic valve level)
Tricuspid valve	Right ventricular (RV) inflow Apical 4-chamber Subcostal 4-chamber and short-axis
Left ventricle (LV)	PLAX PSAX Apical 4-chamber, 2-chamber, long-axis Subcostal 4-chamber and short-axis
Right ventricle	PLAX (RV outflow tract only) RV inflow PSAX (MV and LV levels) Apical 4-chamber Subcostal 4-chamber
Left atrium	PLAX PSAX Apical 4-chamber, 2-chamber, long-axis Subcostal 4-chamber
Right atrium	PSAX (aortic valve level) Apical 4-chamber Subcostal 4-chamber and short-axis
Aorta	
Ascending	High parasternal and standard parasternal long-axis
Arch	Suprasternal notch
Descending thoracic	Suprasternal notch Parasternal with angulation Apical 2-chamber with modification Subcostal
Interatrial septum	Parasternal short-axis Subcostal 4-chamber
Coronary sinus	Parasternal long-axis to RV inflow view (sweep) Apical 4-chamber angulated posteriorly

MV, Mitral valve; LV, left ventricle; PSAX, parasternal short axis; PLAX, parasternal long axis; RV, right ventricle.

TABLE 2-5	

Echocardiographic Findings in Elderly Patients

Echo Format	Findings
2D echo	Left and right atrial enlargement
	Mitral annular calcification
	Aortic valve fibrosis and calcification (usually without significant stenosis)
	Tortuosity of the aorta
	Prominent angle between the base of the septum and aortic root appearing as a "septal knuckle"
Doppler echo	LV inflow pattern with E < A and prolonged deceleration slope
	Pulmonary vein (LA inflow) pattern with increased systolic flow, reduced antegrade diastolic flow and prominent *a*-wave reversal of flow

LV, Left ventricular; LA, left atrial.

moving the transducer cephalad one or two interspaces. The upper limit of normal for aortic root dimensions in adults is $1.6\,cm/m^2$ at the annulus and $2.1\,cm/m^2$ at the aortic leaflet tips in systole.

In the long-axis view, the right coronary cusp of the *aortic valve* is anterior and the noncoronary cusp is posterior (the left coronary cusp is lateral to the image plane). In systole, the thin aortic leaflets open widely, assuming a parallel orientation to the aortic walls. In diastole, the leaflets are closed, with a small obtuse closure angle between the two leaflets. The leaflets appear linear from the closure line to the aortic annulus due to the hemicylindrical shape of the closed leaflets (linear along the length of the cylinder, curved along its short axis). In normal young individuals, the leaflets are so thin that only the apposed portions at the leaflets' closure line are seen. The 3D anatomy of the attachment line of the aortic leaflets to the aortic root is shaped like a crown with the three commissures attached near the tops of the sinuses of Valsalva and the midportion of each leaflet attached near the base of each sinus (Fig. 2–5). This attachment line often is referred to as the aortic "annulus," although there are no distinct tissue characteristics of this attachment zone. Note that there is fibrous continuity between the aortic root and the anterior mitral leaflet. The absence of intervening myocardium between aortic and mitral valves helps identify the anatomic left ventricle in complex congenital disease.

The anterior and posterior *mitral valve* leaflets appear thin and uniform in echogenicity, with chordal attachments leading toward the medial (or posteromedial) papillary muscle seen in the long-axis view, although the papillary muscle itself is slightly medial to the long-axis plane. The anterior mitral leaflet is longer than the posterior leaflet but has a smaller annular length so that the surface areas of the two leaflets are similar (Fig. 2–6). As the mitral leaflets open in diastole, the tips separate and the anterior leaflet touches or comes very close to the ventricular septum. In systole, the leaflets coapt, with some overlap between the leaflets (apposition zone) and a slightly obtuse (>180°) angle relative to the mitral annulus plane. The chordae normally remain posterior to the plane of leaflet coaptation in systole. However, some normal individuals have systolic anterior motion of the chordae, due to mild redundancy of chordal tissue that is not associated with hemodynamic abnormalities. This must be distinguished from the pathologic systolic anterior motion of the mitral leaflets seen in hypertrophic obstructive cardiomyopathy. The mitral annulus (the attachment between the mitral leaflets, left atrium, and left ventricle) is an anatomically well-defined fibrous structure with an elliptical shape. The long-axis view bisects the minor axis of the mitral annulus. (The major axis is seen in the apical four-chamber view.)

The *left atrium* is seen posterior to the aortic root with a similar anteroposterior dimension as the aortic root. The *right pulmonary artery* lies between the aortic root and superior aspect of the left atrium but may not be well seen on transthoracic images. The *coronary sinus* is seen in the atrioventricular groove posterior to the mitral annulus. Dilation of the coronary sinus due to a persistent left superior vena cava (which can be confirmed by echo-contrast injection in a left arm vein) is an occasional incidental finding of no clinical significance that can mimic a left atrial mass.

Posterior to the left atrium, the *descending thoracic aorta* is seen in cross section. A long-axis view of the descending thoracic aorta can be obtained from this window by rotating the transducer counterclockwise. Note that the oblique sinus of the pericardium lies between the left atrium and the descending thoracic aorta so that a pericardial

TABLE 2-6

Selected Normal Echocardiographic Dimensions in Adults

Parameter	Range	Range Indexed to BSA	Upper Limit of Normal
Aorta			
Annulus diameter (cm)	1.4–2.6	$1.3 \pm 0.1\,cm/m^2$	<$1.6\,cm/m^2$ (men and women)
Diameter at leaflet tips (cm)	2.2–3.6	$1.7 \pm 0.2\,cm/m^2$	<$2.1\,cm/m^2$ (men and women)
Ascending aorta diameter (cm)	2.1–3.4	$1.5 \pm 0.2\,cm/m^2$	
Arch diameter (cm)	2.0–3.6		
Left Ventricle			
Short-axis dimension (cm)			
Diastole	3.5–6.0	$2.3–3.1\,cm/m^2$	
Systole	2.1–4.0	$1.4–2.1\,cm/m^2$	
Long-axis dimension (cm)			
Diastole	6.3–10.3	$4.1–5.7\,cm/m^2$	
Systole	4.6–8.4		
End-diastolic volume (mL)			
Men	96–157	$67 \pm 9\,mL$	
Women	59–138	$61 \pm 13\,mL$	
End-systolic volume (mL)			
Men	33–68	$27 \pm 5\,mL$	
Women	18–65	$26 \pm 7\,mL$	
Ejection fraction (%)			
Men	0.59 ± 0.06		
Women	0.58 ± 0.07		
LV-wall thickness (cm) (end-diastole)	0.6–1.1		Men < 1.2 cm
LV-mass (gm)			Women < 1.1 cm
Men	<294 g	<$163\,g/m$*	<$150\,g/m^2$
Women	<198 g	<$121\,g/m$*	<$120\,g/m^2$
Left Atrium			
Anterior-posterior dimension (cm) (PLAX)	2.3–4.5	$1.6–2.4\,cm/m^2$	
Medial-lateral dimension (cm) (A4C)	2.5–4.5	$1.6–2.4\,cm/m^2$	
Superior-inferior dimension (cm) (A4C)	3.4–6.1	$2.3–3.5\,cm/m^2$	
Mitral Annulus			
End-diastole (cm)	2.7 ± 0.4		
End-systole (cm)	2.9 ± 0.3		
Right Ventricle			
Wall thickness (cm)	0.2–0.5	$0.2 \pm 0.05\,cm/m^2$	
Minor dimension (cm)	2.2–4.4	$1.0–2.8\,cm/m^2$	
Length			
Diastole (cm)	5.5–9.5	$3.8–5.3\,cm/m^2$	
Systole (cm)	4.2–8.1		
Pulmonary Artery			
Annulus diameter (cm)	1.0–2.2		
Main PA (cm)	0.9–2.9		
Inferior Vena Cava Diameters			
(at RA junction) (cm)	1.2–2.3		

BSA, Body surface area; LV, left ventricle; PA, pulmonary artery; RA, right atrium.

Refs: Roman et al. AJC 1989 64:507–11   Pini et al. Circ 1989 80:915
    Schnittger et al. JACC 1983 2:934–8   Erbel et al. Dtsch med Wschr 107:1872 (1982)
    Truiulzi et al. Echo 1984 1:403–9   Hahn et al. Z. Kardiol 71:445 (1982)
    Levy et al. AJC 1987 59:936
    Pearlman et al. JACC 1988 12:1432–10
*Indexed for height.

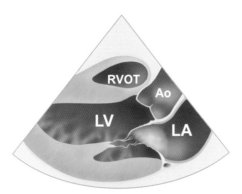

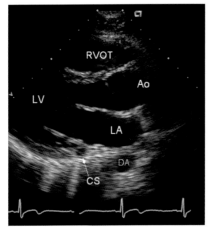 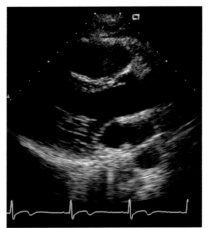

■ **FIGURE 2–4.** The tomographic section from the 3D view of the parasternal long axis view has been rotated into the standard echocardiographic format with the transducer position, or apex of the sector scan, at the top of the image. Corresponding normal parasternal long-axis 2D echo images at end-diastole (*left*) and end-systole (*right*) show the anatomic features. In addition, the descending thoracic aorta (DA) is seen posterior to the left atrium.

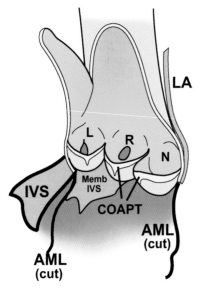

■ **FIGURE 2–5.** Schematic diagram of normal aortic valve anatomy shown in a frontal view with the aortic root "opened" between the left (L) and noncoronary (N) cusps by cutting through the anterior mitral leaflet (AML) to demonstrate the crown-shaped "annulus." The commissures are near the top of each sinus and each leaflet has a hemi-cylindrical shape so that the closed leaflets appear as a straight line in the long-axis view. Each aortic leaflet has a coaptation zone, with overlap between adjacent leaflets and a thicker region, the nodule of Arantius at the center of each cusp. The close anatomic relationships of the aortic valve to the interventricular septum (IVS), membranous septum (MS), mitral valve, and left atrium (LA) can be appreciated.

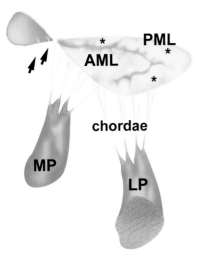

FIGURE 2–6. Schematic diagram of normal mitral valve anatomy. The anterior mitral leaflet (AML) attaches to a smaller portion of the circumference of the annulus than the posterior mitral leaflet (PML) but the anterior leaflet is longer. The posterior leaflet consists of three segments (*asterisks*) designated the medial, central, and lateral scallops. Both leaflets attach to both the medial and lateral papillary muscle (MP and LP). The anterior leaflet has been cut and turned back to show attachments of basal chordae (*arrows*) that attached to the body of the leaflet, rather than at the leaflet edge, as seen with marginal chordae.

effusion can be seen between these two structures, while a pleural effusion will be seen only posterior to the descending thoracic aorta.

The *left ventricular* septum and posterior wall are seen at the base and midventricular level in the long-axis view, allowing assessment of wall thickness, chamber dimensions, endocardial motion, and wall thickening of these myocardial segments. From the parasternal window, the left ventricular apex is not seen—the apparent "apex" usually is an oblique image plane through the anterolateral wall.

A portion of the muscular *right ventricular outflow tract* is seen anteriorly. Unlike the symmetric prolate ellipsoid shape of the left ventricle, the right ventricle does not have an easily defined long or short axis. In effect, the right ventricle is "wrapped around" the left ventricle, with an inflow region, an apical region, and an outflow region forming a somewhat anteroposteriorly flattened U-shaped structure. Most standard image planes result in oblique tomographic sections of the right ventricle, so right ventricular size and systolic function are best evaluated from multiple views, as discussed more fully in Chapter 6.

Right Ventricular Inflow and Outflow Views

In the long-axis plane, the transducer is moved apically and then is angulated medially to obtain

a view of the *right atrium, tricuspid valve,* and *right ventricle* (Fig. 2–7). In this right ventricular inflow view, the septal and anterior leaflets of the tricuspid valve are well seen. The right ventricular apex is heavily trabeculated, while the outflow tract (supracristal region) has a smoother endocardial surface. The moderator band, a prominent muscle trabeculation that traverses the right ventricular apex obliquely and contains the right bundle branch, may be seen in both parasternal and apical views (Fig. 2–8). The papillary muscles are more difficult to identify in the right ventricle than in the left ventricle. Typically, there are two principal papillary muscles (anterior and posterior) with a smaller supracristal (or conus) papillary muscle. The moderator band attaches near the base of the anterior right ventricular papillary muscle.

The *coronary sinus* is identified as it enters the right atrium adjacent to the tricuspid annulus. By slowly scanning back to a left ventricular long-axis view, the coronary sinus can be followed along its length.

Another normal anatomic feature of the right atrium (Fig. 2–9) that may be appreciated on echocardiographic imaging is the *crista terminalis,* a muscular ridge that courses anteriorly from the superior to inferior vena cava and divides the trabeculated anterior portion of the right atrium from the posterior, smooth-walled sinus venosus segment. The right atrial appendage is rarely seen on transthoracic imaging but is a trabeculated protrusion of the right atrium extending anterior to the right atrial free wall and base of the aorta.

The *inferior vena cava* is seen entering the right atrium inferior to the coronary sinus. In some individuals, a prominent Eustachian valve is seen at the junction of the inferior vena cava and right atrium both in this view and from the subcostal window. When a more extensive fenestrated valve is present, it forms a Chiari network extending from the inferior to superior vena cava, attached to the crista terminalis posteriorly and the fossa ovalis medially, with a netlike structure that appears as mobile echos in the right atrium. Both these findings are considered normal variants of no clinical significance.

The interatrial septum is not well seen in the right ventricular inflow view, being just inferior and parallel to the image plane. However, careful angulation between the long axis and right ventricular inflow views allows examination of the atrial septum with recognition of the thick primum septum at its junction with the central fibrous body, the thin fossa ovalis in the central portion of the atrial septum, the ridgelike limbus

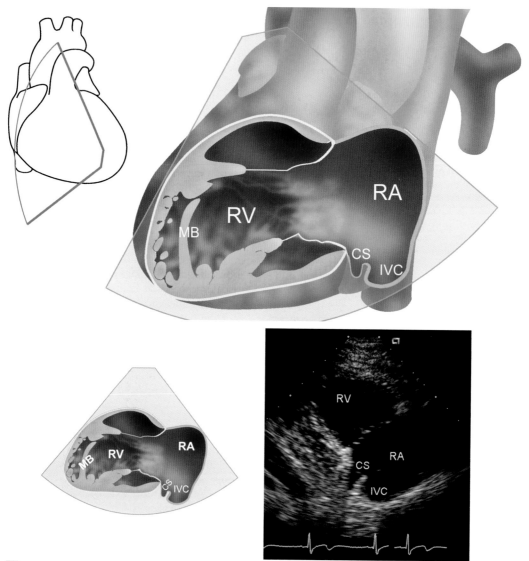

■ **FIGURE 2–7.** Right ventricular inflow view. The position of the image plane is shown on the line drawing with the 3D heart rotated to shown the anatomic details (*top*). The 2D image (*below left*) and tomographic plane (*below right*), shown in the standard orientation, show the right ventricle (RV) and atrium (RA), tricuspid valve (TV), and ostia of the coronary sinus (CS) and inferior vena cava (IVC). In this view, two tricuspid leaflets are seen, typically the anterior and septal leaflets, but the posterior leaflet may be seen depending on the exact image plane and individual variation.

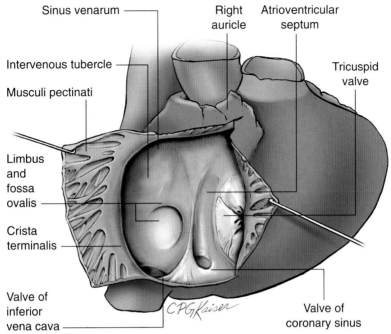

Sinus venarum

Right auricle

Atrioventricular septum

Intervenous tubercle

Tricuspid valve

Musculi pectinati

Limbus and fossa ovalis

Crista terminalis

Valve of inferior vena cava

Valve of coronary sinus

FIGURE 2-8. The interior of the right atrium seen from the right side. The view is toward the interatrial septum. (From Rosse C, Gaddum-Rosse P: Hollinshead's Textbook of Anatomy, 5th ed. Philadelphia: Lippincott-Raven, 1997, p 473. Used with permission.)

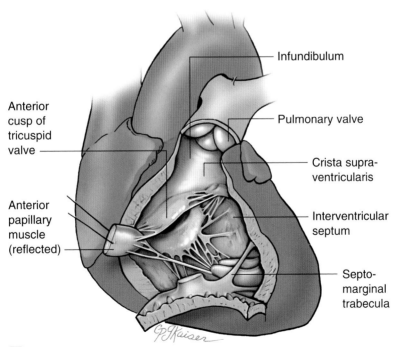

Infundibulum

Anterior cusp of tricuspid valve

Pulmonary valve

Crista supra-ventricularis

Anterior papillary muscle (reflected)

Interventricular septum

Septo-marginal trabecula

FIGURE 2-9. The interior of the right ventricle. The crista supraventricularis separates the inflow part of the ventricle from the infundibulum, or conus arteriosus. Note the great distance between the septal leaflet of the tricuspid valve and the pulmonary valve. (From Rosse C, Gaddum-Rosse P: Hollinshead's Textbook of Anatomy, 5th ed. Philadelphia: Lippincott-Raven, 1997, p 473. Used with permission.)

located superior to the fossa, and the ridge adjacent to the junction with the coronary sinus.

Moving the transducer toward the base and then angulating laterally, a long-axis view of the right ventricular outflow tract, *pulmonic valve,* and pulmonary artery is obtained. This view is particularly useful for recording flow velocities in the right ventricular outflow tract and pulmonary artery.

Short-Axis Views

Short-axis views are obtained from the parasternal window by rotating the transducer clockwise 90° and then angulating the transducer superiorly or inferiorly to obtain specific image planes.

At the *aortic valve* level (Figs. 2–10 and 2–11), the short-axis view demonstrates all three aortic valve leaflets—right, left, and noncoronary cusps. In systole, the aortic leaflets open to a near-circular orifice. In diastole, the typical Y-shaped arrangement of the coaptation lines of the leaflets is seen. Identification of the number of aortic valve leaflets is made most accurately in systole, since a bicuspid valve may appear trileaflet in diastole due to a raphe in the position of a normal commissure. Normally, the aortic valve leaflets are thin at the base with an area of thickening on the ventricular aspect in the middle of the free edge of each cusp, which serves to fill the space at the center of the closed valve. These nodules

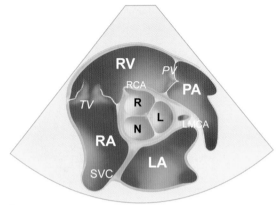

■ **FIGURE 2–10.** Parasternal short-axis view at the aortic valve level showing the relationship between the three cusps of the aortic valve—right coronary cusp (R), noncoronary cusp (N), left coronary cusp (L)—and the left atrium (LA), right atrium (RA), right ventricular outflow tract (RVOT), and the pulmonary artery (PA) with right and left branches. The positions of the right coronary artery (RCA), left main coronary artery (LMCA), superior vena cava (SVC), pulmonic valve, and tricuspid valve are shown.

normally enlarge with age (nodules of Arantius) and can have small mobile filaments attached on the ventricular surface (Lambl's excrescences). These small but normal structures may be seen when echocardiographic images are of high quality and should not be mistaken for pathologic

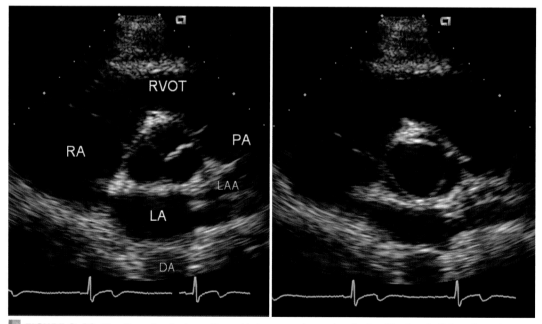

■ **FIGURE 2–11.** Two-dimensional echocardiographic images at the aortic valve level in diastole (*left*) and systole (*right*). Note the three open leaflets of the aortic valve in systole and the normal perpendicular relationship of aortic and pulmonic valves. LAA, left atrial appendage.

conditions. The origins of the left main and right coronary arteries often can be identified in this view.

The aortic and pulmonic valve planes normally lie perpendicular to each other. Thus, when the aortic valve is seen in short axis, the pulmonic valve is seen in long axis. In adults, evaluation of the leaflets of the pulmonic valve is limited; usually only one or two leaflets are seen well, and a short-axis view often is not obtainable.

The close relationship between the aortic valve and other intracardiac structures is apparent in this short-axis view. In addition to the pulmonic valve and right ventricular outflow tract, which are seen anterolaterally adjacent to the left coronary cusp, portions of the tricuspid valve are seen anteriorly and slightly medially, adjacent to the right coronary cusp. The two leaflets of the tricuspid valve seen in this view are the septal and anterior leaflets.

Posteriorly, the right atrium, interatrial septum, and left atrium lie in proximity to the noncoronary cusp of the aortic valve. The left atrial appendage can be better imaged from this view by a slight lateral angulation and superior rotation of the transducer. The central location of the aortic valve illustrates how disease processes can extend from the aortic valve or root into the right ventricular outflow tract, right atrium, or left atrium. Extension of disease processes into the ventricular septum or anterior mitral leaflet also is possible, as evident in the long-axis view.

At the *mitral valve* short-axis level (Fig. 2–12), the thin anterior and posterior mitral leaflets are seen as they open nearly to the full cross-sectional area of the left ventricle in diastole and close in systole. The posterior leaflet consists of three major scallops—medial, central, and lateral—although there is considerable individual variability. The two mitral commissures—the points on the annulus where the anterior and posterior leaflets meet—are located medially and laterally. Note that this parallels the arrangement of the papillary muscles so that chordae from the medial aspects of both anterior and posterior leaflets attach to the medial (or posteromedial) papillary muscle and chordae from the lateral aspects of both leaflets attach to the lateral (or anterolateral) papillary muscle. Chordae branch at three levels (primary, secondary, and tertiary) between the papillary muscle tip and mitral leaflet with a progressive decrease in chordal diameter and increase in the number of chordae from approximately 12 at the papillary muscle to 120 at the mitral leaflet. Most chordae attach at the free edge of the leaflets (called *marginal chordae*), but some (called *basal*

chordae) attach to the left ventricular surface of the leaflet. Occasionally, aberrant chordae to the ventricular septum or other structures are seen in an otherwise normal individual.

At the mid-ventricular (or *papillary muscle* level) short-axis view (Fig. 2–13), the left ventricle is seen in circular cross section. The nomenclature of left ventricular myocardial segments is discussed in Chapter 8, but basically, the ventricle is divided into anterior (septum and free wall), anterolateral, inferolateral (also called posterior), and inferior (free wall and septum) segments for consistent descriptors of the location of abnormalities.

The left ventricle typically appears circular in short axis, so that an elliptical appearance of the chamber usually is due to a nonperpendicular orientation relative to the long axis of the left ventricle. Moving the transducer superiorly with apical angulation resolves this problem. Actual distortion of the circular cross section may be seen in patients with ischemic cardiac disease, prior myocardial infarction, and aneurysm formation. The short-axis view at the papillary muscle level allows measurement of wall thickness and internal dimensions of the left ventricle in systole and diastole from either the 2D image or a 2D-guided M-mode recording. Rotating the transducer between the long- and short-axis views at this level ensures a true short-axis measurement (perpendicular to the long axis). Oblique measurements will result in overestimation of wall thickness and ventricular dimensions.

This view also allows assessment of endocardial motion and wall thickening at the midventricular level in the distribution of the left anterior descending artery (anterior septum and anterior wall), posterior descending artery (inferior septum and inferior wall), and circumflex artery (anterolateral and inferolateral walls) (see Chapter 8). Ventricular septal motion may reflect abnormalities other than coronary disease, including right ventricular volume and/or pressure overload, conduction abnormalities, and the postcardiac-surgery state (see Fig. 6–17).

The medial and lateral papillary muscles are seen in this short-axis plane and serve as landmarks identifying the midventricular level. Rarely, one of the papillary muscles may be bifid, resulting in an appearance of three separate papillary muscles. Note that the apical segments of the left ventricular myocardium are not seen in standard parasternal views. However, in some patients, a short-axis view of the left ventricle near the apex can be obtained by moving the transducer laterally and angling medially.

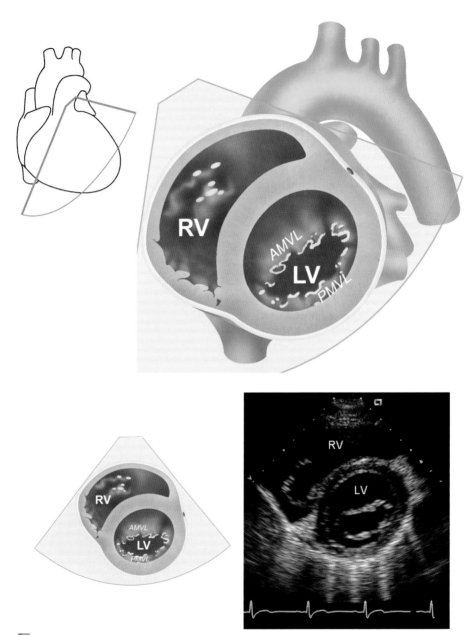

■ **FIGURE 2–12.** Short-axis plane at the mitral valve level. The position of the short-axis plane is shown on the line drawing. The 3D view shown by tilting the apex up to show the cross section of the right and left ventricle with the anterior and posterior mitral valve leaflets (AMVL and PMVL). The tomographic plane has been rotated with the apex of the sector at the top (*bottom left*) to correspond to the 2D echocadiographic image (*bottom right*).

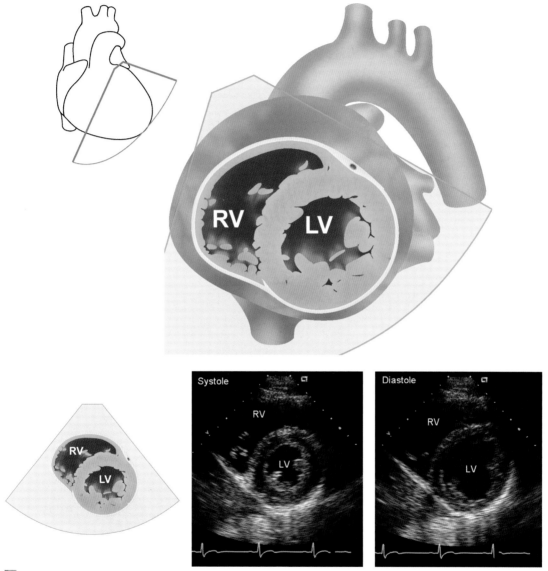

■ **FIGURE 2–13.** Short-axis plane at the papillary muscle level. The position of the short-axis plane is shown on the line drawing. The 3D view shown by tilting the apex up to show the cross section of the right and left ventricle with the medial and lateral papillary muscles. The tomographic plane has been rotated with the apex of the sector at the top (*bottom left*) to corrspond to the 2D echocadiographic images in systole and diastole (*bottom right*). Note the circular shape of the left ventricle with symmetric wall thickening and inward endocardial motion with contraction.

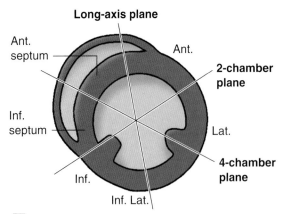

Long-axis plane

Ant. septum

Ant.

2-chamber plane

Inf. septum

Lat.

4-chamber plane

Inf.

Inf. Lat.

■ **FIGURE 2–14.** Relationship between the short-axis plane with left ventricular wall segments indicated, and the apical four-chamber, two-chamber (also called vertical long-axis), and aortic long-axis image planes (perpendicular to the short-axis plane).

Apical Window

The apical window is identified initially by palpation of the left ventricular apex with the patient in a steep left lateral decubitus position. An apical "cutout" in the examination stretcher allows optimal patient positioning and placement of the transducer on the apical impulse. Transducer position then is adjusted as needed to obtain optimal images. The relationship between the three basic apical views and the short-axis plane is shown in Figure 2–14.

Four-Chamber View

In the apical four-chamber view, the length of the *left ventricle* is seen in a plane perpendicular to both the short-axis and long-axis planes (Figs. 2–15 and 2–16). The anterolateral wall, apex, and inferior septum lie in this tomographic plane. The left ven-

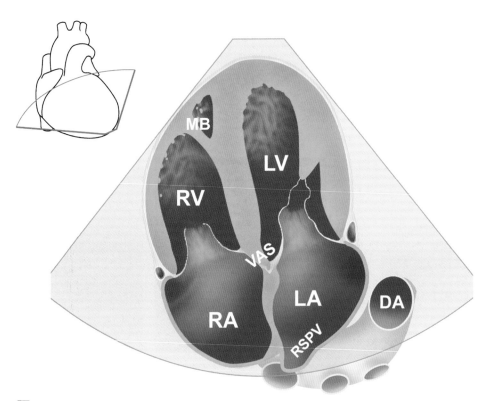

■ **FIGURE 2–15.** Apical four-chamber view. The apical four-chamber view shows the relationships of the left and right ventricles (LV and RV) and atria (LA and RA). In the left ventricle, the papillary muscle, chordae, and anterior and posterior mitral leaflets are seen. The descending aorta (DA) is seen in partial cross section lateral to the left atrium, while the right superior pulmonary vein (RSPV) drains into the left atrium adjacent to the interatrial septum. In the right ventricle, the moderator band (MB) and the anterior and septal tricuspid valve leaflets are seen. Note the ventriculoatrial septum (VAS) separating the left ventricle from the right atrium in association with the normal, slightly more apical position of the tricuspid compared with the mitral valve annulus.

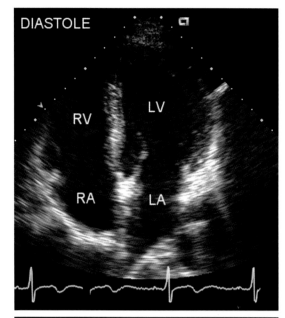

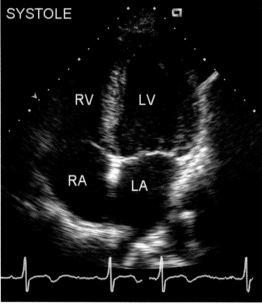

FIGURE 2–16. Two-dimensional echo images in an apical four-chamber view at end-diastole (*above*) and end-systole (*below*). LV and RV, left and right ventricles; LA and RA, left and right atria.

tricle appears as a truncated ellipse with a longer length than width and a tapered but rounded apex. If the transducer is not positioned at the true apex, the left ventricle will appear foreshortened, with a spherical shape and little tapering of the apex. Foreshortening of the long-axis plane must

be distinguished from disease processes, such as chronic aortic regurgitation, which result in increased sphericity of the ventricle. Although the right ventricle is more trabeculated than the left ventricle, prominent trabeculation also can be seen at the left ventricular apex and must be distinguished from apical thrombus. When aberrant left ventricular trabeculae transverse the ventricular chamber, a "chord" or "web" is seen on 2D echo.

Medially, the *right ventricle* is triangular with a cavity about half the area of the left ventricle. The right ventricular apex is less round and more basal than the left ventricular apex. The moderator band often is seen traversing the right ventricle near the apex. The right ventricle can be further evaluated by moving the transducer medially over the right ventricular apex. Considerable individual variability in the shape and wall motion of the right ventricle, particularly at the apex, is seen in healthy individuals, so caution is needed in diagnosing an abnormal right ventricle from any single tomographic plane.

The four-chamber view also shows the mitral annulus in its major dimension, the anterior mitral valve leaflet (located adjacent to the septum), and the posterior mitral valve leaflet (adjacent to the lateral wall), along with chordae and attachments to the lateral papillary muscle. The mitral leaflet tips separate widely in diastole, and in systole the closure plane of the leaflets may appear "flat" (a 180° closure angle) due to the nonplanar "saddle" shape of the annulus, with the four-chamber view bisecting the annulus at its most apical position compared to the more basal annulus segments seen in a long-axis view. However, significant displacement of the leaflets beyond the plane of the mitral annulus is not seen unless the view is foreshortened or mitral valve disease is present.

The tricuspid annulus lies slightly (up to 1.0 cm) closer to the apex than the mitral annulus. The tricuspid leaflets show a wide diastolic opening; thin, uniformly echogenic, leaflets; and normal coaptation in systole. The septal leaflet is imaged adjacent to the septum. The tricuspid leaflet adjacent to the free wall may be either the anterior or posterior leaflet, depending on the exact rotation and angulation of the image plane.

The left and right atria are distal from the apical transducer position. Although a general assessment of size and shape can be made, ultrasound resolution at this depth is poor, and detailed evaluation of atrial tumors or clots often is not possible. The interatrial septum lies parallel to the ultrasound beam in this view, so "dropout" –absence of reflected signal–from the region of the fossa ovalis is common. This should not be mistaken for an atrial septal defect.

The descending thoracic aorta may be seen lateral to the left atrium. The pulmonary veins enter the left atrium posteriorly but may be difficult to image at this depth in adults. If the transducer is angulated posteriorly from the four-chamber view, more posterior portions of the lateral and inferior septal myocardium are seen. In addition, the length of the coronary sinus comes into view in the atrioventricular groove.

Angulating the transducer anteriorly, the aortic valve and root are seen in an oblique long view. This view is sometimes referred to as the apical "five-chamber" view. More anterior portions of the septum and lateral wall are seen, especially at the base, as the transducer is angulated anteriorly. This view of the anterior mitral leaflet, left ventricular outflow tract, and aortic valve is at an angle approximately 60° to 90° from the long-axis view. In some adults, further anterior angulation of the transducer allows visualization of the pulmonary artery arising from the right ventricle. A view of the pulmonic valve from the apical window is more easily obtained in young adults and children.

Two-Chamber View

From the four-chamber view, the transducer is rotated counterclockwise approximately 60° to obtain the two-chamber view of the left ventricle, mitral valve, and left atrium (Fig. 2–17). The apical two-chamber view is used for evaluation of the anterior left ventricular wall (seen to the right of the screen) and the posterior or inferolateral wall (seen on the left). Fine adjustments in transducer position may be needed to depict the anterior wall endocardium due to interference from adjacent lung tissue. To ensure that the proper rotation has been made for a two-chamber view, the transducer is angled posteriorly to intersect both papillary muscles symmetrically. Then the transducer is angled slightly anteriorly so that neither papillary muscle is seen in its long axis in this view. The anterior mitral leaflet is seen en face, so the apparent closure plane of the leaflet relative to the annulus can be misleading. The left atrial appendage may be visualized adjacent to the anterior wall. A long-axis view of the descending thoracic aorta can be obtained by angulating posteriorly and rotating counterclockwise from the two-chamber view.

Long-Axis View

Rotating the transducer another 60° from the two-chamber view (120° from the four-chamber view) yields a long-axis view similar to the parasternal long-axis view (Fig. 2–18). The aortic valve, left ventricular outflow tract, and mitral valve are seen in long axis. The left ventricular walls visualized in this view are the anterior septum (on the right side of the screen) and posterior or inferolateral wall (on the left). Compared with the parasternal long-axis view, the left ventricular apex now is seen, but the aortic and mitral valves are at a greater image depth (with consequent poorer image resolution).

Other Apical Views

Nonstandard short-axis views of the left ventricular apex using a higher frequency transducer (5 or 7.5 MHz) are helpful if a left ventricular apical thrombus is suspected. One useful view is obtained by sliding the transducer medially from the left ventricular apex and then angulating posteriorly.

Subcostal Window

With the patient supine and the legs bent at the knees (if necessary) to relax the abdominal wall musculature, subcostal images of the cardiac structures are obtained. A view of all four chambers shows the right ventricular free wall, the midsection of the interventricular septum, and the anterolateral left ventricular wall (Fig. 2–19). In this view, the interatrial septum is perpendicular to the direction of the ultrasound beam, allowing evaluation of atrial septal defects.

A subcostal short-axis view of the left ventricle allows measurements of left ventricular wall thickness and dimensions that are comparable with dimensions obtained from a parasternal short-axis view, albeit at a greater depth and through different myocardial segments. The subcostal window provides a useful alternative for qualitative and quantitative evaluation of the left ventricle when the parasternal window is inadequate.

Rotating the transducer inferiorly from the subcostal four-chamber view, a long-axis view of the inferior vena cava is obtained as it enters the right atrium. The size of the proximal 2–3 cm of the inferior vena cava at rest and changes in size with respiration are used to estimate right atrial pressure (see Table 6–6). The hepatic veins (particularly the central hepatic vein, which courses parallel to the ultrasound beam in this view) are helpful in assessing right atrial pressure and for recording right atrial Doppler filling patterns. The proximal abdominal aorta is imaged in long axis medial to the inferior vena cava.

Suprasternal Notch Window

With the patient supine and the neck extended, the transducer is positioned in the suprasternal

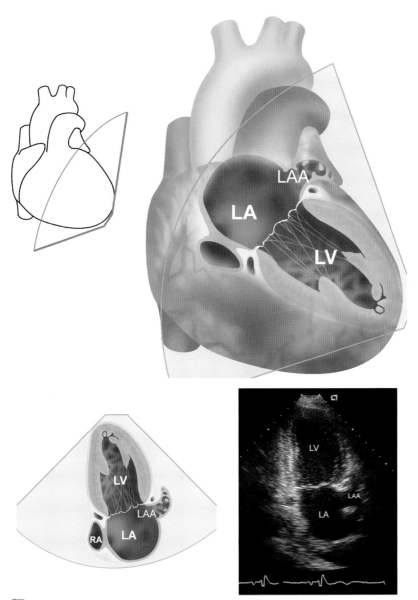

■ **FIGURE 2–17.** Apical two-chamber view. The position of the image plane is shown on the line drawing. The 3D view shows the cross section of the left atrium and ventricle with the left atrial appendage (LAA), coronary sinus in the atrioventricular groove, and the mitral valve. In the two-chamber view, small portions of the posterior mitral leaflet are seen laterally and medially with the anterior leaflet filling most of the annulus area. Part of a papillary muscle has been shown for orientation, but the papillary muscles are seen located symmetrically posterior to the image plane. The tomographic plane has been rotated with the apex of the sector at the top (*bottom left*) to correspond to the 2D echocadiographic image (*bottom right*). In this view, the inferior and anterior left ventricular walls are seen.

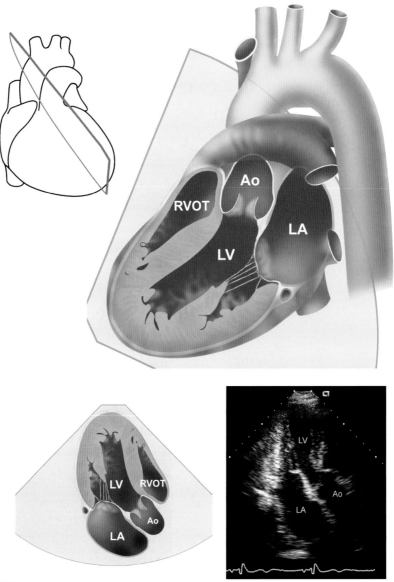

▊ **FIGURE 2–18.** Apical long-axis view. The position of the image plane is shown on the line drawing. The 3D view shows the cross section of the aortic root (Ao), left ventricle (LV), left atrium (LA), and right ventricular outflow tract (RVOT). In the long axis view, the anterior and posterior mitral valve leaflets are seen. The tomographic plane has been rotated with the apex of the sector at the top (*bottom left*) to correspond to the 2D echocardiographic image (*bottom right*). In this view, the anterior septal and posterior (inferolateral) left ventricular walls are seen.

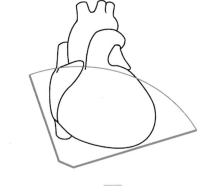

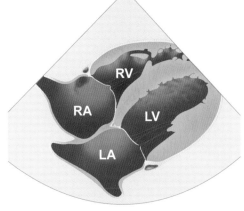

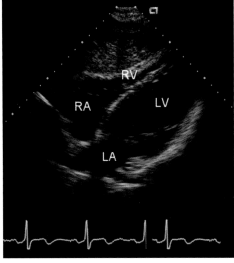

▌ **FIGURE 2–19.** Subcostal four-chamber view. The position of the image plane (*left*), tomographic view rotated with apex of the sector scan at the top of the image (*center*), and corresponding 2D (*right*) subcostal view. The interatrial septum is perpendicular to the ultrasound beam from this window, allowing evaluation for atrial septal defects.

notch or right supraclavicular position to obtain a view of the aortic arch in long and short axis. The long-axis view (with respect to the aortic arch) shows the ascending aorta, arch, proximal descending thoracic aorta, and the origins of the right brachiocephalic and left common carotid and subclavian arteries (Fig. 2–20). The corresponding veins lie superior to the aortic arch, with the superior vena cava lying adjacent to the ascending aorta. The right pulmonary artery is seen "under" the curve of the aortic arch and can be followed to its branch point by rotating the transducer medially.

The short-axis view shows the aortic arch in cross section. The left pulmonary artery can be imaged by rotating slightly laterally. The left atrium lies inferior to the pulmonary arteries in both long- and short-axis views, so it may be possible to evaluate atrial pathology or flow disturbances from this window.

Other Acoustic Windows

In specific cases, other acoustic windows may be needed. For example, a dextropositioned heart would necessitate mirror-image acoustic windows. When a large pleural effusion is present, good-quality images may be obtained in some cases by imaging from the posterior chest wall through the effusion with the patient in a sitting position.

M-MODE RECORDINGS

Although M-mode recordings have largely been replaced by 2D imaging, M-mode recordings still have an important role in evaluation of rapid motion of cardiac structures, because the sampling rate is 1800 frames per second rather than the 30 to 60 frames per second used for 2D imaging. The rapid sampling rate also makes identification of thin moving structures, such as the left

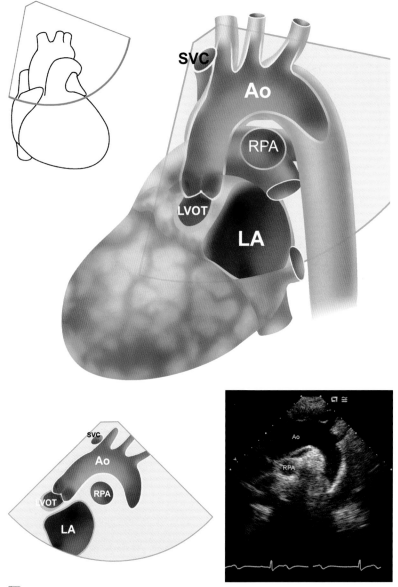

FIGURE 2–20. Suprasternal notch view. The position of the image plane is shown on the line drawing. The 3D view shows the cross-section of the ascending aorta, arch and proximal descending aorta with the origins of the left carotid and subclavian arteries. The right pulmonary artery (RPA) lies immediately inferior to the arch, with the left atrium (LA) and aortic valve sometimes seen from this window.

ventricular endocardium, more accurate and reproducible by showing motion as well as depth of the structure of interest. The potential disadvantage of M-mode data—a nonperpendicular orientation to the structure of interest—can be avoided by using the 2D image in two orthogonal planes to position the M-mode sampling line.

Use of the M-mode feature is most helpful when guided by the 2D image and used either for

■ timing of rapid cardiac motions,
■ precise measurements of cardiac dimensions, or
■ further evaluation of structures seen on 2D imaging (such as suspected vegetations) to aid in their identification.

Aortic Valve and Left Atrium

An M-mode recording through the aortic root at the leaflet tip level shows the parallel walls of the

Aortic Valve and Left Atrial M-mode

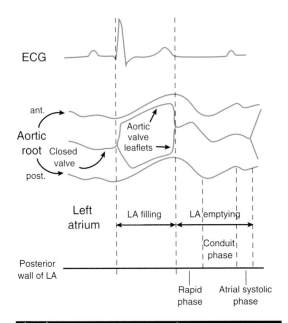

The aortic leaflet coaptation point is seen as a thin line in diastole. In systole, the leaflets separate rapidly and completely, forming a boxlike appearance on the M-mode recording. Fine systolic fluttering of the aortic valve leaflets may be seen in healthy individuals.

Mitral Valve

An M-mode recording at the mitral valve level intercepts the anterior right ventricular wall and chamber, the interventricular septum, the anterior and posterior mitral leaflets, the posterior left ventricular wall, and the pericardium (Fig. 2–22). The coaptation point of the mitral leaflets in systole is seen as a thin line that moves slightly anteriorly during systole, paralleling the motion of the posterior wall. In early diastole, the leaflets separate widely, with the maximum early diastolic motion of the anterior leaflet termed the *E point*. Normally, there is only a small distance between the E point and the maximal posterior motion of the

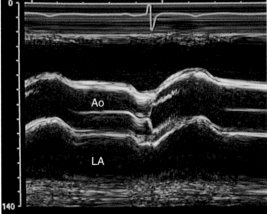

FIGURE 2–21. Schematic (*top*) and M-mode tracing (*bottom*) of a normal aortic valve and left atrium. Ao, aorta; LA, left atrium.

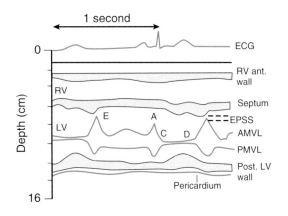

aorta moving anteriorly in systole and posteriorly in diastole (Fig. 2–21). The left atrium is posterior to the aortic root and shows filling in atrial diastole (ventricular systole) and emptying in atrial systole (ventricular diastole). Left atrial filling is largely responsible for the anterior displacement of the aortic root, so aortic root "motion" on M-mode reflects left atrium dimensions. Increased aortic root motion is seen when there is increased left atrial filling and emptying (e.g., with mitral regurgitation). Decreased aortic root motion is seen in low cardiac output states, with corresponding low volumes of atrial filling and emptying.

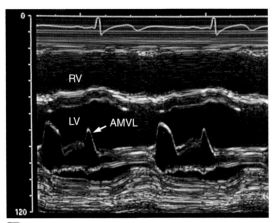

FIGURE 2–22. Schematic (*top*) and M-mode tracing (*bottom*) of a normal mitral valve. AMVL, anterior mitral valve leaflet; PMVL, posterior mitral valve leaflet; EPSS, E-point septal separation; RV, right ventricle; LV, left ventricle.

ventricular septum–E-point septal separation (EPSS). In the absence of mitral stenosis, an increased EPSS indicates left ventricular dilation, systolic dysfunction, or aortic regurgitation.

The leaflets move toward each other in mid-diastole (diastasis) and then separate again with atrial systole, resulting in the late-diastolic peak, the *A point*. The slope of anterior mitral leaflet closure from *A* to the closure point (*C*) is linear unless left ventricular end-diastolic pressure is elevated when a "*B* bump" or "*A-C* shoulder" may be seen on the M-mode recording of mitral valve motion. Fine fluttering of the anterior mitral leaflet is not seen in healthy individuals and usually indicates aortic regurgitation.

Left Ventricle

An M-mode recording perpendicular to the long axis of and through the center of the left ventricle at the papillary muscle level provides standard measurements of systolic and diastolic wall thickness and chamber dimensions (Fig. 2–23). These measurements are limited in that they represent only a single line through the left ventricle and thus do not accurately describe the left ventricle when the disease process is asymmetric, such as with prior myocardial infarction. However, many disease processes do result in symmetric changes in the left ventricle (volume overload, hypertrophy), and the accuracy and reproducibility of these measurements make them useful in patient management. Examples of their use include sequential evaluations of left ventricular end-systolic dimension in patients with chronic asymptomatic aortic regurgitation or assessment of left ventricular hypertrophy in hypertensive patients.

The posterior wall endocardium is identified as the continuous line with the steepest upslope in early systole, taking care to distinguish the endocardium from reflections due to overlying mitral chordal structures. Similarly, the endocardium of the septum is identified as a continuous line with systolic inward motion. Measurements are made (using the ASE recommendations) from the leading edge of the septal endocardial echo to the leading edge of the posterior wall endocardium.

An M-mode recording at this level also may be helpful in timing the motion of the right ventricular free wall when cardiac tamponade is suspected or for detection of a small posterior pericardial effusion.

Other M-Mode Recordings

An M-mode recording through the pulmonic valve is similar to an aortic valve M-mode recording except that usually only one leaflet can be recorded in adults. The slight displacement of the

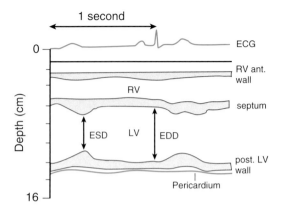

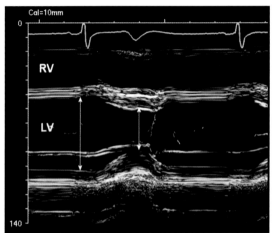

■ FIGURE 2–23. Schematic (*top*) and M-mode tracing (*bottom*) at the left ventricular papillary muscle level. ESD, end systolic dimension; EDD, end diastolic dimension; LV, left ventricle; RV, right ventricle.

leaflet in diastole (after atrial contraction) is called the A wave and is increased (>7 mm) when pulmonic stenosis is present and decreased (<2 mm) when pulmonary hypertension is present. Transient midsystolic closure (or "notching") of the pulmonic valve on M-mode may be seen when pulmonary hypertension is present (Fig. 2–24). An M-mode recording through the tricuspid valve is analogous to a mitral valve recording but rarely is useful clinically.

NORMAL INTRACARDIAC FLOW PATTERNS

Basic Principles

Laminar versus Disturbed Flow

Normal intracardiac flow patterns are characterized by laminar flow (Fig. 2–25). *Laminar flow* is defined as movement of fluid along well-defined parallel stream lines with uniform flow velocities.

M-mode Pulmonic Valve

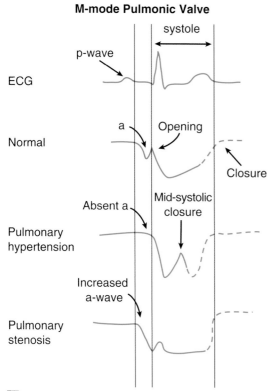

FIGURE 2–24. Patterns of pulmonic valve motion.

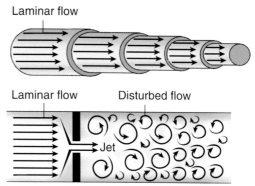

FIGURE 2–25. Laminar flow is characterized by parallel stream lines at uniform velocities with concentric layers of flow, each with a predictable and uniform direction and velocity (*top*). Disturbed flow occurs downstream from areas of narrowing (stenotic orifice, regurgitant orifice, or intracardiac shunt) with blood flow in multiple directions and velocities (*bottom*). In the orifice itself, a laminar high-velocity jet occurs.

In three dimensions, laminar flow consists of concentric layers (or lamina) of flow, each with a predictable and uniform direction and velocity.

Steady laminar flow becomes disturbed when the dimensionless Reynolds number exceeds 2000 to 2500. The Reynolds number (R_e) is directly related to blood flow velocity V, lumen diameter d, and blood density ρ and inversely related to viscosity γ:

$$R_e = (Vd\rho)/\gamma \qquad (2\text{–}1)$$

When blood flow patterns are disturbed, blood cells move in multiple directions at multiple velocities rather than along uniform, parallel stream lines. *Turbulence,* in fluid dynamic terms, refers to the specific situation in which the flow pattern of a particular fluid element is no longer predictable. While intracardiac flow disturbances rarely exhibit true turbulence, this term is used clinically to denote nonlaminar flow.

Flow-Velocity Profiles

The spatial distribution of velocities in cross section at a specific intracardiac location and at a specific time point in the cardiac cycle is known as the *flow-velocity profile* (Fig. 2–26). If all the parallel stream lines in a laminar flow pattern have the same velocity, then the flow-velocity profile is "flat." If velocity is higher in the center of the vessel and lower at the walls of the vessel, the flow profile is "curved" (usually parabolic). While normal flow in peripheral vessels has a curved flow-velocity profile, many intracardiac flows have a relatively flat flow-velocity profile. Factors that tend to equalize the velocity distribution across the cross-sectional area of flow include tapering of the flow stream, acceleration of flow, and an inlet-type geometry. Thus, the proximal aorta and pulmonary artery and the mitral and tricuspid annuli

Flow Velocity Profiles

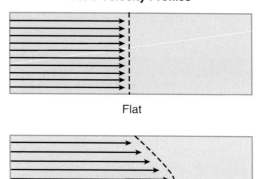

FIGURE 2–26. In a schematic longitudinal cross section of a flow stream, with the length of each arrow proportional to velocity, the difference between a flat and a parabolic flow velocity profile is shown.

have reasonably flat flow-velocity profiles. Downstream, the spatial distribution of flow changes. For example, in the ascending aorta, the flow profile becomes skewed, with higher-velocity flow along the inside curve of the aortic arch and lower velocities along the outer curve. Many Doppler quantitative methods make assumptions about the spatial flow profile at a particular intracardiac site. In some cases, these assumptions can be verified by careful pulsed or color Doppler evaluation.

Clinical Quantitative Doppler Methods

There are three basic principles common to the clinical use of Doppler ultrasound in evaluation of cardiac disease (Table 2–7). These will be presented briefly here and in more detail, including technical aspects and potential pitfalls, in subsequent chapters as follows:

- measurement of volume flow in Chapter 6,
- the relationship between velocity and pressure gradients in Chapter 11, and
- the spatial flow pattern through a small orifice (e.g., regurgitant valve) in Chapter 12.

Measurement of Volume Flow

When blood flow is laminar with a flat flow-velocity profile, it is intuitive that the instantaneous flow rate can be calculated as cross-sectional area or CSA (in cm^2) times flow velocity (in cm/s). Similarly, by integrating flow velocity over the duration of flow, stroke volume, SV (in cm^3) can be calculated as

$$SV\,(cm^3) = CSA\,(cm^2) \times VTI\,(cm) \quad (2\text{–}2)$$

where VTI is the velocity time integral (cm) of the Doppler velocity curve. This method is used clinically to measure stroke volume and cardiac output at rest or after physiologic or pharmacologic interventions, to evaluate the severity of valvular regurgitation, as a component in the equation for valve area calculations, and to quantitate the ratio of pulmonary to systemic blood flow in patients with intracardiac shunts.

Velocity-Pressure Relationships

At any area of significant narrowing in the flow stream—whether a stenotic valve, a ventricular septal defect, or a regurgitant orifice—flow velocity increases in relation to the degree of narrowing; the narrower the opening, the faster is the velocity for a given volume flow rate. In most clinical situations, the velocity in this narrow "jet" through the narrowed orifice is related quantitatively to the pressure gradient across the narrowing, as stated in the simplified Bernoulli equation:

$$\Delta P = 4v^2 \quad (2\text{–}3)$$

where ΔP is the instantaneous pressure gradient (mm Hg), and v is the instantaneous velocity (m/s). This relationship between pressure gradient and velocity is important for quantitation of valve stenosis severity, noninvasive determination of pulmonary artery pressures, and evaluation of other intracardiac hemodynamics (Table 2–8) using continuous-wave Doppler ultrasound.

Spatial Pattern of Flow

Flow through a small orifice is characterized by a

- proximal flow convergence region;
- narrow flow stream through the orifice, called the vena contracta; and a
- downstream flow distrubance.

Each of these components of the spatial flow pattern can be evaluated with color flow imaging,

TABLE 2–7		
Principles of Doppler Quantitation		
Method	**Assumptions/Characteristics**	**Examples of Clinical Applications**
Volume flow $SV = CSA \times VTI$	Laminar flow Flat flow profile Cross-sectional area (CSA) and velocity time integral (VTI) measured at same site	Cardiac output Continuity equation for valve area Regurgitant volume calculations Intracardiac shunts, pulmonary to systemic flow ratio
Velocity-pressure relationship $\Delta P = 4v^2$	Flow limiting orifice CW Doppler signal recorded parallel to flow	Stenotic valve gradients Calculation of pulmonary pressures Left ventricular dP/dt
Spatial flow patterns	Proximal flow convergence region Narrow flow stream in orifice (vena contracta) Downstream flow disturbance	Detection of valve regurgitation and intracardiac shunts Level of obstruction Quantitation of regurgitant severity

TABLE 2–8

Noninvasive Hemodynamic Data Obtained by Echocardiography

Measurement	Chapter
LV systolic function	6
Stroke volume, cardiac output	
LV *dP/dt*	
Pulmonary artery pressures	6
LV diastolic function	7
Relaxation	
Compliance	
Filling pressures	
Valve stenosis	11
Pressure gradients	
Valve areas	
Valve regurgitation	12
Vena contracta	
Proximal isovelocity surface area (PISA)	
Regurgitant orifice area	
Regurgitant volumes	
Shunt calculations	17

LV, Left ventricular; SV, stroke volume; CO, cardiac output; *dP/dt*, rate of change in pressure over time.

which allows real-time demonstrations of flow patterns in each tomographic plane, for example, with valve regurgitation. The proximal flow convergence region allows calculation of volume flow rates. The vena contracta provides a simple measure of regurgitant severity. The downstream flow distrubance allows detection of valvular regurgitation and intracardiac shunts, and determination of the anatomic level of right or left ventricular outflow obstruction. In addition, the 3D shape of the flow disturbance may provide clues as to the etiology of regurgitation.

Normal Antegrade Intracardiac Flows

Normal antegrade intracardiac flows can be evaluated with either pulsed or continuous-wave Doppler ultrasound (Table 2–9). Accurate measurement of antegrade flow velocities is dependent on several technical factors. Most important is a parallel alignment between the ultrasound beam and the direction of blood flow. The ultrasound instrument measures Doppler frequency shifts. The displayed velocities are *calculated* with the Doppler equation based on transducer frequency, the speed of sound in blood, and the angle between the Doppler beam and flow of interest. For intracardiac flows, the 3D direction of flow is difficult to determine, particularly when flow is abnormal, and attempts to "correct" for the presumed intercept angle are likely to increase, rather than decrease, measurement error. Instead, the

examiner positions the ultrasound beam as parallel as possible to the flow of interest based on obtaining the highest calculated velocity with careful transducer positioning and angulation (Table 2–10). In the Doppler equation, cos θ = 1 (and therefore can be ignored) when flow is oriented directly away (intercept angle = 0°) or straight toward (intercept angle = 180°) the ultrasound transducer. Small deviations from a parallel intercept angle (up to 20°) result in only a small error (6%) in velocity calculations (see Fig. 1–31). While this approach generally results in accurate velocity data, the possibility of underestimation of intracardiac velocities due to a nonparallel intercept angle always must be considered in an echocardiographic examination. This potential limitation becomes significant when recording high-velocity flows in valvular stenosis, regurgitation, or intracardiac shunts.

Other technical factors pertinent to recording antegrade flow velocities include the use of an appropriate velocity scale, wall filters, and gain settings. The standard velocity format is to display flows toward the transducer above and flows away from the transducer below the zero baseline. The baseline may be shifted to maximize the flow of interest and the velocity scale adjusted so that the

TABLE 2–9

Normal Antegrade Doppler Flow Velocities

Parameter	Normal Range (m/s)
Ascending aorta	1.0–1.7
LV outflow tract	0.7–1.1
LV inflow	
E-velocity	0.6–1.3 (0.72 ± 0.14)
Deceleration slope	5.0 ± 1.4 m/s
A-velocity	0.2–0.7 (0.47 ± 0.4)
Pulmonary artery	0.5–1.3
RV inflow	
E-velocity	0.3–0.7
RA filling (SVC, HV)	
Systole	0.32–0.69 (0.46 ± 0.08) m/s
Diastole	0.06–0.45 (0.27 ± 0.08) m/s
LA filling (pulmonary vein)	
Systole	0.56 ± 0.13 m/s
Diastole	0.44 ± 0.16 m/s
Atrial reversal	0.32 ± 0.07 m/s

LV, left ventricular; E, early diastolic peak; A, late (atrial) diastolic peak; RV, right ventricular; RA, right atrial; SVC, superior vena cava; HV, hepatic vein; LA, left atrial.
From: Wilson et al: Br Heart J 53:451, 1985; Hatle and Angelsen: Doppler Ultrasound in Cardiology, 2nd ed. Philadelphia: Lea & Febiger, 1985; Van Dam et al: Eur Heart J 8:1221, 1987; 9:165, 1988; Jaffe et al: AJC 68:550, 1991; Appleton et al: JACC 10:1032, 1987.

TABLE 2-10

Transthoracic Views for Normal Antegrade Flow Velocities

Antegrade Flow	View
LV outflow tract	Apical four-chamber (angulated anterior) Apical long-axis
Aorta (ascending)	LV-apex Suprasternal notch (SSN)

Descending aorta
  (thoracic)
  (proximal abdominal)
	SSN
	Subcostal

LV inflow (mitral)	Apical four-chamber or long-axis
RV outflow tract	RV outflow Parasternal short-axis (aortic valve level) Subcostal short-axis
RV inflow (tricuspid)	RV inflow Apical four-chamber
LA inflow (pulmonary vein)	Apical four-chamber
RA inflow	Subcostal (central hepatic vein) SSN (superior vena cava)

LV, left ventricular; RV, right ventricular; LA, left atrial; RA, right atrial; SSN, suprasternal notch.

velocity curve uses the entire displayed range. Wall filters are set as low as possible, without resulting in excessive noise, to allow accurate measurement of time intervals. Gain settings are adjusted to show the peak velocity and velocity curve clearly without excessive background noise. A sample volume length of 5 to 10 mm typically is used to record antegrade flow velocities because this length provides reasonable intracardiac localization with adequate signal strength.

Signal aliasing (as discussed in Chapter 1) occurs even with normal intracardiac flow velocities. Use of the baseline shift can resolve this problem in most cases. If aliasing persists, use of high pulse-repetition frequency or continuous-wave Doppler is needed for unambiguous display of the maximum velocity.

With appropriate instrument setting and attention to technical details, antegrade velocities with pulsed Doppler ultrasound appear as smooth envelopes with a well-defined onset and end of flow, a well-defined maximum velocity, and a thin band of velocities at each time point. The area under the velocity curve is "clear" because the flow velocities at a specific intracardiac site are relatively uniform. Continuous-wave Doppler recordings differ in that the curve is "filled in" due to inclusion of lower velocities along the entire length of the ultrasound beam.

Left Ventricular Outflow

An apical or suprasternal notch window is used to obtain a parallel intercept angle between the ultrasound beam and direction of blood flow in the left ventricular outflow tract and ascending aorta (Fig. 2–27). In general, left ventricular outflow velocities are most accurately recorded from a transthoracic approach, as it is more difficult to obtain a parallel intercept angle from the transesophageal approach. In some cases, a transgastric "apical" approach may be useful but potential underestimation of velocity, due to a nonparallel intercept angle, always should be considered.

With a pulsed Doppler sample volume positioned on the left ventricular side of the aortic valve, an ejection velocity curve is recorded with a steep acceleration slope, a sharply peaked early systolic maximum velocity, and a less steep deceleration slope (Fig. 2–28). Note the narrow band of velocities at any instant in time during acceleration, reflecting the uniformity of blood flow velocity in the outflow tract during acceleration. During deceleration, the range of flow velocities at any instant is slightly wider (spectral broadening) as instability in the flow pattern during deceleration results in slight variation in flow velocities. The aortic valve closing click is seen immediately

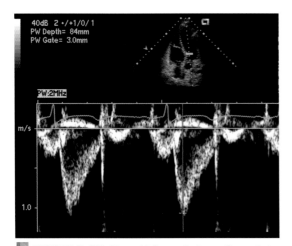

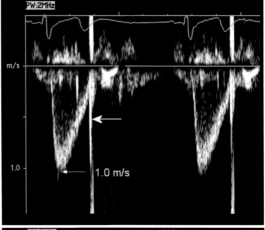

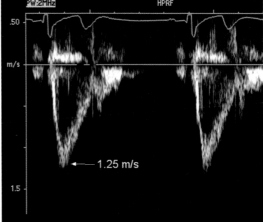

■ **FIGURE 2–27.** Normal left ventricular outflow velocity curve recorded with pulsed Doppler from an anteriorly angulated apical four-chamber view with the sample volume positioned just proximal to the aortic valve (*top*). The spectral display (*bottom*) shows a smooth velocity curve with a well-defined peak of 1.0 m/s and a clear closing click. There is a very narrow velocity curve during acceleration with slight spectral broadening during deceleration due to differences in the uniformity of flow during acceleration and deceleration.

following end-ejection. Flow recordings with pulsed Doppler on the aortic side of the valve appear similar except that the aortic valve opening click is seen, instead of the closing click, and the maximum velocity is slightly higher, by 0.2 to 0.4 m/s, than the outflow tract velocity due to slight narrowing of the cross-sectional area of flow at the aortic leaflet tips.

With continuous-wave Doppler interrogation of the aortic valve, both opening and closing clicks are recorded. The area under the velocity curve is filled in with lower velocity signals because lower velocity blood flow signals that originate in the left ventricle along the length of the ultrasound beam are displayed as well (see Fig. 2–28).

With a normal aortic valve, the area under the velocity curve (the velocity-time integral) reflects stroke volume, which can be calculated by multiplying by cross-sectional area. The normal antegrade maximum velocity across the valve is approximately 1 to 1.2 m/s and is the same whether measured by pulsed or continuous-wave Doppler methods. The normal outflow tract velocity typically is 0.8 to 1 m/s, corresponding to a velocity "step-up" across the valve or ratio of outflow tract to aortic velocity of 0.7 to 1.

The relationship between velocity and pressure gradients across *nonstenotic* valves is somewhat complex and is not fully described by the Bernoulli equation (which applies to areas of narrowing). The period of acceleration corresponds

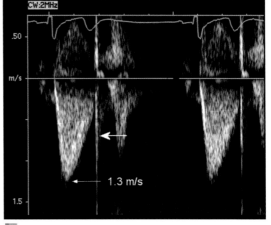

■ **FIGURE 2–28.** Normal left ventricular outflow recorded with pulsed Doppler proximal to the aortic valve (*top*) showing laminar flow with an aortic closing (but not opening) click, distal to the aortic valve (*center*) showing higher velocity laminar flow with no visible valve click, and with continuous-wave Doppler (*bottom*) showing both an opening and closing click and filling in of the velocity curve due to recording velocity along the entire length of the ultrasound beam.

to a slight pressure gradient from the left ventricle to the aorta, with the maximum pressure gradient corresponding to maximum acceleration. Left ventricular pressure falls below aortic pressure in midsystole, and at this point, deceleration of flow occurs. Thus, for the normal valve, maximum velocity occurs at the pressure crossover point (see Fig. 6–1). During deceleration, aortic pressure remains slightly higher than left ventricular pressure until flow decelerates to zero and the valve closes. At this point, left ventricular pressure continues to decline rapidly.

Right Ventricular Outflow

The right ventricular outflow tract and pulmonary artery are studied from a parasternal short-axis or right ventricular outflow tract view. In the healthy individual, the right ventricular ejection curve is similar to the left ventricular ejection curve except that peak velocity is slightly lower (0.8 to 1 m/s), the ejection period is longer, and the velocity curve is more rounded, with the maximum velocity occurring in midsystole. The shapes of the right and left ventricular ejection curves appear to relate to the downstream vascular resistance. The low-resistance pulmonary vasculature results in a slower rate of acceleration of blood flow, with the maximum velocity (and pressure crossover) occurring later in the ejection cycle. When pulmonary vascular resistance is increased, the right ventricular ejection curve resembles left ventricular ejection more closely with a sharper velocity curve and earlier peak velocity.

Left Ventricular Inflow

Diastolic flow across the mitral valve shows two peaks: an early diastolic peak velocity (E wave) reflecting passive early diastolic filling and a late diastolic peak velocity due to atrial contraction (A wave) (Fig. 2–29). The normal E velocity in healthy, young individuals is approximately 1 m/s, with an A velocity of 0.2 to 0.4 m/s, reflecting the normal small contribution of atrial contraction to left ventricular diastolic filling. If diastole is long enough, a period of no flow, or diastasis, between the two flow curves is seen.

Even in normal individuals, the pattern of left ventricular diastolic filling varies with age, loading conditions, heart rate, and PR interval. With age, there is a gradual reduction in E velocity, prolongation in the rate of early diastolic deceleration, and increase in A velocity so that the ratio of E to A velocity changes from greater than 1 in young individuals, to approximately 1 at ages 50 to 60, to less than 1 in older healthy individuals.

Increased preload results in an increase in E velocity, while decreased preload has the opposite effect. When diastole is short (i.e., with a rapid heart rate), the A velocity becomes superimposed (or summated) onto the downslope of the E velocity, resulting in an apparent higher A velocity. At very high heart rates, only a single E/A peak may be seen. Prolongation of the PR interval has a similar effect. These variations in the normal pattern of left ventricular diastolic filling should be recognized to avoid an inappropriate interpretation of an "abnormality."

Typically, left ventricular diastolic filling is recorded from an apical window on transthoracic studies. In addition to the physiologic variability discussed above, the peak E velocity and the ratio of the E to A peaks may differ depending on whether the sample volume is placed at the mitral annulus or at the mitral leaflet tips. Appropriate positioning of the sample volume depends on whether the Doppler curve is used to evaluate diastolic filling of the left ventricle (leaflet tips probably most useful) or transmitral stroke volume (mitral annular level most useful). Continuous-wave Doppler recordings show the highest velocities wherever they occur along the length of the ultrasound beam. Left ventricular diastolic filling is discussed in more detail in Chapter 7.

Right Ventricular Inflow

Right ventricular inflow can be recorded from an apical approach or from the parasternal right ventricular inflow view. The pattern of right ventricular diastolic filling is similar to left ventricular filling, although peak flow velocities are slightly lower with a normal right ventricular inflow E velocity of 0.3 to 0.7 m/s.

Left Atrial Filling

It is technically challenging to record left atrial filling from a transthoracic approach due to suboptimal signal strength at the depth of the pulmonary veins in many adults. However, with careful attention to technical details, this flow curve is obtainable in the right superior pulmonary vein in an apical four-chamber view in approximately 90% of patients. From a transesophageal approach, flow in both right and left pulmonary veins can be recorded, with the most laminar flow signals obtained from the left superior pulmonary vein (see Fig. 2–29).

Atrial contraction results in brief backflow in the pulmonary veins (a wave) followed by a biphasic filling pattern with prominent filling of the atrium (x descent) during ventricular systole, a

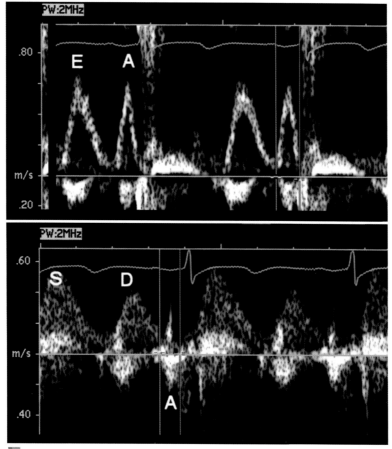

■ FIGURE 2-29. Normal left ventricular inflow velocity curve (*top*) recorded with pulsed Doppler showing rapid early diastolic filling (E) and the atrial (A) contribution to late diastolic filling. Left atrial filling (*bottom*) recorded on transthoracic echocardiography in the right superior pulmonary vein shows systolic (S) and diastolic (D) filling with a small atrial (A) reversal of flow.

second brief reversal of flow (*v* wave) following ventricular contraction, and a second atrial filling curve (*y* descent) during ventricular diastole (see Chapter 7). Abnormalities of left atrial filling can be seen in patients with mitral regurgitation (Chapter 12), constrictive pericarditis (Chapter 10), and restrictive cardiomyopathy (Chapter 9).

Right Atrial Filling

Right atrial filling can be assessed from Doppler recordings of superior vena caval flow (from a suprasternal notch approach) or central hepatic vein flow (which lies parallel to the ultrasound beam from a subcostal window). The pattern of flow again is analogous to the pulsation pattern of the neck veins seen on clinical examination, with an *a* wave, an *x* descent reflecting systolic filling,

a *v* wave, and a *y* descent reflecting diastolic filling of the right atrium (see Fig. 7–5).

Descending Aorta

Flow patterns in the descending aorta are important in the evaluation of cardiac disorders because the downstream flow pattern depends on the presence and severity of specific cardiac lesions. Examples include aortic regurgitation, patent ductus arteriosus, and aortic coarctation. Descending thoracic aorta flow can be recorded from a suprasternal notch approach and shows antegrade flow with a systolic velocity curve, a peak velocity of about 1 m/s, and brief early diastolic flow reversal (see Fig. 16–9). The proximal abdominal aorta recorded from a subcostal approach shows a similar flow pattern (see Fig. 16–12).

Normal Color Doppler Flow Patterns

Impact of Color Doppler Physics on Flow Displays

While spectral Doppler (pulsed or continuous) is preferable for accurate measurement of specific intracardiac blood flow velocities, the overall pattern of intracardiac flow is best evaluated with color flow imaging. Unfortunately, although in theory normal laminar flow should appear as a uniform red or blue color, in fact, color flow display instrumentation results in more complex patterns.

For example, flow in the left ventricular outflow tract is a uniform red color from a parasternal long-axis view because the direction of flow is toward the transducer. The same flow is a uniform *blue* color from an apical approach because now it is directed away from the transducer (Fig. 2-30). This same phenomenon can be seen with flows in a single image plane. For example, antegrade flow in the aortic arch from a suprasternal notch view appears red (toward the transducer) in the more proximal segment and blue (away from the transducer) more distally with a small black area in the center of the image where the ultrasound beam is perpendicular to flow. Similarly, in the abdominal aorta from a subcostal approach, antegrade flow appears alternatively red and then blue as it transverses the image plane (see Fig. 1-34). In these examples, the change in color is due to a change in intercept angle between the ultrasound beam and blood flow at the left versus right edge of the sector.

Less dramatic changes in intercept angle across the 2D image also result in a complex color flow pattern for laminar normal flow. For example, evaluation of the left ventricular outflow tract in an apical long-axis view may show an apparent higher systolic velocity along the ventricular septum than along the anterior mitral leaflet (Fig. 2-31). This appearance results from a more parallel intercept angle between the Doppler beam and blood flow along the septum than adjacent to the mitral valve. The same actual velocities across the outflow tract result in differing Doppler frequency shifts depending on this intercept angle. Because the instrument assumes that $\cos\theta = 1$ for each signal, a falsely low velocity is calculated for nonparallel intercept angles, with the resulting image showing an apparent increase in velocity across the image plane due to differing intercept angles.

In addition to intercept angle, color flow images also are affected by the phenomenon of

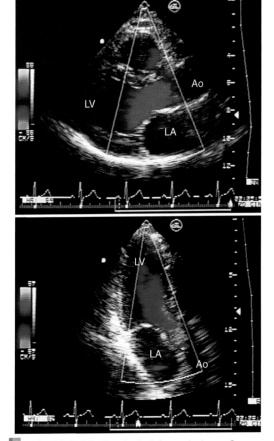

FIGURE 2-30. Flow in the left ventricular outflow tract recorded from a high parasternal position (*top*) is red (toward the transducer), while the same flow from an apical approach (*bottom*) is blue (away from the transducer).

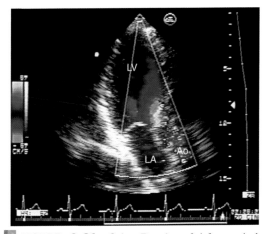

FIGURE 2-31. Color Doppler of left ventricular outflow from an apical long-axis view shows aliasing proximal to the aortic valve due to either a more parallel intercept angle between the Doppler scan line and direction of blood flow *or* a higher velocity near the septum versus adjacent to the anterior mitral valve leaflet.

signal aliasing. The Nyquist limit, as displayed at the top and bottom of the color scale, typically is 60 to 80 cm/s with a 2- or 3-MHz transducer at depths used for transthoracic cardiac imaging. Since normal intracardiac flow velocities often exceed this limit, signal aliasing occurs. Flow toward the transducer is displayed in red at velocities less than the Nyquist limit, but once aliasing occurs, this same flow signal is displayed in blue. Thus, flow toward the transducer is red aliasing to blue, while flow away from the transducer is blue aliasing to red. In fact, multiple aliases can occur with high-velocity flows displayed sequentially as going from red to blue to red and so on. An example of normal aliasing is seen in the left ventricular inflow pattern on the apical four-chamber view, where the red flow toward the apex turns blue as it exceeds the Nyquist limit (see Fig. 1–35). While confusing at first, patterns of signal aliasing can be used to advantage in quantitation of intracardiac flows using the proximal isovelocity surface area approach discussed in Chapter 12.

Another color image pattern seen even with normal intracardiac flows is *variance,* which often is encoded as green on the color display. While the concept of variance is that a single intracardiac site exhibits multiple flow velocities and directions (such as in a regurgitant jet), from the foregoing discussions of intercept angle and aliasing, it is apparent that a normal flow pattern might meet variance criteria. For example, in a region at the aliasing limit, the instrument may sequentially measure flow toward then away from the transducer due to aliasing and then assign variance to that color pixel. Awareness that a color variance pattern can occur with normal intracardiac flows avoids erroneous interpretations.

Normal Ventricular Outflow Patterns

Color flow imaging of left ventricular outflow can be recorded from an apical approach in either an anteriorly angulated four-chamber view or a long-axis view. Flow is laminar, but aliasing typically occurs at this depth, resulting in a complex color pattern. While measurement of stroke volume proximal to the aortic valve, which *assumes* a flat flow velocity profile, has been validated, it remains controversial whether the appearance of aliasing along the ventricular septum in systole is due to a skewed flow profile or to variations in intercept angle across the color sector.

Note that while accurate measurements of antegrade velocities with pulsed or continuous-wave Doppler require a parallel intercept angle, with color flow imaging, the spatial pattern of flow is of interest rather than the absolute velocities. Thus, views with nonparallel intercept angles

often are helpful. For example, left ventricular outflow can be evaluated with color flow imaging in a parasternal long-axis view even though the flow direction is almost perpendicular to the ultrasound beam. As shown in Chapter 12, this view also is useful for evaluation of abnormal flows in the outflow tract, such as aortic regurgitation.

Right ventricular outflow can be depicted from a parasternal short-axis view, from the right ventricular outflow view, or from a subcostal short-axis view. Because velocities are slightly lower and the depth of interrogation is less than for left ventricular outflow, the flow pattern away from the transducer typically shows a uniform blue color.

Normal Ventricular Inflow Patterns

In the apical four-chamber view, left ventricular inflow appears as a broad flow stream extending laterally across the mitral annulus and lengthwise to the left ventricular apex. If the Nyquist limit is exceeded, signal aliasing occurs with a color shift at the aliasing velocity. In real time, the separate flows of early and late diastolic filling may be seen. When ultrasound penetration is optimal, diastolic flow extends from the pulmonary veins to the left ventricular apex. The normal spatial pattern of the left ventricular inflow is directed along the lateral left ventricular wall, in mid-diastole, with blue flow away from the transducer along the ventricular septum consistent with a "vortex" of flow in the left ventricle in diastole (Fig. 2–32). Interestingly, the normal counterclockwise vortex is reversed in patients after mitral valve replacement.

Right ventricular inflow patterns on color flow imaging are analogous to the patterns seen in the

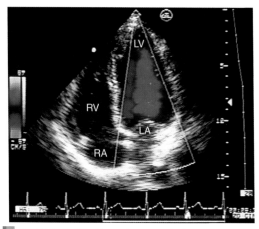

▌ **FIGURE 2–32.** Normal pattern of left ventricular filling in mid-diastole in an apical four-chamber view shows flow toward the apex along the lateral wall simultaneously with flow away from the transducer along the septum.

left ventricle, although a diastolic "vortex" is not as prominent.

Normal Atrial Inflow Patterns

Inflow into the left atrium occurs via the four pulmonary veins. On transthoracic imaging, the right superior pulmonary vein is the easiest to visualize in the apical four-chamber view. Color flow imaging showing the biphasic red inflow from this vein allows correct placement of a pulsed Doppler sample volume for recording the spectral Doppler data. All four pulmonary veins can be depicted on transesophageal echo, but again, use of color flow imaging may facilitate identification of each vein. This approach is particularly helpful with right-sided veins, which may be difficult to recognize on 2D imaging alone.

Inflow into the right atrium occurs via the superior and inferior venae cavae and the coronary sinus. Evaluation may be complicated by some degree of tricuspid regurgitation (present in 80% to 90% of healthy subjects and a higher percentage of patients), which typically is directed along the interatrial septum. Flow from the inferior vena cava and coronary sinus may be seen in the right ventricular inflow view, as well as in the short-axis view at the aortic valve level and in the apical four-chamber view. Superior vena caval flow is seen from the suprasternal notch approach. In the right atrium, recognition of the several normal inflow patterns is important when an atrial septal defect is suspected. Note that 20% of healthy subjects have a patent foramen ovale (demonstrable by intravenous echo contrast during a Valsalva maneuver), but color flow evidence for a patent foramen ovale is present in only approximately 5% of healthy individuals.

Physiologic Valvular Regurgitation

With careful examination techniques, a small amount of mitral and tricuspid regurgitation is detectable in between 70% and 80% of healthy people. In addition, mild pulmonic regurgitation, appearing as a narrow red "flame" in diastole, is an incidental finding (present in 70% to 80% of normal individuals). These physiologic degrees of regurgitation are characterized by a localized signal that often is seen only briefly during the cardiac cycle. Small amounts of mitral, tricuspid, and pulmonic valvular regurgitation are of no apparent clinical significance. In contrast, aortic regurgitation is rarely seen in healthy subjects (5% of individuals) on color flow imaging.

Technical Aspects of Color Flow Imaging

The color flow display is dependent on each specific ultrasound instrument to some extent. However, many parameters are adjustable by the operator, so an optimal examination requires careful attention to instrument settings.

The *color flow map* usually can be varied in terms of

- the color scale used,
- the addition of variance to the color scale, and
- the use of a power scale instead of a color scale.

The specific color scale used is a matter of personal preference, with the diagnostic goal being to optimize the display and recognition of abnormal flow patterns.

The *velocity range* of the color flow map is determined by the Nyquist limit, and as for conventional pulsed Doppler, the range can be altered by shifting the zero baseline, changing the pulse repetition frequency, or altering the depth of the displayed image.

Color Doppler power output and *gain* are adjusted so that gain is just below the level at which random background noise appears. "Wall filters" can be varied to exclude low-velocity signals from the color flow display. In addition, many instruments allow variation in the assignment of a returning signal to 2D or Doppler display (depending on signal strength). One approach to optimizing the color flow display is to reduce the 2D gain, since the instrument does not display flow data on top of "structures" even when the 2D signal is due to excessive gain.

Perhaps the most important technical factor in color flow imaging is optimization *of frame rate*. As discussed in Chapter 1, color flow frame rate depends on sector width, depth, pulse repetition frequency, and the number of samples per sector line. The examiner optimizes frame rate by focusing on the flow of interest, narrowing the sector, and decreasing the depth as much as possible. When frame rate remains inadequate for timing flow abnormalities, a color M-line through the area of interest may be helpful, for example, in assessment of aortic regurgitation.

THE ECHOCARDIOGRAPHIC EXAMINATION

Core Elements

Although the echocardiographic examination should be directed toward the specific clinical question in each individual patient, it is important to use a systematic and consistent format for the examination. The only exceptions to a standarized protocol should be limited follow-up studies in patients with a recent, complete examination. In addition, as the study is in progress, additional imaging and data collection are needed to fully pursue the clinical quesiton or any observed abnormalities.

A suggested set of core elements for diagnostic imaging and Doppler data is shown at the end of this chapter. Although these core elements may differ from laboratory to laboratory, the concept of a standarized examination sequence is critical to ensure that abnormalties are not missed. It is essential that blood pressure and the indication for echocardiography are reviewed prior to beginning the examination. An electocardiographic lead should always be recorded to assist in evaluating timing of cardiac motion and Doppler flows.

The core elements of the examination allow the physician to evaluate the following structures:

Left Ventricle
∎ Internal dimensions and wall thickness,
∎ Segmental wall motion abnormalities,
∎ Overall systolic function (including ejection fraction), and
∎ Diastolic filling.

Aortic Valve and Root
∎ Aortic root dimension and appearance,
∎ Aortic valve anatomy, and
∎ Evidence for regurgitation or stenosis.

Mitral Valve and Left Atrium
∎ Mitral valve anatomy and motion,
∎ Evidence for stenosis or regurgitation, and
∎ Left atrial size.

Right Side of the Heart
∎ Right ventricular size and systolic function (qualitative),
∎ Right atrial size,
∎ Valve anatomy and function, and
∎ Estimated pulmonary artery pressure.

Pericardium
∎ Evidence for thickening or effusion.

Additional Components

If any abnormalities are seen on the core elements, the sonographer records additional components, as detailed in the The Echo Exam: Additional Components (page 69). In addition, the core elements are supplemented with additional components based on the clinical indications for the study. The combination of core elements and additional components then constitutes a complete echocardiographic examination.

An example of findings on the core elements leading to additional data recording is when a calcified aortic valve is present. With this finding, attention is focused first on the precise valve anatomy–bicuspid, calcific, rheumatic–and then on the function of the valve. The degree of stenosis is quantitated from the maximum aortic jet velocity and calculation of valve area (see Chapter 11) and the degree of regurgitation is evaluated with color flow and continuous-wave Doppler techniques (see Chapter 12). Next, the left ventricular response to the pressure load imposed by the abnormal aortic valve is assessed both for systolic function (see Chapter 6) and diastolic function (see Chapter 7).

Another example is evaluation of a patient after myocardial infarction. In this case, attention is focused on the extent and distribution of left ventricular segmental wall motion abnormalities (see Chapter 8). If apical akinesis or dyskinesis is noted, a diligent search for an apical thrombus is indicated (see Chapter 15). If the patient has a new murmur, careful evaluation is performed to evaluate the possibility of mitral regurgitation due to papillary muscle dysfunction or the possibility of a postinfarction ventricular septal defect. Overall left ventricular systolic function is evaluated, as is right ventricular function.

Even if no obvious abnormalities are noted during the basic examination, the study may be focused toward the specific clinical question in that patient. For example, if endocarditis is suspected (see Chapter 14), more attention to valvular anatomy is needed, with careful transducer angulation and nonstandard views to optimize visualization of possible valvular vegetations. Although endocarditis cannot be excluded by echocardiography, a careful and thorough negative examination does decrease the likelihood of disease.

Another example of how the clincial indication affects the examination is the patient referred for heart failure symptoms. Even if the core elements appear normal at the time of recording, a complete evaluation of systolic and diastolic left ventricular function is needed to evaluate for a cardiac cause of the patient's symptoms.

The need to focus the examination on the specific clinical question and at the same time ensure that significant abnormalities are not missed highlights the necessity for appropriate training of both the physician responsible for the examination and the sonographer performing the study, as well as for close interaction between these two individuals during the performance and interpretation of the study. Furthermore, close interaction with the referring physician is needed both before the examination is performed to clarify the differential diagnosis and clinical questions and after the examination to integrate the pretest likelihood with the echocardiographic findings and estimate the probability of any remaining diagnostic problems.

SUGGESTED READING

1. Henry WL, DeMaria A, Gramiak R, et al, and the American Society of Echocardiography, Committee on Nomenclature and Standards: Report on two-dimensional echocardiography. Circulation 62:212–222, 1980.

   Nomenclature standards for image orientation, imaging planes, and transducer location.

   Clear schematic drawings.

2. Cerqueira MD, Weissman NJ, Dilsizian V, et al: Standardized myocardial segmentation and nomenclature for tomographic imaging of the heart: a statement for healthcare professionals from the Cardiac Imaging Committee of the Council on Clinical Cardiology of the American Heart Association. Circulation 105:539–542, 2002.

   Standards for defining cardiac image orientation and myocardial segments that can be used by all imaging modalities to enhance correlation between different approaches. The standard reference for cardiac displays is defined as the long axis of the left ventricle. The names used for image planes are short axis (90° to long axis), vertical long axis (apical two-chamber plane), and horizontal long axis (four-chamber plane). Myocardial segments are defined at the basal and mid-ventricular level (clockwise from the anterior septal insertion) as anterior, anterolateral, inferolateral, inferior, inferoseptal, and anteroseptal. There are four apical segments (anterior, septal, inferior, and lateral).

3. Quinones MA, Otto CM, Stoddard M, et al: Recommendations for quantification of Doppler echocardiography: a report from the Doppler quantification taks force of the nomenclature and standards committee of the American Society of Echocardiography. J Am Soc Echocardiogr 15:167–184, 2002.

   Nomenclature standards for recording, measuring, and reporting Doppler data including pulsed, continuous, and color flow Doppler. Excellent review of normal flow patterns and basic Doppler principles for calcuation of volume flow rate, pressure gradients, and regurgitant valve lesions. 77 references. Useful glossary of Doppler terms.

4. Lentner C (ed): Geigy Scientific Tables, vol 5: Heart and Circulation, 8th ed. Basel, Switzerland: Ciba-Geigy, 1990.

   Excellent reference source summarizing normal values for cardiovascular imaging. Includes invasive and noninvasive normal data. Well referenced.

5. Netter FH: The Heart. Basel, Switzerland: Ciba, 1969.

   Clear illustrations of detailed cardiac anatomy with concise accompanying text on pages 2–12. A useful introduction and review of cardiac structure.

6. Thubriker M: The Aortic Valve. Boca Raton, Florida: CRC Press, 1990.

   Monograph on detailed anatomy, structure, and function of the aortic valve.

7. Roberts WC: Morphologic features of the normal and abnormal mitral valve. Am J Cardiol 51:1005–1028, 1983.

   A review of anatomy and function of the mitral valve based on 1010 autopsy cases. Excellent discussion and illustrations of normal mitral valve anatomy, mitral stenosis, and mitral regurgitation. Both photographs and schematic drawings are included.

8. Schnittger I, Gordon EP, Fitzgerald PJ, Popp RL: Standardized intracardiac measurements of two-dimensional echocardiography. J Am Coll Cardiol 2:934–938, 1983.

   Normal 2D echo intracardiac measurements are described in detail for 35 healthy adults.

9. Triulzi M, Gillam LD, Gentile F, et al: Normal adult cross-sectional echocardiographic values: Linear dimensions and chamber areas. Echocardiography 1:403–426, 1984.

   Tabular presentation of normal echo dimensions in 72 normal adults.

10. Pearlman JD, Triulzi MO, King ME, et al: Limits of normal left ventricular dimensions in growth and development: Analysis of dimensions and variance in the two-dimensional echocardiograms of 268 normal healthy subjects. J Am Coll Cardiol 12:1432–1441, 1988.

    Graphic display of normal echo dimensions in 72 adults and 196 children showing relationship of each dimension to body surface area with mean and 90% tolerance limits.

11. Roman MJ, Devereux RB, Kramer-Fox R, O'Loughlin J: Two-dimensional echocardiographic aortic root dimensions in normal children and adults. Am J Cardiol 64:507–512, 1989.

    Derivation of gender-specific upper limits of normal (indexed to body size) for aortic root dimensions based on 135 adults and 52 children.

12. Benjamin EJ, Levy D, Anderson KM, et al: Determinants of Doppler indexes of left ventricular diastolic function in normal subjects (the Framingham Heart Study). Am J Cardiol 70:508–515, 1992.

    Detailed study of the relationship between age and Doppler measures of left ventricular diastolic filling in the Framingham population after exclusion of subjects with hypertension, cardiac disease, or other organ system disease (n = 1485). E velocity decreased from 0.71 ± 0.14 m/s at ages 20–29 years to 0.53 ± 0.17 m/s for those ~70 years of age. A velocity increased from 0.35 ± 0.06 to 0.64 ± 0.14 m/s in the same groups. The E/A ratio was 1.03 ± 0.26 m/s at ages 60–69.

13. Appleton CP, Hatle LK, Popp RL: Superior vena cava and hepatic vein Doppler echocardiography in healthy adults. J Am Coll Cardiol 10:1032–1039, 1987.

    Normal superior vena cava and hepatic vein Doppler flows show a systolic and diastolic antegrade flow with a reduction or reversal in antegrade flow following atrial systole (a wave). Variation with respiration is prominent in normal healthy adults.

14. Basnight MA, Gonzalez MS, Kershenovich SC, Appleton CP: Pulmonary venous flow velocity: Relation to hemodynamics, mitral flow velocity and left atrial volume, and ejection fraction. J Am Soc Echocardiogr 4:547–558, 1991.

15. Klein AL, Tajik AJ: Doppler assessment of pulmonary venous flow in healthy subjects and in patients with heart disease. J Am Soc Echocardiogr 4:379–392, 1991.

16. Bartzokis T, Lee R, Yeoh TK, et al: Transesophageal echo-Doppler echocardiographic assessment of pulmonary venous flow patterns. J Am Soc Echocardiogr 4:457–464, 1991.

    Each of these three references (14 to 16) provides detailed descriptions of normal pulmonary venous flow patterns and the physiologic variables that affect the flow pattern.

17. Sager KB, Parail AC: Aging changes seen on echocardiography. In: Otto CM (ed): The Practice of Clinical Echocardiography, 2nd ed. Philadelphia: WB Saunders, 2002, pp 797–805.

 Detailed review of the normal cardiac changes with aging as assessed by echocardiography including age-grouped tables of normal values for left ventricular dimensions and function and Doppler flow velocities. 51 references.

18. Gottdiener JS, Diamond JA, Phillips RA: Hypertension: impact of echocaridographic data on the mechanism of hypertension, treatment options, prognosis and assessment of therapy. In: Otto CM (ed): The Practice of Clinical Echocardiography, 2nd ed. Philadelphia: WB Saunders, 2002, pp 705–738.

 In addition to a review of echocardiographic studies in hypertension, this chapter includes a detailed discussion of the issues involved in using echocardiographic data in epidemiologic studies. 315 references.

19. Gardin JM, Adams DB, Douglas PS, et al: Recommendations for a standardized report for adults transthoracic echocardiography: A report from the American Society of Echocardiography's Nomenclature and Standards Committee and Task Force for a Standardized Echocardiography Report. J Am Soc Echocardiogr 15:275–290, 2002.

 Recommendations for performing and reporting transthoracic echocardiography examinations in adults. An excellent resource for developing a standarized echocardigraphy examination in each laboratory.

The Echo Exam *Core Elements*

A complete Echo Exam consists of Core Elements plus Additional Components.

Modality	Window	View/Signal	Measurements
Clinical data		Indication for echo Key history and PE findings Previous cardiac imaging data Blood pressure at time of Echo Exam	
2D imaging	*Parasternal*	Long axis Short axis aortic valve Short axis mitral valve Short axis LV (papillary muscle level) Right ventricular inflow Right ventricular outflow	LV dimensions LV wall thickness Aortic root dimension LA dimension
	Apical	4-chamber Anteriorly angulated 4-chamber 2-chamber Long axis	Visual estimate of ejection fraction
	Subcostal	4-chamber IVC with respiration	
Pulsed Doppler	*Apical*	Left ventricular inflow at leaflet tips	E velocity A velocity
		Left ventricular outflow	LV outflow velocity
Color flow	*Parasternal*	Long axis Short axis of aortic and mitral valves RV inflow and outflow	Color flow to identify regurgitation of all 4 valves. Measure vena contracta if possible
	Apical	4-chamber Long-axis	Mitral, tricuspid and aortic valves
Continuous wave Doppler	*Parasternal*	Tricuspid valve Pulmonic valve	TR-jet velocity
	Apical	Aortic valve Mitral valve Tricuspid valve	Aortic regurgitation Mitral regurgitation TR-jet (PAP)

LV, left ventricle; IVC, inferior vena cava; TR, tricuspid regurgitation; PAP, pulmonary artery pressure.

The Echo Exam *Additional Components*

Abnormality on Core Elements	Additional Echo Exam Components (Chapter)
Reason for Echo	Additional components to address specific clinical question*
Left Ventricle	
Decreased ejection fraction	See Systolic Function and Dilated Cardiomyopathy (6, 9)
Abnormal LV filling velocities	See Diastolic Function (7)
Regional wall motion abnormality	See Ischemic Heart Disease (8)
Increased wall thickness	See Hypertrophic Cardiomyopathy, Restrictive Cardiomyopathy and Hypertensive Heart Disease (9)
Valves	
Imaging evidence for stenosis or an increased antegrade transvalvular velocity	See Valve Stenosis (11)
Regurgitation greater than mild on color flow imaging or CW Doppler	See Valve Regurgitation (12)
Prosthetic valve	See Prosthetic Valves (13)
Valve mass or suspected endocarditis	See Endocarditis and Masses (14, 15)
Right Heart	
Enlarged right ventricle	See Pulmonary Heart Disease and Congenital Heart Disease (9, 17)
Elevated TR-jet velocity	See Pulmonary Pressures (6)
Pericardium	
Pericardial Effusion	See Pericardial Effusion (10)
Pericardial thickening	See Constrictive Pericarditis (10)
Great Vessels	
Enlarged aorta	See Aortic Disease (16)

*The echo exam should always include additional components to address the clinical indication. For example, if the indication is "heart failure," additional components to evaluate systolic and diastolic function are needed even if the Core Elements do not show obvious abnormalities. If the indication is "cardiac source of embolus," the Additional Components for that diagnosis are needed.

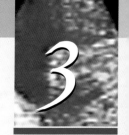

TRANSESOPHAGEAL ECHOCARDIOGRAPHY

3

Transesophageal echocardiography offers the advantages of improved image quality compared to transthoracic images, particularly of posterior structures, such as the pulmonary veins, left atrium, and mitral valve. Image quality is improved both because of the decreased distance between the transducer and the structures of interest and because of the absence of intervening lung or bone tissue. A better signal-to-noise ratio and decreased image depth also allows use of higher frequency (5- and 7-MHz) transducers, which further enhances image quality.

However, transesophageal imaging is more risky than transthoracic imaging due to the insertion of the probe in the esophagus and the need for conscious sedation in most patients. Typically, a transesophageal examination provides additional information but does not replace a transthoracic examination and, in some situations, transthoracic imaging provides better image quality and diagnostic Doppler data. For example, anterior structures, such as a prosthetic aortic valve, may be better imaged from the transthoracic approach. For Doppler velocity measurements, the transthoracic approach offers more acoustic windows with the ability to adjust the transducer angle freely in both the transverse and elevational planes. In contrast, transducer position and angulation are constrained from the transesophageal approach by the relative positions of the esophagus and heart. The inability to align the

Doppler beam parallel to the flow of interest may result in substantial velocity underestimation. In addition, it often is more difficult to obtain standard anatomic measurements from the transesophageal approach due to oblique two-dimensional (2D) image planes. Thus, even when transesophageal imaging is necessary, data from the transthoracic examination are integrated into the final clinical interpretation.

In this chapter, the transesophageal procedure and risks are briefly outlined followed by a description of the standard views obtained from each acoustic window (transesophageal, standard transgastric, transgastric apical, and descending aorta). Sections on the transesophageal 2D and Doppler evaluation of each cardiac valve and chamber are included to guide the reader to the optimal views for each anatomic structure. This chapter focuses on normal anatomy and flow patterns. Clinical indications for transesophageal imaging are discussed in Chapter 5 and pathologic images are included in subsequent chapters.

PROTOCOL AND RISKS

Transesophageal echocardiography is performed by a physician skilled in both echocardiography and the endoscopy procedure, as detailed in published guidelines for physician training. Typically, a cardiac sonographer assists the physician, adjusting instrument settings for optimal image quality and data acquisition. Many physicians use mild conscious sedation, in addition to local anesthesia of the pharynx, to minimize patient discomfort and improve tolerance of the procedure. When conscious sedation is used, a designated, qualified individual (usually a nurse) monitors and documents the patient's blood pressure, heart rate, respiratory rate, arterial oxygen saturation, and level of consciousness throughout the procedure. In addition, the nurse ensures patency of the airway and provides suction of oral secretions as needed (see Suggested Reading 11). The specific protocol, medications used for conscious sedation, and monitoring procedures are dictated by the standards of each institution.

Transesophageal echocardiography has a very low incidence of complications when performed by trained individuals with appropriate patient selection and monitoring. However, this procedure does have known risks, which must be taken into consideration in deciding whether the potential information obtained justifies use of this procedure (Table 3–1). The rate of complications serious enough to interrupt the procedure is less than 1% with a reported mortality rate of fewer than 1 in 10,000 patients. Risks are higher in patients with a history of esophageal disease, impaired respiratory status, or sleep apnea. If the preprocedure history or physical examination suggests an increased risk for conscious sedation, appropriate consultation with anesthesiology is essential. If there is a history of esophageal disease or symptoms related to impaired swallowing, a preprocedure barium swallow or gastroenterology consultation may be needed.

TABLE 3–1		
Risks of Transesophageal Echocardiography		

Risks of Esophageal Intubation

Dental trauma
Esophageal trauma or perforation
Bleeding
Aspiration
Dislodgement of endotracheal tube, especially on probe
  withdrawal
Displacement of nasogastric tubes

Risks of Conscious Sedation

Hypotension
Respiratory depression (hypoxia, respiratory arrest)
Arrhythmias
Bronchospasm
Death

The risk of aspiration is minimized by having the patient fast for several hours before the procedure, use of a left lateral decubitus position during probe insertion, and having the patient continue to fast after the procedure until recovery from the local anesthesia of the pharynx. Esophageal trauma or perforation is unlikely in the absence of a history of esophageal disease or swallowing difficulty, both of which can be ascertained by clinical history. Bleeding complications are rare and usually mild, and the procedure can be safely performed with therapeutic levels of systemic anticoagulation. Initial concern that transesophageal imaging might increase the risk of endocarditis has been alleviated by several studies showing the absence of bacteremia following this procedure so that most physicians do not routinely use antibiotic prophylaxis.

TOMOGRAPHIC VIEWS

The exact views obtained on a transesophageal study vary depending on the relative positions of the heart, esophagus, and diaphragm in each patient. Even though a multiplane probe allows full rotation of the scan plane, the fixed position of the transducer in the esophagus constrains the possible image planes that can be obtained, potentially resulting in oblique image orientations compared with the three-dimensional (3D) reference system used for transthoracic images. The goal on transesophageal echocardiography is to perform a systematic and comprehensive examination, using standard short-axis, long-axis, two-chamber, and four-chamber image planes whenever possible. Standard views then are supplemented with additional image planes to demonstrate the specific pathologic processes in each patient. Three-dimensional echocardiographic techniques will facilitate obtaining the optimal views as this approach becomes more usable and widely available.

A recommended sequence of images comprising a basic complete examination is shown in the Echo Exam section at the end of this chapter. The following sections describe views useful for evaluation of the valves and cardiac chambers that can be used to supplement the basic examination as determined by the specific clinical question.

The position of the tip of the probe is described as esophageal or transgastric and is referenced to the cardiac structures seen in each view. The absolute distance of the transducer from the patient's mouth will vary depending on body size and cardiac position. There also will be variability in the exact degree of rotation, tilt, and angulation needed to obtain the best short-axis, long-axis, two-chamber, and four-chamber views. When standard views are obtained, the images correspond to the anatomy described for the equivalent transthoracic views, with the major difference being image orientation given the transesophageal transducer position.

For transesophageal echocardiograms, transducer motions will be referred to as

■ *repositioning*, defined as movement of the probe up and down in the esophagus;
■ *rotation*, defined as rotating the image plane from 0° to 180° using the multiplane control knob;
■ *turning*, defined as moving the entire transducer in a rotational fashion in the esophagus to show a mediolateral change in image plane;
■ *angulation*, defined as bending and extending the probe so that the image plane is directed superiorly or inferiorly at an angle to the original image plane; and
■ *tilt*, defined as lateral motion of the transducer tip to image different structures in the same image plane (although slight superior motion occurs as well).

From the transesophageal position, most image planes are achieved using repositioning, rotation, and turning of the transducer. The use of angulation is particularly important on transgastric views. An essential principle in using a multiplane probe is that the anatomic area of interest should be centered in the image before rotation to a new view to ensure that the structure of interest remains in the image plane.

Esophageal Position

Four-Chamber Plane

As the transducer is advanced into the esophagus from the mouth toward the stomach, acoustic access is limited by interposition of the air-filled trachea until the transducer passes beyond the trachea at the level of the carina. From a high transesophageal position, with the probe located posterior to the left atrium, a standard four-chamber view usually can be obtained in the 0° position with angulation of the transducer toward the left ventricular apex (Fig. 3–1). As with transthoracic imaging, slight changes in angulation allow imaging of the coronary sinus posteriorly and the left ventricular outflow tract and aortic valve anteriorly (the "five-chamber" view) (Fig. 3–2). In the four-chamber view, the lateral wall and inferior septal segments of the left ventricle are seen. Care is needed to include as much of the full length of the ventricle as possible in this view. Typically, even with optimal positioning and angulation, transesophageal views are somewhat foreshortened compared to the true long-axis views of the ventricle and the apparent apex may

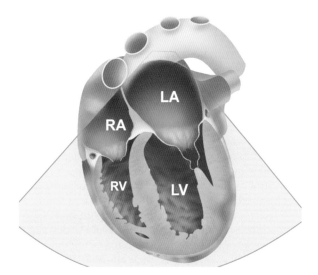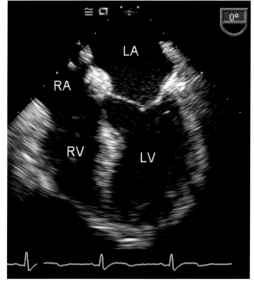

■ **FIGURE 3–1.** Transesophageal four-chamber view. Drawing (*left*) and echocardiographic image (*right*) in a transesophageal four-chamber view is obtained from a high transesophageal position with the multiplane probe at 0° rotation. In this view, the apparent apex may actually represent a segment of the anterior wall because of foreshortening of the long axis of the ventricle.

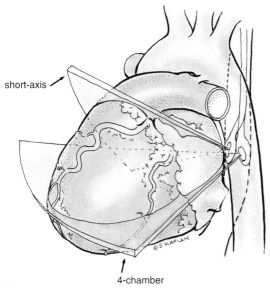

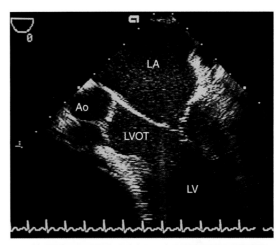

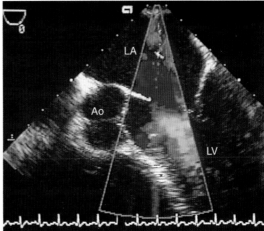

■ **FIGURE 3–2.** Illustration of the use of angulation of the transducer from a high esophageal position with the probe at 0° rotation to obtain a four-chamber view (as shown in Fig. 3–1) or a short-axis view of the left atrial appendage (as shown in Fig. 3–7).

■ **FIGURE 3–3.** Slight anterior angulation from the four-chamber view, midway between the image planes shown in Fig. 3–2, allows visualization of the aortic valve and left ventricular outflow tract (*top*). Color flow shows normal systolic laminar flow in the outflow tract (*bottom*).

actually represent a more proximal segment of the anterior wall. Even so, a biplane ejection fraction can be calculated from end-diastolic and end-systolic endocardial borders traced in the four- and two-chamber transesophageal views.

When the transducer is positioned posterior to the center of the left atrium, the central portions of both the anterior and posterior leaflets of the mitral valve are demonstrated well in the 0° four-chamber view. Anterior angulation provides a view of the left ventricular outflow tract and anterior mitral leaflet analogous to the apical five-chamber view (Fig. 3–3). Posterior angulation provides images of more lateral segments of the valve leaflets with coronary sinus visualized on extreme posterior angulation.

While examining the left atrium in the four-chamber plane, it is helpful to slowly advance and withdraw the transducer to visualize the full superior and inferior extent or to slowly angulate the probe tip to provide sequential cross sections of the left atrium. Because the left atrium is in the near field of the image, careful adjustment of imaging parameters is needed to avoid misinterpretation of near-field artifacts. For this reason, identification of a small thrombus along the posterior left atrial wall is problematic.

In the standard four-chamber transesophageal image, the size, shape, and systolic function of the right ventricle can be assessed by turning the probe toward the patient's right side. This view also provides visualization of the septal and anterior leaflets of the tricuspid valve and the right atrium. The interatrial septum is depicted well with the fossa ovalis and primum septum region clearly identifiable (Fig. 3–4).

Two-Chamber Plane

After ensuring that the left ventricular apex is in the center of the image in a four-chamber view, the image plane is slowly rotated to approximately 60° to obtain a two-chamber view (Fig. 3–5). Because the apex often is not exactly centered in three dimensions, the position and angulation of the transducer may need adjustment to obtain a two-chamber view that includes the full length of the left ventricle (Fig. 3–6). In this view, the

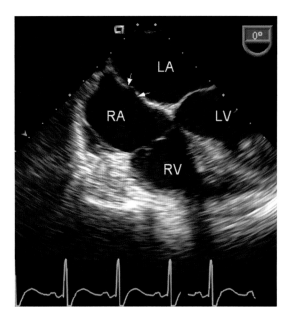

■ **FIGURE 3–4.** A view of the tricuspid valve and interatrial septum is obtained by turning the transducer from the four-chamber view toward the patient's right side. The thin central region of the interatrial septum known as the fossa ovalis is between the *arrowheads*.

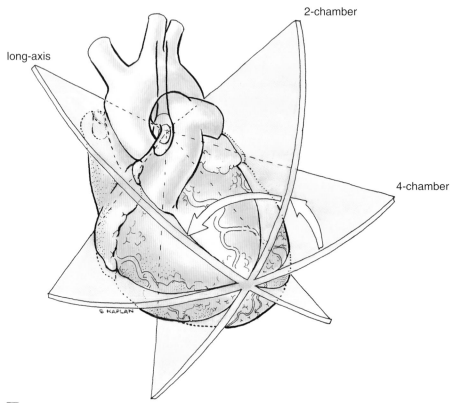

■ **FIGURE 3–5.** Rotation of the image plane starting from the four-chamber view, with the left ventricular apex centered in the image, allows a two-chamber view (see Fig. 3–6) at approximately 60° rotation and a long-axis view (see Fig. 3–8) at approximately 120° rotation. Slight repositioning and angulation of the transducer may be needed as the image plane is rotated to ensure inclusion of the left ventricular apex in the image.

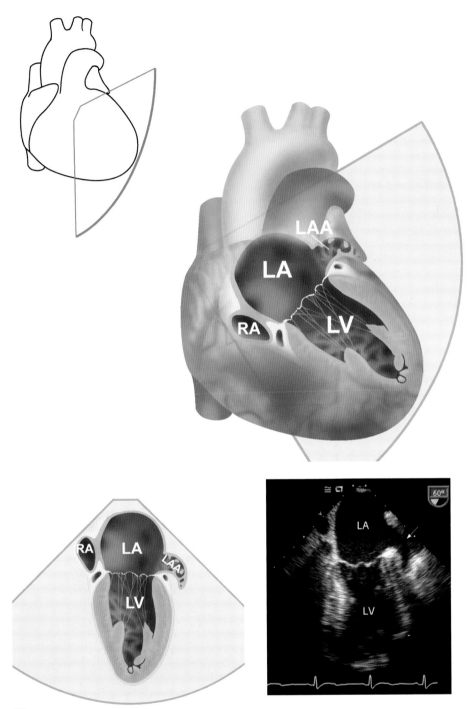

■ **FIGURE 3–6.** Transesophageal two-chamber view. The position of the image plane is shown on the line drawing. This image plane is equivalent to the vertical long-axis plane with other tomographic imaging modalities. Typically, the image plane is rotated to approximately 60 degrees, with adjustments to transducer position and flexion, although there is individual variation. The 3D view shows the cross-section of the left atrium and ventricle with the left atrial appendage (LAA), coronary sinus in the atrioventricular groove, and the mitral valve. In the two-chamber view, small portions of the posterior mitral leaflet are seen laterally and medially with the anterior leaflet filling most of the annulus area. Part of a papillary muscle has been shown for orientation, but the papillary muscles are seen located symmetrically posterior to the image plane. The tomographic plane has been rotated with the apex of the sector at the top (*bottom left*) to correspond to the 2D echocadiographic image (*bottom right*).

inferior and anterior left ventricular walls of the left ventricle are seen allowing assessment of regional function and providing the orthogonal plane (along with the four-chamber view) for calculation of ejection fraction. With further rotation to about 90°, the left atrial appendage is depicted in a view approximately perpendicular to that obtained in the transverse plane (Fig. 3–7). The left superior pulmonary vein can be seen entering the left atrium by slightly withdrawing and turning the probe laterally. In the two-chamber view, typically only the anterior leaflet of the mitral valve is seen so that it is difficult to evaluate leaflet prolapse in this view.

Long-Axis Left Ventricular Plane

With the transducer positioned in the high esophagus, posterior to the left atrium, further rotation of the image plane to approximately 120° results in a long-axis view of the left ventricle and aorta (Fig. 3–8). Again, slight adjustment of transducer position and angulation may be needed to obtain a view that includes the left ventricular apex. Similar to a transthoracic long-axis view, the proximal ascending aorta, sinuses of Valsalva, and right and noncoronary leaflets of the aortic valve are depicted well. Scanning between this view and the 90° image planes allows appreciation of the perpendicular relationship between aortic and

pulmonic valve planes and the slightly more cephalad position of the pulmonic valve. The long-axis view is particularly helpful in evaluating for ascending aortic dissection, subaortic membrane, supracristal ventricular septal defect, sinus of Valsalva aneurysm, aortic valve vegetations, and abscess formation. Note that in the esophageal long-axis plane, withdrawing the transducer in the esophagus results in more cephalad images of the ascending aorta with the superior limit of imaging determined by the interposed air-filled bronchus (Fig. 3–9).

The anterior and posterior mitral leaflets are seen in a long-axis orientation and the coronary sinus can be identified in cross section in the atrioventricular groove. The right pulmonary artery is visualized posterior to the aortic root at the superior aspect of the left atrium. In the long-axis view, the anterior septum and posterior wall of the left ventricle are seen. In addition, a portion of the right ventricular outflow tract is seen anterior to the aortic valve (in the far field of the image).

Other Long-Axis Image Planes

At a rotation angle of 90°, the probe can be turned from the left ventricular long-axis view toward the patient's left side to obtain a long-axis view of the pulmonic valve and right ventricular outflow tract

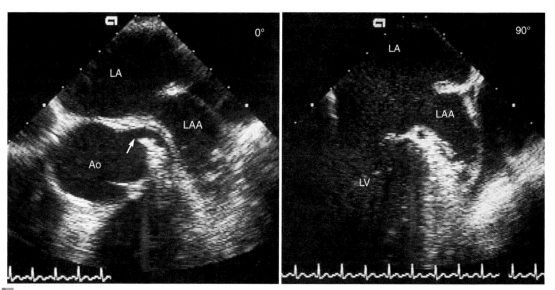

■ **FIGURE 3–7.** *Left*: Left atrial appendage seen in the 0° image plane obtained from the four-chamber view by slight withdrawal and anterior angulation of the transducer. Note the normal trabeculation in the atrial appendage and the left main coronary artery (*arrow*) arising from the aortic root. *Right*: Orthogonal view of the atrial appendage obtained by rotation to 90°. Both these images were obtained with a 7.0-MHz transducer to optimize detection of atrial appendage thrombus.

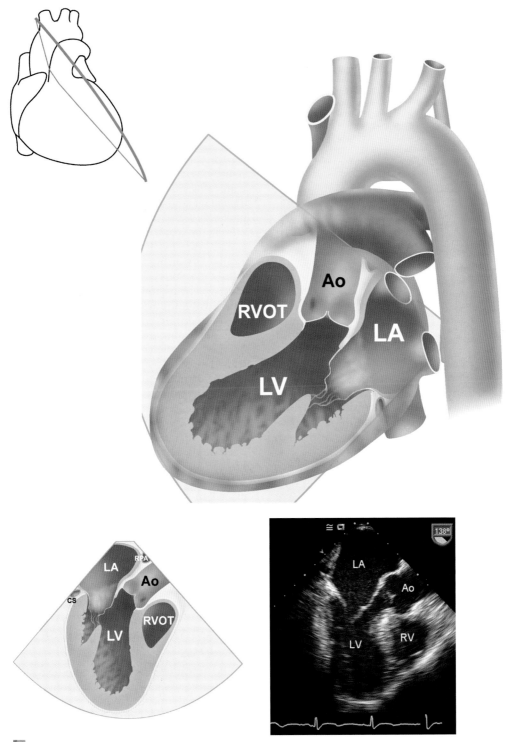

▌ FIGURE 3–8. Transesophageal long axis view. The position of the image plane is shown on the line drawing. This view typically is obtained at approximately 120° rotation, but there is considerable individual variability in the exact image plane needed to show the aorta and left ventricle in a long-axis orientation. The 3D view shows the cross-section of the aortic root (Ao), left ventricle (LV), left atrium (LA), and right ventricular outflow tract (RVOT). In the long-axis view, the anterior and posterior mitral valve leaflets are seen. The tomographic plane has been rotated with the apex of the sector at the top (*bottom left*) to correspond to the 2D echocardiographic image (*bottom right*).

■ **FIGURE 3–9.** From the transesophageal long-axis view, further cephalad segments of the ascending aorta can be seen by slight withdrawal of the transducer in the esophagus.

(Fig. 3–10). In this view, the pulmonic valve is in the far field of the image and may be shadowed by the aortic valve and root if calcification is present. Portions of the right ventricle and tricuspid valve are seen, depending on the exact position of the heart relative to the esophagus in each patient.

At a 90° rotation, when the probe is turned toward the patient's right side images of the right ventricle and tricuspid valve in an inflow view are obtained. If the probe is turned further to the right, a long-axis view of the right atrium is obtained with the superior vena cava entering from the right side of the screen and the inferior vena cava on the left (Fig. 3–11). In some individuals, a Eustachian valve at the inferior caval-atrial junction is seen. The trabeculated right atrial appendage often can be seen with slight medial rotation from this view.

Minor changes in the rotation angle may be needed to optimize each view. As with the left ventricular long-axis view, adjustment of transducer position (advancement and withdrawal) allows imaging of much of the cephalad to caudal extent of the cardiac structures in each of these tomographic planes.

Short-Axis Plane

A short-axis view at the aortic valve level can be obtained by rotating the image plane to between 30° and 45° and withdrawing the probe in the esophagus to the level of the aortic valve. Visualization of aortic valve anatomy is excellent,

showing the three leaflets and sinuses of Valsalva (Fig. 3–12). The origin of the left main coronary artery is easily identified after minor adjustments in the depth and tilt of the image plane. The right coronary artery is more difficult to visualize and is clearly identified in only a minority of patients. The interatrial septum is depicted well, with the fossa ovalis clearly defined.

By turning the transducer laterally and angulating superiorly from the 0° esophageal position, the left atrial appendage and left superior pulmonary vein are seen (see Fig. 3–7). Prominent features include normal trabeculation of the atrial appendage and a variably prominent ridge at the junction of the anteriorly directed left superior pulmonary vein and the left atrial appendage. The laterally directed left inferior pulmonary vein is seen by advancing the transducer and angulating slightly inferiorly. The right pulmonary veins can be imaged by rotating the transducer medially and withdrawing the transducer cephalad (to see the anteriorly directed right superior pulmonary vein) or by angulating the transducer inferiorly (to see the medially directed right inferior pulmonary vein). The pulmonary veins also can be identified in the 90° image plane, turning the transducer toward the patient's right to show the right pulmonary veins and to the left for the left pulmonary veins. Again, color flow imaging often facilitates identification of the pulmonary veins based on the characteristic venous inflow patterns (Fig. 3–13).

In many patients, the pulmonary artery can be imaged in the 0° image plane by further withdrawing the probe in the esophagus to obtain a view straight down the main pulmonary artery from the bifurcation to the valve level. In some cases, this view is limited by the position of the air-filled bronchus and some patients may find the probe uncomfortable when positioned at this level in the esophagus.

Standard Transgastric Position

Short-Axis Plane

As the transducer is passed into the stomach, slight resistance may be encountered at the gastroesophageal junction. With the probe tip in the stomach, superior angulation (flexing the scope) in the 0° image plane results in a short-axis view of the left ventricle at the papillary muscle level (Fig. 3–14). In this view, global left ventricular systolic function, left ventricular dimensions and wall thickness, and regional left ventricular function can be evaluated (Fig. 3–15).

Depending on the position of the patient's heart with respect to the diaphragm, a short-axis

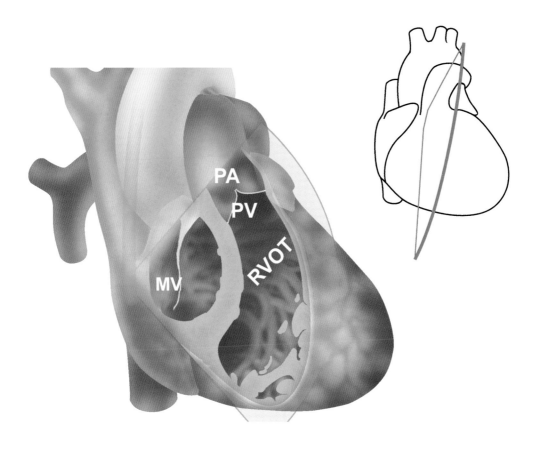

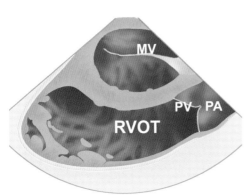

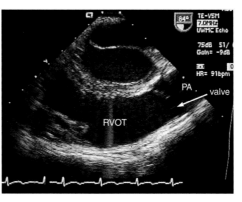

■ **FIGURE 3–10.** Transesophageal right ventricular outflow tract view. In the 90° transesophageal image plane, the right ventricular outflow tract (RVOT), pulmonic valve (PV), and pulmonary artery (PA) can be demonstrated with the probe turned toward the patient's left side (*top*). The tomographic plane has been rotated with the apex of the sector scan at the top (*bottom left*) to correspond to the echocardiographic image (*bottom right*).

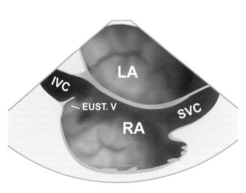

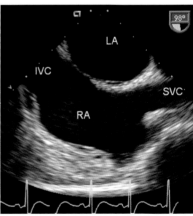

■ **FIGURE 3–11.** Transesophageal right atrial view. With the probe turned toward the patient's right side, the right atrium and superior and inferior vena cava can be visualized in the 90° transesophageal image plane as shown in the drawing (*top*) with visulization of the superior and inferior vena cava (SVC and IVC), left and right atrium (LA and RA). A Eusthasian valve often is present at the IVC-RA junction. The tomographic plane has been rotated with the apex of the sector scan at the top (*bottom left*) to correspond to the echocardiographic image (*bottom right*). Part of the trabeculated right atrial appendage is seen adjaceent to the superior vena cava (SVC).

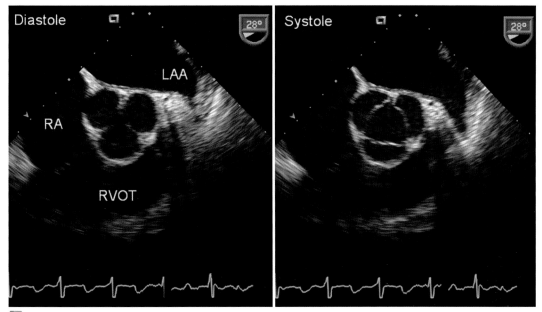

FIGURE 3–12. A short-axis view of the aortic valve in diastole (*left*) and systole (*right*) is seen in a transesophageal view at 28° rotation. The degree of rotation needed to obtain this short-axis view varies from approximately 30° to 50°; the images themselves should be used to ensure a true short-axis image. Oblique image planes may result in artifactual distortion of the valve apparatus.

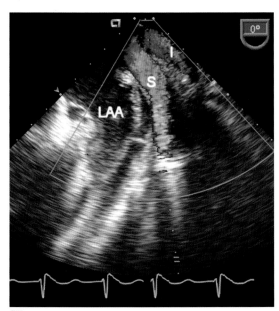

FIGURE 3–13. The left superior (S) and inferior pulmonary veins (I) are seen in the 0° plane with the probe at the level of the left atrial appendage (LAA). Color flow imaging facilitates identification of the pulmonary views as they enter the left atrium.

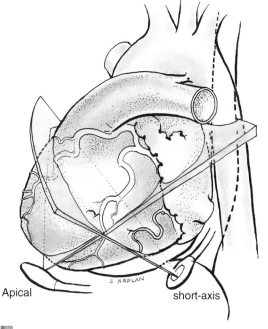

FIGURE 3–14. From the transgastric position, the probe can be positioned near the gastroesophageal junction to obtain a short-axis view of the left ventricle or can be advanced into the stomach to obtain an "apical" view. Transgastric apical images may show a foreshortened left ventricle because the true left ventricular apex often does not lie on the diaphragm.

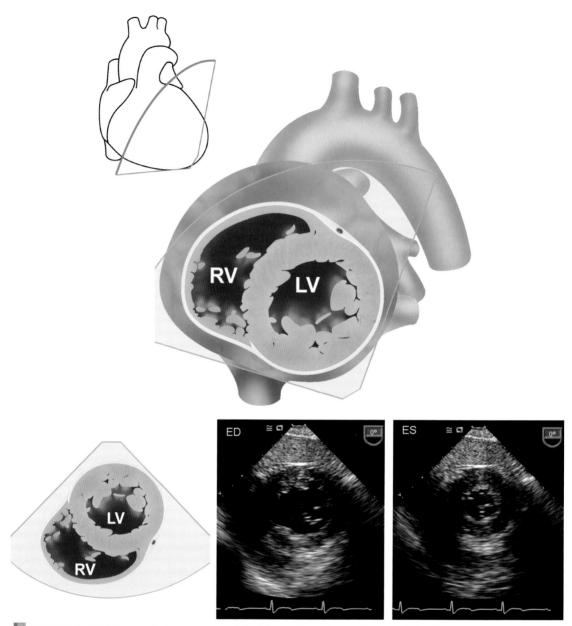

FIGURE 3–15. Transgastric short-axis view of the left ventricle at the papillary muscle level (*top*) is obtained by retroflexion of the transducer from a transgastric position. This view is particularly valuable for intraoperative monitoring of left ventricular size and global and regional systolic function. The tomographic plane has been rotated with the apex of the sector at the top (*bottom left*) to correspond to the end-diastolic (ED) and end-systolic (ES) echocardiographic images (*bottom center and right*).

view at the mitral valve level may be obtainable by slight withdrawal of the transducer toward the esophagus (Fig. 3–16). The transgastric short-axis view at the mitral valve level is helpful in precise definition of the mitral valve apparatus anatomy in patients with valve dysfunction.

Two-Chamber Plane

A two-chamber view of the left ventricle can be obtained from the transgastric position by rotating the image plane to the 90° position (Fig. 3–17). From this two-chamber view, turning the entire

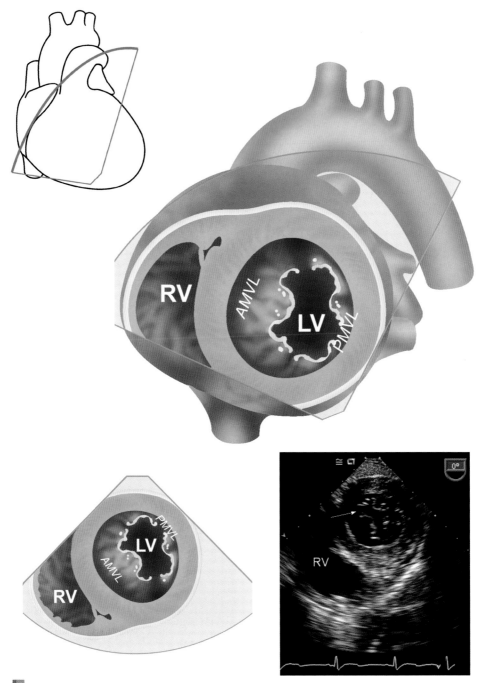

■ **FIGURE 3–16.** Transgastric short axis at the mitral valve level. From the transgastric short-axis view of the left ventricle, slight withdrawal of the probe toward the gastroesophageal junction may allow a short-axis view of the mitral valve with definition of the anterior (AMLV) and posterior mitral valve leaflets (PMVL). The tomographic plane has been rotated with the apex of the sector scan at the top (*bottom left*) to correspond to the echocardiographic image (*bottom right*).

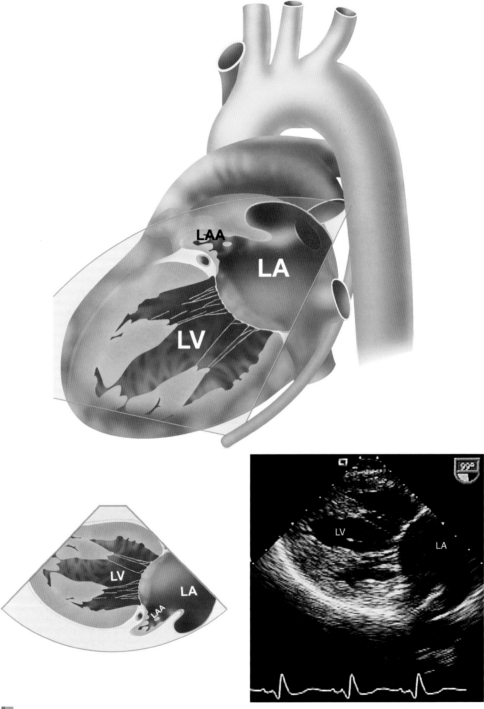

■ **FIGURE 3–17.** Transgastric two-chamber view. From the transgastric short-axis view, 90° rotation provides a two-chamber view of the left ventricle, atrium, and atrial appendage (*top*). The tomographic image plane has been rotated with the apex of the sector at the top to correspond with the echocardiographic image (*bottom right*). Turning the transducer toward the patient's right side from this view provides a two-chamber view of the right atrium and right ventricle, analogous to a transthoracic right ventricular inflow view.

probe toward the patient's right side results in a view of the right atrium, tricuspid valve, and right ventricle similar to a transthoracic right ventricular inflow view. In some individuals, the right ventricular outflow tract and pulmonic valve also can be demonstrated.

Transgastric Apical Position

Four-Chamber Plane

From the transgastric short-axis view, the transducer is further advanced into the fundus of the stomach. In most individuals, an "apical" four-chamber view can be obtained using the 0° image plane of the probe if the left ventricle lies on the diaphragm, without intervening lung. Note that the transducer may not be on the true left ventricular apex, so this view typically is foreshortened. Anterior angulation shows the aortic valve in a view similar to the transthoracic anteriorly angulated four-chamber view, which allows Doppler interrogation of the left ventricular outflow tract and valve (Fig. 3–18).

Long-Axis Plane

From the transgastric apical four-chamber plane, rotation of the image plane to 120° results in a long-axis view of the left ventricular outflow tract, providing a more parallel intercept angle for Doppler study of outflow tract and aortic velocities. However, this view cannot be obtained in all patients, particularly if the transducer is not on the true left ventricular apex, because lung tissue is interposed between the transducer and cardiac structures as the image plane is rotated.

Descending Thoracic Aorta

From the transesophageal or transgastric position, the transducer is turned (either direction) until the image plane is directed slightly left of the patient's spine to obtain a short-axis view of the descending thoracic aorta. The aorta appears circular and shows normal systolic pulsations (Fig. 3–19). The descending thoracic aorta can be depicted in sequential short-axis views from its postgastric position to the junction with the aortic arch as the probe is slowly withdrawn in the esophagus. When the transducer reaches the level of the arch, turning the transducer medially, with inferior angulation, allows a long-axis view of the arch itself. The descending thoracic aorta also can be depicted in a long-axis plane by centering the aorta in the 2D sector and rotating the image plane to 90°. This long-axis view complements the short-axis view of the descending aorta in evaluation of aortic dissections, aneurysms, and

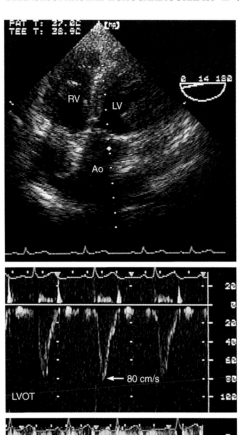

■ **FIGURE 3–18.** Transgastric apical view angulated anteriorly to include the aortic root (*top*). This view allows recording of left ventricular outflow tract velocity with pulsed Doppler (*middle*), and aortic jet velocity with 2D-guided continuous-wave Doppler ultrasound (*bottom*). When a high-velocity jet is suspected, careful angulation and positioning of the transducer is needed to obtain the highest velocity signal. Because of the constraints on transducer positioning and the lack of a view equivalent to the transthoracic suprasternal notch view, the possibility of velocity underestimation should be considered.

atheromas and improves the differentiation of ultrasound artifacts from anatomic abnormalities. The 90° image plane also allows identification of the origin of the left subclavian artery, which is important for describing the proximal extent of

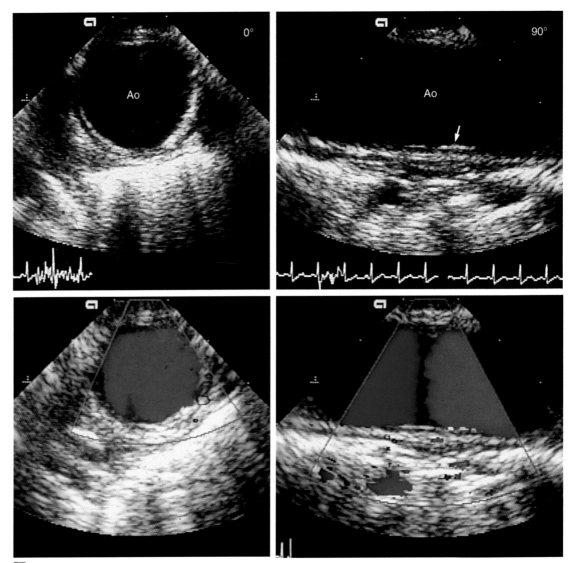

■ FIGURE 3–19. Transesophageal 2D and color flow images of the descending thoracic aorta in short-axis (*left*) (0° rotation) and long-axis (*right*) (90° rotation) views on 2D echo (*top*) and with color flow imaging (*bottom*). Mild atherosclerosis is present (*arrow*).

dissection and for placement of an intraaortic balloon pump (see Chapter 16).

VALVE ANATOMY AND NORMAL DOPPLER FLOWS

Optimal evaluation of valve anatomy and function on transesophageal echocardiography includes the use of at least two standard orthogonal imaging planes (Table 3–2). This approach provides a reasonably complete evaluation of valve anatomy and aids recognition of ultrasound artifacts. Continuous-wave and pulsed Doppler velocities should be recorded with the ultrasound

beam aligned parallel to the flow stream. However, a parallel intercept angle may be difficult to achieve given the constraints on transducer position from the transesophageal approach. As with transthoracic imaging, color Doppler is helpful for evaluation of abnormal flow patterns even at nonparallel intercept angles.

Left Ventricular Outflow and Aortic Valve

The aortic valve and left ventricular outflow tract can be imaged by anterior angulation from the 0° four-chamber view obtained with the transducer positioned posterior to the left atrium. This view

TABLE 3–2			
Transesophageal Views for Cardiac Valves			
Valve	**View**	**Probe position**	**Rotation Angle**
Aortic	Long-axis	High esophageal	~120–130°
		or	
		Transgastric	~90° (turn probe to visualize LVOT)
	Short-axis	High esophageal	~30–50°
	"Five-chamber"	High esophageal	0° (anteriorly angulated)
		or	
		Transgastric apical	
Mitral	Long-axis	High esophageal	~120–130°
		Transgastric	90°
	Short-axis	Transgastric (at GE junction)	May be obtained in some patients at 0° with probe flexed
	Four-chamber	High esophageal	0°
		or	
		Transgastric apical	
Pulmonic	Long-axis	Very high esophageal	0° (looking straight down PA from bifurcation)
	Outflow view	High esophageal	~90° (turn probe to left)
Tricuspid	Four-chamber	High esophageal	0°
	RV-inflow (esophageal)	High esophageal	~90° (turn probe to right)
	RV-inflow (transgastric)	Transgastric	~90° (turn probe to right)

PA, pulmonary artery; RV, right ventricular; GE, gastroesophageal; LVOT, left ventricular outflow tract.

is analogous to a transthoracic anteriorly angulated four-chamber view. Rotation of the image plane to approximately 45° provides a short-axis view of the aortic valve with clear delineation of the valve leaflets in systole and diastole. Slight withdrawal of the probe shows the sinuses of Valsalva and left main coronary artery while slight advancement provides a short-axis view of the left ventricular outflow tract. A long-axis view is obtained by rotating the image plane to approximately 120° (Fig. 3–20). In both the short- and long-axis views, image quality is optimized by use of a high transducer frequency and adjustment of the depth to maximize the valve image. The aortic valve also can be imaged in a five-chamber view from a transesophageal position with anterior angulation from the four-chamber view at 0° rotation.

Doppler evaluation of the aortic valve on transesophageal echocardiography is problematic with color flow imaging for valvular regurgitation being the most helpful approach. With the probe positioned in the high esophagus (posterior to the left atrium), color flow imaging can be used to evaluate the flow disturbance due to aortic regurgitation in the anteriorly angulated four-chamber and long-axis views. In addition, the cross-sectional area of the aortic regurgitant jet can be evaluated starting in a short-axis view of the aortic valve and slowly advancing the probe in the esophagus to obtain a short-axis view of the outflow tract. As with transthoracic imaging, the short-axis jet area relative to outflow tract area is a reliable color flow measure of regurgitant severity.

Accurate antegrade velocity measurements across the aortic valve may not be possible because of the nonparallel intercept angle between the ultrasound beam and the direction of blood flow from the transesophageal position. In many patients, a transgastric apical view allows recording of pulsed and continuous-wave Doppler flow velocities proximal to and across the aortic valve (see Fig. 3–18). However, caution is needed in interpretation of the Doppler data, because unlike a transthoracic examination, a high-velocity signal across the aortic valve cannot be studied from multiple windows with careful transducer angulation to ensure that a parallel intercept angle has been obtained. If aortic valve pathology is present, transthoracic recording of antegrade velocities is most accurate and should be performed in all cases.

Left Ventricular Inflow and Mitral Valve

The mitral valve leaflets are evaluated by slow rotation from the transesophageal four-chamber

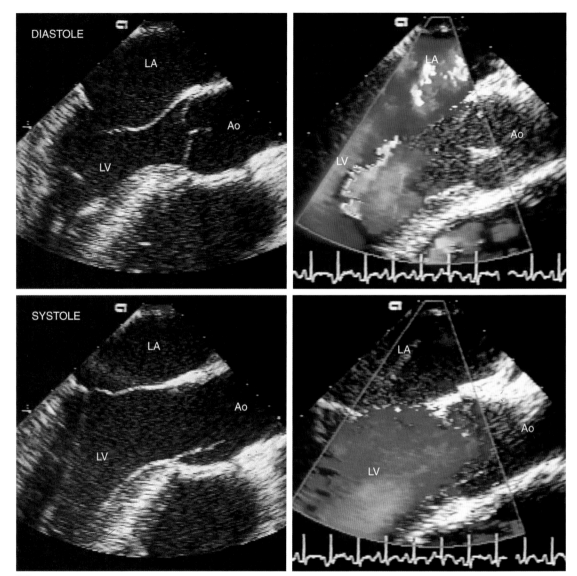

▌ FIGURE 3–20. Long-axis images of the aortic and mitral valve with the depth adjusted to optimize evaluation of valve anatomy and motion. The 2D images (*left*) in diastole (*top*) and systole (*bottom*) show normal aortic and mitral opening and closure. The color flow images (*right*) show normal left ventricular inflow with no aortic regurgitation in diastole (*top*) and normal antegrade flow in the left ventricular outflow tract and no mitral regurgitation in systole (*bottom*).

view to the long-axis view with frequent image recording. Again, adjusting the transducer frequency, image depth, and other instrument parameters are needed for optimal image quality. Adjustments in transducer angulation and position may be needed to fully evaluate pathologic findings. The subvalvular apparatus usually is well seen in these views unless there is valve calcification with shadowing of distal structures. If additional views are needed, the examiner should obtain transgastric short-axis and two-chamber

views of the mitral valve. Other useful views include the transgastric apical view, although image quality may be suboptimal at the depth of the mitral valve.

The pattern of antegrade flow across the mitral valve (left ventricular diastolic filling) can be recorded with pulsed Doppler in the four-chamber or long-axis view at a parallel intercept angle (Fig. 3–21). Because the flow is directly away from the transducer, the velocity curve with the typical early diastolic peak (E) and late dias-

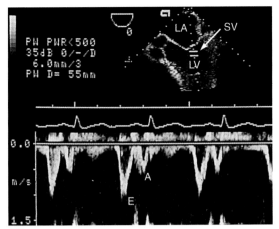

FIGURE 3–21. Left ventricular inflow recorded with pulsed Doppler with the sample volume positioned at the mitral leaflet tips from an anteriorly angulated transesophageal four-chamber view. The flow pattern is similar to a transthoracic recording of left ventricular inflow, albeit inverted as the flow is directed away from the transducer.

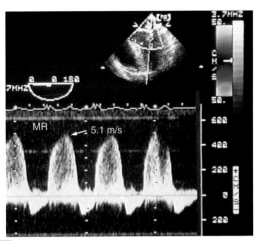

FIGURE 3–22. Continuous-wave Doppler recording of mitral regurgitation from a transesophageal four-chamber view. Color flow was used to identify the vena contracta of the regurgitant jet for the initial positioning of the continuous-wave Doppler beam. Transducer position and angulation then were modified as needed to obtain a clear signal with the highest flow velocity.

tolic peak (*A*) velocities is shown below the baseline. Color Doppler can be used to evaluate for mitral regurgitation as the image plane is slowly rotated from the four-chamber to two-chamber to long-axis view. Alternatively, transmitral flow can be recorded from the transgastric apical approach, although signal strength is lower due to the greater depth of the mitral valve from this position. Mitral regurgitation can be evaluated with continuous-wave Doppler from the high esophageal position, using the color flow signal to align the continuous-wave Doppler beam with the vena contracta of the regurgitant jet (Fig. 3–22).

Right Ventricular Outflow and Pulmonic Valve

The right ventricular outflow tract is best imaged from a high esophageal position at 0° rotation with a long-axis view of the pulmonary artery from the valve plane to its bifurcation. Doppler velocities can be recorded from this position at a parallel intercept angle as flow is directed straight toward the transducer (Fig. 3–23). The pulmonic valve also may be visualized in the 90° long-axis plane with the pulmonic valve seen in its perpendicular relationship to the aortic valve in the far field of the image (see Fig. 3–10). However, velocities cannot be recorded from this approach due to a nonparallel intercept angle. In some patients, the pulmonic valve also can be imaged from the transgastric position either in the 90° image plane including the tricuspid valve or in a very anteriorly angulated apical four-chamber view.

Right Ventricular Inflow and Tricuspid Valve

The tricuspid valve is well imaged in the standard four-chamber views, both from the transesophageal position and from the transgastric apical view. Other useful views include the transesophageal right ventricular inflow view and the transgastric two-chamber view turned to show the right heart structures. In a transgastric view obtained close to the diaphragm, the entry of the coronary sinus into the right atrium adjacent to the tricuspid valve can be seen. Further advancement of the transducer often allows a short-axis view of the tricuspid valve.

The tricuspid regurgitant jet may be recorded from either transesophageal or transgastric views; however, underestimation of velocity should be considered given the limited ability to vary transducer position to ensure a parallel intercept angle. If high pulmonary pressures are suspected, transthoracic continuous-wave Doppler recordings or invasive measures of pulmonary pressure should be obtained.

CHAMBER ANATOMY AND ATRIAL INFLOW

Left Ventricle

Standard views of the left ventricle are obtained from the transesophageal position in four-

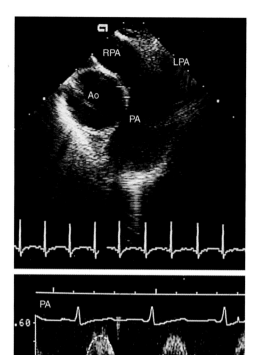

FIGURE 3–23. A very high transesophageal position provides a long-axis view (*top*) of the main pulmonary artery and its bifurcation into right and left pulmonary arteries. The ascending aorta is seen in short axis. This view allows recording of flow in the pulmonary artery at a parallel intercept angle because flow is directly toward the transducer (*above*).

each myocardial segment with a high degree of interobserver reproducibility for grading of wall motion in standard segments. In the transgastric short-axis view, the wall segments are the same as in a transthoracic short-axis view, *except* that the entire image has been rotated approximately 180° clockwise (if standard display format is used). Compared with a transthoracic subcostal short-axis view, the image is rotated 90° clockwise (see Fig. 8–7).

Left Atrium

The location and flow patterns of the pulmonary veins are readily assessed by transesophageal echocardiography. The flow pattern is most easily recorded in the left superior pulmonary vein where the typical systolic and diastolic antegrade flows and the reversal after atrial contraction can be appreciated (Fig. 3–25). Although flow tends to be more laminar with a narrow band on velocities on the spectral display in the left, compared to right, superior pulmonary vein, in general flow patterns are similar in all four pulmonary veins. However, exceptions do occur as, for example, when mitral regurgitation is present. In this situation, the regurgitant jet may be directed eccentrically, altering flow patterns in some, but not all, pulmonary veins.

If left atrial thrombus is suspected, the atrial appendage should be examined in at least two orthogonal views. Recognition of low flow (spontaneous contrast) and appendage thrombi are enhanced by use of a high transducer frequency (7 MHz). Care is needed to distinguish normal trabeculation from localized thrombus formation. Trabeculae tend to be more linear and are continuous with the atrial wall in more than one view. Thrombi typically protrude into the appendage, often with independent motion.

The flow pattern in the left atrial appendage can be recorded with pulsed Doppler ultrasound with the sample volume positioned in the appendage, approximately 1 cm from the junction with the body of the left atrium. The normal flow pattern (see Fig. 15–21) is characterized by ejection of blood from the appendage following atrial contraction at a velocity greater than 40 cm/s. Abnormal flow patterns are seen with atrial fibrillation, atrial flutter, and other tachyarrhythmias.

The interatrial septum is depicted well in the standard four-chamber view and can be evaluated in detail by centering the septum in the image and then slowly rotating the image plane with continuous recording of images. The fossa ovalis and primum septum are clearly demarcated, and the "flap valve" of a patent foramen ovale often can be identified on 2D imaging, before confirmation

chamber, two-chamber, and long-axis views (Table 3–3). A standard short-axis view is obtained from the transgastric position. These views allow calculation of left ventricular volumes and ejection fraction. Comparisons with radionuclide and contrast angiography have shown that transesophageal calculation of ejection fraction is both accurate and reproducible (Fig. 3–24). End-diastolic and end-systolic volumes often are underestimated because the image plane does not include the full long axis of the ventricle. However, transesophageal echocardiography remains accurate for evaluation of relative changes in ventricular volumes based on short-axis area changes in an individual patient. Left ventricular volume status can be assessed during surgery using a combination of these views, or using a single view, such as the transgastric short-axis view for continuous monitoring.

Standard views of the left ventricle also allow evaluation of regional ventricular function for

TABLE 3–3

Transesophageal Views for Evaluation of Cardiac Chambers

Chamber	View	Probe Position	Rotation Angle
Left ventricle	Four-chamber	High esophageal	0°
	Two-chamber	High esophageal	60°
		Transgastric	90°
	Long-axis	High esophageal	120°
	Short-axis	Transgastric	0° with angulation of the probe tip
Left atrium	Four-chamber	High esophageal	0°, Also allows assessment of all 4 pulmonary veins with medial and lateral turning and slight angulation of the transducer
	Two-chamber	High esophageal	60°
	Long-axis	High esophageal	120°
Right ventricle	Four-chamber	High esophageal	0°
	Right ventricular inflow view	High esophageal	90° with probe turned toward patient's right side
		or	
		Transgastric	90° with probe turned toward patient's right side
Right atrium	Four-chamber	High esophageal	0° with posterior angulation to visualize coronary sinus
	Right atrial view	High esophageal	90° with probe turned toward patient's right side
	Low atrial view	Gastroesophageal junction	0° to visualize entry of coronary sinus into right atrium

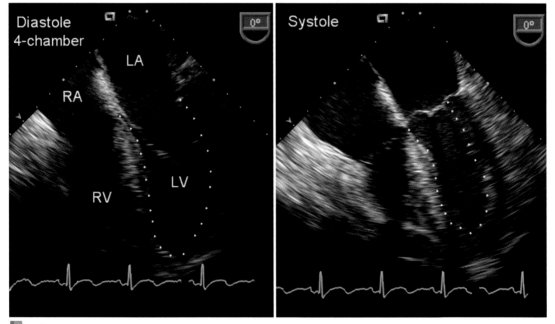

■ **FIGURE 3–24.** Examples of endocardial border tracings at end-diastole and end-systole in a transesophageal four-chamber for calculation of left ventricular ejection fraction. Borders are also traced in the two-chamber view at 60° of rotation.

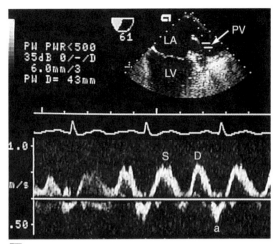

■ **FIGURE 3-25.** Pulsed Doppler recording of normal flow in the left superior pulmonary vein shows systolic (S) and diastolic (D) inflow with a small atrial (a) reversal signal.

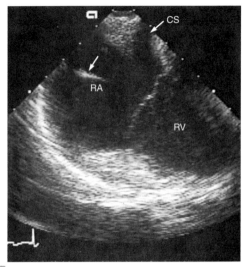

■ **FIGURE 3-26.** Low transesophageal view of the right heart showing the entry of the coronary sinus (CS) into the right atrium. A central venous catheter (*arrow*) is present with the tip in the right atrium.

with color Doppler or an intravenous contrast injection (see Fig. 15–24).

Right Ventricle

As with transthoracic echocardiography, quantitation of right ventricular size and systolic function is difficult due to the complex geometry of this chamber. Qualitative assessment of size and function is made from the transesophageal four-chamber and apical short-axis views. In the future, 3D echocardiography may allow more precise quantitation of right ventricular geometry and function.

Right Atrium

The body of the right atrium is best imaged in the transesophageal four-chamber view. In addition, the long-axis view of the right atrium obtained with the image plane at 90° and the probe rotated toward the right with the probe tip at the left atrial level allows visualization of the atrial appendage (with normal trabeculation) and the junctions of the superior and inferior vena cava with the right atrium. Movement of the probe up in the esophagus allows evaluation of the cephalad extent of the superior vena cava, while movement toward the stomach provides additional views of the inferior vena cava.

The coronary sinus can be identified in a posteriorly angled four-chamber view. The entry of the coronary sinus into the right atrium is best seen in the 0° image plane with the transducer positioned near the gastroesophageal junction and angulated superiorly (Fig. 3–26).

SUGGESTED READING

1. Burwash IG, Chan KW: Transesophageal echocardiography: Indications, procedure, image planes and Doppler flows. In: Otto CM (ed): The Practice of Clinical Echocardiography, 2nd ed. Philadelphia: WB Saunders, 2002, pp 1–22.

   Detailed chapter on performance of transesophageal echocardiography, standard image planes, Doppler flows, and indications. 170 references.

2. Oxorn DC: Monitoring ventricular function in the operating room: impact on clinical outcomes. In: Otto CM (ed): The Practice of Clinical Echocardiography, 2nd ed. Philadelphia: WB Saunders, 2002, pp 23–45.

   Review of the use of transesophageal echocardiography by a cardiac anesthsiologist for monitoring ventricular function in the operating room. This chapter also have detailed sections on special situations including separation from cardiopulmonary bypass, off-pump coronary bypass surgery, positioning of intravascular devices, and transplant surgery. 132 references.

3. Sidebotham D, Merry A, Legget M: Practical Perioperative Transesophageal Echocardiography. New York: Butterworth-Heinemann, 2003.

   A very useful concise book summarizing the use of intraoperative echocardiography. A nice handbook for quick reference by cardiologists and anesthioligists. Includes a CD with video clips of intraoperative studies.

4. Johnson SB, Sisley AC: The surgeon's use of transesophageal echocardiography. Surg Clin North Am 78:311–336, 1998.

   Brief review of the basic views obtained on transesophageal echocardiography followed by a discussion of the use of transesophageal echocardiography in patients with cardiac or aortic trauma, in the critical care unit, and in patients with suspected aortic dissection. 72 references.

6. De Simone R, Paolella RG: Interactive Atlas of Transesophageal Color Doppler Echocardiography on CD-ROM for Windows/MAC, 2nd ed. New York: Springer, Heidelberg, 1997.

Well-organized CD-ROM atlas of transesophageal echocardiographic images.

7. Konstadt SN, Shernan S, Oka Y: Clinical Transesophageal Echocardiography: A Problem-Oriented Approach. Philadelphia: Lippincott Williams & Wilkins, 2003.

Multiauthor textbook on transesophageal echocardiography with chapters arranged by disease process in patients undergoing cardiac surgery (e.g., mitral stenosis, myxomatous mitral valve, aortic dissection) and noncardiac surgery (e.g., liver transplantation, trauma, hemodynamic monitoring).

8. Nanda NC, Domanski MJ: Atlas of Transesophageal Echocardiography. Baltimore: Williams & Wilkins, 1998.

This 520-page atlas includes numerous transesophageal images with detailed figure legends. Some schematic diagrams and pathologic correlations are included. The sections on congenital heart disease are especially helpful.

9. Oxorn D, Otto CM: Atlas of Intraoperative Echocardiography: Clinical, Surgical and Pathologic Correlation. Philadelphia: WB Saunders. In press.

This text and CD-ROM includes over 100 intraoperative transesophageal cases with surgical photographs and video-clips and examples of pathology, in addition to still images and video clips of the transesophageal examination. Each case is accompanied by a clinical vignette, brief discussion, and suggested reading.

10. Daniel WG, Erbel R, Kasper W, et al: Safety of transesophageal echocardiography: A multicenter survey of 10,419 examinations. Circulation 83:817–821, 1991.

In 10,419 transesophageal examinations performed at 15 European centers over 1 year, probe insertion was unsuccessful in only 2% of attempted studies and the procedure had to be interrupted in only 1% of cases. Reasons for interrupting the procedure included intolerance of the endoscope, pulmonary, cardiac, and bleeding complications. There was 1 death (1/10,000) due to bleeding from a lung tumor with esophageal infiltration. Since nearly all these studies were performed without conscious sedation, the additional risk associated with sedative medications must be considered. The percentage of transesophageal compared to transthoracic studies in this registry averaged 9% but varied from 1.4% to 23.6% between institutions.

11. Practice guidelines for sedation and analgesia by non-anesthesiologists: A report by the American Society of Anesthesiologists Task Force on Sedation and Analgesia by Non-Anesthesiologists. Anesthesiology 84:459–471, 1996.

Consensus statement detailing the clinical standards for conscious sedation including patient evaluation, preprocedure preparation, monitoring (level of consciousness, ventilation, oxygenation, and hemodynamics), data recording, and availability of emergency equipment. The importance of having a staff person dedicated solely to patient monitoring and safety is emphasized, and the appropriate training of personnel is discussed.

12. Smith MD, MacPhail B, Harrison MR, Lenhoff SJ, DeMaria AN: Value and limitations of transesophageal echocardiography in determination of left ventricular volumes and ejection fraction. J Am Coll Cardiol 19:1213–1222, 1992.

In 36 patients undergoing left ventriculography, various transesophageal echocardiographic methods for calculation of left ventricular ejection fraction and volumes were compared with ventriculography. Ejection fraction was most accurately evaluated with the biplane Simpson's rule method (r = 0.85). However, ventricular volumes and length were consistently underestimated by transesophageal echocardiography, suggesting that foreshortening of the long axis of the ventricle occurs with transesophageal images.

13. Ryan T, Burwash I, Lu J, Otto C, et al: The agreement between ventricular volumes and ejection fraction by transesophageal echocardiography or a combined radionuclear and thermodilution technique in patients after coronary artery surgery. J Cardiothorac Vasc Anesth 10:323–328, 1996.

Three sets of measurements of radionuclide and transesophageal echocardiographic measurement of left ventricular volumes and ejection fraction were made after coronary artery bypass grafting surgery. Ejection fraction measured by transesophageal echocardiography using Simpson's rule or the area-length method was accurate and reproducible. However, agreement for measurement of ventricular volumes was poor.

14. Julius M. Gardin, MD, David B, et al: Recommendations for a standardized report for adult transthoracic echocardiography: A report from the American Society of Echocardiography's Nomenclature and Standards Committee and Task Force for a Standardized Echocardiography Report. J Am Soc Echocardiogr 15:275–290, 2002.

Position statement on the components of a complete echocardiograhy examination and the format and terminology for reporting echocardiographic results. The detailed outline is a useful reference for echocardiography laboratories and physicians in developing an examination protocol and in developing a library of terms for echocardiography reports.

The Echo Exam *Basic Transesophageal Exam*

Probe Position		View	Focus on
High Esophageal Set depth to include LV apex	0°	4-chamber	LV size and function (septum and lateral walls) RV size and systolic function LA and RA size Withdraw probe to see LA appendage Mitral and tricuspid valves Angulate anteriorly to see aortic valve
	~60°	2-chamber	LV size and function (inferior and anterior walls) LA and LA appendage Mitral valve
	~120°	Long-axis	LV size and function (anterior septum and posterior walls) LA size Mitral and aortic valves Withdraw probe to see ascending aorta
High Esophageal ↓ depth to optimize valves	~120°	Long-axis	Mitral valve anatomy and function Color Doppler for mitral regurgitation Antegrade mitral flow with pulsed Doppler Aortic valve anatomy and color flow
	~60°	2-chamber	Mitral valve anatomy and function Color Doppler for mitral regurgitation LA appendage imaging and Doppler flow
	0°	4-chamber	Mitral valve anatomy and function Color Doppler for mitral regurgitation Aortic valve (angulate anteriorly to "5-chamber" view) for anatomy and color flow Atrial septum
Transgastric	0°	Short-axis	LV wall motion, wall thickness, chamber dimensions RV size and function
	90°	Long-axis	LV and mitral valve Turn medially to image RV and tricuspid valve
Transgastric apical	0°	4-chamber	Useful for antegrade aortic flow but may still be non-parallel intercept angle
Transgastric to high esophageal	0°	Short axis descending aorta	Image aorta from the diaphragm to aortic arch

LV, left ventricular; RV, right ventricular; LA, left atrial; RA, right atrial.

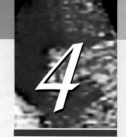

OTHER ECHOCARDIOGRAPHIC MODALITIES

Transthoracic and transesophageal echocardiography are standard clinical diagnostic modalities that are widely available and used by most cardiologists. In addition, other echocardiographic modalities in clinical practice include

■ stress echocardiography,
■ contrast echocardiography, and
■ three-dimensional echocardiography.

Stress echocardiography now is a standard approach in most echocardiography laboratories. Contrast echocardiography is increasingly used, particularly at academic medical centers. Three-dimensional (3D) echocardiography is still in development but soon will become a practical clinical modality.

In addition, several newer applications of cardiac ultrasound are used in specific clinical settings by physicians with special expertise in areas other than echocardiography. In many cases, these ultrasound examinations are performed as part of another diagnostic or therapeutic procedure and the primary physician may be an anesthesiologist, an interventional cardiologist, an electrophysiolo-

gist, an emergency room physician, or a general internist. These procedures include

■ intraoperative transesophageal echocardiography,
■ intracardiac echocardiography,
■ intravascular ultrasound, and
■ hand-held echocardiography.

As detailed in Chapter 5, appropriate education and training in cardiac ultrasound is needed by these physicians. However, the cardiac sonographer and physician often are involved in ensuring optimal data acquisition and interpretation of these examinations. This chapter provides an introduction to each of these other echocardiographic modalities. Advanced echocardiographers will want to read further on these topics as indicated in the Suggested Readings.

STRESS ECHOCARDIOGRAPHY

Basic Principles

Stress echocardiography is based on the concept that an increased cardiac workload is needed to elicit signs of physiologic dysfunction in many types of cardiac disease. For example, in patients with coronary artery disease, resting myocardial blood flow is adequate so that myocardial function, seen on echocardiography as wall thicken-ing and endocardial motion, is normal at rest. However, when cardiac workload is increased, the increased oxygen demands of the myocardium cannot be balanced by an increase in flow in the coronary artery, resulting in ischemia with impairment of myocardial thickening and endocardial motion (Fig. 4–1). Stress testing with imaging of myocardial function is more sensitive and specific for detection of coronary artery disease than stress testing with electrocardiography (ECG) (see Chapter 8).

An increase in cardiac workload can be achieved by having the patient exercise, either on a supine bicycle or an upright treadmill, or by infusion of a pharmacologic agent, such as dobutamine, that increases heart rate. In addition to echocardiographic imaging, key elements in interpretation of stress test results include

■ duration of exercise,
■ maximum workload (approximated by heart rate–blood pressure product),
■ symptoms,
■ blood pressure response,
■ arrhythmias, and
■ ST-segment changes on ECG.

Image Acquisition

The basic principles of image acquisition for stress echocardiography are to use standard image planes, ensure that all myocardial segments are visualized in at least one (and preferably two views), to use comparable views at rest and stress, and to record images in a digital cine loop format with side-by-side display of rest and stress images (Fig. 4–2). The cine loop format is essential as otherwise the change in heart rate between rest and stress makes interpretation of wall motion difficult.

For evaluation of regional ventricular function, optimal endocardial definition is essential. When endocardial definition remains suboptimal despite careful patient positioning, use of harmonic imaging and other imaging adjustments, contrast echocardiography, or a nonechocardiographic imaging approach should be considered.

The sensitivity of stress echocardiography for detection of coronary disease depends on acquiring stress images at the maximal cardiac workload. With pharmacologic stress testing, this is rarely an issue as the stress level can be maintained until image acquisition is complete. However, with exercise stress, the workload declines rapidly on cessation of exercise so that images must be acquired as quickly as possible after exercise. Both the time from stopping exercise and the heart rate at the time of image acquisition compared to maximum heart rate are recorded as indicators of workload. Three-dimensional echocardiographic acquisition systems that allow simultaneous real-time imaging in multiple image planes offer the promise of faster acquisition times at peak stress, with the potential for improved diagnostic sensitivity.

Applications

The use of stress echocardiography in patients with known or suspected coronary artery disease is discussed in detail in Chapter 8 and includes

■ detection of coronary artery disease,
■ assessment of the area of myocardium-at-risk,
■ risk stratification after myocardial infarction,
■ evaluation after revascularization, and
■ detection of myocardial viability.

Stress echocardiography is particularly useful for detection of coronary artery disease in specific patient groups including

■ women with chest pain symptoms and/or cardiac risk factors,
■ patients after heart transplantation,
■ patients being considered for renal transplantation, and
■ patients undergoing vascular surgery.

Stress echocardiography also can be used to evaluate changes in cardiac hemodynamics including valve gradients and areas, regurgitant severity,

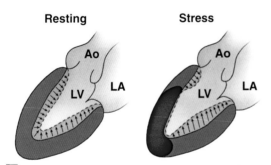

Resting   **Stress**

■ **FIGURE 4–1.** Diagram illustrating the concept of stress echocardiography in a patient with a 70% stenosis in the proximal third of the left anterior descending (LAD) coronary artery. At rest (*left*), endocardial motion and wall thickening are normal. After stress (*right*), either exercise or pharmacologic, the middle and apical segments of the anterior wall become ischemic, showing reduced endocardial wall motion and wall thickening. If the LAD extends around the apex, the apical segment of the posterior wall also will be affected, as shown here. The normal segment of the posterior wall shows compensatory hyperkinesis.

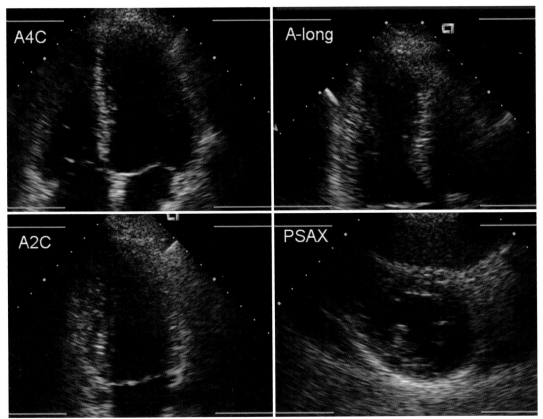

■ **FIGURE 4–2.** Example of the standard image planes used for stress echocardiography: apical four-chamber (A4C), apical two-chamber (A2C), apical long axis (A-long), and parasternal short axis (PSAX). Images are acquired in a digital cine loop format at each stress stage and then re-sorted to show the baseline and peak stress images side by side for each view. Images are gated to show only systole so that endocardial motion and wall thickening appear to occur at same period, although there is a substantial difference in heart rate between baseline and peak stress.

and pulmonary pressures. As discussed in subsequent chapters, echocardiography is used in patients with valvular or congenital heart disease for evaluation of changes with stress in

- aortic valve area in calcific aortic stenosis,
- mitral regurgitant severity in myxomatous mitral valve disease,
- pulmonary pressures in mitral stenosis or regurgitation,
- aortic coarctation pressure gradients, and
- dynamic outflow obstruction in hypertrophic cardiomyopathy.

Limitations

Direct assessment of detailed coronary anatomy requires coronary angiography. Stress echocardiography provides assessment of the functional consequences of coronary artery disuse on myocardial function. The major limitations of stress echocardiography are failure to achieve an adequate workload and poor endocardial definition. Optimally, the method of stress is chosen to allow an adequate workload in that patient, with pharmacologic testing used in those who cannot exercise to a maximal workload due to orthopedic, neurologic, pulmonary, or other conditions. The choice of imaging modality (echocardiography versus radionuclide) also is chosen based on image quality in each patient. Evaluation of myocardial viability remains a challenge and other approaches, such as enhanced magnetic resonance imaging or positron emission tomography are more accurate than stress echocardiography and are likely to become more widely available.

CONTRAST ECHOCARDIOGRAPHY

Contrast echocardiography refers to the injection into the bloodstream of an agent that results in increased echogenicity of the blood or myocardium on ultrasound imaging, producing opacification of the cardiac chambers or an increase in echo-density of the myocardium. Ultrasound "contrast" is generated by the presence of microbubbles in the ultrasound field. At low ultrasound power outputs, microbubbles scatter ultrasound at the gas/liquid interface resulting in detection of a strong signal by the transducer. Fundamental ultrasound imaging is based on detection of this signal reflected from the fluid-gas interface. In addition, ultrasound causes compression and expansion (e.g., oscillation) of microbubbles with the resonant frequency of a microbubble inversely related to its diameter. Harmonic imaging detects this nonlinear resonant signal. However, at higher power outputs, ultrasound results in microbubble destruction. Thus, careful adjustment of instrument power outputs is needed during contrast imaging.

Contrast Agents

There are two types of echo-contrast agents, those that opacify the right heart and those that opacify the left heart and myocardium. When the size of the microbubbles is greater than the lung capillary diameter, the microbubbles are trapped in the pulmonary capillaries so that no contrast material is seen in the left side of the heart in the absence of an intracardiac right-to-left communication (Fig. 4–3). Left heart contrast is achieved with microbubbles in the 1- to 5-μm range, which traverse the pulmonary bed. Microbubbles in this size range resonate at a frequency of 1.5 to 7 MHz, corresponding to clinical transducer frequencies.

The most widely used agent for right heart contrast is agitated saline. A simple approach is to rapidly push 5 mL of sterile saline, with a small amount (approximately 0.2 mL) of air between two syringes connected with a three-way stopcock. This results in the production of large

microbubbles that do not pass through the pulmonary vascular bed. When the saline appears opaque, it is injected rapidly into a peripheral vein during echocardiographic imaging with the total volume and rate of injection adjusted based on image quality. The contrast effect may be enhanced by following the contrast injection with 10 mL of nonagitated saline. Care is taken to ensure that there is no visible free air in the injection system. In addition, agitated saline should not be used in patients with known significant right-to-left shunts.

Commercially available left heart contrast agents consist of air or low-solubility fluorocarbon gas in stabilized microbubbles encapsulated with denatured albumin, monosaccharides, or other formulations. These agents typically are prepared just before injection with specific directions for preparation and use of each agent. Some require resuspension before each bolus intravenous injection. Others are diluted and given as a continuous infusion. Microbubbles are fragile so careful handling and infusion techniques are needed for diagnostic results. The optimal volume and rate of infusion depend on the specific contrast agent used with the objective being to provide full opacification, while minimizing attenuation due to excess microbubble density.

Instrument settings are adjusted to optimize image quality during contrast opacification of the left ventricle including a decrease in the overall power output (usually to a mechanical index of approximately 0.5), a focal depth setting at the mid or near field, a lower transducer frequency and an increase in overall gain and dynamic range.

Applications

Contrast echocardiography has four proposed diagnostic applications:

- Detection of intracardiac shunts
- Enhancement of Doppler signals
- Left ventricular opacification
- Myocardial perfusion

Right heart contrast allows detection of right-to-left intracardiac shunts by the appearance of contrast in the left heart within one to two beats of contrast appearance in the right heart. With a patent foramen ovale, right-to-left shunting may be present only after Valsalva maneuver because of the transient increase in right atrial, compared to left atrial, pressure (see Chapter 15). Even with predominant left-to-right shunts (for example, with an atrial-septal defect) there usually is a small amount of right-to-left shunting when the pressures on both sides of the defect are similar,

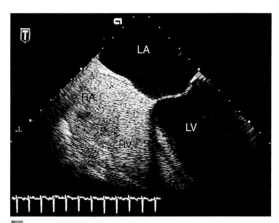

FIGURE 4–3. Transesophageal view showing dense opacification of the right atrium following a peripheral venous injection of agitated saline solution, which does not pass through the pulmonary vascular bed.

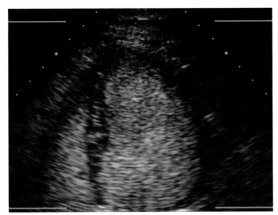

FIGURE 4–4. Example of the use of a commercially available contrast agent that passes through the pulmonary bed after an intravenous injection. In this dobutamine stress echocardiographic examination, the resting image in an apical four-chamber view with opacification of the left ventricular chamber enhances recognition of the endocardial border, thereby improving assessment of regional wall motion.

allowing detection of shunting with right heart contrast. Other examples of the use of right heart contrast include identification of a persistent left superior vena cava or identification of the systemic venous inflow pathway in complex congenital heart disease.

Contrast has been used at some centers to increase Doppler signal strength, for example, the tricuspid regurgitant jet. However, the effect of contrast on the Doppler signal varies with instrument parameters and this approach has not gained widespread use.

Left ventricular opacification in patients with poor image quality either on resting studies or during stress echocardiography enhances recognition of segmental wall motion abnormalities and overall left ventricular systolic function (see Chapter 8). Most centers now routinely perform contrast enhancement during stress studies when endocardial definition is suboptimal (Fig. 4–4).

Assessment of myocardial perfusion with contrast echocardiography is technically challenging. Only approximately 6% of the stroke volume perfuses the myocardium, so the relative number of microbubbles in the coronary circulation is small. Mechanical and ultrasound destruction of microbubbles further limits the contrast effect. Thus, special imaging modes, such as intermittent imaging, pulse inversion, or power modulation imaging, are needed for myocardial contrast imaging. Further studies are needed before myocardial contrast perfusion imaging becomes a routine clinical test (Fig. 4–5).

Limitations

Right heart contrast to detect large intracardiac shunts is needed infrequently given the sensitivity and specificity of color Doppler and transesophageal imaging. The primary use of right heart contrast is for detection of a patent foramen ovale. A small ventricular septal defect usually will not be detected with a right heart contrast injection because there is little right-to-left shunting.

The use of left heart contrast requires considerable experience to judge the infusion rate and volume needed to optimally opacify the left ventricle. When the microbubble density is too high, an excessive contrast effect at the apex results in attenuation of the signal or "shadowing" of the rest of the left ventricle. A swirling appearance may be seen with too little contrast or in low flow

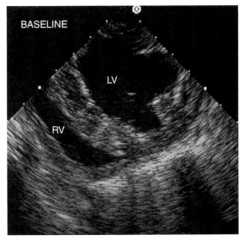
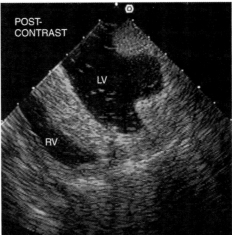

FIGURE 4–5. Epicardial images of the left ventricle in an experimental model showing myocardial opacification after injection of echo contrast material directly into the aortic root, thus bypassing the pulmonary vascular bed.

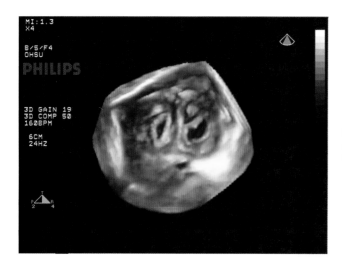

FIGURE 4–6. Real-time 3D image showing the tricuspid and mitral valves from the perspective of the left and right atrium. Courtesy of Phillips Ultrasound, Andover, Mass.

states. Bubble destruction due to a high mechanical index also results in a swirling pattern with inadequate ventricular opacification.

The addition of a contrast injection to the echocardiographic examination increases the cost and risk of the procedure. Although major adverse reactions to contrast agents are rare, patients may experience nausea/vomiting, headache, flushing, or dizziness. Hypersensitivity reactions can occur. In addition, the added time and personnel needed for placement of an intravenous line during a standard echocardiographic examination or exercise stress study make this approach impractical in many laboratories.

THREE-DIMENSIONAL ECHOCARDIOGRAPHY

The term *three-dimensional (3D) echocardiography* refers broadly to several approaches for acquisition and display of cardiac ultrasound images. All of these approaches are similar in that cardiac structures are shown in relationship to each other in all three spatial dimensions and in that structures can be rotated or viewed from different orientations, even after image acquisition. In addition to 3D spatial accuracy, cardiac imaging also requires high time resolution for clinical utility. It is likely that cardiac ultrasound will become fully 3D in the future, but the exact implementation of the optimal 3D approach is in evolution.

Acquisition

There are two basic approaches to acquisition of echocardiographic data in a 3D format: volumetric ultrasound imaging, or two-dimensional (2D) imaging in multiple planes with a known 3D location.

Volumetric imaging uses a complex multiarray transducer that simultaneously acquires ultrasound data from a 3D pyramidal volume. Rapid parallel image processing provides ultrasound images that can be viewed in real time in any orientation on the screen (Fig. 4–6). Alternatively, a volumetric transducer allows simultaneous display of more than one tomographic image plane (Fig. 4–7).

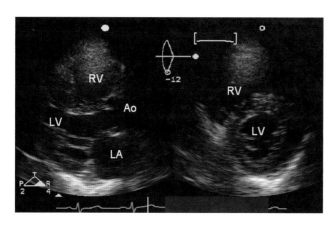

FIGURE 4–7. Simultaneous images are obtained in a parasternal long-axis and short-axis view using a volumetric real-time 3D transducer. The angle between the two simultaneous image planes can be adjusted as shown by the circle in the center of the image.

Advantages of volumetric ultrasound image acquisition include real-time image formation and rapid acquisition. The disadvantage of volumetric imaging is that it is difficult to optimize image quality for all structures in the 3D volume simultaneously. Even when technical issues related to beam focusing and image quality are resolved, the direction of the ultrasound beam relative to the structure of interest affects image quality, that is, the issue of axial versus lateral resolution. In addition, ultrasound artifacts, such as shadowing, reverberations, and poor penetration, may affect the image, as with any ultrasound modality.

Three-dimensional echocardiography also can be performed with image acquisition in multiple 2D image planes, as long as the position of each image plane in 3D space is known and linked to the 2D image. This approach can be used with rotational image acquisition, such as on transesophageal echocardiography, from a single transducer location. Alternatively, images can be acquired from multiple transducer positions when combined with a magnetic locator system that records the position and angle of each image plane (Fig. 4–8). The advantages of 2D acquisition for 3D images are that image quality can be optimized in each image plane and data from multiple image planes can be combined to produce a fuller data set than from a single volumetric transducer location. Disadvantages include misregistration of images if the transducer (with rotational scanning) or the patient (with multiple image planes) moves during the acquisition period and the time needed to reconstruct the 3D image from nonsimultaneous 2D image planes.

Display

There are three basic approaches to display of 3D echocardiographic data:

- Real-time "3D" display
- Simultaneous 2D image planes
- Border reconstructions

The most intuitive display format for 3D echocardiography is a 3D image that can be rotated and viewed from multiple perspectives in real-time. Current display formats suffer from attempting to show 3D images on 2D displays; this limitation should be resolved as 3D display systems become more widely available. The real-time 3D display also can be "cropped" to show different views of the interior structures of the heart. For example, the mitral valve can be viewed from the perspective of the left atrium; this provides a compelling view of prolapsing segments of the valve in patients with myxomatous mitral valve disease. The image can then be rotated and recropped to show a long-axis type image of the mitral valve. Similarly, the aortic valve can be viewed en face from the perspective of the aorta, a view that correlates closely with the surgical view of valve anatomy, from the left ventricular side of the valve or in a long-axis orientation (Fig. 4–9). As 3D display systems improve, it may be possible to "travel" through the heart, for example following the path of blood flow in a patient with complex congenital heart disease.

The 3D echocardiographic data set also can be used to generate multiple 2D image planes. Volumetric scanning allows simultaneous display of multiple image planes (Fig. 4–10). The ability to acquire left ventricular images in multiple planes simultaneously should speed image acquisition during stress echocardiography, potentially improving diagnostic accuracy. In addition, the ability to "move through" a 3D data set in any 2D image plane will allow better appreciation of cardiac anatomy in patients with complex structural heart disease and allow precise localization of abnormalities.

As with 2D echocardiography, quantitation from 3D data requires tracing cardiac borders. Border tracing from 3D data sets provides very accurate left ventricular volume measurements and display systems that provide semiautomated border tracing in 3D have been developed (Figs. 4–11 and 4–12). Three-dimensional reconstructions of the left ventricle also allow detailed assessment of wall motion and endocardial thickening and left ventricular shape (see Chapter 6). In addition, right ventricular size and function can be quantitated by 3D echocardiography. Quantitative 3D measurements of the mitral valve apparatus have provided insight into the mechanisms of mitral regurgitation. However, quantitative 3D echocardiography based on reconstructions of borders is limited by the need for border tracing and the time needed for reconstruction. As automated edge detection programs improve and analysis times decrease, these approaches will become more widely used.

Clinical Utility

The clinical role of 3D echocardiography will continue to evolve as this technology matures. In addition to providing more detailed anatomic relationships and more accurate quantitation, 3D images are more intuitive than 2D images, allowing quicker appreciation of cardiac anatomy by more health care providers. Potentially, 3D echocardiography could be faster than 2D scanning and could reduce variability in image acquisition. Currently, specialized centers are using 3D echocardiography for patients with complex

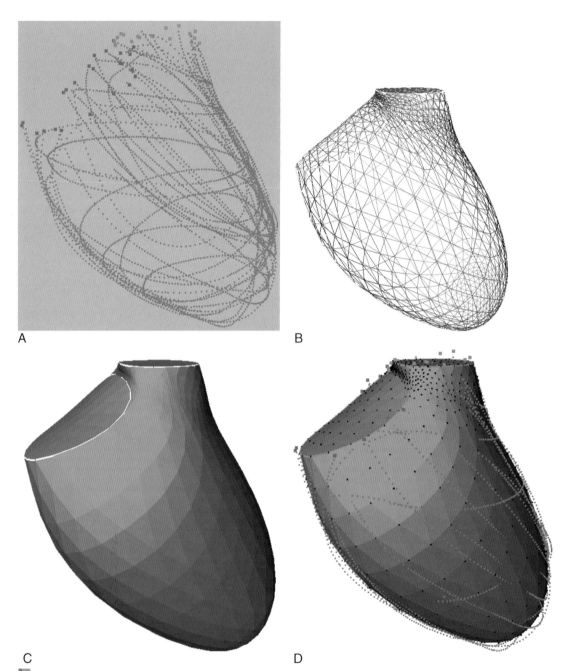

FIGURE 4–8. In vivo reconstruction of the left ventricular cavity at end-diastole. *A:* Traced borders using freehand transthoracic scanning from multiple acoutic windows including short axis and apical rotational views, registered in 3D using a magnetic locator system. The aortic annulus is indicated in red and the mitral annulus in green points. *B:* Using the piece-wise smooth subdivision method for 3D reconstruction, the second-subdivision mesh (520 faces) is fit to the traced border points with reconstruction of the aortic and mitral annulus. *C:* Final reconstructed surface of the left ventricle at end-diastole. *D:* Superimposed actual traced borders and points on the reconstructed surface. (Courtesy of Florence Sheehan, MD.)

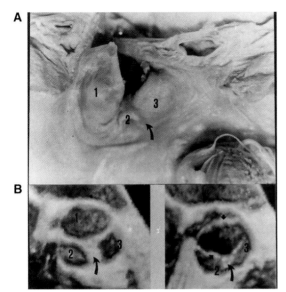

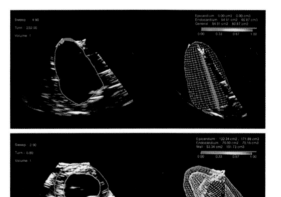

A

B

■ **FIGURE 4–9.** Pathologic specimen showing the ventricular side of a bicuspid aortic valve with fusion of leaflets 2 and 3 (A) corresponding closely with images obtained by 3D echocardiography in diastole and systole (B). (Reprinted from Espinola-Zavaleta N, et al: Anatomic three-dimensional echocardiographic correlation of bicuspid aortic valve. J Am Soc Echocardiogr 16:46–53, 2003; Fig. 8. With permission from American Society for Echocardiography.)

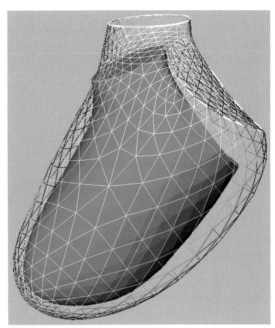

■ **FIGURE 4–11.** In vivo reconstruction of the left ventricular cavity at end-diastole (*outer mesh*) and end-systole (*solid surface*) allows accurate calculation of end-diastolic and end-systolic volumes, even when ventricular shape is distorted. (Courtesy of Florence Sheehan, MD.)

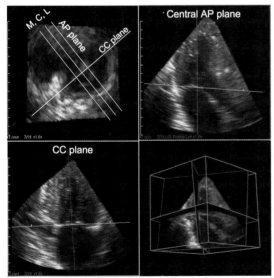

■ **FIGURE 4–10.** Volumetric imaging was used to obtain an image planes from the medial commissure to lateral commissure (CC) of the mitral valve and three anteroposterior (AP) image planes perpendicular to the CC plane, through the medial (M), central (C) and lateral (L) segments of the mitral valve appartus. (From Kwan J, Shiota T, Agler DA, et al: Geometric differences of the mitral apparatus between ischemic and dilated cardiomyopathy with significant mitral regurgitation: real-time three-dimensional echocardiographic study. Circulation 107:1135–1140, 2003; Fig. 1. Used with permission.)

■ **FIGURE 4–12.** The use of an interactively aided algorithm for calculation of left ventricular volume and mass is illustrated. The slice view is shown on the left for a long axis image (*top*) and short axis image (*bottom*) with the operator traced endocardial and epicardial borders shown. Using these operator-traced borders, the computer instantly generates a meshlike cast of the ventricle, which is superimposed on the image (*right*). These images can be freely rotated to allow the operator to evaluate, and modify as needed, the correspondence between the computer generated cast and the left ventricular surface. (Reprinted from Schmidt MA, Freidlin RZ, Ohazama CJ, et al: J Am Soc Echocardiogr 14:1–10, 2001; Fig. 1. With permission from American Society for Echocardiography.)

structural disease. However, because instrumentation is in development, 3D echocardiography is not yet a standard part of the routine clinical examination.

INTRACARDIAC ECHOCARDIOGRAPHY

Instrumentation

Intracardiac echocardiography (ICE) uses a catheter-like ultrasound probe that is passed into the right heart chambers from the femoral vein (Fig. 4–13). The transducer frequency is variable from 5 to 10 MHz to provide adequate penetration to image structures at distances up to 10 cm from the transducer and to provide optimal image resolution. Current devices provide single-plane imaging, pulsed and color Doppler, with a steerable probe connected to a standard ultrasound imaging system.

Technique

Typically, the 10F 90-cm long disposable probe is inserted via a venous sheath as part of an invasive

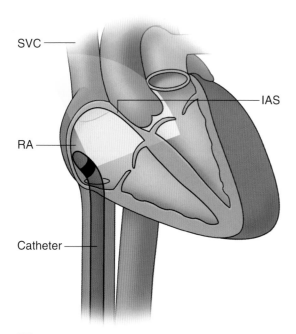

■ **FIGURE 4–13.** Intracardiac echocardiography is performed by advancing the probe from the inferior vena cava to the right atrium (RA). The probe is retroflexed to image the interatrial septum (IAS). SVC, superior vena cava. (Reprinted from Bartel T, Muller S, Caspari G, Erbel R: Intracardiac and intraluminal echocardiography: indications and standard approaches. Ultrasound Med Biol 28(8):997–1003, 2002; Fig. 2. With permission from World Federation for Ultrasound in Medicine and Biology.)

cardiac procedure in the cardiac catheterization or electrophysiology laboratory. The physician performing the interventional or electrophysiologic procedure often also acquires the cardiac images because expertise in intracardiac manipulation of catheters is needed for this procedure. Fluoroscopy is used for placement of the probe because it does not accommodate a guidewire. The tip of the probe can be tilted and flexed using dials at the base of the probe and the image plane can be adjusted by advancing, withdrawing, or rotating the probe, similar to a single plane transesophageal transducer. The transducer can be positioned in the

- inferior vena cava,
- right atrium, or
- right ventricle.

The right atrial location is most useful for monitoring invasive procedures.

From the inferior vena cava, the transducer is turned to visualize the abdominal aorta. From the right atrial position, the following views are obtained:

- Short-axis aortic valve
- Tricuspid valve and right ventricle
- Mitral valve and left ventricle
- Interatrial septum
- Left atrium and left pulmonary veins

The interatrial septum is seen from a right atrial position with the catheter retroflexed to show the fossa ovalis, septum primum, and right and left atrium. The aortic valve is demonstrated by straightening and slightly anteflexing the probe and turning it toward the aorta (Fig. 4–14). The tricuspid valve and right ventricle are best viewed by anteflexing the probe after positioning the tip superiorly in the right atrium. From this position, turning the probe posteriorly allows visualization of the mitral valve and left ventricle. The left pulmonary veins are demonstrated by angulation from the atrial septal view inferiorly to image the left atrial appendage, and then the pulmonary views (Fig. 4–15). From this position, the probe is turned clockwise and advanced superiorly in the atrium to show the two right pulmonary veins. These views allow diameter measurements and pulsed and color Doppler interrogation of all four pulmonary veins (Fig. 4–16).

From the right ventricle, a view of the outflow tract and pulmonary artery can be obtained. The left ventricle also can be evaluated, but care in interpretation of wall motion is needed if the catheter is moving in the right ventricle.

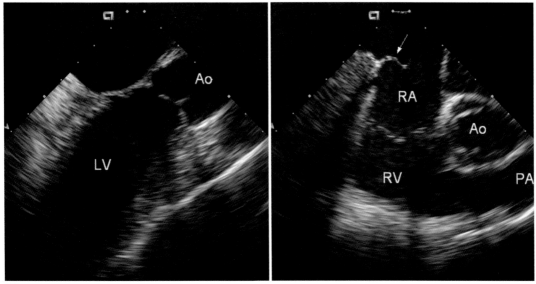

■ **FIGURE 4-14.** Intracardiac view of the aortic valve in a short-axis (*right*) and long-axis (*left*) orientation obtained with the transducer tip in the right atrium. A valve at the junction of the inferior vena cava and right atrium (*arrow*) is seen. RA, right atrium; RV, right ventricle; Ao, aorta; PA, pulmonary artery.

Applications

ICE is primarily used for monitoring invasive procedures, although the diagnostic potential of this modality has not been fully evaluated. In a patient undergoing an invasive cardiac procedure, image quality is usually inadequate on transthoracic imaging and transesophageal imaging typically requires general anesthesia, given the duration of the procedure. ICE is well tolerated, provides accurate information, and provides continuous imaging data to the physician performing the procedure.

The primary applications of intracardiac echocardiography are monitoring of percutaneous defect closures and valvuloplasty, and arrhythmia catheter ablation procedures.

In the cardiac catheterization laboratory, ICE at baseline before closure of an atrial septal defect allows evaluation of the atrial septal defect size and position and identification of adjacent structures

■ **FIGURE 4-15.** Intracardiac image of the left superior and inferior pulmonary veins during an electrophysiology abalation procedure with measurement of the diameter of the pulmonary vein orifice. LA, left atrium; LIPV, left inferior pulmonary vein; LSPV, left superior pulmonary vein.

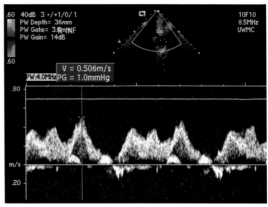

■ **FIGURE 4-16.** Intracardiac echocardiographic recording of pulmonary vein flow using pulsed Doppler ultrasound.

including the pulmonary veins and coronary sinus. During the procedure, intracardiac imaging allows optimal positioning of the device at each stage of the procedure (Fig. 4–17). After the device is deployed, color flow intracardiac imaging allows evaluation for any residual shunt.

For an electrophysiology procedure, ICE is used to monitor the

■ transseptal puncture,
■ detailed evaluation of left atrial and pulmonary vein anatomy,

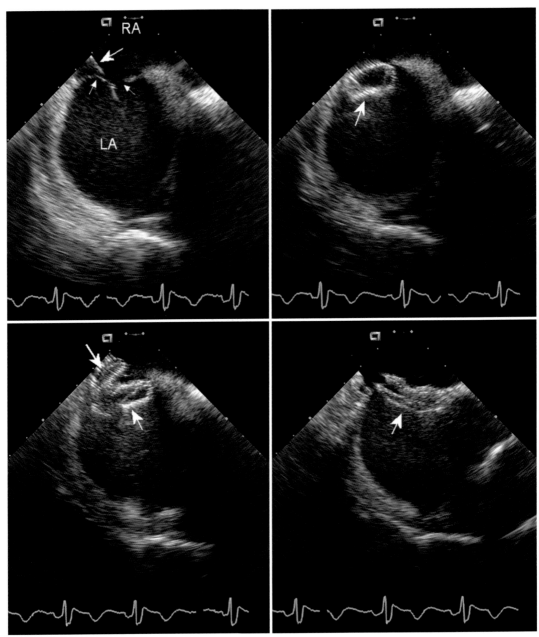

■ **FIGURE 4–17.** Intracardiac echocardiographic guidance during placement of an Amplatzer atrial septal closure device. The catheter is guided across the atrial septal defect (*top left*) and the left atrial side of the device is deployed first (*top right*), followed by deployment of the right atrial side of the device (*bottom left*). When the device is correctly positioned, the guiding catheter is detached with flattening the two sides of the device to close the atrial septal defect (*bottom right*). (Images courtesy of Steve Goldberg, MD.)

- placement of the radiofrequency ablation probe with optimal probe-tissue contact,
- development of spontaneous contrast during the ablation, and
- detection of any complications of the procedure.

Visualization of the "tenting" of the atrial septum produced by the transseptal catheter when correctly positioned improves the safety of this procedure. Potential complications that can be detected immediately with ICE include intracardiac thrombus formation (Fig. 4–18), pericardial effusion, and pulmonary vein obstruction.

Limitations

The major limitations of ICE are cost and the risks of an invasive procedure. However, because most patients undergo ICE as part of an invasive therapeutic procedure, there is little additional risk. The current cost of the disposable catheter is substantial, which limits use of this technology for diagnostic purposes. The single-plane probe design is adequate, but a biplane or multiplane probe would improve image acquisition.

INTRAVASCULAR ULTRASOUND

Instrumentation and Technique

Intravascular ultrasound uses a 30- to 50-MHz transducer on a steerable catheter that is positioned within the coronary arteries during interventional coronary procedures. This transducer provides an image depth of 2 to 3 cm with high resolution of the vessel wall and atherosclerotic plaques (Fig. 4–19). Catheter positioning and image acquisition are performed by the interventional cardiologist as part of the therapeutic procedure. Image acquisition typically is performed with a small, dedicated ultrasound system.

Applications

Intravascular ultrasound is used when standard angiographic and pressure data are inadequate to evaluate the length and severity of coronary artery narrowing and composition of the atherosclerotic plaque.

These data then are used to guide the therapeutic approach by the interventional cardiologist.

HAND-HELD ECHOCARDIOGRAPHY

Instrumentation

The term "hand-held" echocardiography refers to the bedside use of small, lightweight ultrasound systems that often have limited capabilities compared to standard ultrasound systems. Several models are available, ranging in size from ones comparable to a briefcase to some that fit in a pocket (Fig. 4–20). Some have a single transducer and are capable of only 2D and color flow imaging with a limited number of instrument controls. Others support multiple transducers and have many of the functions of a larger instrument. Cost tends to parallel the number of features and transducer types.

Applications

These ultrasound systems are useful for rapid triage of patients in the emergency department and intensive care unit as they allow evaluation for pericardial effusion, overall left and right ventricular systolic function, and segmental wall motion abnormalities.

In addition, they may identify valve abnormalities such as aortic valve calcification on 2D imaging or mitral regurgitation on color flow imaging. However, in general, evaluation of valve disease, diastolic function, suspected aortic dissection, and congenital heart disease requires a full echocardiographic examination with a standard ultrasound system. An example of the use of hand-held ultrasound includes the patient with chest pain and a nondiagnostic ECG; an akinetic anterior wall indicates coronary disease whereas a pericardial effusion suggests pericarditis. Another example is the hypotensive patient; severe global left ventricular hypokinesis indicates heart failure,

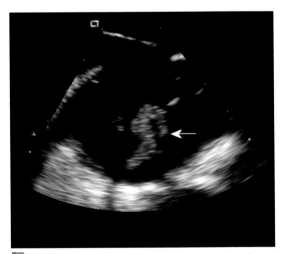

■ **FIGURE 4–18.** Intracardiac echocardiography allowed the rapid recognition of thrombus associated with a catheter in the right atrium during an electrophysiologic procedure. The patient was promptly treated with increased anticoagulation and catheter removal of the thrombus with no clinical complications. (Image courtesy of Robert Rho, MD.)

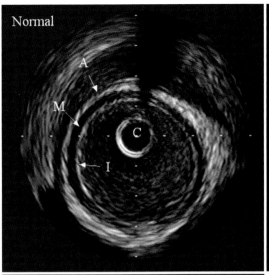

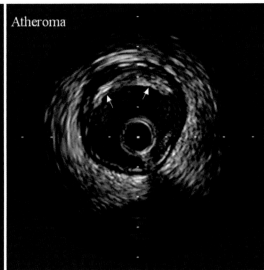

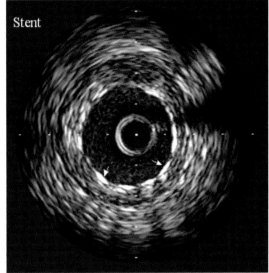

FIGURE 4–19. Intravascular ultrasound images of the left anterior descending coronary artery. A normal proximal segment of the vessle shows the normal thin bright layer representing the intima (I), the darker region corresponding to the media (M) and the adventia (A) surrounding the artery wall. In a more distal segment of the vessel (note the smaller vessel diameter), an atheroma is present with the typical eccentric crescent shaped lesions extending from 10 o'clock to 2 o'clock (*arrows*) in the artery. A region with a stent shows the close apposition between the stent (*arrows*) and vessel wall.

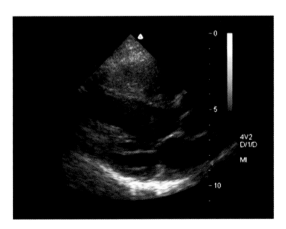

FIGURE 4–20. Parasternal long axis image obtained with the Terason "hand-held" ultrasound system that is based on signal processing in a small box integrated into the transducer cable, which is connected to a standard laptop computer with custom software.

while a small hyperdynamic left ventricle suggests an alternate diagnosis, such as septic shock. In many cases, hand-held echocardiography supplements the physical examination and will be increasingly utilized as small, low-cost devices become available.

Limitations

Accurate use of these imaging devices requires appropriate training and experience in cardiac ultrasound. The greatest limitation of these instruments is a missed diagnosis due to an inexperienced operator or suboptimal image quality. Whenever hand-held images suggest a new cardiac diagnosis or when diagnostic images cannot be obtained, a complete echocardiographic examination is needed. In many cases, hand-held echocardiography supplements the physical examination and will be increasingly utilized as small, low-cost devices become available.

SUGGESTED READING

Stress Echocardiography (see Chapter 8)

Contrast Echocardiography

1. Porter TR, Noll D, Xie F: Myocardial contrast echocardiography: methods, analysis, and applications. In: Otto CM (ed): The Practice of Clinical Echocardiography, 2nd ed. Philadelphia: WB Saunders, 2002, pp 159–182.
   Review of the methods for performing and analyzing contrast echocardiography plus a review of the current and potential clinical applications of this technique. 151 references.

2. A Series on Contrast Echocardiography in the Journal of the American Society of Echocardiography 2000–2002:
   a. Moos S, Odabashian J, Jasper S, et al: Incorporating ultrasound contrast in the laboratory. J Am Soc Echocardiogr 13:240–247, 2000.
   b. Burgess P, Moore V, Bednarz J, et al: Performing an echocardiographic examination with a contrast agent. J Am Soc Echocardiogr 13:629–636, 2000.
   c. McCulloch M, Gresser C, Mooset S, et al: Ultrasound contrast physics. J Am Soc Echocardiogr 13:959–967, 2000.
   d. Witt SA, McCulloch M, Sisk E, et al: Achieving a diagnostic contrast enhanced echocardiogram. J Am Soc Echocardiogr 14:327–334, 2001.
   e. Bednarz J, Waggoner A, Moos S, et al: Myocardial contrast echocardiography. J Am Soc Echocardiogr 15:1111–1119, 2002.
   A series of articles by sonographers for sonographers with both background information and practical details on doing contrast echocardiography. Highly recommended for all sonographers and physicians who plan to do contrast studies.

3. Yong Y, Wu D, Fernandes V, et al: Diagnostic accuracy and cost-effectiveness of contrast echocardiography on evaluation of cardiac function in technically very difficult patients in the intensive care unit. Am J Cardiol 89: 711–718, 2002.
   In 32 consecutive intensive care unit patients with technically difficult transthoracic images, adequate endocardial definition for evaluation of wall motion was seen in 13% of segments on standard imaging, 34% on harmonic imaging, 87% with contrast echocardiography, and 90% on transesophageal imaging. In addition, ejection fraction calculated from contrast images correlated best with transesophageal ejection fraction (r = 0.91).

4. Stewart MJ: Contrast echocardiography. Heart 89:342–348, 2003.
   Review of the principles of contrast echocardiography, indications for right heart contrast, left ventricular opacification, and myocardial perfusion imaging. 20 annotated references. Clear illustrations.

3D Echocardiography

5. Sheehan FS: Three-dimensional echocardiography: approaches and applications. In: Otto CM (ed): The Practice of Clinical Echocardiography, 2nd ed. Philadelphia: WB Saunders, 2002, pp 202–234.
   Detailed review of the modes of 3D image acquisition, quantitative analysis of 3D data sets, visual displays of 3D images, and clinical applications. 180 references.

6. Lange A, Palka P, Burstow DJ, Godman MJ: Three-dimensional echocardiography: historical development and current application. J Am Soc Echocardiogr 12:403–412, 2001.
   Review of the method and feasibility of 3D grey scale imaging, including visualization of valve anatomy and congenital heart disease. 3D color flow of mitral regurgitant jets also is illustrated.

7. Binder TM, Rosenhek R, Porenta G, et al: Improved assessment of mitral valve stenosis by volumetric real-time three-dimensional echocardiography. J Am Coll Cardiol 36:1355–1361, 2000.
   Compared to 2D imaging, real-time volumetric 3D echocardiography provided a faster, easier, and more accurate approach for identification and measurement of the mitral valve orifice in rheumatic mitral stenosis.

8. Wong SP, Johnson RK, Sheehan FH: Rapid and accurate left ventricular surface generation from three-dimensional echocardiography by a catalog based method. Int J Cardiovasc Imaging 19:9–17, 2003.
   Validation of a method for rapidly generating a quantitative analysis of left ventricular volumes, mass, and ejection from 3D images. Rapid quantitation of 3D images is needed for this approach to be clinically useful.

9. Kwan J, Shiota T, Agler DA, et al: Geometric differences of the mitral apparatus between ischemic and dilated cardiomyopathy with significant mitral regurgitation: real-time three-dimensional echocardiographic study. Circulation 107:1135–1140, 2003.
   3D imaging was used to generate an image plane aligned to intersect both mitral commissures, and 3 perpendicular anterior-posterior planes to display the medial, central and lateral aspects of the leaflets as shown in Figure 4–10. These unique views derived from the 3D data set allowed quantitative analysis of the anatomy of the mitral apparatus.

10. Handke M, Jahnke C, Heinrichs G, et al: New three-dimensional echocardiographic system using digital radiofrequency data: visualization and quantitative analysis of aortic valve dynamics with high resolution: methods, feasibility and initial clinical experience. Circulation 107:2876–2879, 2003.

An approach to 3D imaging that provides higher time resolution (frame rates of 168 Hz instead of 25 Hz with conventional 3D imaging) allows detailed evaluation of rapidly moving cardiac structures such as the aortic valve.

Intracardiac Echocardiography

11. Bartel T, Muller S, Caspari G, Erbel R: Intracardiac and intraluminal echocardiography: indications and standard approaches. Ultrasound Med Biol 28(8):997–1003, 2002.

    Review with diagrams and clear descriptions of how to obtain standard views on intracardiac echocardiography.

12. Bruce CJ, Packer DL, Belohlavek M, Seward JB: Intracardiac echocardiography: newest technology. J Am Soc Echocardiogr 12:788–795, 2000.

    Summary of the development of intracardiac echocardiography with some nice illustrations of intracardiac images and Doppler data. 42 references.

13. Mullen MJ, Dias BF, Walker F, et al: Intracardiac echocardiography guided device closure of atrial septal defects. J Am Coll Cardiol 41:285–292, 2003.

    Both intracardiac and transesophageal echocardiography were performed in 24 patients undergoing percutaneous atrial septal defect closure. Intracardiac echocardiography was feasible and provided all the needed images in 96% of cases.

14. Bartel T, Konorza T, Arjumand J, et al: Intracardiac echocardiography is superior to conventional monitoring for guiding device closure of interatrial communications. Circulation 107:795–797, 2003.

    In a randomized study of transesophageal versus intracardiac echocardiography in 44 patients undergoing percutaneous atrial septal defect or patent foramen ovale closure, there were no complications in either group. However, fluoroscopy and procedure time were shorter and general anesthesia was not needed in the intracardiac ultrasound group.

15. Bruce CJ, Friedman PA: Intracardiac echocardiography. Eur J Echocardiogr 2:234–244, 2001.

    Intracardiac echocardiography during invasive electrophysiologic procedures allows guidance of the transseptal puncture, visualization of pulmonary veins, ensures ablation electrode tissue contact, and allows rapid identification of procedural complications.

Intravascular Echocardiography

16. Linker DT: Principles of intravasular ultrasound. In: Otto CM (ed): The Practice of Clinical Echocardiography, 2nd ed. Philadelphia: WB Saunders, Philadelphia, pp 340–348.

    Review of the special characteristics of intravascular ultrasound imaging, catheter design, and clinical implications.

17. Kitamura K, Yock PG, Fitzgerald PJ: Intravascular ultrasound: histologic correlation and clinical applications. In: Otto CM (ed): The Practice of Clinical Echocardiography, 2nd ed. Philadelphia: WB Saunders, 2002, pp 349–366.

The correlation between intravascular ultrasound images of coronary atherosclerosis and histopathology is discussed along with an overview of the clinical applications of intravascular ultrasound. 181 references.

Hand-held Echocardiography

18. Seward JB, Douglas PS, Erbel R, et al: Hand-carried cardiac ultrasound (HCU) device: recommendations regarding new technology. A report from the Echocardiography Task Force on New Technology of the Nomenclature and Standards Committee of the American Society of Echocardiography. J Am Soc Echocardiogr 15:369–373, 2002.

    The ASE recommends that hand-held ultrasound as an extension of the physical examination should be performed only by health professionals with at least Level 1 training (see Chapter 5) in echocardiography.

19. Kimura BJ, Blanchard DB, Willis CL, DeMaria AN: Limited cardiac ultrasound examination for cost-effective echocardiography referral. J Am Soc Echocariogr 15:640–646, 2002.

    Although this study was performed with a conventional full-function echocardiographic system, it illustrates how a limited examination can be cost-effective in carefully selected subsets of patients.

20. Spencer KT, Anderson AS, Bhargava A, et al: Physician-performed point-of-care echocardiography using a laptop platform compared with physical examination in the cardiovascular patient. J Am Coll Cardiol 37:2013–2018, 2001.

    Hand-held echocardiography was superior to physical examination for detection of abnormal cardiac findings with physical examination missing 43% of major findings compared to 21% missed with hand-held echocardiography, using a complete echocardiographic examination with a standard instrument as the standard of reference. Major findings were defined as moderate or severe regurgitation, moderate or severe ventricular dysfunction, hypertrophic cardiomyopathy, mitral valve prolapse, and ventricular septal defect.

21. Godkin GM, Spevack DM, Tunick PA, Kronzon I: How useful is hand-carried bedside echocardiography in critically ill patients? J Am Coll Cardiol 37:2019–2022, 2001.

    Hand-held ultrasound was compared with a conventional echocardiographic examination in 80 critically ill patients. Hand-held ultrasound missed a finding related to the reason for referral in 31% of patients and missed an additional 19% of other clinically important abnormalities.

22. Quiles J, Barcia-Fernandez MA, Almeida PB, et al: Portable spectral Doppler echocardiographic device: overcoming limitations. Heart 89:1014–1018, 2003.

    In a comparison of hand-held and conventional ultrasound instrument Doppler measurements in 98 consecutive patients, the hand-held data was accurate for evaluation of diastolic function. However, the tricuspid regurgitant jet velocity could not be measured in many patients, resulting in a missed diagnosis of pulmonary hypertension in 8 patients.

The Echo Exam *Other Echocardiographic Modalities*

Modality	Instrumentation	Indications	Special Training
Intraoperative TEE	Transesophageal echo in the OR	Monitoring ventricular function Evaluation of valve repair and other complex procedures	Anesthesiologists with training in echocardiography
Stress echo	Digital cine loop image acquisition Exercise or pharmacologic stress	Suspected or known coronary diease Myocardial viability Valve and structural heart disease	Performance, risks and interpretation of stress studies
Contrast echo	Microbubbles for right or left heart contrast	Detection of patent foramen ovale LV endocardial definition	Intravenous administration of contrast agents
3D echo	Volumetric or 2D image acquisition Various display formats	Congenital heart disease, Rapid acquisition for LV regional function	Image acquisition and analysis
Intracardiac echo (ICE)	5–10 MHz catheter like intracardiac probe	Interventional procedures (ASD closure) EP procedures	Invasive cardiology training and experience
Intravascular ultrasound (IVUS)	30–50 MHz intracoronary catheter	Degree of coronary narrowing and plaque morphology training	Interventional cardiology
Hand-held ultrasound	Small, inexpensive ultrasound instruments	Beside evaluation by MD for pericardial effusion, LV global and regional function	At least level 1 echo training

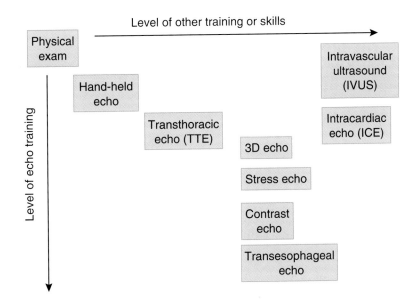

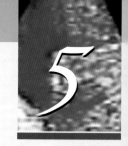

CLINICAL INDICATIONS AND QUALITY ASSURANCE

APPROACH TO THE DIAGNOSTIC USE OF ECHOCARDIOGRAPHY

Accuracy of a Diagnostic Test

The first level of analysis in evaluating a diagnostic test is to consider its accuracy. The clinical utility of any diagnostic test, including echocardiography, depends, in large part, on the certainty with which a specific diagnosis can be confirmed or excluded based on the test results (Fig. 5–1). Test results are defined as true positive (TP) and true negative (TN) when the test result correctly identifies the disease state and as false positive (FP) or false negative (FN) when the true result is discordant with the disease state.

The sensitivity of a test is the degree to which it identifies all patients with the disease. The specificity of a test is the degree to which it identifies all patients without the disease.

- Sensitivity = TP/(TP + FN)
- Specificity = TN/(TN + FP)

Sensitivity and specificity are related inversely to each other; in general, the higher the sensitivity, the lower is the specificity and vice versa. Whether a higher sensitivity is preferable to a higher specificity depends on the clinical question.

If the goal of the test is identification of all patients with the disease, a high sensitivity is preferable. If the goal is confirmation of the diagnosis in an individual patient, a high specificity is preferable. The relationship between sensitivity and specificity can be evaluated quantitatively for any given diagnostic test using receiver-operator curve (ROC) analysis (Fig. 5–2). Accuracy indicates the percentage of patients in whom the test results are correct in identifying the presence or absence of disease.

- Accuracy = (TP + TN)/all tests

A major limitation of applying sensitivity/specificity data to an individual patient is the problem of whether a particular patient has a "true" or a "false" test result. At first glance, it might seem that use of positive and negative predictive values would be more useful in the clinical setting. Predictive values indicate the percentage of patients with a positive test result who have the suspected disease and the percentage with a negative test result who do not have the suspected disease.

- Positive predictive value = true positives divided by all positives
- Negative predictive value = true negatives divided by all negatives

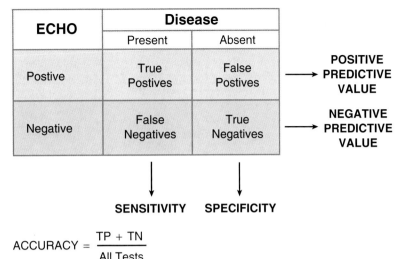

FIGURE 5-1. Sensitivity and specificity in comparison with positive and negative predictive value. Note that predictive values are dependent on the prevalence of the disease in the study population and thus cannot be extrapolated to other patient groups (TP = true positives; TN = true negatives).

$$ACCURACY = \frac{TP + TN}{All\ Tests}$$

However, the absolute number of patients with false-positive or false-negative test results depends on the prevalence of disease in the population studied as well as the sensitivity and specificity of the test. Intuitively, this is obvious comparing the use of echocardiography to "screen" healthy young subjects for endocarditis (many false-positive results due to ultrasound imaging artifacts) versus the same test in patients who have a new murmur, fever, and positive blood culture results. The finding of a valvular vegetation on echocardiography in the latter group has a much higher predictive value for a diagnosis of endocarditis than in the healthy subjects, even though the sensitivity and specificity of echocardiography for diagnosing endocarditis are the same in both groups. Thus, the positive or negative predictive value of a test reflects disease prevalence as well as test accuracy.

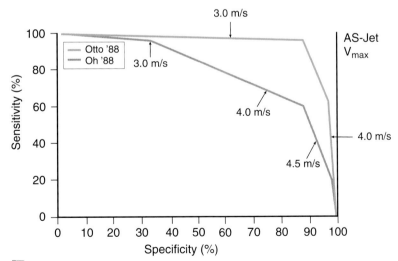

FIGURE 5-2. Graph of sensitivity versus specificity, known as a receiver-operator curve, comparing the studies of Otto and Pearlman[9] and Oh et al.[10] In the first study, a clinical decision rule was proposed for timing of valve replacement in aortic stenosis based on jet velocity breakpoints at 3 and 4 m/s. In the second study, a single breakpoint at 4.5 m/s was suggested, but the data show that a two-breakpoint approach at 3 and 4.5 m/s also would be appropriate. Patients with jet velocities between these breakpoints require calculation of aortic valve area and assessment of coexisting aortic regurgitation.

Integration of Clinical Data and Test Results

A better approach to the use of sensitivity/ specificity data in patient treatment is to consider relevant clinical data along with the test result. The value of a diagnostic test increases when the pretest likelihood of disease is integrated with the test results to derive a posttest likelihood of disease. This approach is known as Bayesian analysis. For example, the pretest likelihood of severe aortic stenosis in an asymptomatic 30-year-old woman with no systolic murmur on careful auscultation is very low. An echocardiogram purporting to show severe aortic stenosis most likely is an erroneous interpretation (a false-positive test result). In this setting, the result does not increase the posttest likelihood of disease very much. In contrast, in an elderly man with a 4/6 aortic stenosis murmur and symptoms of angina, syncope, and heart failure, the diagnosis of severe valvular aortic stenosis can be made with a high level of certainty even before any test is performed. The echocardiogram serves only to confirm the diagnosis and define the severity of obstruction. In general, diagnostic tests are most helpful when the pretest likelihood of disease is intermediate so that the test result will substantially change the posttest likelihood of disease (Fig. 5–3).

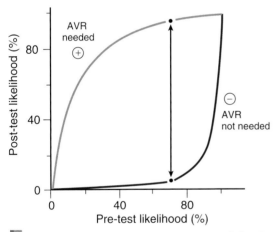

FIGURE 5–3. Bayesian analysis has been applied to the use of echocardiography for diagnosis of severe aortic stenosis requiring valve replacement. The posttest likelihood (*y* axis) of need for aortic valve replacement (AVR) was calculated for each hypothetical pretest likelihood (*x* axis). Pretest and corresponding posttest likelihoods for the study population are indicated by the arrow. (Reprinted with permission from Otto CM, Pearlman AS: Doppler echocardiography in adults with symptomatic aortic stenosis. Arch Intern Med 148:2553–2560, 1988; copyright 1988, American Medical Association.)

The Threshold Approach to Clinical Decision Analysis

The most comprehensive approach to evaluation of a diagnostic test is clinical decision analysis. Clinical decision analysis incorporates several rigorous approaches to the problem of clinical prediction, with the method most applicable to a diagnostic test, such as echocardiography, being the threshold approach. The basic tenet of clinical decision analysis as applied to a diagnostic test is that the test results should have an impact on patient care by either

- prompting a change in therapy, or
- leading to a change in the subsequent diagnostic strategy in that patient.

This basic assumption is formalized in the threshold model of decision analysis. In this approach, two disease probability thresholds are defined for the diagnostic test:

- a lower threshold below which the risk of the test is greater than the risk of not treating the patient, and
- an upper threshold above which treating the patient is lower risk than performing the test.

The intermediate range–where the risk of treating or not treating the patient is greater than the risk of the diagnostic test–is known as the testing zone (Fig. 5–4). For any specific indication, the testing zone for echocardiography generally is wide because of the low risk and high accuracy of this technique. However, both an upper and lower threshold still are definable for echocardiography. The upper threshold is reached in situations in which the diagnosis is clear, and echocardiographic examination would only delay appropriate treatment. For example, a patient with a classic presentation of an ascending aortic dissection (chest pain, wide mediastinum, peripheral pulse loss) requires prompt surgery. Any delay due to unnecessary diagnostic testing could result in additional morbidity or mortality.

It is tempting to assume that there is no lower end to the test zone for echocardiography given the absence of known adverse biologic effects of this procedure. However, the risk of the test also includes the risks of additional diagnostic tests or even erroneous treatment choices resulting from a false-positive or false-negative echocardiographic finding. For example, an echocardiogram is not indicated to evaluate for aortic dissection in a young patient with atypical chest pain and a normal physical examination, electrocardiogram, and chest radiograph. If a false-positive echocar-

Threshold Approach to Clinical Decision Making

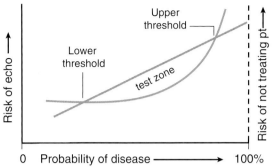

FIGURE 5–4. Diagram illustrating the threshold approach to clinical decision making. The risk of the diagnostic test–in this case, echocardiography–is shown in the blue line (*left y axis*) with the risk of not treating the patient for the suspected disease shown in the grey line (*right y axis*). The probability of disease based on the clinical presentation is shown from 0% to 100% on the *x* axis. The lower threshold is the point at which the risk of not treating the patient is greater than the risk of echocardiography. The upper threshold is the point at which the risk of echocardiography (including false-negative results, delay in treatment) is greater than the risk of not treating the patient. The test zone is the pretest likelihood of disease between these two thresholds.

diographic diagnosis leads to further evaluation with cardiac catheterization, any complications from the invasive procedure ultimately can be considered a consequence of the echocardiographic results. Thus, a lower limit to the test zone does exist for echocardiography and can be defined for each specific diagnostic indication by applying decision analysis techniques.

Other clinical decision analysis approaches have been applied to specific clinical problems that use echocardiographic data as a branch point in the decision analysis tree. One example is the problem of timing of valve replacement in chronic asymptomatic aortic regurgitation (see Suggested Reading 7).

Cost-Effectiveness

An additional consideration in medical practice is the cost-effectiveness of a diagnostic procedure. Note that this term includes not only the cost of the test (echocardiography compares favorably with other cardiac diagnostic tests) but also the effectiveness of the test–that is, test accuracy and its impact on patient management. This type of analysis has been applied to some echocardiographic diagnostic issues, but more widespread use of this approach is needed.

Clinical Outcome

The most important measure of the value of a diagnostic test is its impact on subsequent clinical outcome (Fig. 5–5). While the first step in evaluation of the clinical utility of a test includes various measures of diagnostic accuracy in comparison to some accepted standard, the more important assessment is whether the diagnostic test changes the subsequent diagnostic or therapeutic plan in each patient. Finally, the clinical utility of the test depends on its ability to predict prognosis; for example, survival in patients with dilated cardiomyopathy, timing of valve surgery in patients

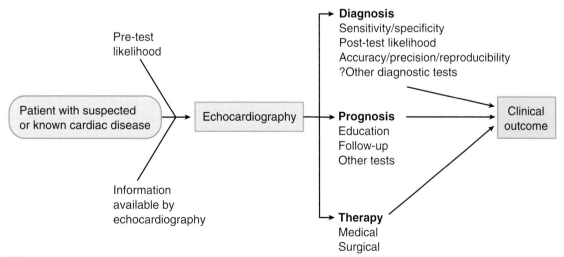

FIGURE 5–5. Flow chart illustrating the importance of the impact of the echocardiographic results on diagnosis, prognosis, and therapy. Ultimately, the effect of the echocardiographic examination on clinical outcome is the best measure of the usefulness of the test result.

with chronic regurgitation, or the rate of hemodynamic progression in patients with valvular stenosis. Now that the accuracy and reliability of echocardiographic techniques have been well established, echocardiographic data are increasingly used in clinical outcome studies, as referenced in the Suggested Readings throughout this textbook.

Implications for Diagnostic Use of Echocardiography

Thus, it no longer is acceptable to consider only sensitivity and specificity in the decision whether to perform a diagnostic test. The echocardiogram request should indicate an appropriate clinical question (not "evaluate heart") with an estimate of the probability of the diagnosis in that patient. Next, the reliability of echocardiography for that diagnosis is considered, and most important, the likelihood that the echocardiographic results will alter patient management is formulated before performing the study. Often it is helpful to consider the specific branch point in the diagnostic/therapeutic plans that the echocardiographic results will be applied to in the clinical decision process.

With these considerations in mind, there are certain situations in which the use of echocardiography clearly changes patient treatment:

■ Making the correct anatomic diagnosis. For example, differentiating a primary valvular problem from systolic left ventricular dysfunction in a patient with heart failure symptoms.
■ Providing important prognostic data in a patient with a known anatomic diagnosis. For example, vegetation size in endocarditis or left ventricular ejection fraction in cardiomyopathy.
■ Identifying complications of a known diagnosis. For example, paravalvular abscess in endocarditis or left ventricular thrombus in cardiomyopathy.

In addition, there are numerous other settings in which echocardiography is considered to be clinically indicated. Whether all these situations meet the strict criteria of the clinical threshold model requires ongoing appraisal.

Throughout this text, the accuracy (sensitivity and specificity) of echocardiography for each specific diagnosis will be indicated, if known. The clinician then should integrate these data with the pretest likelihood of disease in each patient. Critical evaluations of the diagnostic utility of echocardiography in specific patient populations and clinical settings will be highlighted, including evaluation of chest pain in the emergency department (Chapter 8), decision making in adults with aortic stenosis (Chapter 11), and aortic regurgitation (Chapter 12), intraoperative assessment of mitral valve repair (Chapter 12), and the diagnosis and prognosis of endocarditis (Chapter 14).

TRANSTHORACIC ECHOCARDIOGRAPHY

Indications

By Clinical Signs and Symptoms

An echocardiogram often is requested to evaluate a specific clinical sign or symptom such as chest pain, heart failure symptoms (Fig. 5–6), a murmur, or cardiomegaly on chest radiography (Fig. 5–7). When the echocardiographer evaluates a patient with one of these indications, it is important that the differential diagnosis is considered and each possibility excluded or confirmed during the course of the examination. For example, a patient with a systolic murmur may have valvular aortic stenosis, a subaortic membrane, hypertrophic cardiomyopathy, mitral regurgitation, a ventricular septal defect, pulmonic stenosis, or tricuspid regurgitation. With two-dimensional (2D) imaging and Doppler evaluation, each of these possible diagnoses can be evaluated. If a careful examination reveals none of these abnormalities, it may be concluded that the murmur is a benign "flow" murmur (Fig. 5–8).

Similarly, in the echocardiographic examination of a patient with chest pain, even if the referring physician has made a presumptive diagnosis of coronary artery disease, the echocardiographer should be alert to any findings suggesting other causes for chest pain such as left ventricular outflow obstruction (valvular aortic stenosis or hypertrophic cardiomyopathy), aortic dissection, or pericarditis. The echocardiographic differential diagnosis for common symptoms is shown in

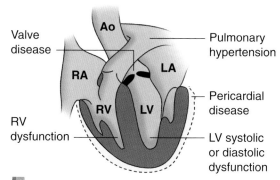

■ **FIGURE 5–6.** Diagram illustrating some of the more common causes of heart failure that should be actively excluded or confirmed during echocardiographic examination.

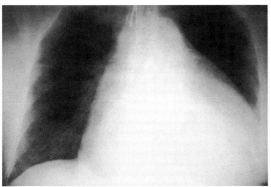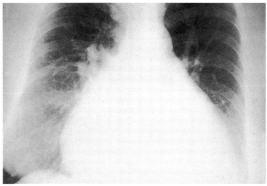

▌ **FIGURE 5-7.** Chest radiographs demonstrating cardiomegaly due to a large pericardial effusion (*left*) and cardiomegaly due to multivalve disease with four-chamber enlargement *(right)*.

Table 5-1 and for common physical signs in Table 5-2. These examples are not meant to be an exhaustive list of the possibilities but rather represent an illustration of the types of conditions the echocardiographer should consider in performing and interpreting the examination.

By Anatomic Diagnosis

In many patients referred for echocardiography, a definite or presumptive anatomic diagnosis has been made. In these patients, the echocardiographer needs to be aware of the information that can be obtained by echocardiography, the limitations of echocardiography, and alternative diagnostic approaches.

For example, in a patient with a systolic murmur known to be due to valvular aortic stenosis, the echocardiogram may be requested to evaluate the severity of obstruction, the degree of coexisting aortic regurgitation, the presence of left ventricular hypertrophy, and the status of left ventricular systolic function, as well as to detect any associated valvular abnormalities (e.g., mitral regurgitation). Usually echocardiography provides all the needed information for clinical decision making other than coronary artery anatomy, but the echocardiographer must acknowledge that stenosis severity may have been underestimated if there was a nonparallel intercept angle between the direction of the aortic jet and the ultrasound beam. In cases where the echocardiographic results appear to be discordant with

TABLE 5-1	
Differential Diagnosis for the Echocardiographer: Common Symptoms	
Reason for Echo	**Differential Diagnosis**
Chest pain	Coronary artery disease: acute myocardial infarction or angina
	Aortic dissection
	Pericarditis
	Valvular aortic stenosis
	Hypertrophic cardiomyopathy
Heart failure	Left ventricular systolic dysfunction (global or segmental)
	Valvular heart disease
	Left ventricular diastolic dysfunction
	Pericardial disease
	Right ventricular dysfunction
Palpitations	Left ventricular systolic dysfunction
	Mitral valve disease
	Congenital heart disease (e.g., ASD, Ebstein's anomaly)
	Pericarditis
	No structural cardiac disease

ASD, atrial septal defect.

Pulmonic stenosis — Ao — Aortic stenosis — PA — Tricuspid regurgitation — LV — Mitral regurgitation — Ventricular septal defect

▌ **FIGURE 5-8.** Diagram illustrating the more common etiologies for a systolic murmur. If an echocardiogram is requested for this indication, the sonographer should focus the examination toward confirmation or exclusion of each of these possibilities.

TABLE 5–2

Differential Diagnosis for the Echocardiographer: Common Signs

Reason for Echo	Differential Diagnosis: Common Signs
Cardiac murmur	
Systolic	Flow murmur (no valve abnormality)
	Aortic stenosis, subaortic obstruction, hypertrophic obstructive cardiomyopathy
	Mitral regurgitation
	Ventricular septal defect
	Pulmonic stenosis
	Tricuspid regurgitation
Diastolic	Mitral stenosis
	Aortic regurgitation
	Pulmonic regurgitation
	Tricuspid stenosis
Cardiomegaly on chest radiography	Pericardial effusion
	Dilated cardiomyopathy
	Specific chamber enlargement (e.g., left ventricle in chronic aortic regurgitation)
Systemic embolic event	Left ventricular systolic function and segmental wall motion abnormalities (aneurysms)
	Left ventricular thrombus
	Aortic valve disease
	Mitral valve disease
	Left atrial thrombus (TTE has low sensitivity)
	Patent foramen ovale

TTE, transthoracic echocardiography.

the clinical impression, alternate diagnostic tests such as cardiac catheterization may be needed.

Echocardiography in a patient with endocarditis is a second, more complex example. On the one hand, echocardiography can detect valvular vegetations, identify the specific valves involved, evaluate the presence and degree of valve dysfunction, and measure associated chamber enlargement. Both left and right ventricular systolic function can be qualitatively and quantitatively evaluated. In addition, abscess formation may be identified. While the potential prognostic value of measuring vegetation size remains controversial, many clinicians find this information of clinical value. On the other hand, a definite diagnosis of endocarditis requires the presence of both echocardiographic and bacteriologic criteria.

When echocardiographic findings are atypical, additional clinical criteria must be present to make the diagnosis. The sensitivity of echocardiography for detection of valvular vegetations varies with image quality; conversely, a healed valvular vegetation may persist after a previous episode of endocarditis. Transesophageal echocardiography is more sensitive for diagnosing valvular vegetations and should be considered if the clinical suspicion of endocarditis is moderate to high and the transthoracic study does not show typical vegetations. Transesophageal echocardiography also is much more sensitive for the diagnosis of paravalvular abscesses and for evaluation of prosthetic valve endocarditis.

In the Echo Exam section at the end of this chapter, the key echocardiographic findings, limitations of echocardiography, and alternate diagnostic approaches for several anatomic diagnoses are indicated. Each of these topics is covered in detail in subsequent chapters.

By Clinical Setting

The third category of indications for echocardiography is the examination requested because the patient is a member of a clinical group in whom "routine" echocardiographic studies are thought to be clinically valuable (Table 5–3). These examinations fall into one of four categories:

■ Screening examinations to detect cardiac abnormalities in a group of patients with a high prevalence of disease
■ Monitoring examinations performed as part of a therapeutic procedure
■ Evaluation before and after a therapeutic intervention to assess the effect of the intervention and detect possible complications and
■ Baseline studies performed in patients at risk for subsequent cardiac disease or progression of preexisting cardiac disease

Screening examinations are performed in first-degree family members of patients with genetically transmitted cardiac diseases, such as Marfan's syndrome or hypertrophic cardiomyopathy, to detect possible cardiac involvement in those individuals. In patients with positive blood cultures and/or a fever of unexplained etiology, an echocardiogram may be ordered to detect possible endocarditis. Similarly, in patients with cerebrovascular events that may be embolic in origin, an echocardiogram is requested to identify any potential cardiac sources of emboli. The value of echocardiography for the last two indications is low if the prevalence of disease in the population is low. A potential cardiac source of emboli is unlikely to be found in patients with a known

TABLE 5-3

Other Clinical Settings in Which Echocardiography Often Is Indicated

Screening Examinations

First-degree relatives of patients with genetic
 cardiovascular diseases
Patients with fevers, positive blood cultures, and
 suspected endocarditis
Patients with cerebrovascular events for possible cardiac
 "source of embolus"
Patients with arrhythmia

Monitoring Studies

Intraoperative evaluation of LV function in high-risk
 patients
LV size and systolic function in patients with chronic
 valvular regurgitation
LV hypertrophy in hypertensive patients

Pre-/Postintervention Echocardiography

Possible procedural complications
Electrophysiologic studies
Endomyocardial biopsy
Effect of intervention
Revascularization (wall motion and thickening)
Pharmacologic therapy (heart failure, hypertension,
 HOCM)
Valve repair or commissurotomy

Baseline Studies

After valve replacement
Before chemotherapy (cardiotoxic)

LV, left ventricular; HOCM, hypertrophic obstructive
cardiomyopathy.

noncardiac cause of the neurologic disorder. Conversely, the likelihood of identifying a potential source of embolus is high in younger patients (age <45 years) or in those with a cardiac history (e.g., left ventricular apical thrombus in a patient with previous myocardial infarction) or pertinent physical findings (e.g., mitral valve disease). Furthermore, the value of the test is directly related to the impact of the test results on the patient's subsequent medical treatment. If the results of the echocardiogram will not alter therapy or the subsequent diagnostic strategy, then the echocardiogram is of little value.

Screening examinations often are requested in patients with cardiac arrhythmias to identify underlying structural abnormalities. For supraventricular arrhythmias without other evidence of underlying heart disease or a family history of a genetic disorder, the likelihood of a structural abnormality is low. Although most patients with ventricular arrhythmias will have

significant structural disease, including left ventricular systolic dysfunction and/or segmental wall motion abnormalities, these diagnoses usually are known on clinical grounds or on the basis of other diagnostic tests before echocardiography.

The use of echocardiography as a low-yield screening examination can have a major negative impact on the diagnostic use of this technique if only a limited number of echocardiographic studies can be performed (depending on the number of instruments, sonographers, and physicians available). In this situation, unnecessary examinations may delay or prevent diagnosis and subsequent therapy in patients with higher-priority indications for echocardiography. For example, an inpatient echocardiogram performed urgently for "source of embolus" in a patient with a low likelihood of disease may delay scheduling of an "elective" outpatient study in a patient with dyspnea. Delay in diagnosis and treatment of a patient with heart failure may result in an adverse medical outcome. Use of practice guidelines, as suggested by the American College of Cardiology and the American Heart Association (see Suggested Readings) or triage of requested studies based on diagnostic yield and urgency, as suggested in Table 5–4, helps to formalize the process of prioritizing requests for echocardiographic examinations.

Monitoring examinations may be performed sequentially over brief or prolonged periods. Intraoperative monitoring of left ventricular size and systolic function by transesophageal echocardiography is useful in cardiac patients undergoing noncardiac surgery to optimize ventricular preload and for early identification of ischemia, thus preventing perioperative myocardial infarction. Monitoring of left ventricular size and systolic function over many years is performed in patients with chronic valvular regurgitation to determine the optimal timing of surgical intervention. In hypertensive patients, monitoring of left ventricular wall thickness and mass allows assessment of the effect of long-term antihypertensive therapy on end-organ damage (in this case, the left ventricle).

Preintervention and postintervention echocardiography may be used to detect possible procedural complications (e.g., pericardial effusion after electrophysiologic catheter studies or after endomyocardial biopsy). In addition, echocardiography may be used to assess the effect of the intervention by comparing preprocedure and postprocedure studies (e.g., in patients undergoing coronary revascularization procedures, percutaneous mitral balloon commissurotomy, or surgical mitral valve repair). The effects of phar-

TABLE 5–4

An Example of How the Priority of Requested Echocardiographic Studies Might Be Grouped

1. High Diagnostic Yield, Emergency Indications

Hypotension–suspected pericardial tamponade
Chest pain–suspected acute aortic dissection or acute myocardial infarction (nondiagnostic ECG)
Heart failure–severe, unknown etiology
Complications of acute MI
Complications of endocarditis–new murmur, heart failure, prolonged PR-interval
Decompensated congenital heart disease

2. High Diagnostic Yield, Nonemergency

Cardiac murmur–stable patient with suspected significant valvular disease
Clinical diagnosis of endocarditis–stable patient with definite clinical criteria for endocarditis
Congestive heart failure–stable patient with new diagnosis of heart failure or change in clinical status
Suspected prosthetic valve dysfunction–currently stable patient with suspected valve dysfunction
Congenital heart disease–patient with new diagnosis or previous surgery
Coronary artery disease–stress echo for diagnosis or follow-up
Chronic aortic root dilation
Pulmonary heart disease or recurrent pulmonary emboli

3. High Diagnostic Yield but Can Be Scheduled Electively

Known valvular heart disease–follow-up studies for ventricular size and systolic function with no interim change in
    clinical symptoms
Preoperative assessment for elective surgery of patients with suspected cardiac dysfunction
Baseline studies after cardiac surgery or valve replacement
"Source of embolus" evaluation in patient <45 years old or in patients with suspected cardiac disease
Family history of inherited cardiac disease
Suspected cardiac mass
Hypertension

4. Moderate to Low Diagnostic Yield

Cardiac "source of embolus" in patient >45 years of age with no evidence of cardiac disease
"Screening" examinations in arrhythmia patients, organ-transplant donors or recipients, or "routine" preoperative
    patients

MI, myocardial infarction; ECG, electrocardiogram.

macologic therapy on a specific endpoint of interest also may be evaluated. Examples include the changes in stroke volume with vasodilator therapy in a patient with dilated cardiomyopathy or changes in the pattern of left ventricular diastolic filling after beta blockade in a patient with hypertrophic cardiomyopathy.

Baseline echocardiographic studies serve as a reference point in patients with a high likelihood of subsequent cardiac dysfunction. In a patient with a prosthetic valve, a baseline study performed when the patient is asymptomatic and clinically stable provides the normal antegrade velocity across the valve in that individual; the degree of normal prosthetic valve regurgitation; the state of the left ventricle with respect to residual dilation, hypertrophy, or systolic dysfunction; and an estimate of postoperative pulmonary artery pressure. If the patient subsequently pres-

ents with suspected valve dysfunction, a more complete and sensitive assessment is possible by comparison with the baseline study than if no previous examination were available. Another example of the value of a baseline study is assessment of left ventricular systolic function before starting a potentially cardiotoxic chemotherapeutic regimen. A baseline study allows differentiation of subtle early systolic dysfunction due to chemotherapy from mild dysfunction that may be at the lower limits of the normal range.

TRANSESOPHAGEAL ECHOCARDIOGRAPHY

The indications for transesophageal echocardiography are based on its superior image quality compared with transthoracic imaging, particularly of posterior cardiac structures (Table 5–5). Several

TABLE 5–5
Some Indications for Transesophageal Echocardiography

Endocarditis with suspected paravalvular abscess
Suspected endocarditis when TTE nondiagnostic
Suspected prosthetic (especially mitral) valve dysfunction
Perioperative evaluation of MV anatomy and function before and after MV repair
Evaluation of posterior structures (e.g., interatrial baffle, sinus venosus ASD) in congenital heart disease
Suspected aortic dissection
Detection of left atrial thrombus (e.g., before catheter balloon mitral commissurotomy)
Search for cardiac "source of embolus" (including patent foramen ovale) in patients with an unexplained systemic
    embolic event
Whenever transthoracic images are nondiagnostic and echocardiography is indicated (e.g., LV function postcardiac
    surgery)

MV, mitral valve; ASD, atrial septal defect; LV, left ventricular; TTE, transthoracic echocardiography.

definite indications for transesophageal echocardiography are apparent when the limitations of transthoracic imaging are considered. The improved sensitivity of transesophageal versus transthoracic echocardiography for detection of paravalvular abscess in patients with endocarditis has been demonstrated convincingly (see Chapter 14). Transesophageal echocardiography clearly is indicated for evaluation of prosthetic mitral valve dysfunction because the shadows and reverberations from the prosthetic valve no longer obscure the left atrium from this approach as they do on transthoracic images (Fig. 5–9) (see also Chapter 13). Abnormalities of the posterior aspect of a prosthetic aortic valve also will be seen well with the transesophageal approach, although the anterior portion of the paravalvular region will be shadowed by the posterior aspect of the prosthetic valve.

Improved evaluation of mitral valve anatomy and the degree of mitral regurgitation are especially useful in the perioperative evaluation of patients undergoing surgical mitral valve repair (see Chapter 12). In patients with congenital heart disease, transesophageal imaging improves diagnostic certainty, particularly in evaluation of posterior structures such as an interatrial baffle surgical repair or a sinus venosus atrial septal defect. The sensitivity of transesophageal echocardiography for detection of left atrial thrombus far exceeds transthoracic imaging. Finally, excellent images of the thoracic aorta, arch, and ascending aorta allow accurate diagnosis of aortic dissection by transesophageal echocardiography.

Other indications for transesophageal echocardiography include evaluation for a patent foramen ovale in patients with a systemic embolic event, and exclusion of endocarditis when this diagnosis is a possibility. Some echocardiographers advocate

the use of transesophageal imaging whenever transthoracic images are nondiagnostic. However, given that the threshold approach to clinical testing predicts a narrower test window as the risk of the test increases, it is appropriate to consider transesophageal studies somewhat more critically. The indications for a transesophageal study should be discussed with the referring physician on a case-by-case basis to determine if the information potentially obtainable justifies the slight but definite risk of the transesophageal approach.

STRESS ECHOCARDIOGRAPHY

In many cardiac conditions, abnormalities of cardiac function are manifested only when increased oxygen consumption results in increased cardiac demands that cannot be met

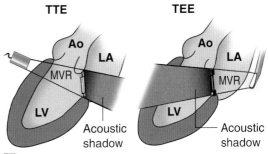

■ **FIGURE 5–9.** Diagram illustrating the problem of acoustic shadowing from a prosthetic mitral valve. On the left, with transthoracic echocardiography (TTE), the acoustic shadow obscures the left atrium, limiting assessment of valvular incompetence by Doppler techniques. On the right, with transesophageal echocardiography (TEE), the left atrium now can be evaluated for valvular incompetence. However, the acoustic shadow now obscures the left ventricular outflow tract.

by the usual compensatory changes. This basic concept has led to the widespread use of stress testing in patients with cardiovascular disease. Increased cardiac demand can be induced by exercise or with appropriate pharmacologic interventions (Table 5–6). The risk of this approach is related to the risk of stress testing with no significant additive effect of echocardiographic imaging.

Exercise echocardiography is performed by recording images of the left ventricle immediately before and immediately after treadmill exercise testing or by recording images during supine or upright bicycle exercise. The most common indication for exercise echocardiography is suspected or known coronary artery disease. At rest, left ventricular endocardial motion and wall thickening are normal, even if significant coronary disease is present, unless there has been prior myocardial infarction. Increased myocardial oxygen demands, such as with exercise, result in ischemia when significant stenosis of an epicardial coronary artery is present. This results sequentially in myocardial metabolic changes, decreased wall thickening and endocardial motion, electrocardiographic changes, and angina, in that order.

Echocardiographic images recorded during ischemia show abnormalities of wall motion, allowing detection of significant coronary artery disease. The specific coronary arteries involved can be identified by the anatomic pattern of induced wall motion abnormalities. Exercise echocardiography, as discussed in detail in Chapter 8, has been found to be more sensitive than exercise electrocardiography (and as sensitive as thallium imaging) for detection of significant coronary artery disease. Exercise echocardiography is particularly helpful in patients with an abnormal resting electrocardiogram (such as bundle branch block or left ventricular hypertrophy). It also has been used to assess the extent of disease, to document functional improvement after revascularization, and to detect restenosis after angioplasty.

In addition to changes in segmental wall motion with exercise stress testing, parameters of global ventricular function, including ventricular volumes, ejection fraction, and the Doppler left ventricular ejection velocity curve, can be evaluated. Other Doppler parameters may be helpful in specific settings. For example, a patient with mitral stenosis will show an excessive rise in pulmonary artery systolic pressure (estimated from the tricuspid regurgitant jet) with exercise. In a patient with aortic coarctation, the increase in gradient across the coarctation with exercise can be demonstrated with Doppler recordings.

Pharmacologic stress echocardiography replaces exercise testing when the patient is unable to exercise (e.g., peripheral vascular disease, musculoskeletal limitations). It also is an attractive alternate to exercise testing when recording of 2D and Doppler data at sequential stages of increased cardiac demand provides useful clinical data. In fact, it can be argued that pharmacologic stress testing is preferable in that the patient can be monitored carefully by echocardiography as the dose is increased, allowing termination of the "stress" as soon as a wall motion abnormality is seen. Pharmacologic stress testing most often is performed using a beta agonist, such as dobutamine, which increases myocardial contractility, myocardial oxygen demands, and the degree of peripheral vasodilation. An alternate pharmacologic agent used in some centers is adenosine, which vasodilates normal coronary vessels, thus "stealing" blood from stenosed vessels resulting in ischemia.

OTHER MODALITIES

Contrast Echocardiography

Contrast studies with agitated saline to opacify the right heart are performed to document an atrial septal defect (Chapter 17), patent foramen ovale (Chapter 15), or persistent left superior vena cava

---

TABLE 5–6

Indications for Stress Echocardiography

Exercise Echocardiography

Coronary artery disease
  Diagnosis
  Extent of disease and vessels involved
  After revascularization
Valvular heart disease
  PA pressures in mitral stenosis patients
Congenital disease
  Aortic coarctation

Pharmacologic Stress Echo

Same indications as exercise echocardiography in patients unable to exercise due to:
  Peripheral vascular disease
  Musculoskeletal limitations
  Or as an alternate to exercise stress
Image acquisition during therapeutic pharmacologic intervention
Valvular heart disease
  Change in valve area with stress in aortic stenosis

PA, pulmonary artery.

TABLE 5-7
Indications for Contrast Echocardiography

Standard IV Contrast (e.g., Agitated Saline Solution)

Detection of atrial septal defects and patent foramen ovale

Doumentation of persistent left superior vena cava

IV Contrast Agents with Pulmonary Transit

Enhancement of contrast between LV chamber and endocardium (improved border recognition)

Myocardial perfusion

Intracoronary Contrast

Opacification of myocardium perfused by injected vessel (e.g., during catheter ablation for hypertrophic cardiomyopathy)

Detection of myocardial ischemia

IV, intravenous; LV, left ventricular.

(Chapter 15) (Table 5–7). Commercially available contrast agents provide smaller microbubbles (4 to 10 μm in diameter) that are injected intravenously but traverse the pulmonary capillary bed. These microbubbles both provide opacification of the left ventricular chamber, which enhances endocardial definition for evaluation of global and regional ventricular function. Contrast enhancement is indicated on both resting and stress echocardiographic studies when image quality is suboptimal and evaluation of ventricular function is needed. Contrast agents also can be injected directly into a coronary artery to define the area perfused by that vessel, for example at the time of percutaneous septal ablation for hypertrophic cardiomyopathy.

Three-dimensional Echocardiography

Three-dimensional (3D) echocardiographic techniques are likely to become more widely used as the technology becomes easier to use and is integrated into standard ultrasound systems. Voxel reconstructions are most useful for demonstrating complex intracardiac 3D relationships, particularly in cases of valvular and congenital heart disease. Disadvantages of gray-scale voxel reconstructions are that the data are only qualitative and optimal display is dependent on the operator's choice of image plane, thus requiring considerable experience both with the 3D technique and with the anatomy of complex cardiac abnormalities.

Three-dimensional reconstructions based on tracing intracardiac borders allow highly accurate measurements of ventricular volumes and systolic function, as discussed in Chapter 6. However, this approach will remain limited to research applications until reliable methods for automatic edge detection are available.

Hand-held Ultrasound

Small, relatively inexpensive, portable or "hand-held" echocardiography instruments now are available. These instruments are of great clinical utility in the emergency department, coronary care unit, and cardiology clinic for triage of acutely ill patients. Indications for hand-held ultrasound are in evolution but these instruments appear to be most useful for evaluation of overall and regional ventricular function and detection of pericardial fluid. For example, a hand-held echocardiogram in a patient with chest pain and a nondiagnostic electrocardiograph that shows akinesis of the anterior wall indicates the need for prompt coronary intervention. Conversely, the finding of large pericardial effusion leads to a different diagnostic and therapeutic pathway. However, caution is needed in the use of these instruments. As with any ultrasound imaging technique, accurate diagnosis depends on the training and experience of the examiner. In addition, image quality and instrument functions are limited on these small devices compared to standard ultrasound systems. Each medical center will need to carefully evaluate the use of these devices and monitor diagnostic accuracy.

QUALITY ASSURANCE IN ECHOCARDIOGRAPHY

There are several steps to ensuring that high-quality echocardiographic studies are provided to our patients. These include documentation of sonographer and physician competency, appropriate laboratory standards, and procedures and continuous quality improvement measures. Documentation of competency typically is based on

■ accreditation–endorsement of a training program or laboratory by a recognized national accrediting agency,

■ certification–documentation of appropriate training and successful completion of an examination in the area of expertise by each physician and sonographer,

■ credentialing–standards set by each health care organization for health care professionals providing patient care at that institution.

In addition, innovative approaches to quality assurance based on statistical analysis of physician or laboratory performance have been proposed.

Statistical database approaches will be increasingly useful as medical record systems are computerized.

Sonographer Education and Training

The sonographer must be familiar with patterns of disease in clinical cardiology, as well as with the technical aspects of performing the examination. Thus, sonographer education and training must include a knowledge base of cardiac anatomy and physiology, cardiac pathology, and clinical cardiology, in addition to ultrasound physics and the echocardiographic examination. Training also includes patient interaction skills, basic medical procedures (such as sterile technique), patient privacy, and so forth.

Guidelines for education and training of cardiac sonographers have been published by the American Society of Echocardiography and are periodically updated. Education and training in an accredited program is recommended with accreditation for cardiac sonographer programs provided by two Joint Review Commissions (JRCs) under the auspices of the Commission on Accreditation of Allied Health Educational Programs: the JRC-Diagnostic Medical Sonography (JRC-DMS) and the JRC-Cardiovascular Technology (JRC-CVT). Education and training includes acquistion of both cognitive and technical skills with demonstration of competancy in each area. After completion of training, sonographers can be credentialed by the American Registry of Diagnostic Medical Sonographers, with separate examinations for adult and pediatric echocardiography, or by Cardiovascular Credentialing International. Cardiac sonographers must attend formal continuing medical education meetings to maintain these credentials.

Physician Education and Training

The physician must have expertise in the technical aspects of the examination, as well as the expected findings in each disease state, in order to guide the sonographer in optimizing data quality and to interpret the recorded data correctly. Details such as transducer frequency, gain controls, processing curves, and depth settings significantly affect 2D image quality. The appropriate choice of Doppler modality for the flow of interest—pulsed, color flow, or continuous-wave Doppler—affects the data obtained. Factors such as wall filters, gain, sample volume size, and color sector width also significantly affect data collection. Knowledge of how these factors affect data quality and knowledge of which views and approaches yield optimal data allow the physician to assess the reliability of recorded data, to suspect abnormalities that may not have been noted explicitly during the examination, to recognize imaging and flow artifacts, and to direct the sonographer in optimal data acquisition.

Physician education and training in echocardiography most often takes place during Cardiology Fellowship Training, in a program accredited by the American Council of Graduate Medical Education. In addition, specific recommendations for training in echocardiography have been published, and are periodically updated, by the American College of Cardiology and American Heart Association. These recommendations divide training into three levels of expertise:

■ Level 1: Basic introduction to echocardiography needed by all cardiologists
■ Level 2: Qualified to independently interpret echocardiographic studies
■ Level 3: Additional qualifications to supervise an echocardiography laboratory

It is recommended that Level 2 training in transthoracic echocardiography be achieved before training in advanced procedures, including transesophageal and stress echocardiography. Recommended numbers of procedures during training are indicated in Table 5–8.

Most physicians completing a 3- or 4-year program in cardiology will have achieved level 2 training. Successful completion of the American Board of Internal Medicine examination in Cardiovascular Disease, in conjunction with at least level 2 training, certifies competence in transthoracic echocardiography.

Other physicians may achieve competency in echocardiography based on the same training guidelines recommended for cardiology trainees. Physicians who receive echocardiography training outside of Cardiology Fellowship Programs have the option of taking the examination provided by the National Board of Echocardiography (NBE) to document competency. In addition, specific guidelines for training of cardiovascular anesthesiologists in echocardiography have been published by the American Society of Echocardiography focusing on expertise in transesophageal and intraoperative echocardiography. The NBE offers a special examination for echocardiography competence by cardiovascular anesthesiologists.

In order to maintain competency in echocardiography, physicians should document Continuing Medical Education and should interpret a minimum of 300 studies per year for level 2 and 500 studies per year for level 3, with performance of some studies recommended. For maintaining competency in transesophageal echocardiogra-

TABLE 5–8				
Summary of ACC/AHA Recommendations for Physician Training in Echocardiography				
Level of Expertise	Cumulative Duration (mo)	Cumulation Number of Studies Performed	Cumulative Number of Studies Interpreted	Annual Studies to Maintain Competace
1	3	75	150	
2	6	150	300	300
3	12	300	750	500
Stress echo		100		100
TEE		50		25–50

phy, 25 to 50 studies should be performed and interpreted annually, with 100 studies per year recommended for stress echocardiography.

Echocardiography Reporting

It is essential that sonographers relay technical concerns to the physician and direct attention to abnormalities noted during the examination. Conversely, the physician should give feedback to the sonographer about the completeness and quality of data recorded and offer suggestions for future patient studies. The physician review also may indicate that additional echocardiographic recordings are needed, either before the patient leaves the laboratory or at a later examination.

The echocardiographic report serves at least two purposes: (1) it conveys the results of the test to the referring physician, and (2) it serves as a narrative summary of the echocardiographic examination for comparison with future studies. Given the wide variety of views and flows that can be recorded, it is helpful for the report to document the structures imaged (even if normal), the flow signals recorded, the different Doppler modalities used, and the overall quality of the study. Any areas of limitation in the study are noted.

In each patient, the various echocardiographic findings then are integrated with each other in the final interpretation. For example, a report describing mitral regurgitation also would include a clear description of valve anatomy with an indication of the most likely etiology of regurgitation or the differential diagnosis if the etiology were unclear. Mitral regurgitant severity is estimated and the method(s) used to generate this estimate are indicated. In addition, the degrees of left atrial and left ventricular dilation are described, with attention to serial changes if previous studies are available. Left ventricular systolic function is quantitated, and the degree of pulmonary hypertension is esti-

mated. All these findings fit together physiologically and thus can be reported in a logical integration of the data. For example, significant mitral regurgitation results in left ventricular and left atrial enlargement due to volume overload, while the chronically elevated left atrial pressure leads to pulmonary hypertension.

Finally, these findings are reviewed in the context of the patient's clinical presentation, potential implications of the findings are discussed with the referring physician, and additional diagnostic tests or follow-up studies are recommended as clinically indicated. If principles of clinical decision analysis are being used in patient management, the pretest and posttest likelihood of disease can be estimated. Ideally, the overall impact of the echocardiographic findings on the patient's therapy or subsequent diagnostic evaluation is reviewed with the referring physician both before and after the examination. Specific comments about endocarditis prophylaxis, periodic echocardiography, or referral to a cardiologist also may be appropriate. Of course, any unexpected or serious findings on echocardiography should promptly be relayed to the referring physician. In some cases, the echocardiography attending may need to assume immediate care of the patient, for example with persistent abnormalities after stress testing or with the unexpected finding of an aortic dissection.

Echocardiography Laboratory Accreditation

Accreditation of echocardiography laboratories is available through the Intersocietal Commission for the Accreditation of Echocardiography Laboratories (ICAEL). This accreditation process reviews all aspects of the echocardiographic examination including

■ physician training and experience,
■ sonographer training and experience,

■ continuing medical education of physicians and sonographers,

■ physical facilities (instruments, examination area, etc.),

■ echocardiography performance,

■ laboratory procedures and protocols,

■ echocardiographic reporting and data storage,

■ quality assurance measures.

The detailed recommendations of the ICAEL provide a useful starting point for laboratory policies and procedures that then can be modified as needed for each institution. The recommendations also include the essential components of transthoracic, transesophageal, and stress echocardiography examinations.

SUGGESTED READING

1. Sox HC Jr, Blatt MA, Higgins MC, Martin KI: Medical Decision Making. Stoneham, Massachusetts, Butterworth-Heinemann, 1988.

    A readable concise textbook summarizing the entire spectrum of medical decision making from sensitivity/specificity to cost-benefit analysis.

2. Diamond GA, Forrester JS: Analysis of probability as an aid in the clinical diagnosis of coronary-artery disease. N Engl J Med 300:1350–1358, 1979.

    Classic article on use of Bayes' theorem to determine posttest likelihood based on pretest likelihood and test results using the example of exercise electrocardiography for diagnosis of coronary artery disease.

3. Patterson RE, Horowitz SF: Importance of epidemiology and biostatistics in deciding clinical strategies for using diagnostic tests: a simplified approach using examples from coronary artery disease. J Am Coll Cardiol 13: 1653–1665, 1989.

    Emphasizes integration of test results in overall patient management.

4. Wasson JH, Sox HC, Neff RK, Goldman L: Clinical prediction rules. Applications and methodological standards. N Engl J Med 313:793–799, 1985.

    Defines approach to developing and validating new clinical prediction rules. This article will be of particular value to individuals proposing new diagnostic approaches based on echocardiographic data.

5. Pauker SG, Kassirer JP: The threshold approach to clinical decision making. N Engl J Med 302:1109–1117, 1980.

    Clear and concise discussion of the concepts of decision analysis focusing on the threshold approach.

6. Pauker SG, Kassirer JP: Decision analysis. N Engl J Med 316:250–258, 1987.

    Review of decision analysis including Bayes' rule, decision trees, and outcome measures. 52 references.

7. Biem HJ, Detsky AS, Armstrong PW: Management of asymptomatic chronic aortic regurgitation with left ventricular dysfunction: a decision analysis. J Gen Intern Med 5:394–401, 1990.

    Example of the application of clinical decision methods to a clinical problem (timing of valve replacement in chronic aortic regurgitation) in which echocardiographic data (left ventricular size and systolic function) are critical to patient management.

8. Detsky AS, Naglie IG: A clinician's guide to cost-effectiveness analysis. Ann Intern Med 113:147–154, 1990.

    Outlines simplified models for cost-effectiveness analysis that should be applicable to comparisons of the use of different diagnostic tests in a specific clinical setting. Provides guidelines for setting priorities within a health care organization based on cost-effectiveness analysis.

9. Otto CM, Pearlman AS: Doppler echocardiography in adults with symptomatic aortic stenosis. Arch Intern Med 148:2553–2560, 1988.

    An example of development and validation of a clinical prediction rule for timing of valve replacement in symptomatic aortic stenosis based on Doppler echo data. Maximum aortic jet velocity (V_{max}) breakpoints are proposed at >4 m/s (valve replacement indicated), <3 m/s (valve replacement not needed), and between 3 and 4 m/s (evaluation of valve area and coexisting aortic regurgitation needed). Simple cost analysis compares noninvasive with invasive diagnostic approach.

10. Oh JK, Taliercio CP, Holmes DR Jr, et al: Prediction of the severity of aortic stenosis by Doppler aortic valve area determination: Prospective Doppler-catheterization correlation in 100 patients. J Am Coll Cardiol 11:1227–1234, 1988.

    Evaluation of Doppler data for diagnosis of severe aortic stenosis. Proposed single maximum aortic jet velocity breakpoint at 4.5 m/s with a sensitivity of 44% and a specificity of 93% for diagnosis of severe stenosis.

11. Cheitlin MD, Alpert JS, Armstrong WF, Aurigemma GP, Beller GA, Bierman FZ, et al: ACC/AHA/ASE 2003 Guidelines Update for the Clinical Application of Echocardiography: Summary Article. A Report of the American College of Cardiology/American Heart Association Task Force on Practice Guidelines. Circulation 108:1146–1162, 2003.

    Task force guidelines on indications for echocardiography divided into class I indications (general agreement that echocardiography is important), class II (divergence of opinions), and class III (not appropriate).

12. Quinones MA, Douglas, PA, Foster E, Gorcsan J, Lewis JF, Pearlman AS, et al. American College of Cardiology/American Heart Association Clinical Competence Statement on Echocardiography: A report of the American College of Cardiology/American Heart Association/American College of Physicians-American Society of Internal Medicine Task Force on Clinical Competence. Circulation 107:1068–1089, 2003.

    Detailed recommendations for physician education and training and maintenance of competency in echocardiography. This document includes sections on transthoracic echocardiography, transesophageal echocardiography, perioperative echocardiography, stress echocardiography, congenital heart disease, fetal echocardiography, and new technologies (hand-held devices, contrast, intracoronary, and intracardiac ultrasound).

13. Cahalan MK, Stewart W, Pearlman A, et al: American Society of Echocardiography and Society for Cardiovascular Anesthesiologists Task Force Guidelines for Training in Perioperative Echocardiography. J Am Soc Echocardiogr 15:647–652, 2002.

Training guidelines for anesthesiologists using echocardiography are proposed with a distinction between Basic Training (use of echocardiography for monitoring and screening) and Advanced Training (use of echocardiography for diagnosis and quantitation of cardiac disease).

14. Ehler D, Carney DK, Dempsey AL, et al: American Society of Echocardiography Sonographer Training and Education Committee. Guidelines for cardiac sonographer education: recommendations of the American Society of Echocardiography Sonographer Training and Education Committee. J Am Soc Echocardiogr 14:77–84, 2001.

   Detailed summary of the educational requirements for education in cardiac sonography. A useful outline for training programs for curriculum development. Physicians should review these guidelines to ensure appropriate education of sonographers performing studies under their supervision.

15. Gibbons EF, Kraft C: Education and training of physicians and sonongraphers. In: Otto CM (ed): The Practice of Clinical Echocardiography, 2nd ed. Philadelphia: WB Saunders, 2003, pp 923–937.

   Detailed review of accreditation and credentialing for physician and sonographers with a discussion of the cognitive and technical skills needed for echocardiography. 97 references.

16. Byrd BF: Maintaining quality in the echocardiography laboratory. In: Otto CM (ed): The Practice of Clinical Echocardiography, 2nd ed. Philadelphia: WB Saunders, 2003, pp 938–946.

   Summary of recommendations for echocardiography laboratory accreditation.

17. Segar DS: The digital echocardiography laboratory. In: Otto CM (ed): The Practice of Clinical Echocardiography, 2nd ed. Philadelphia: WB Saunders, 2003, pp 947–958.

   Review of how to set up and maintain a digital echocardiography laboratory. Extensive glossary of terms used in digital echocardiography is very helpful for communicating with your computer experts.

18. Berger AK, Gottdiener JS, Yohe MA, Guerrero JL: Epidemiological approach to quality assessment in echocardiographic diagnosis. J Am Coll Cardiol 34(6):1831–1836, 1999. Comment in: J Am Coll Cardiol 34(6):1837–1838, 1999.

   The authors propose a unique approach to quality improvement based on statistical analysis of computerized clinical database to assess for reader variability in echocardiography interpretation. This type of approach promises to become standard as our medical centers become fully computer based.

Useful Web Sites
Professional Organizations

American College of Cardiology: www.acc.org
American Heart Association: www.americanheart.org

Society for Diagnostic Medical Sonography: www.sdms.org
American Society of Echocardiography: www.asecho.org
European Society of Cardiology: www.escardio.org

All of these professional organizations have guidelines for training and education and for the indications for echocardiography that are posted on the web sites and periodically updated.

Accreditation

Accreditation Council on Graduate Medical Education: www.acgme.org

Provides the requirements and procedures for accreditation of physician training programs, including Fellowship in Cardiovascular Disease.

Commission on Accreditation of Allied Health Education Programs: www.caahep.org

Includes Essentials and Guidelines for accreditation of programs in cardiac sonography by the Joint Review Commission for Diagnostic Medical Sonography (JRC-DMS) and the Joint Review Commission for Cardiovascular Technology (JRC-CVT). Also includes lists of accredited programs. Currently, the JRC-DMS provides accreditation to a total of 99 programs, with 31 echocardiography programs. The JRC-CVT provides accreditation to a total of 25 programs, with 12 noninvasive cardiology programs.

Intersocietal Commission for Accreditation of Echocardiography Laboratories: www.icael.org

Details of the requirements and procedures for accreditation of echocardiography laboratories. This web site has a wealth of detail that will be useful to any laboratory seeking to establish protocols and procedures.

Credentialing

American Registry of Diagnostic Medical Sonography (ARDMS): www.ardms.org

The ARDMS offers four credentials, one of which is Registered Diagnostic Cardiac Sonographer with examination options in adult and pediatric echocardiography.

Cardiovascular Credentialing International: www.cci-online.org

CCI offers three examinations, one of which is noninvasive/echocardiography leading to credentialing as a Registered Cardiac Sonographer.

American Board of Internal Medicine: www.abim.org

Policies for physician credentials in Internal Medicine and its subspecialties, including cardiovascular disease, with examination dates and registration. An index provides verification of physician status on these examinations.

National Board of Echocardiography: www.echoboards.org

The National Board of Echocardiography offers two examinations: Examination of Special Competency in Adult Echocardiography (ASCeXAM) and Examination of Special Competency in Perioperative Transesophageal Echocardiography (PTEeXAM). Certification is based on documentation of training and experience and passing the examination.

The Echo Exam *Indications for Transthoracic Echocardiography*

Clinical Diagnosis	Key Echo Findings	Limitations of Echo	Alternate Approaches
Valvular Heart Disease			
Valve stenosis	Etiology of stenosis, valve anatomy Transvalvular ΔP, valve area Chamber enlargement and hypertrophy LV and RV systolic function Associated valvular regurgitation	Possible underestimation of stenosis severity Possible coexisting coronary artery disease	Cardiac cath MRI
Valve regurgitation	Mechanism and etiology of regurgitation Severity of regurgitation Chamber enlargement LV and RV systolic function PA pressure estimate	TEE may be needed to evaluate mitral regurgitant severity and valve anatomy (esp. before MV repair)	Cardiac cath MRI
Prosthetic valve function	Evidence for stenosis Detection of regurgitation Chamber enlargement Ventricular function PA pressure estimate	Imaging prosthetic valves is limited by shadowing and reverberations TEE is needed for suspected prosthetic MR due to "masking" of the LA on TTE	Cardiac cath
Endocarditis	Detection of vegetations (TTE sensitivity 70–85%) Presence and degree of valve dysfunction Chamber enlargement and function Detection of abscess Possible prognostic implications	TEE more sensitive for detection of vegetations (>90%) A definite diagnosis of endocarditis also depends on bacteriologic criteria TEE more sensitive for abscess detection	Blood cultures and clinical findings also are diagnostic criteria for endocarditis
Coronary Artery Disease			

Acute myocardial infarction	Segmental wall motion abnormality reflects "myocardium at risk"
	Global LV function (EF)
	Complications:
	  Acute MR vs. VSD
	  Pericarditis
	  LV thrombus, aneurysm
	  RV infarct
		Coronary artery anatomy itself not directly visualized	Coronary angio
			Radionuclide LV angio
			Cardiac cath

Angina	Global and segmental LV systolic function Exclude other causes of angina (e.g., AS, HOCM)	Resting wall motion may be normal despite significant CAD Stress echo needed to induce ischemia and wall motion abnormality	Coronary angio Stress thallium ETT
Pre-/post-revascularization	Assess wall thickening and endocardial motion at baseline Improvement in segmental function post-procedure	Dobutamine stress and/or contrast echo needed to detect viable but non-functioning myocardium	MRI PET Thallium ETT Contrast echocardiography
End-stage ischemic disease	Overall LV systolic function (EF) PA pressures Associated MR LV thrombus RV systolic function		Coronary angio Radionuclide EF

Clinical Diagnosis	Key Echo Findings	Limitations of Echo	Alternate Approaches
Cardiomyopathy			
Dilated	Chamber dilation (all four) LV and RV systolic function (qualitative and EF) Coexisting atrioventricular valve regurgitation PA systolic pressure LV thrombus	Indirect measures of LVEDP Accurate EF may be difficult if image quality poor.	Radionuclide EF LV and RV angiography
Restrictive	LV wall thickness LV systolic function LV diastolic function PA systolic pressure	Must be distinguished from constrictive pericarditis	Cardiac cath with direct, simultaneous RV and LV pressure measurement after volume loading
Hypertrophic	Pattern and extent of LV hypertrophy Dynamic LVOT obstruction (imaging and Doppler) Coexisting MR Diastolic LV dysfunction		
Hypertension	LV wall thickness and chamber dimensions LV mass LV systolic function Aortic root dilation, AR		
Pericardial Disease	Pericardial thickening Detection, size, and location of PE 2D signs of tamponade physiology Doppler signs of tamponade physiology	Diagnosis of tamponade is a hemodynamic and clinical diagnosis Constrictive pericarditis is a difficult diagnosis Not all patients with pericarditis have an effusion	Intracardiac pressure measurements for tamponade or constriction MRI or CT to detect pericardial thickening
Aortic Disease			
Aortic root dilation	Etiology of aortic dilation Aortic root diameter measurements Anatomy of sinuses of Valsalva (esp. Marfan's syndrome) Associated aortic regurgitation	May not visualize entire ascending aorta	CT, MRI Aortography, TEE
Aortic dissection	2D images of ascending aorta (PLAX, PSAX), aortic arch (SSN), descending thoracic (A2C), and proximal abdominal (SC) aorta Imaging of dissection "flap" Associated aortic regurgitation Ventricular function	TEE more sensitive (97%) and specific (100%) Cannot assess distal vascular beds	Aortography CT MRI TEE

Continued

Clinical Diagnosis	Key Echo Findings	Limitations of Echo	Alternate Approaches
Cardiac Masses			
LV thrombus	High sensitivity and specificity for diagnosis of LV thrombus Suspect with apical wall motion abnormality or diffuse LV systolic dysfunction	Technical artifacts can be misleading 5-MHz or higher frequency transducer and angulated apical views needed	LV thrombus may not be recognized on radionuclide or contrast angiography
LA thrombus	Low sensitivity for detection of LA thrombus, although specificity is high Suspect with LA enlargement, MV Disease	TEE is needed to detect LA thrombus reliability	TEE
Cardiac tumors	Size, location, and physiologic consequences of tumor mass	Extracardiac involvement not well seen Cannot distinguish benign from malignant, or tumor from thrombus	TEE CT MRI (with cardiac gating) Intracardiac echo
Pulmonary Hypertension			
	Estimate of PA pressure Evidence of left-sided heart disease to account for increased PA pressures RV size and systolic function (cor pulmonale) Associated TR	Indirect PA pressure measurement Unable to determine pulmonary vascular resistance accurately	Cardiac cath
Congenital Heart Disease			
	Detection and assessment of anatomic abnormalities Quantitation of physiologic abnormalities Chamber enlargement Ventricular function	No direct intracardiac pressure measurements Complicated anatomy may be difficult to evaluate if image quality is poor (TEE helpful)	MRI with 3D reconstruction Cardiac cath TEE 3D Echo

A2C, Apical two-chamber; Angio, angiography; AS, aortic stenosis; CAD, coronary artery disease; Cath, catheterization; CT, computed tomography; EF, ejection fraction; ETT, exercise treadmill test; HOCM, hypertrophic obstructive cardiomyopathy; LA, left atrial; LV, left ventricular; LVEDP, left ventricular end-diastolic pressure; LVOT, left ventricular outflow tract; MHz, megahertz; MR, mitral regurgitation; MRI, magnetic resonance imaging; MV, mitral valve; AP, pressure gradient; PA, pulmonary artery; PE, pericardial effusion; PET, position emission tomography; PLAX, parasternal long-axis; PSAX, parasternal short-axis; RV, right ventricular; SC, subcostal; SSN, suprasternal notch; 2D, two-dimensional; TEE, transesophageal echocardiography; TR, tricuspid regurgitation; TTE, transthoracic echocardiography; VSD, ventricular septal defect.

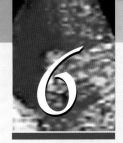

LEFT AND RIGHT VENTRICULAR SYSTOLIC FUNCTION

6

The degree of left ventricular systolic dysfunction is a potent predictor of clinical outcome for a wide range of cardiovascular disease, including ischemic cardiac disease, cardiomyopathies, valvular heart disease, and congenital heart disease. Echocardiography provides both qualitative and quantitative measures of systolic function. Visual estimates of global and regional function from echocardiographic images, quantitative ventricular volumes and ejection fractions based on endocardial border tracing, and Doppler echocardiographic ejection phase indices all are valuable clinical tools.

Evaluation of ventricular systolic function is the most important application of echocardiography, so that even when evaluation of ventricular systolic function is not the focus of the examination, it plays an essential role in every study. For research applications, echocardio-

graphic measures of left ventricular systolic function provide important baseline data on disease severity. In addition, these data can serve as a sensitive and reliable surrogate endpoint for intervention trials in patients with ventricular dysfunction.

BASIC PRINCIPLES

Cardiac Cycle

Systole typically is defined as the segment of the cardiac cycle from mitral valve closure to aortic valve closure (Fig. 6–1). The onset of systole is defined by the electrocardiogram (ECG) as ventricular depolarization (onset of the QRS complex), with the end of systole occurring after repolarization (end of T wave). In terms of ventricular pressure and volume curves over time,

131

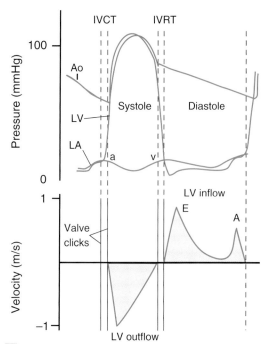

FIGURE 6–1. The cardiac cycle. Left ventricular (LV), aortic (Ao), and left atrial (LA) pressures are shown with the corresponding Doppler left ventricular outflow and inflow velocity curves. The isovolumic contraction time (IVCT) represents the time between mitral valve closure and aortic valve opening, while the isovolumic relaxation time (IVRT) represents the time between aortic valve closure and mitral valve opening.

systole begins when left ventricular diastolic pressure exceeds left atrial pressure, resulting in closure of the mitral valve. Mitral valve closure is followed by isovolumic contraction, during which the cardiac muscle depolarizes, calcium influx and myosin-actin shortening occur, and ventricular pressure increases rapidly at a constant ventricular volume (although shape changes may occur). When ventricular pressure exceeds aortic pressure, the aortic valve opens. During ejection (aortic valve opening to closing), left ventricular volume falls rapidly as blood flows from the left ventricle to the aorta. Left ventricular pressure exceeds aortic pressure for approximately the first half of systole, corresponding to rapid acceleration of blood flow and a small pressure difference from the ventricle to the aorta. In the normal heart, pressure crossover occurs in midsystole, so during the second half of systole, aortic pressure exceeds left ventricular pressure, resulting in continued forward blood flow but at progressively slower velocities (deceleration). Aortic valve closure occurs at the dicrotic notch of the aortic pressure tracing, immediately following end-ejection. In

sum, systole includes isovolumic contraction and ventricular ejection (acceleration and deceleration phases). Ventricular volume ranges from a maximum at end-diastole (or onset of systole) to a minimum at end-systole.

Physiology of Systolic Function

Fundamentally, ventricular systolic function is best described by contractility: the basic ability of the myocardium to contract. However, contractility is affected by several physiologic parameters, including

- heart rate,
- coupling interval,
- metabolic factors, and
- pharmacologic agents.

In addition, for a given degree of contractility, ventricular ejection performance can vary depending on

- preload (initial ventricular volume or pressure), and
- afterload (aortic resistance/impedance or end-systolic wall stress).

Evaluation of contractility itself thus requires measurement of ventricular ejection performance under different loading conditions. Experimentally, contractility often is described by the slope of the end-systolic pressure-volume relationship (E_{max}). To derive this value, left ventricular pressure is graphed on the vertical axis, with volume on the horizontal axis, rather than graphing both as a function of time (Fig. 6–2). This pressure-volume "loop" then represents a single cardiac cycle, with different pressure-volume loops for the same ventricle representing different loading conditions (such as increasing or decreasing ventricular end-diastolic volume or changing afterload). E_{max} is the slope of the line that intersects the end-systolic pressure-volume point for each curve (Fig. 6–3).

The effect of preload on ventricular ejection performance is summarized by the Frank-Starling curve showing ventricular end-diastolic volume (or pressure) on the horizontal axis and stroke volume on the vertical axis (Fig. 6–4). For a given degree of contractility, there is a curvilinear relationship between these variables such that increasing end-diastolic volume results in a greater stroke volume. An increase in contractility shifts this curve up and to the left; conversely, a decrease in contractility shifts it downward and to the right.

Afterload, defined by resistance or impedance, has an inverse relationship with stroke volume such that increasing vascular resistance results in a decreased stroke volume (see Fig. 6–4). An increase

Pressure-volume Loop

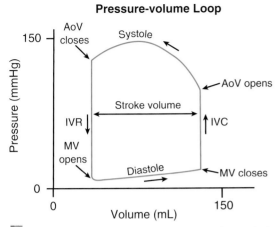

FIGURE 6–2. Pressure-volume loop. Left ventricular volume is graphed on the horizontal axis, with pressure on the vertical axis. The temporal direction of pressure-volume changes is shown by the arrows. During diastole, volume increases with little rise in pressure. After mitral valve (MV) closure, isovolumic contraction (IVC) results in a rapid rise in pressure with no change in volume. At the onset of ejection, the aortic valve (AoV) opens with a rapid decrease in left ventricular volume during systole. Aortic valve closure is followed by isovolumic relaxation (IVR).

Preload

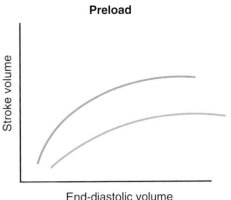

Afterload

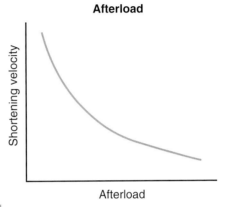

FIGURE 6–4. *Top:* The relationship between end-diastolic volume and stroke volume is shown for a normal (*blue*) and failing (*tan*) left ventricle. *Bottom:* The inverse relationship between afterload and left ventricular myocardial shortening velocity is shown.

in contractility shifts this curve upward and to the right; a decrease in contractility shifts it to the left.

Measurement of left ventricular systolic function independent of loading conditions is difficult using echocardiographic or other clinical approaches. It rarely is possible to construct

pressure-volume loops under different loading conditions due to the problem of measuring instantaneous left ventricular volumes and the potential risk of altering loading conditions in ill patients. Thus, clinical evaluation of ventricular function has focused on measurements of cardiac output, ejection fraction, and end-systolic dimension or volume, even though the load dependence of these measures is a clearly acknowledged limitation.

Ventricular Volumes and Geometry

The normal shape of the left ventricle is symmetric with two relatively equal short axes and with the long axis running from the base (mitral annulus) to the apex. In long-axis views, the apex is slightly rounded, so the apical half of the ventricle resembles a hemiellipse. The basal half of the ventricle is more cylindrical, so the ventricle appears circular in short-axis views. Various assumptions about left ventricular shape have

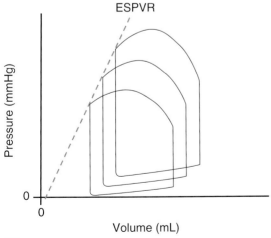

FIGURE 6–3. Pressure-volume loops at different loading conditions (e.g., increasing end-diastolic volumes) are used to derive a line describing end-systolic pressure-volume relationship (ESPVR), also known as elastance (E_{max}). This measure of left ventricular contractility is insensitive to changes in loading conditions.

been used to derive formulas for calculating ventricular volumes from linear dimensions (M-mode), cross-sectional areas (two-dimensional [2D] echo) or three-dimensional (3D) volumes. Formulas using linear or cross-sectional measurements are simplifications to greater or lesser degrees, and there is variability among patients in the shape of the ventricle.

While ventricular volumes instantaneously throughout the cardiac cycle are of interest, usually only end-diastolic volume (EDV) and end-systolic volume (ESV) are measured in the clinical setting. Ejection fraction (EF) is

$$EF(\%) = (SV/EDV) \times 100\% \qquad (6-1)$$

where stroke volume (SV) is calculated as

$$SV = EDV - ESV \qquad (6-2)$$

with cardiac output obtained by multiplying stroke volume by heart rate.

Other useful parameters of ventricular function include (1) wall stress and (2) left ventricular mass. Wall stress is the force per unit area exerted on the myocardium. Wall stress is dependent on

- cavity dimensions, or radius (R),
- pressure (P), and
- wall thickness (Th).

The basic equation for wall stress (σ) is

$$\sigma = PR/2Th \qquad (6-3)$$

Wall stress can be described in three dimensions as circumferential, meridional (longitudinal), or radial. Typically, end-systolic calculations of circumferential and meridional wall stress are used clinically. Left ventricular mass is the total weight of the myocardium, derived by multiplying the volume of myocardium times the specific density of cardiac muscle.

Cardiac Output

The basic function of the heart is as a pump, so that measurements of cardiac output are useful in routine day-to-day patient treatment. Cardiac output is the volume of blood pumped by the heart per minute, with stroke volume being the amount pumped on a single beat. While cardiac output can be derived from ventricular volumes, as described above, a variety of other approaches to measurement are available, including indicator dilation methods (Fick, thermodilution), Doppler velocity data, ventricular impedance, and radionuclide methods.

Response to Exercise

Ventricular systolic function and cardiac output are dynamic, responding rapidly to the metabolic demands of the individual. Cardiac output increases from a mean of 6 L/min at rest to 18 L/min with exercise in young, healthy adults. Most of this increase in cardiac output is mediated by an increase in heart rate. With supine exercise, there is only a minimal increase in stroke volume (approximately 10%), whereas with upright exercise, the increase in stroke volume is approximately 20% to 35%. With exercise, end-diastolic volume is unchanged or slightly decreased, but ejection fraction increases and end-systolic volume decreases. With imaging techniques, endocardial motion and myocardial wall thickening are augmented with an appearance of "hypercontractility" during and immediately following exercise.

IMAGING OF THE LEFT VENTRICLE

Qualitative Evaluation of Systolic Function

Both global and regional ventricular function can be evaluated with 2D echocardiography on a semiquantitative scale by an experienced observer. Overall left ventricular systolic function is evaluated best from multiple tomographic planes, typically

- parasternal long-axis,
- parasternal short-axis,
- apical four-chamber,
- apical two-chamber, and
- apical long-axis views.

Attention to image acquisition is needed to obtain adequate endocardial definition. The echocardiographer then integrates the degree of endocardial motion and wall thickening from these views to classify overall systolic function as normal, mildly reduced, moderately reduced, or severely reduced. Some experienced observers can estimate ejection fraction visually from 2D images with a reasonable correlation with ejection fractions measured quantitatively by echocardiography or other techniques. Typically, ejection fraction is estimated in intervals of 5% to 10% (i.e., 20%, 30%, 40%, and so on) or an estimated ejection fraction range is reported (e.g., 20% to 30%).

There are several other imaging parameters that are provide a qualitative measure of left ventricular systolic function. M-mode signs include

- the separation between the maximum anterior motion of the mitral leaflet and maximum posterior motion of the ventricular septum (E-point septal separation), and
- the degree of anteroposterior motion of the aortic root.

With normal systolic function, the anterior mitral leaflet opens to nearly fill the ventricular chamber resulting in little (0–5 mm) E-point septal separation. With systolic dysfunction, this distance is increased due to a combination of left ventricular dilation and reduced motion of the mitral valve because of low transmitral volume flow. Similarly, left ventricular systolic dysfunction results in reduced left atrial filling and emptying (low cardiac output), seen on M-mode as reduced anteroposterior motion of the aortic root.

On 2D echocardiography, the mitral annulus moves toward the ventricular apex in systole, with the magnitude of this motion proportional to the extent of shortening in ventricular length—a useful measure of overall left ventricular systolic function. Normal subjects have motion of the mitral annulus toward the apex ≥8 mm, with a mean value of 12 ± 2 mm in both four- and two-chamber views. The sensitivity of mitral annulus motion < 8 mm is 98% with a specificity of 82% for identification of an ejection fraction < 50%.

Qualitative evaluation of overall systolic function is a simple and highly predictive index that is of great clinical utility. On the other hand, several factors can limit the usefulness of this evaluation. First, the accuracy of the estimated ejection fraction is dependent on the experience of each observer. Second, inadequate endocardial definition can result in incorrect estimates of systolic function. Third, integration of data from multiple tomographic images can be difficult when the pattern of contraction is asynchronous (with conduction defects, pacers, postoperative septal motion) or when the pattern of contraction is asymmetric (with prior myocardial infarction or with ischemia), especially when dyskinesis is present. To some extent, these limitations are minimized by an experienced observer, optimal endocardial definition, and integration of data from multiple views. However, when possible, it is preferable to avoid the limitations of estimates of systolic function by performing quantitative measurements.

Regional ventricular function also can be evaluated by imaging in multiple tomographic planes. Most often, regional function is evaluated qualitatively by dividing the ventricle into segments corresponding to the coronary artery anatomy and then grading wall motion on a 1 to 4+ scale as normal (score = 1), hypokinetic (score = 2), akinetic (score = 3), or dyskinetic (score = 4). In some cases, hyperkinesis—that is, a compensatory increase in wall motion in regions remote from an acute myocardial infarction or the normal increase seen with exercise—also is scored. Evaluation of segmental wall motion is discussed in detail in Chapter 8.

Quantitative Evaluation of Left Ventricular Systolic Function

Dimensions and Volumes

Left ventricular short-axis dimensions and wall thickness are most accurately measured using 2D-guided M-mode echocardiography. The major advantage of M-mode echocardiography is high time resolution, which facilitates recognition of endocardial motion. Starting in a long-axis view, left ventricular measurements are made with the M-mode beam positioned just beyond the mitral leaflet tips (mitral chordal level), perpendicular to the long axis of the ventricle in a long-axis view, and centered in the short-axis view. The left ventricular posterior wall endocardium is identified on the M-mode recording as the most continuous line with the steepest systolic motion. The posterior wall epicardium is identified as the echo reflection immediately anterior to the pericardium. The septal endocardium again is identified as the steepest motion in systole with a continuous reflection through the cycle (see Fig. 2–22). On the right ventricular side of the septum, it is important to exclude any reflections due to right ventricular trabeculations. Conversely, a dark "midseptal" stripe often is noted and should not be confused with the endocardial borders. M-mode measurements are more accurate than 2D measurements because identification of the endocardial border on a still frame 2D image may be difficult.

Left ventricular wall thickness and dimensions are measured from the leading edge to leading edge of each interface of interest (American Society of Echocardiography recommendations) for optimal measurement accuracy. For example, ventricular internal dimensions are measured from the leading edge of the septal endocardium to the leading edge of the posterior wall endocardium. Normal values for these measurements are indicated in Table 6–2.

In addition to left ventricular wall thickness and internal dimensions (LVID) at end-diastole (d) and end-systole (s), fractional shortening can be calculated as

$$\text{Fractional shortening (\%)}$$
$$= (\text{LVID}_d - \text{LVID}_s)/\text{LVID}_d \times 100\% \tag{6-4}$$

Fractional shortening is a rough measurement of left ventricular systolic function, with the normal range being 25% to 45% (95% confidence limits).

A potential disadvantage of M-mode dimensions is that overestimation will occur if the beam

TABLE 6–1

Selected Studies Validating 2D-Echocardiographic LV Volume Measurements

First Author/Year	Volume/Method	n	r	Regression Equation	SEE	Standard of Reference
Teicholz/1974	Ejection fraction $V = [7.0/(2.4 + D)] \times D^3$	25	0.87	Echo = 0.61 angio + 0.01 mL		Biplane LV-angio
Schiller/1979	Modified Simpson's rule	30				
	Diastolic volume		0.80	Echo = 0.7 angio − 1 mL	15 mL	
	Systolic volume		0.90	Echo = 0.7 angio − 2 mL	8.5 mL	
	Ejection fraction		0.87	Echo = angio + 5	7.6%	
Folland/1979	Modified Simpson's rule	35				Single-plane angio
	Ejection fraction		0.78	Angio = 1.01 echo + 0.04	9.7%	Radionuclide
	Ejection fraction		0.75	Radionuclide = 0.75 echo + 0.07	8.7%	
Parisi/1979	Modified Simpson's rule	50				Single-plane angio
	Diastolic volume		0.82	Angio = 1.08 echo + 30 mL	39 mL	
	Systolic volume		0.90		29 mL	
	Ejection fraction		0.80		9%	
Gueret/1980	Modified Simpson's rule	11				Cineangiography in closed-chest dogs
	Diastolic volume		0.89	Cine = 0.88 echo + 22 mL	10 mL	1h S/P LAD occlusion
	Systolic volume		0.86	Cine = 0.95 echo + 11 mL	9 mL	
	Ejection fraction		0.92	Cine = 1.13 echo − 7.5%	5%	
Silverman/1980	Biplane area-length	20				Biplane angio
	Diastolic volume		0.96	Echo = 1.05 angio − 3.64		
	Systolic volume		0.91	Echo = 1.37 angio − 1.37		
	Ejection fraction		0.82	Echo = 0.82 angio + 0		
Wyatt/1980	Modified Simpson's rule	21				Directly measured fluid volume in fixed hearts
	2/3 area length		0.98	Echo = 1.0x − 0.7 mL	6.6 mL	
	Area-length (cylinder)		0.97	Echo = 1.0x − 8.9 mL	8.6 mL	
	Hemiellipsoid (bullet)		0.97	Echo = 1.49x − 13.4 mL	12.8 mL	
			0.97	Echo = 1.25x − 11.1 mL	10.9 mL	
Starling/1980	Simpson's rule	70				Single or biplane (n = 30) LV angio
	Diastolic rule		0.80	Echo = 0.66 angio + 42 mL	34 mL	
	Systolic volume		0.88	Echo = 0.72 angio + 18 mL	27 mL	
	Ejection fraction		0.90	Echo = 0.76 angio + 12%	7%	

Source/Year	Method	n	r	Regression equation	SEE	Comparison method
Quinones/1981	Simplified method	55	0.93		6.7%	Radionuclide
	Ejection fraction		0.91		7.4%	Angio
Tortoledo/1983	Simplified method	52				Single-plane angio
	Diastolic volume		0.88	Angio = 1.07 echo − 7.3 mL	28 mL	
	Systolic volume		0.94	Angio = 1.0 echo + 1.3 mL	19 mL	
	Ejection fraction		0.92	Angio = 0.93 echo + 3.5 mL	7%	
Weiss/1983	Modified Simpson's rule (15–19 "slices")	52	0.97		6.6% (mean % error)	Direct volume measurement in isolated ejecting dog hearts
Erbel/1985	Simpson's rule	46				Single-plane angio
	Diastolic volume		0.91	Echo = 0.66 angio + 0.8 mL	26 mL	
	Systolic volume		0.94	Echo = 0.57 angio + 18 mL	19 mL	
	Ejection fraction		0.80	Echo = 0.61 angio + 13%	9%	
Zoghbi/1990	Echo-tilt method	24				Biplane angio
	Diastolic volume		0.92	Angio = 0.80 echo + 37 mL	23 mL	
	Systolic volume		0.96	Angio = 0.97 echo − 1 mL	16 mL	
	Ejection fraction		0.82	Angio = 1.17 echo − 4	10%	
Smith/1992	TEE Simpson's rule	36				LV angio (single-plane)
	Diastolic volume		0.85	Echo = 0.75 angio + 0.2 mL	42 mL	
	Systolic volume		0.94	Echo = 0.78 angio − 3.5 mL	22 mL	
	Ejection fraction		0.85	Echo = 0.82 angio + 9.0 mL	8%	
Zile/1992	Prolate ellipsoid using constant long-axis/short-axis ratio	25				LV angio in dog model
	Diastolic volume		0.96	Echo = 1.0 angio − 1.8 mL		
	Systolic volume		0.95	Echo = 0.98 angio − 0.65 mL		

Data from Teicholz LE et al: N Engl J Med 291:1220–1226, 1974; Schiller NB et al: Circulation 60:547–555, 1979; Folland ED et al: Circulation 60:760–766, 1979; Parisi AF et al: Clin Cardiol 2:257–263, 1979; Gueret P et al: Circulation 62:1308–1318, 1980; Silverman NH et al: Circulation 62:548–557, 1980; Wyatt HL et al: Circulation 61:1119–1125, 1980; Starling MR et al: Circulation 63:1075–1084, 1981; Quinones MA et al: Circulation 64:744–753, 1981; Tortoledo FA et al: Circulation 67:579–584, 1983; Weiss JL et al: Circulation 67:889–895, 1983; Erbel R et al: Circulation 67:205–215, 1983; Zoghbi WA et al: J Am Coll Cardiol 15:610–617, 1990; Smith MD et al: J Am Coll Cardiol 19:1213–1222, 1992; Zile MR et al: J Am Coll Cardiol 20:986–993, 1992.

SEE, standard error of the estimate; angio, left ventricular angiography; LAD, left anterior descending coronary artery.

TABLE 6-2

Selected Studies Validating 3D-Echocardiographic LV Volume Measurements

First Author/Year	Method	n	r	Regression Equation	SEE	Standard of Reference
Nessly/1991	Canine model	33	0.86	Echo = 0.83 RN + 4 mL	6 mL	RN angiography
Kuroda/1991	In vitro phantom					
	Pull-back reconstruction		0.99	Echo = 1.1x − 10 mL	5.8 mL	True volume by weight
	Rotational reconstruction		0.99	Echo = 1.0x − 7 mL	6.5 mL	
Handschumacher/1993	Ventricular phantoms		0.99	Echo = 0.96x + 2.2 mL	2.7 mL	Direct volumes
	Gel-filled excised ventricles		0.99	Echo = 0.99x + 0.11 mL	5.9 mL	
Gopal/1993	Normal adults	15	EDV 0.92	Echo = 0.84 MRI + 22 mL	7 mL	MRI
			ESV 0.81	Echo = 0.51 MRI + 18 mL	4 mL	
Sapin/1993	Excised porcine hearts	25	0.99	y = 1.02 Echo + 3.7 mL	7.1 mL	Direct volumes
Sapin/1994	Patients (mean age 48 yr)	35	EDV 0.97		11.0 mL	LV angiography
			ESV 0.98		10.2 mL	
Jiang/1995	In vitro phantoms	10	0.99		3.2–6.1 mL	Direct volumes
	Autopsy hearts with LV aneurysms	12	0.99		3.4–4.2 mL	
	Canine LV aneurysm model	19	EDV 0.99	4.3 mL		
			ESV 0.99		3.5 mL	
Gopal/1997	Patients with abnormal LV	30	EDV 0.90		31.8 mL	MRI
			ESV 0.93		24.1 mL	
Altmann/1997	Children	12	EDV 0.98		8.7 mL	MRI
			ESV 0.98		5.6 mL	
Leotta/1997	In vitro phantom	12	1.00	y = 1.00x − 0.6 mL	1.3 mL	Direct volumes
	In vitro heart	5	1.00	y = 1.02x − 1.3 mL	0.4 mL	Direct volumes
	In vivo (human)	20	0.99	3D-SV = 1.18DOP − 17.9 mL	2.8 mL	Doppler SV

First author/year	Subjects	N	Correlation	Regression equation	Result	Modality
Kuehl/1998	Patients	24	EDV 0.9 ESV 0.94 EF 0.93	$y = 0.87x + 2.2$ $y = 0.96x - 0.6$ $y = 0.96x - 2.0$	23.9 17.2 7.0 mL	Angio
Mele/1998	Patients	50	EDV 0.95 ESV 0.96 EF 0.92	$y = 0.93x + 9.1$ $y = 0.94x + 4.3$ $y = 0.90x + 4.1$	15.2 11.4 6.2 mL	Angio, RN angiography, MRI
Nosir/1998	Patients	41	EF 0.99			RN angiography
Qin/2000	Patients (13 with LV aneurysms)	29	LV Volumes r = 0.97		Mean difference −28 mL	MRI
Teupe/2001	Fixed pig hearts	20	LV Volumes r = 0.99		3.0–5.5 mL	Anatomic volumes
Schmidt/2001	Explanted sheep hearts	11	LV Volumes r = 0.99	$Y = 1.31 + 0.98x$	2.2 mL	Known volumes
Lee/2003	Patients	25	EDV 0.99 ESV 0.99 EF 0.92		11.3 mL 10.2 mL 6%	MRI
Kawai/2003	Patients	15	EDV 0.94 ESV 0.96 EF 0.93	$y = 0.82x + 5.1$	EDV 21.6 mL ESV 14.8 mL EF 7.6%	SPECT

Data from Nessly ML et al: J Cardiothorac Vasc Anesth 5:40–45, 1991; Kuroda T et al: J Echocardiography 4:475–484, 1991; Handschumacher MD et al: J Am Coll Cardiol 21:743–753, 1993; Gopal AS et al: J Am Coll Cardiol 22:258–270, 1993; Sapin PM et al: J Am Coll Cardiol 22:1530, 1993; Sapin PM et al: J Am Coll Cardiol 24:1054, 1994; Jiang L et al: Circulation 91:222, 1995; Gopal AS et al: J Am Soc Echocardiogr, 10:853, 1997; Altman K et al: Am J Cardiol 80:1060–1065, 1997; Leotta DF et al: J Am Soc Echocardiogr 10:830, 1997; Kuehl et al: J Am Soc Echocardiogr 11:1113, 1998; Mele et al: 11:1001, 1998. Nosir et al: J Am Soc Echocardiogr 11:620, 1998; Qin JX et al: J Am Coll Cardiol 36: 900–907, 2000; Teupe C et al: Int J Cardiovasc Imagin 17:99–105, 2001; Schmidt MA et al: J Am Soc Echocardiogr 14:1–10, 2001; Lee D et al: J Am Soc Echocardiogr 14:1001–1009, 2001; Kawai J et al: J Am Soc Echocardiogr 16:110–115, 2003.

SV. Stroke volume; MRI, magnetic resonance imaging; IV, left ventricle; DOP, Doppler; RN, radionuclide; EDV, end-diastolic volume; ESV, end-systolic volume; SPECT, single-photon emission computed tomography.

is oblique with respect to the long or short axis of the ventricle. On the other hand, underestimation can occur if the M-line is not centered in the ventricular chamber. Both these potential errors can be avoided by using 2D imaging in both long- and short-axis planes to verify the M-mode beam orientation. With nonsymmetric disease processes (ischemic cardiac disease) or with alterations in left ventricular shape (dilated cardiomyopathy), M-mode measurements at the base may not be representative of overall left ventricular dimensions or function.

Two-dimensional echocardiographic calculation of ventricular volumes is based on endocardial border tracing at end-diastole and end-systole in one or more tomographic planes (Table 6–1). Prerequisites for quantitative evaluation with 2D echocardiography are

■ nonoblique standard image planes or image planes of known orientation relative to the long and short axis of the left ventricle,
■ inclusion of the apex of the ventricle,
■ adequate endocardial definition, and
■ accurate identification of the endocardial borders.

In some patients, image quality is inadequate for endocardial definition. Even when image quality is adequate, endocardial borders must be traced manually by an experienced physician or sonographer for accurate quantitation of left ventricular systolic function by echocardiography. Because 2D echocardiography is a tomographic technique, left ventricular volume calculations are based on geometric assumptions about the shape of the left ventricle. Obviously, accuracy in individual patients will be highest with methods that have the fewest geometric assumptions and that use data from multiple tomographic images.

The greatest accuracy would be expected with three-dimensional (3D) reconstructions that use data from multiple tomographic images of known orientation and make no geometric assumptions (Table 6–2). However, current disadvantages of 3D echocardiography include acquisition times, the need for manual border tracing, and either an incomplete data set that does not include the entire left ventricle or cumbersome 3D locator systems, limiting widespread clinical utility for quantitative data analysis (see Suggested Readings 6–9). Simpler methods, based on one to three image planes, provide reasonably accurate information with less time-consuming data collection. These simpler methods are the current standard for clinical practice.

The geometric assumptions for calculating left ventricular volumes from tomographic data range from a simple ellipsoid shape to complex hemicylindrical hemiellipsoid shapes (Fig. 6–5). For each approach, left ventricular end-diastolic and end-systolic volumes are calculated from the corresponding tracings at that phase of the cardiac cycle. The single-plane ellipsoid method uses the length L and 2D area A of a single long-axis view. Left ventricular volume is calculated assuming an ellipsoid shape as:

Single-Plane Ellipsoid

$$V = 8A^2/3\pi L \qquad (6\text{–}5)$$

This formula also can be written as

$$V = 0.85A^2/L \qquad (6\text{–}6)$$

or

Area-Length Method

$$V = \left(\frac{5}{6}A^2\right)\Big/L \qquad (6\text{–}7)$$

The biplane ellipsoid model uses a long-axis view only for length L and area A_L, and incorporates an orthogonal short-axis diameter D and area A_s:

Biplane Ellipsoid

$$V = (\pi L/6)(4A_s/\pi D)(4A_L/\pi L) \qquad (6\text{–}8)$$

or

$$V = (\pi/6)D_1 D_2 L \qquad (6\text{–}9)$$

where D_1 and D_2 are orthogonal short-axis diameters. The hemicylindrical hemiellipsoid model assumes that the base of the ventricle is approximated by a cylinder and the apex by an ellipsoid. Volume is calculated from a long-axis length L and the cross-sectional area A_m of an orthogonal short-axis view at the midpapillary level:

Hemisphere Cylinder

$$V = [(A_m)(L/2)] + [(2/3)(A_m)(L/2)] \qquad (6\text{–}10)$$

or

"Bullet" Formula

$$V = 5/6 \times AL \qquad (6\text{–}11)$$

In the presence of regional wall motion abnormalities, all these methods will be less accurate, since if the region of abnormal wall motion is included in the dimension or area measurements, volumes will be overestimated. Apical biplane methods are more robust in this setting, using summation of a series of disks from apex to base (often called Simpson's rule):

Simpson's Rule

$$V = \sum_{n=20} [\text{area} \times (L/20)] \qquad (6\text{–}12)$$

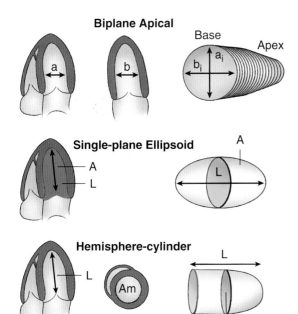

Biplane Apical

a   b

Base   Apex
a_i b_i

Single-plane Ellipsoid

A
L

A
L

Hemisphere-cylinder

L

Am

L

Am

FIGURE 6–5. Examples of three formulas for left ventricular volume calculations showing the 2D echocardiographic views and measurements on the left and the geometric model on the right. For the biplane apical method, endocardial borders are traced in apical four-chamber and two-chamber views which are used to define a series of orthogonal diameters (*a* and *b*). A "Simpson's rule" assumption based on stacked disks is used to calculate volume. The single-plane ellipsoid method uses the 2D area (A) and length (L) in a single (usually apical four-chamber) view. The hemisphere-cylinder method uses a short-axis endocardial area at the midventricular level (Am) and a long-axis length (L). For each method, both end-diastolic and end-systolic measurements are needed for calculation of end-diastolic and end-systolic volumes, respectively, and for ejection fraction determination.

or a modified Simpson's rule approximation, which uses three parallel "slices" of the ventricle to obtain volume:

Modified Simpson's Rule

$$V = (A_1 + A_2)h + (A_3 h/2) + (\pi h^3/6) \quad (6\text{–}13)$$

where $h = L/3$, A_1 = mitral valve short-axis area, A_2 = papillary muscle level area, and A_3 = apex short-axis area.

Ejection Fraction

For each of these formulas, end-diastolic volume is calculated from end-diastolic images and end-systolic volumes from end-systolic images. Stroke volume, then, is the difference between EDV and ESV [Eq. (6–2)], while ejection fraction (EF) is calculated with Eq. (6–1).

Other modifications and simplifications of left ventricular volume formulas have been suggested

(see Table 6–1 and Suggested Reading). The ASE recommends use of biplane apical views with a modified Simpson's rule approach:

Biplane Apical Volume

$$V = (\pi/4)\sum_{i=1}^{20} a_i b_i \times (L/20) \quad (6\text{–}14)$$

where the length L of the ventricle is divided into 20 disks ($i = 1$ to $i = 20$) from base to apex with a diameter of each disk determined in two apical views (*a* and *b*). The recommended alternate approach (when two views are not available) is the single-plane ellipsoid formula, Eq. (6–5). An example of the 2D images needed for left ventricular volume calculation is shown in Figure 6–6.

Left Ventricular Mass

Left ventricular mass can be estimated from M-mode dimensions of septal thickness (ST), posterior wall thickness (PWT), and left ventricular internal dimensions (LVID) at end-diastole. Note that the original description of this method by Reichek and Devereux used PENN convention measurements with the endocardial echos included in wall thickness and excluded from chamber dimensions (rather than leading edge to leading edge). If the ASE recommended diastolic measurements are used, a correction factor is needed. The formula then is

Left ventricular mass = $0.80 \times$
$$\left[1.04(ST + PWT + LVID)^3 - LVID^3\right]$$
$$+ 0.6\,g \quad (6\text{–}15)$$

On 2D or 3D echocardiography, left ventricular mass theoretically can be determined by tracing epicardial borders to calculate the total ventricular volume (walls plus chamber), subtracting the volumes determined from endocardial border tracing, and then multiplying by the specific density of myocardium:

LV mass =
1.05(total volume – chamber volume)
$$(6\text{–}16)$$

However, epicardial definition rarely is adequate for this approach. Instead, mean wall thickness is calculated from epicardial (A_1) and endocardial (A_2) cross-sectional areas in a short-axis view at the papillary muscle level. The short-axis radius b is calculated as

$$b = \sqrt{A_2/\pi} \quad (6\text{–}17)$$

Mean wall thickness t, then, is

$$t = \left(\sqrt{A_1/\pi}\right) - b \quad (6\text{–}18)$$

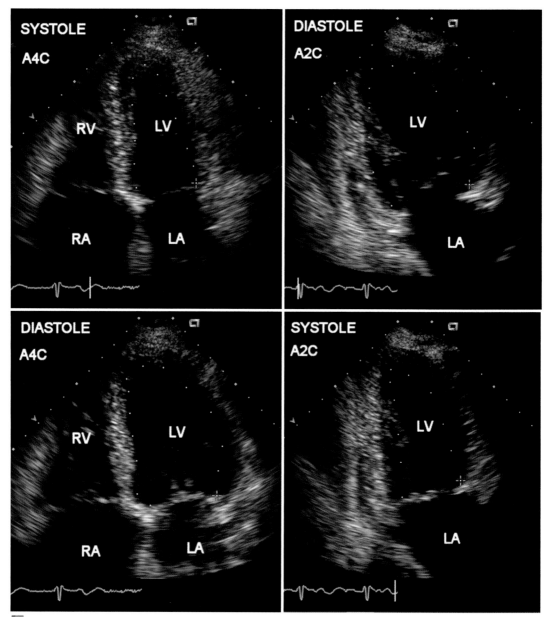

FIGURE 6–6. Examples of apical four-chamber (*left*) and two-chamber (*right*) views at end-diastole (*top*) and end-systole (*bottom*), showing the traced endocardial borders for calculation of ventricular volumes.

and the cross-sectional area of the myocardium (Am) in this short-axis view is

$$Am = A_1 - A_2 \qquad (6\text{–}19)$$

Myocardial mass is calculated from these measurements plus the left ventricular length L from the level of the short-axis plane to the base (d) and to the apex (a) such that $d + a = L$. Using an area-length formula, as

$$\text{LV mass} = 1.05\left\{\left[\frac{5}{6} A_1 (a + d + t)\right]\right.$$
$$\left. - \left[\frac{5}{6} A_2 (a + d)\right]\right\} \qquad (6\text{–}20)$$

The images needed for LV mass calculation are shown in Figure 6–7.

Left Ventricular Wall Stress

Estimates of left ventricular wall stress can be calculated from M-mode data in combination with pressure data. Meridional stress σ_m is

$$\sigma_m = P(LVID)/[4PWT(1 + LVID/PWT)] \tag{6-21}$$

where P = left ventricular pressure, LVID = left ventricular internal dimensions, and PWT = posterior wall thickness. A simpler approach to estimating wall stress is to calculate the relative wall thickness (RWT):

$$RWT = (2 \times PWT)/LVID \tag{6-22}$$

which is a useful index for evaluation of patients with left ventricular hypertrophy.

In addition, both meridional and circumferential stress can be calculated from 2D echocardiographic images in combination with ventricular pressure measurements. Meridional wall stress σ_m is calculated from left ventricular peak pressure P, the myocardial area A_m, and cavity area A_c in a short-axis view at the papillary muscle level as (Fig. 6–8):

$$\sigma_m = 1.33P(A_m/A_c) \times 10^3 \, dyn/cm^2 \tag{6-23}$$

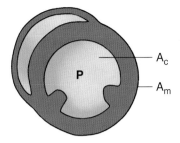

$$\sigma_m = 1.33P(A_m/A_c) \times 10^3 \, dynes/cm^2$$

▐ **FIGURE 6–8.** Schematic diagram of the measurements needed for calculation of meridional wall stress or σ_m. In a short-axis view at the papillary muscle level, the cavity area (Ac), and myocardial area (Am) at end-systole are measured in combination with left ventricular pressure (P).

Circumferential stress σ_c can be calculated using these variables plus ventricular length L from an apical four-chamber view as

$$\sigma_c = \frac{1.33P\sqrt{A_c}}{\sqrt{A_m + A_c} - \sqrt{A_c}} \left[\frac{\frac{4(A_c)^{3/2}}{\pi L^2}}{\sqrt{A_m + A_c} - \sqrt{A_c}} \right] \tag{6-24}$$

Measures of wall stress are most useful in ventricular pressure or volume overload states (such as hypertension, aortic stenosis, aortic or mitral regurgitation) to evaluate left ventricular systolic function.

Technical Aspects

Endocardial Definition

Accurate identification of the ventricular endocardium is key in the echocardiographic evaluation of left ventricular systolic function. Endocardial definition is affected by the physics of ultrasound instrumentation, by anatomic factors, and by technical factors, including the skill of the sonographer. The endocardial-ventricular cavity interface is curved from any imaging window, so the endocardium appears as a thin, bright line where it is perpendicular to the ultrasound beam (axial resolution) but as a broad, "blurred" line where the beam is parallel to the endocardial-ventricular cavity interface (lateral resolution). As for other ultrasound targets, lateral resolution is depth-dependent. In addition, there may be "dropout" of signals due to attenuation, a parallel intercept angle, acoustic shadowing, or reverberations.

Anatomically, the endocardium is not a smooth surface but has numerous trabeculations that are

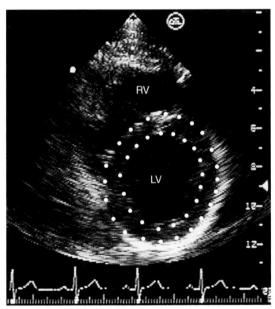

▐ **FIGURE 6–7.** Parasternal short-axis view at the papillary muscle level with tracing of epicardial and endocardial borders at end-diastole for calculation of left ventricular mass, in combination with a left ventricular length measurement from an apical approach.

most prominent at the left ventricular apex. The ultrasound beam is reflected from the inner edge of these trabeculations so that the "endocardium" identified by echocardiography differs from the "endocardium" identified by contrast ventriculography, in which contrast material fills these trabeculations, outlining their outer edge.

Several technical factors affect endocardial definition during image acquisition, and meticulous examination technique is needed for optimal image quality. First, acoustic access can be optimizing by

▪ patient positioning,
▪ use of an echo stretcher with an apical cut-out,
▪ having the patient suspend respiration, and
▪ careful adjustment of transducer position.

Instrument settings can dramatically affect image quality, including

▪ transducer frequency,
▪ gain,
▪ gray-scale settings,
▪ focal depth, and
▪ tissue harmonic imaging.

Endocardial borders are traced from digitally acquired images using the real-time motion of the images to aid in identification of the endocardial border during the tracing process. End-diastolic and end-systolic images are traced on the same cardiac cycle with end-diastole defined as onset of the QRS complex and end-systole defined as minimal ventricular volume. For the apical biplane approach, the patient is positioned in a steep left lateral position, using a stretcher with an apical cut-out, to avoid foreshortening the ventricular apex. A higher-frequency transducer is used for optimal image quality, provided penetration is adequate, and the focal depth of the transducer is adjusted to the depth of interest. The sector depth and width should be adjusted to maximize the size of the left ventricle on the screen and to optimize frame rate. Tissue harmonic imaging improves endocardial definition in most patients. In addition, the patient is asked to suspend respiration, while avoiding a Valsalva maneuver, at the phase of respiration where image quality is optimal. When endocardial definition remains poor despite these measures, use of an intravenous contrast agent to opacify the left ventricle should be considered.

The trained human observer remains the most accurate means for endocardial border tracing, limiting the wide application of quantitative methods because manual tracing of endocardial borders at end-diastole and end-systole in at least two views remains a tedious and time-consuming task. In many cases, identification of the endo-cardium requires analysis of the moving image using both the cine-loop and frame-by-frame features of the system to assist in identification of the border as the bright linear echo reflection that moves with the cardiac cycle and is spatially continuous. In the future, automatic edge-detection programs or other approaches to determination of area changes may alleviate this problem.

Geometric Assumptions

In addition to the geometric assumptions of the mathematical models themselves, quantitation of left ventricular volumes depends on accurate measurement of ventricular lengths, diameters, and cross-sectional areas. Two-dimensional echo views that foreshorten the left ventricle will result in underestimation of left ventricular length, whereas oblique short-axis views will overestimate the cross-sectional area of the chamber. Adequate apical views require a steep left lateral decubitus position with an apical cutout in the echo-stretcher mattress to obtain the true long axis of the chamber. Short-axis views should appear circular if perpendicular to the long axis of the left ventricle.

Respiratory motion and cardiac motion within the chest during the cardiac cycle further confound the geometric assumptions of left ventricular volume calculations. The effect of respiratory motion of the heart relative to the transducer can be avoided by measuring beats at the same phase of respiration or by having the patient briefly suspend respiration during data acquisition. In some cases, optimal images are obtained when the patient suspends respiration after taking in a small breath, rather than at end-expiration. It is more difficult to correct for the motion of the heart itself using a tomographic imaging procedure. Cardiac translation (movement of the heart in the chest), rotation (movement around the long axis of the heart), and torsion (unequal rotational motion of the heart) can result in images of different segments of the left ventricle during systole and diastole, even with a fixed image plane. While cardiac motion has only a limited effect on the accuracy of left ventricular volume calculations, it can have a pronounced effect on quantitative evaluation of regional ventricular function, as discussed in Chapter 8.

Accuracy and Reproducibility

Qualitative comparison of left ventricular systolic function from different studies on the same patient is facilitated by the digital cine-loop side-by-side format used in most laboratories. With this approach, a single high-quality beat is captured in digital format (either the entire cardiac cycle or just the systolic phase). The study to be compared is captured similarly with the same number of frames in the cine-loop so that when the images are played side by side, heart rates are "matched" temporally. The advantage of this approach is that the same view can be examined as long as is needed for careful qualitative (or quantitative) evaluation. This approach is particularly useful for evaluation of regional ventricular function. Of course, the influence of loading conditions on left ventricular systolic function still must be considered when comparing studies performed at different time points in a patient's clinical course.

In most reported series, intraobserver variability for left ventricular volumes ranges from 5% to 10%. Interobserver variability is greater, ranging from 7% to 25% for ventricular volumes. Since ejection fraction is a calculated percentage, reproducibility is better, with variability of approximately 10%. These values are similar to reported variability for ventricular volumes and ejection fraction determined by contrast or radionuclide ventriculography. Note that variability between studies in an individual patient includes

- physiologic variability (loading condition, heart rate, volume states),
- image acquisition variability (endocardial definition, image orientation), and
- measurement variability in tracing the endothelial borders.

In a careful study designed to assess measurement variability for 2D echo left ventricular volumes, it was concluded that a significant change between studies is a change in ejection fraction >2%, end-diastolic volume >2%, and end-systolic volume >5% (see Suggested Reading 5).

DOPPLER EVALUATION OF LEFT VENTRICULAR SYSTOLIC FUNCTION

Stroke Volume Calculation

Doppler echocardiographic evaluation of left ventricular systolic function usually is based on calculation of stroke volume and cardiac output (Table 6–3). Using Doppler and 2D echo data, stroke volume (SV in cubic centimeters or milliliters) is calculated as cross-sectional area (CSA in cm^2) of flow times the velocity-time integral (VTI in cm) of flow through that region:

$$SV = CSA \times VTI \qquad (6\text{--}25)$$

Conceptually, the left ventricle ejects a volume of blood into the cylindrical aorta on each beat (Fig. 6–9). The base of this cylinder is the systolic cross-sectional area of the outflow tract, while its height is the distance the average blood cell traveled during ejection for that beat. This distance is

expressed as the integral of the Doppler systolic velocity-time curve, since velocity is the first derivative of distance. Alternatively, this distance also can be thought of as mean velocity (cm/s) multiplied by ejection duration(s). Again, since the volume of a cylinder is base times height, stroke volume is cross-sectional area multiplied by the velocity-time integral.

This approach to stroke volume calculation depends on several basic assumptions.

First, the cross-sectional area must be measured accurately. Typically, diameter is measured and 2D area calculated as $\pi(D/2)^2$ based on the assumption of a circular geometry. Deviations from a circular geometry or changes in cross-sectional area during the flow period will result in inaccuracies unless appropriate corrections are included in the calculations. Small errors in 2D diameter measurements become large errors in cross-sectional area calculations because of the quadratic relationship between these variables. Using a transducer orientation and instrument settings that maximize image quality, performing measurements based on axial (rather than lateral) resolution, performing diameter measurements in two orthogonal planes (when possible), and averaging several beats can help minimize this source of error.

Second, the pattern of flow is assumed to be laminar, and (in most clinical applications) the spatial flow profile across the flow stream is assumed to be relatively flat. These assumptions ensure that the velocity curve represents the spatial (as well as temporal) average flow in that region. The validity of the assumption of laminar flow in the great vessels and across normal cardiac valves is demonstrated by the narrow band of velocities and smooth spectral signal seen on pulsed Doppler echo recordings. A flat-flow profile also is a reasonable assumption at the inlet to the great vessels and across the valve planes due to the effects of geometric convergence and acceleration. A flat-flow velocity profile can be confirmed by moving the sample volume across the flow stream in two orthogonal views to demonstrate uniform velocities at the center and the edges of the flow stream.

Third, the Doppler signal is assumed to have been recorded at a parallel intercept angle to flow, resulting in an accurate velocity measurement (based on a $\cos\theta = 1$ in the Doppler equation). In practical terms, the sonographer aligns the Doppler beam in the presumed direction of flow and then carefully moves the ultrasound beam across the image plane and in the elevational plane to obtain the highest-velocity signal, indicating the most parallel alignment with flow. Note that the

TABLE 6–3

Selected Studies Validating Doppler Volume Flow Measurement

First Author/ Year	Volume Flow Site/Method	n	r	Regression Equation	SEE	Standard of Reference
Huntsman/ 1983	Ascending aorta	100	0.94	DOP = 0.95x + 0.38	0.58 L/min	TD CO
Fisher/1983	Mitral leaflets	52	0.97	DOP = 0.98x + 0.02	0.23 L/min	Roller pump
Meijboom/ 1983	Mitral leaflets	26	0.99	DOP = 0.97x + 0.07	0.13 L/min	EM flow
	RVOT	26	0.99	DOP = 0.96x + 0.11	0.16 L/min	Roller pump
Lewis/1984	Mitral annulus	35	0.96	TD = 0.91x + 5.1	5.9 mL	TD SV
	LVOT	39	0.95	TD = 0.91x + 7.8	6.4 mL	TD SV
Stewart/1985	Mitral leaflets	29	0.97	DOP = 0.98x + 0.3	0.3 L/min	Roller pump
	Aortic annulus	33	0.98	DOP = 1.06x + 0.2	0.3 L/min	Roller pump
	Pulmonary annulus	30	0.93	DOP = 0.89x + 0.4	0.5 L/min	Roller pump
Bouchard/ 1987	Aortic leaflets	41	0.95	DOP = 0.97x + 1.7	7 mL	TD SV
Dittmann/1987	Mitral annulus	40	0.86	DOP = 0.88 + 1.75	0.80 L/min	TD CO
	LVOT (M-mode)	40	0.93	DOP = 0.94x + 0.44	0.59 L/min	TD CO
DeZuttere/ 1988	Mitral orifice (instantaneous)	30	0.91	DOP = 0.92x + 0.35	0.53 L/min	TD CO
Hoit/1988	Mitral leaflets	48	0.93	DOP = 1.1x − 0.45	0.36 L/min	TD CO
Otto/1988	LVOT (proximal to stenotic aortic valve	52	0.91	DOP = 1.0x + 0.03	0.25 L/min	EM flow and timed collection
Burwash/1993	LVOT (proximal to aortic stenosis	75	0.86	CO = 0.92 DOP + 0.26	0.50 L/min	Transit-time flow probe
Lefrant/2000	Ascending aorta	58 pts (314 paired data)	0.84	DOP = 0.84TD + 1.39		TD CO
Gentles/2001	Ascending aorta	20 children with complex CHD	0.96	DOP = 0.98Fick − 0.08 mL		Fick CO
Chandraratna/ 2002	Pulmonary artery (continuous)	50 ICU pts	0.92	DOP = 0.93TD + 0.60	0.7 L/min	TD CO

Data from Huntsman et al: Circulation 67:593–601, 1983; Fisher et al: Circulation 67:872–877, 1983; Meijboom et al: Circulation 68:437–445, 1983; Lewis et al: Circulation 70:425–431, 1984; Stewart et al: J Am Coll Cardiol 6:653–662, 1985; Bouchard et al: J Am Coll Cardiol 9:75–83, 1987; Dittman et al: J Am Coll Cardiol 10:818–823, 1987; DeZuttere et al: J Am Coll Cardiol 11:343–350, 1988; Hoit et al: Am J Cardiol 62:131–135, 1988; Otto et al: Circulation 78:435–441, 1988; Burwash et al: Am J Physiol 265 (Heart Circ Physiol 34):1734, 1993; Lefrant et al: Intensive Care Med 26: 693–697, 2000; Gentles et al: J Ultrasound Med 20: 365–370, 2001; Chandraratna PA et al: J Am Soc Echocardiogr 15:1381–1386, 2002. RVOT, right ventricular outflow tract; LVOT, left ventricular outflow tract; CO, cardiac output; EM, electromagnetic; TD, thermodilution; DOP, Doppler; SEE, standard error of the estimate.

optimal window for Doppler interrogation is when the ultrasound beam and flow stream are parallel, while the optimal window for diameter measurement is when the ultrasound beam and tissue-blood interfaces are perpendicular.

Fourth, it is crucial that the diameter and velocity measurements be made at the same anatomic site since the cross-sectional area and flow velocity curves must be temporally and spatially congruent for accurate volume flow rate calculations. As the cross-sectional area of flow narrows or expands, flow velocity will increase or decrease correspondingly so that conjoining information from two different anatomic sites will result in erroneous stroke volume data. Similarly, dynamic changes in stroke volume occur with changes in

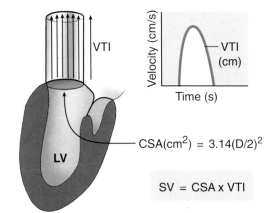

$$CSA(cm^2) = 3.14(D/2)^2$$

$$SV = CSA \times VTI$$

▌ **FIGURE 6–9.** Doppler stroke volume calculation. The cross-sectional area (CSA) of flow is calculated as a circle based on a 2D echo diameter (D) measurement. The length of the cylinder of blood ejected through this cross-sectional area on a single beat is the velocity-time integral (VTI) of the Doppler curve. Stroke volume (SV) then is calculated as CSA × VTI.

heart rate, loading conditions, exercise, etc. so that measurements made at disparate times cannot be combined. In clinical practice, diameter and velocity recordings are made in close sequence and are repeated if there is any question of an interval physiologic change.

Sites for Stroke Volume Measurement

Stroke volume can be measured by this approach at any intracardiac site where both cross-sectional area and the flow velocity integral can be recorded given the assumptions of laminar flow and a flat flow profile.

Left Ventricular Outflow

Left ventricular stroke volume can be measured in the aorta either at the aortic valve leaflet tips or in the ascending aorta. While some would argue which anatomic level (ascending aorta or leaflet tips) should be used, measurements at each of these levels can be accurate provided that diameter and flow velocity are measured at the same anatomic site. Ascending aortic diameter is measured from a parasternal long-axis view, and the flow velocity curve is recorded from either an apical or a suprasternal notch window. If continuous-wave Doppler ultrasound is used, the highest velocities along the path of the beam will be recorded, so the narrowest segment of the aorta (the sinotubular junction) should be used for diameter measurements. Alternatively, a circular orifice area can be calculated from an M-mode diameter of aortic leaflet opening, and pulsed

Doppler can be used to record the flow velocity in the aortic orifice itself. Note that if aortic valve disease is present, stroke volume measurement in the ascending aorta will be inaccurate due to non-laminar flow distal to the valve.

Measurement of stroke volume in the left ventricular outflow tract, at the aortic annulus just proximal to the valve leaflets, offers the advantages that (1) flow remains laminar proximal to a stenosis (allowing transaortic stroke volume calculations in patients with aortic valve disease) and (2) the needed data can be recorded in nearly all patients. Left ventricular outflow tract diameter is measured in a parasternal long-axis view parallel and immediately adjacent to the aortic valve, in midsystole, from the septal endocardium to the leading edge of the anterior mitral leaflet (Fig. 6–10). Pulsed Doppler is used from an apical approach to record the velocity curve, using the closing click of the aortic valve to ensure that the sample volume is located at the annulus (the same site as the diameter measurement). When aortic stenosis is present, the small region of flow convergence proximal to the narrowed aortic valve is avoided by moving the sample volume slightly apically until a narrow spectral width is seen at the velocity peak.

Mitral Valve

Transmitral stroke volume can be calculated by one of two basic approaches. The standard approach to transmitral stroke volume determination postulates that the mitral annulus is the limiting cross-sectional flow area, with the leaflets moving passively in response to the flow stream. Transmitral stroke volume is calculated as the product of the cross-sectional annulus area and the velocity-time integral of flow recorded at the mitral annulus level (Fig. 6–11). The mitral annulus is assumed to be circular, using a parasternal long-axis diameter, or, more accurately, elliptical, using an apical four-chamber view for the major axis of the ellipse and the long-axis view for the minor axis.

An alternate approach, given the complex motion of the mitral leaflets in diastole, is to use a "mean" mitral orifice area derived from the maximal 2D opening of the mitral valve in early diastole corrected for the mean degree of M-mode leaflet separation throughout diastole. Transmitral flow is recorded with pulsed Doppler at the leaflet tips. Although accurate, this approach is tedious to perform in the clinical setting and is rarely used.

Right Side of the Heart

In the right side of the heart, stroke volume can be calculated by analogous methods in the

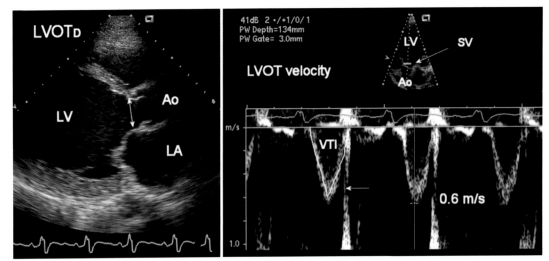

■ **FIGURE 6–10.** Examples of left ventricular outflow tract diameter measurement from a parasternal long-axis view (*left*) and the pulsed Doppler recording of left ventricular outflow just proximal to the aortic valve from an apical approach (*right*) for stroke volume calculation in a patient with dilated cardiomyopathy. The aortic valve closing click (*arrow*) on the outflow tract velocity recording ensures that the sample volume (SV) location is immediately adjacent to the valve, corresponding with the site of outflow tract diameter measurement.

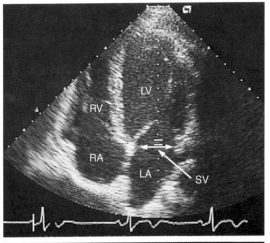

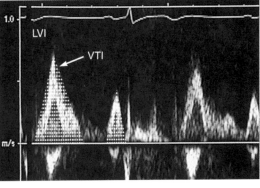

■ **FIGURE 6–11.** *Top:* Example of mitral annulus diameter measurement (*arrow*) in an apical four-chamber view with the sample volume (SV) positioned at the mitral annulus. *Bottom:* The pulsed Doppler left ventricular inflow signal is recorded for transmitral stroke volume calculation.

pulmonary artery or across the tricuspid valve (Fig. 6–12). In adult patients, use of the pulmonary artery site may be limited by poor image quality resulting in unobtainable or inaccurate pulmonary artery diameter measurements. However, from a transesophageal echocardiography approach, pulmonary artery flow and diameter often can be measured.

Differences in Transvalvular Volume Flow Rates

In a normal heart, stroke volume across each of the four valves is equal, and measurement at more than one site only serves as an internal accuracy check. However, in the presence of valvular regurgitation or an intracardiac shunt, calculation of stroke volume at two intracardiac sites allows quantitation of the degree of regurgitation or pulmonic-to-systemic shunt ratio, as detailed in Chapters 12 and 17.

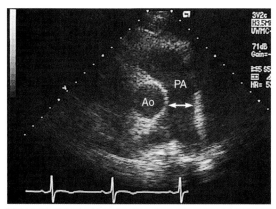

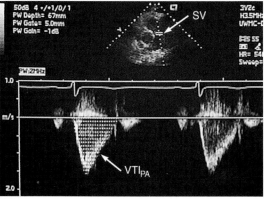

▐ **FIGURE 6–12.** Examples of pulmonary artery diameter measurement in a parasternal right ventricular outflow view (*top*) and pulsed Doppler pulmonary artery flow recorded from a parasternal approach (*bottom*) for transpulmonic stroke volume calculation

Other Doppler Measures of Left Ventricular Systolic Function

Ejection Acceleration Times

In addition to stroke volume calculations, the shape of the Doppler ejection curve may provide information about ventricular function. When systolic function is normal, the isovolumic contraction period is short, and the rate of pressure rise in early systole is rapid. These features are reflected in the Doppler velocity curve, which shows a short isovolumic contraction time, a rapid acceleration of blood in early systole, and a short interval from the onset of flow to maximum velocity. With impaired left ventricular systolic function, the isovolumic contraction time (also known as the preejection period) becomes progressively longer, the rate of acceleration diminishes, and the time to maximum velocity increases, with all these changes mirrored in the Doppler velocity curve. In addition to measuring these variables at rest, some centers have found evaluation of aortic ejection curves with exercise useful in detection of left ventricular systolic dysfunction.

Rate of Ventricular Pressure Rise

When mitral regurgitation is present, the continuous-wave Doppler velocity curve indicates the instantaneous pressure difference between the left ventricle and the left atrium in systole, assuming a constant intercept angle between the mitral regurgitant jet and the ultrasound beam. Given the rapid rate of rise of left ventricular pressure with normal systolic function (and the low left atrial pressure), mitral regurgitation typically shows a rapid rise to maximum velocity as per the Bernoulli equation. If the rate of rise in ventricular pressure is reduced due to left ventricular systolic dysfunction, the rate of increase in velocity of the mitral regurgitant jet also is reduced. For example, in patients with premature ventricular beats, the altered contractility of the premature beat will be evidenced by a marked difference in the rate of velocity increase of the mitral regurgitant jet. The slope of the mitral regurgitant jet can be quantitated as the rate of change in pressure over time (dP/dt) by measuring the time interval between the mitral regurgitant jet velocity at 1 and at 3 m/s (Figs. 6–13 and 6–14). At each velocity, the corresponding pressure gradient is $4v^2$ per the Bernoulli equation. Then,

$$dP/dt = \left[4(3)^2\right] - \left[4(1)^2\right]/\text{time interval}$$
$$= 32\,\text{mm Hg}/\text{time interval} \qquad (6\text{–}26)$$

Thus, a longer time interval indicates a depressed dP/dt, and vice versa. Of course, the calculation of

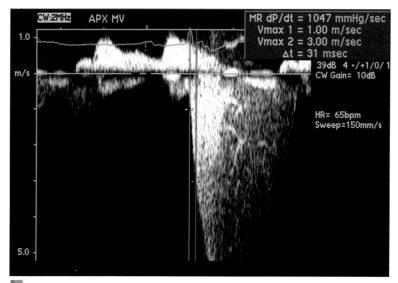

■ **FIGURE 6–13.** Left ventricular *dP/dt* can be calculated from the mitral regurgitant jet based on the interval between 1 and 3 m/s on the velocity curve. In this example of normal ventricular systolic function (*dP/dt* > 1000 mm Hg/s), the scale has been expanded to optimize the accuracy of the measurement.

dP/dt can be performed only when a recordable mitral regurgitant jet is present and assumes a constant (and parallel) intercept angle between the mitral regurgitant jet and the ultrasound beam during the measurement period.

Limitations and Technical Considerations

The major limitation of Doppler evaluation of left ventricular systolic function in adults is accurate diameter measurement for cross-sectional area calculations. While Doppler velocity curves can be recorded consistently with little interobserver measurement variability (2% to 5%), the variability of 2D diameter measurements is significantly greater (8% to 12%). For Doppler velocity data, the major source of measurement variability is data recording, given the critical importance of obtaining a parallel intercept angle between the ultrasound beam and the flow of interest. For 2D

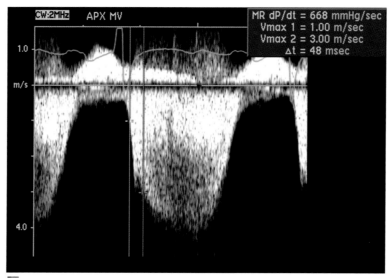

■ **FIGURE 6–14.** Example of the slow rate of rise in mitral regurgitant velocity in a patient with dilated cardiomyopathy, corresponding to a dP/dt of 668 mm Hg/s, as shown by the parallel vertical lines.

diameters, the major source of variability is measuring the 2D images, particularly when image quality is suboptimal or when lateral resolution limits accurate border recognition. Despite these potential limitations, Doppler measurement of stroke volume has been well validated in a variety of clinical and research settings.

Measurement of *dP/dt* is limited by the need for enough mitral regurgitation to generate a Doppler signal with a well-defined velocity curve. Changes during ejection in the intercept angle between the ultrasound beam and the regurgitant jet will result in an erroneous measurement, because the assumption that $\cos\theta = 1$ in the Doppler equation will not be valid.

ECHO APPROACH TO RIGHT VENTRICULAR SYSTOLIC FUNCTION

Imaging of the Right Ventricle

Qualitative Evaluation

The right ventricle is evaluated qualitatively by 2D imaging (Fig. 6–15) from several different windows:

- parasternal long- and short-axis,
- right ventricular inflow,
- apical four-chamber, and
- subcostal four-chamber views.

In each view, evaluation of the right ventricle includes

- area of the chamber (relative to the left ventricular chamber),
- shape of the right ventricular cavity,
- wall thickness,
- motion of the right ventricular free wall, and
- pattern of ventricular septal motion.

The normal shape of the right ventricle is complex in three dimensions, with the inflow segment located medial to the left ventricle, the body and apex located anterior to the left ventricle, and the right ventricular outflow tract located superior to the left ventricle and aortic valve. There is no simple geometric shape that approximates the right ventricular chamber; rather, it is "wrapped around" the left ventricle in a U-shaped fashion. Because echocardiographic long- and short-axis views are oriented with respect to the left ventricle, the right ventricle may appear abnormal in some individuals due to the position of the right ventricle relative to the image plane. This occurs most often in parasternal views, where the right ventricle may be imaged in an oblique orientation. Both subcostal

and apical four-chamber windows tend to offer more consistent views of the right ventricle, with the right ventricle appearing somewhat triangular with a broad base and narrow apex. The right ventricular apex is slightly closer to the base than the left ventricular apex (by about one third of the left ventricular length) in normal individuals.

With right ventricular dilation, the right ventricular outflow tract may be enlarged in the parasternal long-axis view. On apical and subcostal views, the right ventricular chamber will be larger and the right ventricular apex is either closer to or encompasses the left ventricular apex. The degree of right ventricular dilation is best evaluated in the apical or subcostal four-chamber view in relation to the size of the left ventricle (LV), taking into consideration the left ventricular size. Right ventricular (RV) size is described as

- normal (smaller than LV with RV apex more basal than LV apex),
- mildly dilated (enlarged but a RV < LV area),
- moderately dilated (RV = LV area), or
- severely dilated (RV > LV area).

Right ventricular dilation is the normal response of the ventricle to volume overload, and its presence mandates a careful search for etiology, such as an atrial septal defect, tricuspid regurgitation, or pulmonic regurgitation. Pressure overload of the right ventricle also leads to dilation so that evaluation of pulmonary pressures is mandatory when the right ventricle is abnormal.

Right ventricular systolic function is evaluated qualitatively as

- normal,
- mildly reduced,
- moderately reduced, or
- severely reduced.

When ventricular systolic function is normal, the relative function of the two ventricles can be compared. When left ventricular systolic function is depressed, the severity of left ventricular dysfunction should be used as an index of right ventricular function; e.g., a normal right ventricle compared to a reduced left ventricular ejection fraction appears hyperdynamic. If both ventricles have a similar qualitative pattern of contraction, the degree of right ventricular dysfunction is similar to the degree of left ventricular dysfunction.

Right ventricular hypertrophy is manifested as increased thickness of the right ventricular free

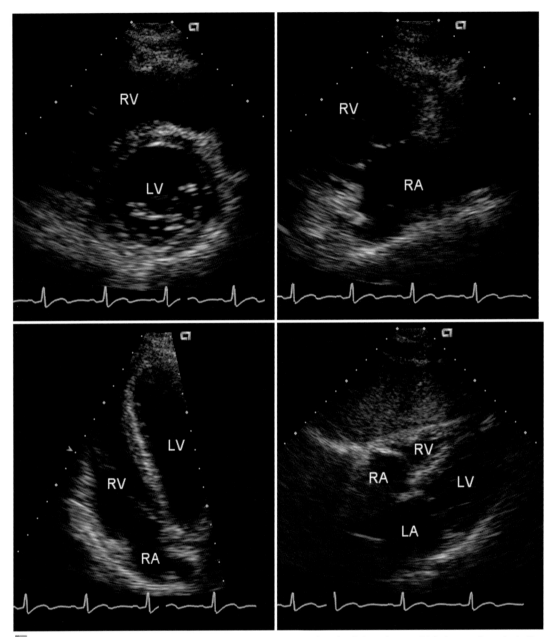

■ **FIGURE 6–15.** Evaluation of right ventricular size and systolic function is based on multiple image planes including parasternal short-axis (*top, left*), right ventricular inflow (*top, right*), apical four-chamber with optimization of the right ventricle (*bottom, left*), and subcostal four-chamber (*bottom, right*) views.

wall as seen on 2D images or by M-mode, with a wall thickness >0.5 cm being abnormal in adults. The presence of right ventricular hypertrophy suggests right ventricular pressure overload and should prompt a search for evidence of elevated pulmonary pressures or pulmonic valve stenosis. Increased thickness of the right ventricular free wall also may be seen in some infiltrative cardiomyopathies or in hypertrophic cardiomyopathy.

Quantitative Evaluation

Quantitative evaluation of right ventricular systolic function by 2D/M-mode echo is difficult. Standard geometric formulas for volume calculations have only limited applicability given the shape of the right ventricle, and while 3D reconstructions have been shown to be accurate, the need for tedious endocardial border tracing and extensive data analysis has restricted its use to the research setting. In most cases, qualitative evaluation is sufficient for clinical decision making.

Technical Considerations

Evaluation of right ventricular systolic function may be limited by poor ultrasound tissue penetration in some individuals. With careful patient positioning and a search from multiple windows, the right ventricle usually can be demonstrated, but endocardial definition may be suboptimal. If clinically indicated, transesophageal echo offers superior images of the right ventricle both in the high esophageal four-chamber view and from a transgastric approach.

Patterns of Ventricular Septal Motion

The interventricular septum functions as part of the left ventricle in the normal heart. During diastole, the left ventricle is circular in a short-axis view, with the normal septal curvature convex toward the right ventricle and concave toward the left ventricle. With the onset of systole, the septal myocardium thickens, and the septal endocardium moves toward the center of the left ventricle such that at end-systole the short-axis image shows a circular left ventricular chamber.

A number of cardiac disorders alter the pattern of ventricular septal motion, the most prominent being right ventricular pressure and volume overload. The basic principle underlying the pattern of septal motion with right ventricular dilation or hypertrophy is that the septum moves toward the center of mass of the entire heart. Normally, the center of cardiac mass coincides with the center of the left ventricle. When right and left ventricular masses are equal, septal motion will be "flat" (on M-mode) or minimal (on 2D echo). When right ventricular mass exceeds left ventricular mass, the septum moves "paradoxically" anterior in systole (on M-mode) and flattens or reverses its curvature in diastole (on 2D echo) (Fig. 6–16).

On 2D echocardiography, pressure overload of the right ventricle (increased mass due to increased wall thickness with a nondilated chamber) results in a leftward shift of septal motion throughout the cardiac cycle with the maximum reversed curvature at end-systole. With predominant right ventricular volume overload, the maximum reversed curvature is seen in mid-diastole with normalization of curvature in systole (see Suggested Reading 22). With increased right ventricular mass due to volume overload, the additional factor of increased right ventricular filling and emptying accentuates the diastolic reverse motion of the septum (due to rapid right ventricular diastolic filling), resulting in a D shape

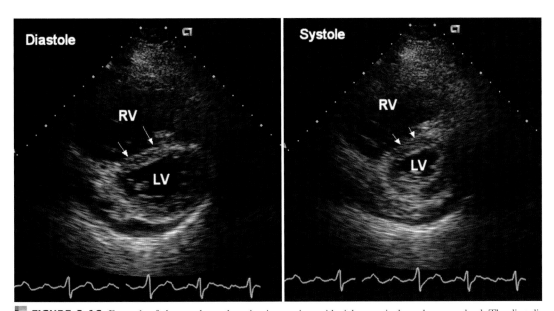

■ **FIGURE 6–16.** Example of abnormal septal motion in a patient with right ventricular volume overload. The diastolic image (*left*) in a parasternal short-axis view shows a markedly dilated right ventricle with flattening of the normal septal contour (*arrows*). The systolic image (*right*) shows persistent slight flattening of the septal contour, suggesting a component of pressure overload.

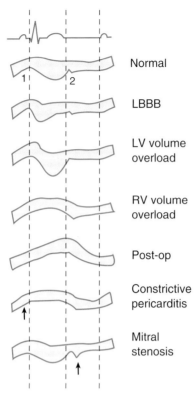

FIGURE 6–17. Schematic diagram of different patterns of septal motion on M-mode echocardiography. The normal pattern is characterized by systolic brief anterior motion (*1*) followed by posterior motion and myocardial thickening. In diastole, a small diastolic dip (*2*) following mitral valve opening may be seen. Left bundle branch block (LBBB) is characterized by systolic rapid downward septal motion. Left ventricular (LV) volume overload results in exaggerated septal (and posterior wall) motion. Right ventricular (RV) volume overload results in paradoxical anterior motion of the septum in systole. A similar pattern is seen in patients after cardiac surgery (Post-op). Constrictive pericarditis is characterized by anterior motion of the septum with atrial filling (before the QRS), while mitral stenosis typically shows a prominent early diastolic dip.

of the left ventricular chamber in early diastole, with the reversed curvature of the septum persisting throughout diastole. Anterior motion with systole may appear less prominent than with isolated pressure overload as the septum moves from its abnormal diastolic position back toward the center of the heart, resulting in a more convex curve relative to the right ventricular chamber. Often, the observation of abnormal septal motion during the examination is the first clue of right ventricular pressure and/or volume overload.

Other abnormalities that affect the pattern of ventricular septal motion are summarized in Figure 6–17. Conduction defects affect the pattern

of motion by altering the sequence of right and left ventricular contraction. Valvular disease can affect the timing of right ventricular versus left ventricular diastolic filling, particularly in early diastole. Pericardial tamponade or constriction results in a fixed total cardiac volume so that respiratory changes in right ventricular filling result in respiratory shifts in the pattern of septal motion.

An abnormal pattern of septal motion may be appreciated on 2D imaging; however, M-mode echo offers more detailed time resolution for studying the pattern of motion. Abnormal septal motion rarely is diagnostic in and of itself, but it may raise a diagnostic possibility that had not been considered previously or may support a suspected diagnosis. For example, a pattern of paradoxical septal motion in association with right ventricular and right atrial enlargement suggests the possibility of an atrial septal defect. This possibility then can be specifically excluded (or confirmed) during the echocardiographic examination. Another example is the patient with a pericardial effusion; in this situation, a changing pattern of septal motion with respiration supports a diagnosis of tamponade physiology.

Pulmonary Artery Pressure Estimates

Clinically, one of the most important quantitative parameters of right ventricular systolic function is an estimate of pulmonary artery pressures. Pulmonary hypertension often occurs in response to chronic left-sided heart diseases, such as mitral stenosis, mitral regurgitation, cardiomyopathy, and ischemic cardiac disease. Knowledge of the degree of pulmonary pressure elevation is critical in patient management (Table 6–2).

Tricuspid Regurgitant Jet Plus Right Atrial Pressure

The most reliable method for estimating pulmonary artery pressures noninvasively is based on measurement of the velocity in the tricuspid regurgitant jet (Table 6–4). This velocity V_{TR} reflects the right ventricular (RV) to right atrial (RA) pressure difference ΔP, as stated in the Bernoulli equation (Fig. 6–20):

$$\Delta P_{RV-RA} = 4(V_{TR})^2 \qquad (6\text{–}27)$$

When added to an estimate of right atrial pressure, right ventricular systolic pressure (RVP) is obtained:

$$RVP = \Delta P_{RV-RA} + RAP \qquad (6\text{–}28)$$

In the absence of pulmonic stenosis (which is rare in adults), right ventricular systolic pressure

TABLE 6–4

Doppler Echo Methods for Pulmonary Artery Pressure Estimation

Method	Advantages	Potential Limitations
Tricuspid regurgitant jet: $PA_{systolic} = 4(V_{TR})^2 + RAP$	Accurate Measurable in a high percentage of patients overall (90%)	Nonparallel intercept angle between jet and ultrasound beam Misidentification of jet signal Right atrial pressure estimate needed Presence of pulmonic stenosis Inadequate signal in some patients with chronic lung disease
Pulmonary artery flow: Time to peak velocity	Readily measured in nearly all patients, including patients with chronic lung disease Estimates *mean* pulmonary artery pressure	Skewed flow profile in pulmonary artery Measurement variability
PR end-diastolic velocity: $PA_{diastolic} = 4(V_{PR})^2 + RAP$	Reflects pulmonary diastolic pressure Adequate signal in 85% of patients. Can be recorded continuously with a transthoracic tranducer	Nonparallel intercept angle between jet and ultrasound beam Right atrial pressure estimate needed

PA, pulmonary artery; RAP, right atrial pressure; PR, pulmonic regurgitation; TR, tricuspid regurgitant.

equals pulmonary artery systolic pressure (Figs. 6–18 and 6–19), so that

$$PAP_{systolic} = 4(V_{TR})^2 + RAP \quad (6\text{-}29)$$

This method has been shown to be highly accurate compared with invasive measurements of pulmonary artery pressure over a wide range of values (Table 6–5). Of course, the reliability of this approach is dependent on obtaining a parallel intercept angle between the tricuspid regurgitant jet and the ultrasound beam. Most often, the apical or right ventricular inflow view yields the highest-velocity signal given careful angulation of the ultrasound beam in three dimensions (Fig. 6–20). Occasionally, the highest-velocity tricuspid regurgitant jet is recorded from a subcostal

approach. Although this method requires the presence of tricuspid regurgitation, this rarely is a limitation, because approximately 90% of normal individuals and patients have some degree of tricuspid regurgitation.

The same concept can be applied to the pulmonic regurgitant velocity curve. The end-diastolic pulmonic regurgitant velocity reflects the pulmonary artery to right ventricular end-diastolic pressure gradient per the Bernoulli equation. When added to an estimate of right atrial pressure, this provides a noninvasive estimate of diastolic pulmonary artery pressure (Fig. 6–21).

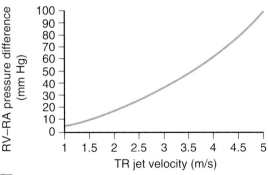

FIGURE 6–18. Relationship between the velocity in the tricuspid regurgitant (TR) jet and the right ventricular–right atrial (RV–RA) pressure difference as calculated with the simplified Bernoulli relationship.

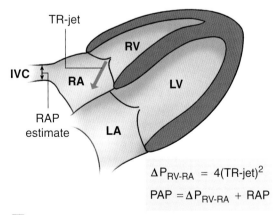

$$\Delta P_{RV\text{-}RA} = 4(TR\text{-}jet)^2$$
$$PAP = \Delta P_{RV\text{-}RA} + RAP$$

FIGURE 6–19. Pulmonary artery pressure (PAP) can be calculated noninvasively based on the velocity in the tricuspid regurgitant (TR) jet and the respiratory variation in inferior vena cava (IVC) size as an estimate of right atrial pressure (RAP).

TABLE 6–5

Selected Studies Validating Noninvasive Pulmonary Artery Pressure Measurement

First Author/Year	Method	n	r	Regression Equation	SEE
Kitabatake/1983	TPV (RVOT)	33	−0.88	Log (mean PAP) = 0.0068 (AcT) + 2.1 mm Hg	–
Stevenson/1989	TR-jet	50	0.96		6.9 mm Hg
	TPV (PA)		0.63		16.4 mm Hg
	IVRT		0.97		5.4 mm Hg
	PR		0.96		4.5 mm Hg
Yock/1984	TR-jet	62	0.95	Doppler RV-RA ΔP = 1.03ΔP + 0.71 mm Hg	7 mm Hg
Berger/1985	TR-jet	69	0.97	Systolic PAP = 1.23 (Doppler ΔP) − 0.09 mm Hg	4.9 mm Hg
Currie/1985	TR-jet	12 7	0.96	Doppler RV-RA ΔP = 0.88ΔP + 2.2 mm Hg	7 mm Hg
Lee/1989	PR	29	0.94	Diastolic PAP (echo) = 0.95 (cath) − 1.0 mm Hg	Mean diff: 3.3 ± 2.2 mm Hg
Chandraratna/2002	PR	50	0.91	Doppler = 0.82Inv + 0.96	3.3 mm Hg

Data from Kitabatake A et al: Circulation 68:302–309, 1983; Stevenson JG et al: J Am Soc Echocardiogr 2:157–171, 1989; Yock PG, Popp RL: Circulation 70:657–662, 1984; Berger M et al: J Am Coll Cardiol 6:359–365, 1985; Curtie PJ et al: J Am Coll Cardiol 6:750–756, 1985; Lee RT et al: Am J Cardiol 64:1366–1370, 1989; Chandraratna et al: J Am Soc Echocardiogr 15:1381–1386, 2002.

RVOT, right ventricular outflow tract; TPV, time to peak flow; TR, tricuspid regurgitation; PR, pulmonic regurgitation; SEE, standard error of the estimate; INV, invasive; IVRT, isovolumic relaxation time.

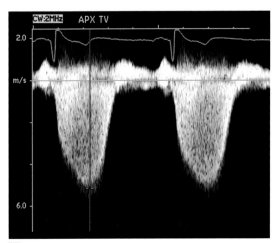

■ **FIGURE 6–20.** Tricuspid regurgitant jet in a patient with severe pulmonary hypertension. The maximum jet velocity of 5 m/s corresponds to a 100 mm Hg pressure difference between the right ventricle and right atrium in systole.

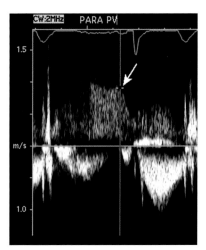

■ **FIGURE 6–21.** Pulmonic regurgitation recorded from a parasternal approach with continuous wave Doppler shows an end-diastolic velocity of 0.8 m/s, indicating low diastolic pulmonary pressures.

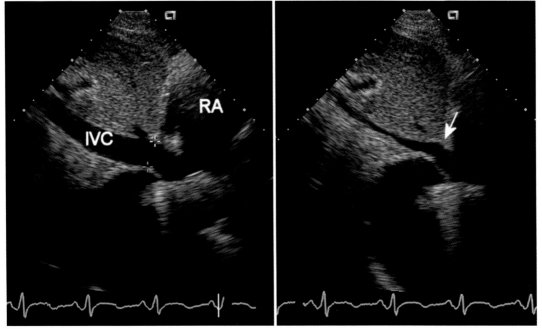

■ **FIGURE 6–22.** Subcostal view of the junction between the inferior vena cava (IVC) and the right atrium (RA) during normal expiration (*top*) and inspiration (*bottom*).

Right atrial pressure is best estimated from evaluation of the inferior vena cava during respiration (Fig. 6–22). From a subcostal window, this segment of the inferior vena cava is imaged during quiet respiration. If the inferior vena caval diameter is normal (1.5 to 2.5 cm) and the segment adjacent to the right atrium collapses by at least 50% with respiration, then right atrial pressure is equal to normal intrathoracic pressures (i.e., 5 to 10 mmHg). Failure to collapse with respiration and/or dilation of the inferior vena cava and hepatic veins is associated with higher right atrial pressures (Table 6–6). When no response is noted with normal respiration, the patient is asked to "sniff." This generates a sudden decrease in intrathoracic pressure, normally resulting in a decrease in inferior vena cava diameter.

An alternate approach to estimation of right atrial pressure is clinical examination of the degree of jugular venous distension. However, while this approach is reliable in distinguishing changes (increases or decreases) over time in filling pressures in an individual patient, it is less accurate in determining the absolute right atrial pressure.

Pulmonary Artery Velocity Curve

Another approach to estimating pulmonary pressure is based on the shape of the pulmonary artery Doppler velocity curve. Comparison of the normal left ventricular and right ventricular ejec-

TABLE 6–6		
Estimation of Right Atrial Pressure		
Inferior Vena Cava	**Change with Respiration or "Sniff"**	**Estimated Right Atrial Pressure (mm Hg)**
Small (<1.5 cm)	Collapse	0–5
Normal (1.5–2.5 cm)	Decrease by >50%	5–10
Normal	Decrease by <50%	10–15
Dilated (>2.5 cm)	Decrease <50%	15–20
Dilated with dilated hepatic veins	No change	>20

tion curves reveals that left ventricular ejection shows very rapid acceleration with a short time from flow onset to maximum velocity, whereas right ventricular ejection shows a slower acceleration, a longer time from onset of flow to peak flow, and a more "rounded" velocity curve. As pulmonary vascular resistance increases, the shape of the right ventricular ejection curve more closely approximates the left ventricular ejection curve, suggesting that the shapes of these velocity curves are related to the downstream resistance or impedance.

The time to peak velocity estimates of pulmonary artery pressure are not as reliable as tricuspid regurgitant jet estimates for two reasons. First, this method depends on measurement of a relatively short time interval, so measurement error is high and reproducibility is low. Second, the spatial flow velocity profile in the pulmonary artery is skewed, with higher acceleration and velocity along the inner edge of the curvature. Even when the sample volume appears positioned in the center of the vessel in a 2D image plane, it may be near the inner wall in the elevational plane, since this curvature is 3D. Thus, the shape of the pulmonary artery velocity curve is most helpful when it is normal. An apparent short time to peak velocity can be due to measurement variability or to the nonuniform spatial flow velocity distribution in the vessel.

Isovolumic Relaxation Time

Pulmonary hypertension is associated with prolongation of the right ventricular isovolumic relaxation time (IVRT). This time can be measured as the interval between pulmonic valve closure and tricuspid valve opening, recorded either with M-mode echocardiography (showing leaflet closure) or Doppler echo (showing the valve "clicks"). Nomograms relating the right ventricular IVRT to the degree of pulmonary hypertension have been shown to be accurate in pediatric populations. In adults, this approach is rarely used because of the difficulty in recording pulmonic valve closure given suboptimal acoustic access in many patients. In addition, as with the time to peak velocity in the pulmonary artery velocity curve, the IVRT is a short interval that is subject to considerable measurement variability.

Limitations and Technical Considerations

Determination of pulmonary artery systolic pressure derived from the continuous-wave Doppler tricuspid regurgitant jet velocity is only as accurate as the primary data. Underestimation of tricuspid regurgitant jet velocity due to a non-parallel intercept angle between the jet and the ultrasound beam results in underestimation of pulmonary artery pressures. Overestimation of pulmonary artery pressures can occur if the mitral regurgitant jet is mistaken for tricuspid regurgitation. Although both signals occur in systole and are directed away from the left ventricular apex, the duration of tricuspid regurgitation is slightly longer than mitral regurgitation (when right and left ventricular systolic function are normal) due to a slightly longer right ventricular systolic ejection period (see Fig. 11–11). The shapes of the velocity curves tend to differ as well, with tricuspid regurgitation having a slower upstroke and a peak later in systole, although the shapes of both velocity curves are affected by changes in ventricular function or atrial pressure. Note that the velocity of mitral regurgitation always is high, because it reflects the systolic left ventricular (approximately 100 mm Hg) to left atrial (approximately 10 mm Hg) pressure difference. With normal pulmonary artery pressures, tricuspid regurgitant jet velocity is 2 to 2.5 m/s. With pulmonary hypertension, pulmonary pressure may approach systemic pressures, with a corresponding tricuspid regurgitant jet velocity in the range of 5 m/s.

It is important to keep separate the concepts of regurgitant *volume flow rate*–which relates to regurgitant severity–and regurgitant jet *velocity*–which reflects the instantaneous pressure gradient across the valve. Severe pulmonary hypertension (with a high tricuspid jet velocity) may occur with only mild tricuspid regurgitation.

The tricuspid regurgitant jet can be used to estimate pulmonary artery pressure when right ventricular and pulmonary artery systolic pressures are equal, specifically in the absence of pulmonic stenosis. *When pulmonic stenosis is present*, pulmonary pressures can be estimated by subtracting the right ventricle to pulmonary artery pressure difference derived from the pulmonic stenotic jet velocity (V_{PS}) from the estimated right ventricular systolic pressure:

$$PAP = \left[4(V_{TR})^2 + RAP \right] - \left[4(V_{PS})^2 \right] \quad (6\text{--}30)$$

The estimate of right atrial pressure from the appearance of the inferior vena cava also can affect the accuracy of Doppler echo pulmonary artery pressure estimates. The importance of this source of error is greatest at intermediate tricuspid regurgitant jet velocities: A tricuspid regurgitant jet velocity of 2.5 m/s with a right atrial pressure of 5 mm Hg indicates a pulmonary artery pressure of only 30 mm Hg (normal to mildly elevated), but if right atrial pressure is 20 mm Hg, then pulmonary artery pressure is 45 mm Hg (moderate pulmonary hypertension). At the extreme (i.e., a tricuspid regurgitant jet of 5 m/s), pulmonary hypertension clearly is severe regardless of the right atrial pressure estimate.

If images of the inferior vena cava are suboptimal, or if the degree of change with respiration is equivocal, it is appropriate to report the range of possible pulmonary artery pressures or to indicate that the right ventricle to right atrial pressure gradient should be added to a clinical estimate of right atrial pressure. Evaluation of respiratory variation in inferior vena cava diameter can be confounded by respiratory motion in the position of the inferior vena cava such that the center of the vessel moves in and out of the image plane. Of course, evaluation of inferior vena cava size and respiratory variation is not helpful in patients supported by positive-pressure ventilation, because intrathoracic pressures are abnormal.

The time to peak velocity in the pulmonary artery can appear short when the Doppler sample volume is positioned along the inner curve of the pulmonary artery. Conversely, impaired right ventricular systolic function may result in an apparently normal time to peak velocity even in the presence of pulmonary hypertension.

ALTERNATE APPROACHES

Left Ventricular Systolic Function

Available alternate approaches to measurement of left ventricular volumes and ejection fraction are contrast angiography in the cardiac catheterization laboratory (Fig. 6–23) and radionuclide ventriculography (Fig. 6–24). Both computed tomography and magnetic resonance imaging are capable of left ventricular volume calculation, although they may not be available routinely. The choice of imaging technique in an individual patient will depend on what other clinical questions are present (e.g., possible valvular disease) as well as availability and cost.

The standard approach to evaluation of cardiac output both in the catheterization laboratory and in the coronary care unit is by the thermodilution technique with an indwelling right-sided heart catheter. Thermodilution outputs offer the advantages that measurements can be repeated frequently by the nurse caring for the patient and pulmonary artery pressures can be monitored continuously as well. Disadvantages of this approach are that it is invasive (risks, discomfort) and it provides only a volumetric flow rate, without direct visualization of ventricular function. Stroke volume can be maintained despite a

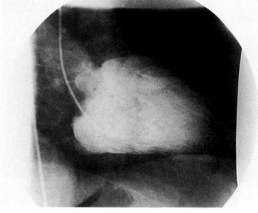
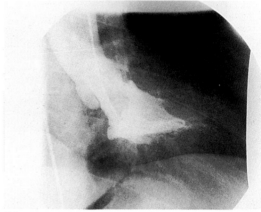

■ **FIGURE 6–23.** Left ventricular angiography is an alternate approach to evaluation of left ventricular systolic function, which is performed most often in patients undergoing cardiac catheterization for other indications, such as coronary artery disease. End-diastolic (*top*) and end-systolic (*bottom*) frames are shown.

low ejection fraction due to compensatory left ventricular dilation. For example, the same stroke volume of 60 mL may result from an ejection fraction of 20% with a left ventricular end-diastolic volume of 300 mL or from a normal ejection fraction (60%) with a smaller left ventricular end-diastolic volume (100 mL).

Right Ventricular Systolic Function

Right ventricular contrast angiography can be performed at catheterization, but there is wide variability in the appearance of the normal right ventricle. Radionuclide ventriculography can be used to derive a right ventricular ejection fraction. The right ventricle also can be imaged on computed tomography or magnetic resonance imaging scanning, and cine-views may be helpful, when available, for evaluation of systolic function.

The alternative to noninvasive Doppler echo estimate of pulmonary artery pressures is direct

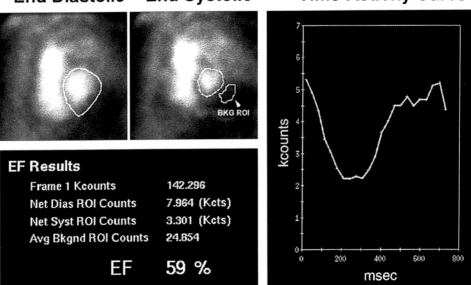

Regions of Interest

End Diastolic   End Systolic   Time-Activity Curve

EF Results

Frame 1 Kcounts	142.296
Net Dias ROI Counts	7.964 (Kcts)
Net Syst ROI Counts	3.301 (Kcts)
Avg Bkgnd ROI Counts	24.854

EF   59 %

■ **FIGURE 6–24.** A radionuclide ventriculogram. Standard view radionuclide ventriculographic images at end-diastole (dias) and end-systole (syst) in a patient with normal cardiac chamber size and global function of both ventricles. The region of interest (ROI) and background region (BKG) for measurement of counts and calculation of ejection fraction is shown. The time-activity curve in kilo-counts per millisecond is graphed.

measurement in the coronary care unit or cardiac catheterization laboratory with a pulmonary artery (Swan-Ganz) catheter. This approach has the advantages of precision, a high degree of accuracy (assuming appropriate transducer calibration and balancing), and the ability to continuously record measurements over several days. In addition, pulmonary vascular resistance can be measured based on invasive measurement of cardiac output and pulmonary pressures. Disadvantages are its costs, potential complications of line placement, and the difficulty of performing repeat measures over longer time intervals. Noninvasive Doppler approaches for continuous pulmonary pressure recording and for estimation of pulmonary vascular resistance are in development (see Suggested Readings 17, 18, 26, and 27).

SUGGESTED READING

Imaging of the Left Ventricle

1. American Society of Echocardiography Committee on Standards, Subcommittee on Quantitation of Two-Dimensional Echocardiograms: Recommendations for quantitation of the left ventricle by two-dimensional echocardiography. J Am Soc Echocardiogr 2:361–367, 1989.

   Clear description of methods for quantitation of left ventricular systolic function by 2D echocardiography as recommended by the American Society of Echocardiography. Technical details of image acquisition, diagrams illustrating quantitative techniques, and tables of normal values are included.

2. Aurigemma GP, Douglas PS, Gaasch WH: Quantitative evaluation of left ventricular structure, wall stress and systolic function. In: Otto CM (ed): The Practice of Clinical Echocardiography, 2nd ed. Philadelphia, WB Saunders, 2002, pp 65–87.

   Two-dimensional echocardiography allows sophisticated evaluation of left ventricular geometry and systolic function. This chapter provides a detailed and critical discussion of approaches to measurement of wall stress and systolic performance. The calculation of circumferential as well as meridional stress is described; 145 references.

3. Folland ED, Parisi AF, Moynihan PF, et al: Assessment of left ventricular ejection fraction and volumes by real-time, two-dimensional echocardiography. A comparison of cineangiographic and radionuclide techniques. Circulation 60:760–766, 1979.

   Key paper comparing five different algorithms for determining left ventricular volumes by 2D echocardiography in comparison with both radionuclide ventriculography and contrast angiography.

4. Smith MD, MacPhail B, Harrison MR, et al: Value and limitations of transesophageal echocardiography in determination of left ventricular volumes and ejection fraction. J Am Coll Cardiol 19:1213–1222, 1992.

Calculation of left ventricular volumes using a modified Simpson's rule can be made from transesophageal images using short-axis views at the mitral valve, papillary muscle, and apical levels plus left ventricular length measured in the four-chamber view. Underestimation of left ventricular length on transesophageal echocardiographic images results in smaller calculated left ventricular volumes than angiographic measurements.

5. Gordon EP, Schnittger I, Fitzgerald PJ, et al: Reproducibility of left ventricular volumes by two-dimensional echocardiography. J Am Coll Cardiol 2:506–513, 1983.

   Repeat recordings and measurement of left ventricular volumes by 2D echocardiography showed 95% confidence limits for individual subjects' measurements of ±15% for end-diastolic volume, ±25% for end-systolic volume, and ±10% for ejection fraction.

6. Thomson HL, Basmadjian AJ, Rainbird AJ, et al: Contrast echocardiography improves the accuracy and reproducibility of left vnetriucular remodeling measurements: A prospective, randomly assigned, blinded study. J Am Coll Cardiol 38:867–875, 2001.

   Accuracy and reproducibility of ventricular volumes and ejection fraction measurements by 2D echocardiography were improved when harmonic imaging and contrast injection, compared to electron beam computed tomography in 26 patients.

Three-dimensional Echocardiography

7. Sheehan FH: Three-dimensional echocardiography. In: Otto CM (ed): The Practice of Clinical Echocardiography, 2nd ed. Philadelphia, WB Saunders, 2002, pp 202–234.

   This chapter reviews the basic principles of the acquisition, display, and clinical applications of quantitative 3D echocardiography. Systems for image acquisition and quantitative analysis of the ventricle are discussed. Quantitative applications of 3D echocardiography include measurement of left ventricular volumes, ejection fraction, and mass. Evaluation of valve anatomy and the right heart chambers also is reviewed; 180 references.

8. Mele D, Fehske W, Maehle J, et al: A simplified, practical echocardiographic approach for 3-dimensional surfacing and quantitation of the left ventricle: Clinical applications in patients with abnormally shaped hearts. J Am Soc Echocardiogr 11:1001–1012, 1998

   In 50 patients with abnormal left ventricles, 3D echocardiographic volumes were calcuated from endocardial border tracing in three apical views obtained by rotational 2D scanning. Ejection fraction by 3D echo was compared to MR imaging in 20 patients, angiography in 22 patients, and radionuclide imaging in 8 patients (r = 0.92, SEE = 6.2%) with an intraobserver variabilty <6% for 3D volumes and ejection fraction.

9. Mondelli JA, Di Luzio S, Nagaraj A, et al: The validation of volumetric real-time 3-dimensional echocaridography for the determination of left ventricular function. J Am Soc Echocardiogr 14:994–1000, 2001.

   A 3D volumetric echocardiographic system was with manual tracing of endocardial borders at end-diastole and end-systole in 6 uniformly spaced apical images at 30 degree intervals. 3D echocardiographic stroke volume correlated well (r=0.93) compared to electromagnetic flow probe in an animal model. In human subjects, ejection fractions by 3D echo and radionuclide angiography showed a closer correlation (r = 0.94) than for 2D ejection fraction (r = 0.85).

10. Hubka M, Bolson EL, McDonald JA, et al: Three-dimensional echocardiographic measurement of left and right ventricular mass and volume: In vitro validation. Int J Cardiovasc Imaging 18:111–118, 2002.

    3D echo scans of in vitro left and right ventricles correlated closely with laser scanned data both for ventricular volumes and ventricular shape.

11. Wong SP, Johnson RK, Sheehan FH: Rapid and accurate left ventricular surface generation from three-dimensional echocardiography by a catalog based method. Int J Cardiovasc Imaging 19:9–17, 2003.

    A rapid method for quantitation of 3D echocardiography using a catalog fit method based on identification of key anatomic features in five standard echocardiographic views of the left ventricle. Compared to manual tracing, the automated method is accurate (r – 0.99) with an average time for generation of an LV surface of 3 ± 0.5 min.

Other Imaging Measures of Systolic Function

12. Simonson JS, Schiller NB: Descent of the base of the left ventricle: An echocardiographic index of left ventricular function. J Am Soc Echocardiogr 2:25–35, 1989.

    The motion of the mitral annulus toward the ventricular apex in systole (lengthwise ventricular shortening) provides a simple method for quantitation of left ventricular systolic function. Average motion in normal individuals was 12 ± 2 mm, with motion <8 mm sensitive (98%) and specific (82%) for diagnosis of an ejection fraction of less than 50%.

13. Zeidan Z, Erbel R, Barkhausen J, et al: Analysis of global systolic and diastolic left ventricular performance using volume-time curves by real-time three-dimensional echocardiography. J Am Soc Echocardiogr 16:29–37, 2003.

    Volumetric scanning with semiautomated endocardial border tracing in 11 equidistant parallel short-axis planes was used to determine ventricular volumes at 40- to 55-msec intervals. These data were used to generate a ventricular volume-time curve allowing measurement of both ejection phase and filling parameters of left ventricular function.

Doppler Evaluation of Systolic Function

14. Lewis JF, Kuo LC, Nelson JG, et al: Pulsed Doppler echocardiographic determination of stroke volume and cardiac output: Clinical validation of two new methods using the apical window. Circulation 70:425–431, 1984.

    Description of left ventricular outflow tract and mitral annulus methods for stroke volume calculation. Validation in 39 patients versus thermodilution cardiac output and application of Doppler stroke volume measurement at two intracardiac sites to calculation of regurgitant volume is described. Interobserver variability for stroke volume or cardiac output (mean percentage error ± 1 SD) was 16.4% ± 13% for the mitral annulus method and 6.8% ± 5% for the left ventricular outflow method.

15. Otto CM, Pearlman AS, Gardner CL, et al: Experimental validation of Doppler echocardiographic measurement of volume flow through the stenotic aortic valve. Circulation 78:435–441, 1988.

    Validation of left ventricular outflow tract method for measurement of stroke volume proximal to a stenotic aortic valve. Repeat measurement of left ventricular outflow tract diameter showed a mean coefficient of variation of 2%.

16. Goldman JH, Schiller NB, Lim DC, et al: Usefulness of stroke distance by echocardiography as a surrogate marker of cardiac output that is independent of gender and size in a normal population. Am J Cardiol 15:499–502, 2001.

The velocity time integral of antegrade flow in the left ventricular outflow tract provides a simplified estimate of forward cardiac output. This approach is similar to calculation of stroke volume except that measurement of outflow tract diameter is eliminated. Thus, this measure represents "stroke distance" and is effectively indexed for body size. The normal range for stroke distance is 18 to 22 cm.

17. Lefrant JY, Benbabaali M, Ripart J, et al: CO assessment by suprasternal Doppler in critically ill patients: comparison with thermodilution. Intensive Care Med 26:693–697, 2000.

In 65 intensive care unit patients, Doppler cardiac output could be measured in 58 (89%) using suprasternal notch continuous wave Doppler and a nomogram for estimation of aortic diameter. For 314 paired measurements, the correlation between Doppler and thermodilution cardiac outputs was 0.84 with a mean time for Doppler measurement of 1.2 ± 0.8 minutes.

18. Gentles TL, Neutze JM, Caulder AL, Greene ER: Cardiac output measurements in congential heart disease: validation of a simple, portable Doppler method. J Ultrasound Med 20:365–370, 2001.

In 20 children with complex congenital heart disease, cardiac output was calculated using a nonimaging suprasternal notch pulsed Doppler system, that uses an operator selected estimate of aortic diameter (derived from angiographic or 2D echo data). Doppler cardiac output correlated well (r = 0.96) with Fick cardiac output with 95% confidence intervals <35% of the mean value of the two methods.

19. Chandraratna PA, Brar R, Vijayasekaran S, et al: Continuous recording of pulmonary artery diastolic pressure and cardiac output using a novel ultrasound transducer. J Am Soc Echocardiogr 15:1381–1386, 2002.

A small steerable transthoracic transducer that attaches to the chest wall was used to continuously measure cardiac output and pulmonary artery diastolic pressure in 50 patients in the intensive care unit. Adequate signals were obtained in 86% for calculation of cardiac output based on pulmonary artery diameter, flow and heart rate, and pulmonary diastolic pressure based on the end-diastolic velocity of the pulmonic regurgitant jet and estimated right atrial pressure. Correlation of Doppler and invasive data was excellent for cardiac output (r = 0.90) and pulmonary artery diastolic pressure (r = 0.92).

20. Chen C, Rodriguez L, Guerrero JL, et al: Noninvasive estimation of the instantaneous first derivative of left ventricular pressure using continuous-wave Doppler echocardiography. Circulation 83:2101–2110, 1991.

The rate of ventricular pressure rise in early systole (dP/dt) can be calculated from the mitral regurgitant jet velocity curve. Both dP/dt$_{max}$ and –dP/dt$_{max}$ can be determined accurately and reliably.

21. Chung N, Nishimura RA, Holmes DR Jr, Tajik AJ: Measurement of left ventricular dP/dt by simultaneous Doppler echocardiography and cardiac catheterization. J Am Soc Echocardiogr 5:147–152, 1992.

Doppler measurement of left ventricular dP/dt from the mitral regurgitant velocity curve was most accurate using the interval from 1 to 3 m/s on the velocity curve.

Right Ventricular Systolic Function

22. Louie EK, Rich S, Levitsky S, Brundage BH: Doppler echocardiographic demonstration of the differential effects of right ventricular pressure and volume overload on left ventricular geometry and filling. J Am Coll Cardiol 19:84–90, 1992.

Right ventricular pressure overload results in a leftward septal shift on 2D echocardiography that is maximal at end-systole and in early diastole. In contrast, right ventricular volume overload results in the maximal leftward septal shift at end-diastole with a relatively normal septal contour at end-systole and early diastole. Recognition of these differing patterns of septal motion focuses the examination on the relevant differential diagnosis.

Noninvasive Pulmonary Pressures

23. Yock PG, Popp RL: Noninvasive estimation of right ventricular systolic pressure by Doppler ultrasound in patients with tricuspid regurgitation. Circulation 70:657–662, 1984.

Description and validation of calculating the right ventricular to right atrial maximum systolic pressure difference from the maximum tricuspid regurgitant jet velocity using the simplified Bernoulli equation. While the Doppler and invasive pressure gradient correlated well (r = 0.95), clinical estimates of right atrial pressure from the degree of jugular venous distension correlated only modestly with measured right atrial pressure (r = 0.80).

24. Currie PJ, Seward JB, Chart K-L, et al: Continuous-wave Doppler determination of right ventricular pressure: a simultaneous Doppler-catheterization study in 127 patients. J Am Coll Cardiol 6:750–756, 1985.

Further validation of the use of tricuspid regurgitant jet velocity to estimate right ventricular systolic pressure in a larger series of patients. An adequate tricuspid regurgitant jet velocity signal was obtained in 111 of 127 (87%) of patients. The average coefficient of variation for measurement of maximum velocity was 2% (range 0 to 18%).

25. Kitabatake A, Inoue M, Asao M, et al: Noninvasive evaluation of pulmonary hypertension by a pulsed Doppler technique. Circulation 58:302–309, 1983.

Pulmonary artery can be estimated from the ratio of right ventricular outflow tract mean pressure acceleration time to total ejection time (r = –0.90). In patients with a normal pulmonary pressure (mean pressure <20 mm Hg) the average time from onset of flow to peak flow velocity (acceleration time) was 137 ± 24 ms. Pulmonary hypertension is associated with a shortened acceleration time and a mid-systolic notch on the deceleration segment of the velocity curve.

26. Scapellato F, Temporelli PL, Eleuteri E, Corra U, Imparato A, Giannuzzi P: Accurate noninvasive estimation of pulmonary vascular resistance by Doppler echocardiography in patients with chronic heart failure. J Am Coll Cardiol 37:1813–1819, 2001.

In 63 patients with heart failure, invasively determined pulmonary vascular resistance (PVR in Wood units) was compared with Doppler measures derived from the tricuspid regurgitant jet and antegrade pulmonary artery flow. A regression equation was derived based on the pre-ejection period (PEP), measured at the time interval from onset of tricuspid regurgitation to onset of antegrade pulmonary flow, acceleration time (AcT), measured at the time from onset to peak pulmonary flow and total systolic time (TT), the sum of PEP and systolic ejection time:

$$PVR = -0.156 + 1.154[(PEP/AcT)/TT]$$

This equation accurately predicted PVR (r = 0.94) after medical therapy to change loading conditions.

27. Abbas AE, Fortuin D, Schiller NB, et al: A simple method for noninvasive estimation of pulmonary vascular resistance. J Am Coll Cardiol 41:1021–1027, 2003.

In 44 patients with simultaneous Doppler and right heart catheterization, the ratio of tricuspid regurgitant velocity (V_{TR}) to the time velocity integral of antegrade flow in the right ventricular outflow tract (VTI_{RVOT}) correlated well (r = 0.93) with invasive measurement of pulmonary vascular resistance (PVR in Wood units):

$$PVR = 10(V_{TR}/VTI_{RVOT}) + 0.16$$

Prospective validation of this proposed approach is needed.

The Echo Exam *Systolic Function*

Global LV function	Wall thickness
	Internal dimensions/ volumes
	dP/dt
	Ejection Fraction
Regional LV function	Segmental wall motion
Global RV function	RV size
	RV systolic function
Pulmonary pressures	Pulmonary systolic pressure
Cardiac output	Stroke volume (SV) and Cardiac output (CO)

Example

A 57-year-old man with a recent inferior myocardial infarction now is hypotensive. Echocardiography shows:

LV wall thickness (diastole)	7 mm
LV end-diastolic dimension	57 mm
LV end-systolic dimension	38 mm
Apical biplane ejection fraction	52%
Time interval between 1 and 3 m/s on MR-Jet	30 msec
Segmental wall motion	Akinesis of basal and mid-LV segments of inferior and infero-lateral walls
RV size	Moderately increased
RV systolic function	Severely decreased
TR-jet velocity (V_{TR})	2.6 m/s
Inferior vena cava	Normal diameter with inspiratory change <50%
LV outflow tract diameter ($LVOT_D$)	2.4 cm
LVOT velocity time integral ($LV1_{LVOT}$)	10 cm
Heart rate (HR)	85 bpm

Discussion

The left ventricle is at the upper limits of normal in size with a mildly reduced ejection fraction and regional wall motion abnormalities consistent with a recent inferior myocardial infarction. Ejection fraction is evaluated qualitatively only when image quality is too poor for tracing endocardial borders for a biplane ejection fraction calculation.

Left ventricular dP/dt is calculated from the interval between 1 and 3 m/s on the MR jet signal (*dt*) as:

$$dP/dt = [4(V_2)^2 - 4(V_1)^2]/dt = [4(3)^2 - 4(1)^2]/dt$$
$$= [36 - 4\,\text{mm Hg}]/.030\,\text{s} = 1067\,\text{mm Hg/s}$$

which is at the lower limits of normal (>1000 mm Hg/s).

RV size and systolic function are graded qualitatively. The findings of a moderately dilated RV with severe systolic dysfunction in this patient are consistent with right ventricular infarction accompanying the inferior LV infarction, as the coronary artery that supplies the LV inferior wall also often supplies the RV free wall.

Right atrial pressure is mildly elevated (estimate 10–15 mm Hg) as shown by the <50% change in the diameter of a non-dilated inferior vena cava with respiration.

Pulmonary systolic pressure (PAP) is calculated from the tricuspid regurgitant jet velocity (V_{TR}) and estimate of right atrial pressure (RAP) as:

$$PAP = 4(V_{TR})^2 + RAP = 4(2.6)^2 + 10 = 27 + 10 = 37\,\text{mm Hg}$$

This is consistent with mild pulmonary hypertension.

Cardiac output (CO) is calculated using the LVOT diameter to calculate the circular cross sectional areas of flow:

$$CSA_{LVOT} = \pi(LVOT_D/2)^2 = 3.14(2.4/2)^2 = 4.5\,\text{cm}^2$$

Stroke volume across the aortic valve (cm³ = mL), then is:

$$SV_{LVOT} = (CSA_{LVOT} \times VTI_{LVOT}) = 4.5\,\text{cm}^2 \times 10\,\text{cm} = 45\,\text{cm}^3$$

Cardiac output is:

$$CO = SV \times HR$$
$$= 45\,\text{mL} \times 85\,\text{beats/min} = 3830\,\text{mL/min or } 3.83\,\text{L/min}$$

This low cardiac output is due to the right ventricular infarction and explains his hypotension.

Quantitation of Left and Right Ventricular Systolic Function

Parameter	Modality	View	Recording	Measurements
Ejection fraction	2D	Apical four-chamber and two-chamber	Adjust depth, optimize endocardial definition, harmonic imaging, contrast if needed	Careful tracing of endocardial borders at end-diastole and end-systole in both views
dP/dt	CW Doppler	MR jet, usually from apex	Pt positioning and transducer angulation to obtain highest velocity MR jet, decrease velocity scale, increased sweep speed	Time interval between 1 m/s and 3 m/s on Doppler MR velocity curve
PA pressures	CW Doppler	Parasternal and apical	Pt positioning and transducer angulation to obtain highest velocity TR jet	Estimate of RA pressure from size and appearance of IVC
Cardiac output	2D and pulsed Doppler	Parasternal LVOT diameter	Ultrasound beam perpendicular to LVOT with depth decreased and gain adjusted to see mid-systolic diameter.	LVOT diameter from inner edge to inner edge in mid-systole, adjacent and parallel to aortic valve.
		Apical LVOT velocity time integral	LVOT velocity from ant. angulated A4C view with sample volume just on LV side of aortic valve	Trace modal velocity of LVOT spectral Doppler envelope.

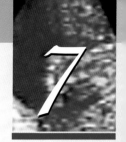

VENTRICULAR DIASTOLIC FILLING AND FUNCTION

There has been increasing recognition that *diastolic* ventricular function often plays an essential role in the clinical manifestations of disease in patients with a wide range of cardiac disorders. For example, many patients with clinical heart failure have normal systolic function with predominant diastolic dysfunction. Diastolic dysfunction may be an early sign of cardiac diseases (as in hypertension), often antedating clinical or echocardiographic evidence of systolic dysfunction. In addition, the degree of diastolic dysfunction may explain the difference in clinical symptoms between patients with similar degrees of systolic dysfunction.

Echocardiographic techniques allow evaluation of right and left ventricular diastolic filling patterns and right and left atrial filling patterns. The relationship between these noninvasive measures and ventricular diastolic function and the utility of these measures in patient evaluation are discussed in this chapter.

BASIC PRINCIPLES

Phases of Diastole

Although several different definitions of diastole have been proposed, the most widely accepted clinical definition is the interval from aortic valve closure (end-systole) to mitral valve closure (end-diastole) (Fig. 7–1). The isovolumic contraction period, from mitral valve closure to aortic valve opening, typically is considered as part of systole.

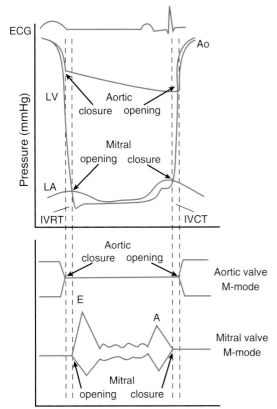

FIGURE 7–1. The relationship between left ventricular (LV), left atrial (LA), and aortic (Ao) pressures and M-mode tracings of the aortic and mitral valve is shown. The isovolumic relaxation time (IVRT) is the interval from aortic valve closure to mitral valve opening. During this interval, left ventricular pressure declines rapidly. A rapid rise in left ventricular pressure occurs during the isovolumic contraction time (IVCT), the interval between mitral valve closure and aortic valve opening.

Diastole can be divided into four phases:

■ isovolumic relaxation,
■ the early rapid diastolic filling phase,
■ diastasis, and
■ late diastolic filling due to atrial contraction.

During the isovolumic relaxation interval, left ventricular pressure falls rapidly following aortic valve closure. At the point where left ventricular pressure falls below left atrial pressure, the mitral valve opens, ending the isovolumic relaxation period. With mitral valve opening, blood flows from the left atrium to the left ventricle, with the rate and time course of flow being determined by several factors, including the pressure difference along the flow path, ventricular relaxation, and the relative compliances of the two chambers. Maximal opening of the mitral leaflets typically

occurs rapidly, within $100 \pm 10\,\mathrm{ms}$ of valve opening, in normal individuals.

As the ventricle fills, pressures between the atrium and ventricle equalize, resulting in a period of *diastasis*, during which there is little movement of blood between the chambers and the mitral leaflets remain in a semiopen position. The duration of diastasis is heart rate–dependent, being longer at slow heart rates and entirely absent at faster heart rates. With atrial contraction, left atrial pressure again exceeds left ventricular pressure, resulting in mitral leaflet opening and a second pulse of left ventricular filling. In normal individuals, the atrial contribution to ventricular filling typically is small, comprising only approximately 20% of total ventricular filling (Fig. 7–2).

The phases of diastole for the right ventricle are analogous to those described for the left ventricle, with the difference that the total duration of diastole is slightly shorter in normal individuals due to a slightly longer right ventricular systolic ejection period.

Parameters of Diastolic Function

There are several physiologic parameters that can be used to describe different aspects of diastolic

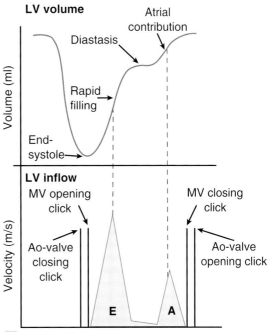

FIGURE 7–2. The relationship between left ventricular volume and the diastolic left ventricular Doppler filling pattern is shown. Early rapid filling coincides with the *E* velocity, followed by diastasis, with little or no flow from left atrium to left ventricle, and atrial contraction, which coincides with the late diastolic *A* velocity. The Doppler velocity curve, in effect, is the first derivative of the left ventricular volume curve.

function, but there is no single measure of overall diastolic function. The most clinically relevant parameters of diastolic function are

- ■ ventricular relaxation,
- ■ myocardial or chamber compliance, and
- ■ filling pressures.

Additional parameters of interest include elastic recoil of the ventricle and the effect of pericardial constraint, but the importance of these factors in normal diastolic ventricular function remains controversial.

Ventricular Relaxation

Left ventricular relaxation, occurring during isovolumic relaxation and the early diastolic filling period, is an active process involving use of energy by the myocardium. Factors affecting isovolumic relaxation include internal loading forces (cardiac fiber), external loading conditions (wall stress, arterial impedance), inactivation of myocardial contraction (metabolic, neurohumoral, and pharmacologic), and nonuniformity in the spatial and temporal patterns of these factors. Abnormal relaxation results in prolongation of the isovolumic relaxation time, a slower rate of decline in ventricular pressure, and a consequent reduction in the early peak filling rate (due to a smaller pressure difference between the atrium and the ventricle when the atrioventricular valve opens). Measures of left ventricular relaxation include the isovolumic relaxation time (IVRT), the maximum rate of pressure decline ($-dP/dt$), and the time constant of relaxation (tau or τ). There are several different mathematical approaches to calculation of tau; basically, it reflects the rate of pressure decline from the point of maximum $-dP/dt$ to mitral valve opening. Although peak rapid filling rate is affected by ventricular relaxation, it is only an indirect measure of this physiologic parameter, because several other factors also affect peak filling (Fig. 7–3).

Ventricular Compliance

Compliance is the ratio of change in volume to change in pressure (dV/dP). Stiffness is the inverse of compliance: the ratio of change in pressure to change in volume (dP/dV). Conceptually, compliance can be divided into myocardial (the characteristics of the isolated myocardium) and chamber (the characteristics of the entire chamber) components. Chamber compliance is influenced by ventricular size and shape, as well as by the characteristics of the myocardium. Extrinsic factors also may affect measurement of compliance, including the pericardium, right ventricular

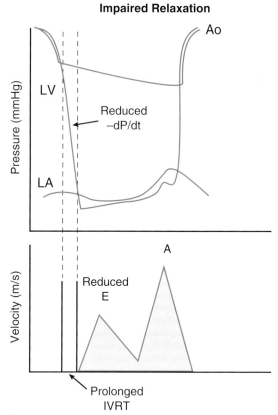

FIGURE 7–3. Impaired left ventricular relaxation is described by a reduced $-dP/dt$, and a prolonged time constant of relaxation. The Doppler velocity curve shows a prolonged IVRT, reduced E velocity (corresponding to a low left atrial–left ventricular gradient at mitral valve opening), and an increased A velocity.

volume, and pleural pressure. Evaluation of ventricular compliance is based on diastolic passive pressure-volume curves showing the degree to which pressure and volume change in relation to each other over the physiologic range of pressures and volumes (Fig. 7–4).

Ventricular Diastolic Pressures

Clinically, evaluation of diastolic pressures alone often is used in patient management. Diastolic filling pressures include left ventricular end-diastolic pressure (LV-EDP) and mean left atrial pressure (LAP). LV-EDP reflects ventricular pressure after filling is complete, while LAP reflects the average pressure in the left atrium during diastole. Clinically, LAP is estimated by the pulmonary artery wedge pressure (PAWP) either at a single time point in the cardiac catheterization laboratory or at many time points with an

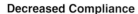

Decreased Compliance

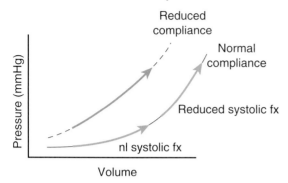

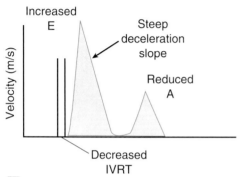

FIGURE 7–4. Reduced diastolic compliance is described by a steeper passive pressure-volume relationship of the left ventricle. As left ventricular volume increases in diastole, pressure rises rapidly, resulting in an initial high left atrial–left ventricular pressure gradient with a rapid decrease in the filling gradient during diastole. The Doppler velocity curve shows a decreased IVRT, steep deceleration slope, and reduced *A* velocity. Note that even with normal compliance, reduced systolic function results in a rightward shift along the normal pressure-volume relationship, resulting in a pattern of diastolic filling similar to decreased compliance.

indwelling right heart (Swan-Ganz) catheter in the intensive care unit.

Ventricular Diastolic Filling (Volume) Curves

Another clinically available measure related to diastolic function is the time course of ventricular filling: the ventricular diastolic filling curve. Experimentally, filling curves can be measured on a beat-to-beat basis from implanted sonocrystal-derived ventricular dimensions or from imped-ance catheter data. Clinically, filling curves can be generated for an individual cardiac cycle from frame-by-frame measurements of ventricular volumes using angiographic, computed tomo-graphy, magnetic resonance, or echocardio-graphic images or from high-temporal-resolution radionuclide studies. Doppler echocardiography offers the ability to measure left ventricular

diastolic filling, noninvasively, on a beat-to-beat basis.

Unfortunately, while ventricular *diastolic function* is one of the major factors affecting the pattern of *diastolic filling*, these two concepts are not identical. Several physiologic parameters other than dia-stolic function affect diastolic filling. Given no change in diastolic function (i.e., relaxation, com-pliance, etc.), the peak early diastolic filling rate will be affected by

■ changes in preload that affect the pressure dif-ference between the ventricle and the atrium (e.g., increased with volume loading, decreased with volume depletion),
■ a change in transmitral volume flow rate (e.g., increased with coexisting mitral regurgitation), or
■ a change in atrial pressure (e.g., elevated left ventricular end-diastolic pressure or a *v* wave due to mitral regurgitation).

Late diastolic filling is affected by

■ cardiac rhythm,
■ atrial contractile function,
■ ventricular end-diastolic pressure,
■ heart rate, and
■ the timing of atrial contraction (PR interval), as well as by
■ ventricular diastolic function.

The importance of considering the influence of these factors on the pattern of diastolic filling as assessed by Doppler echocardiography is discussed in more detail in the following sections. In addition, it is obvious that the utility of ventricular diastolic filling patterns for assessing diastolic function is valid only in the absence of obstruction at the atrioventricular valve level (i.e., mitral stenosis). In patients with rhythms other than normal sinus rhythm (e.g., atrial fibrillation), evaluation of diastolic function with Doppler is limited.

Atrial Pressures and Filling Curves

Another component of the evaluation of ventric-ular diastolic function is measurement of atrial filling patterns and pressures. Elevations in ven-tricular diastolic pressures will be reflected in elevated pressures in the atrium and atrial filling patterns obviously are closely linked with diastolic ventricular function, especially in early diastole, when the atrioventricular valve is open, since the atrium serves as a "conduit" for flow from the venous circulation to the ventricle (Fig. 7–5).

Right atrial pressures normally are quite low (0 to 5 mm Hg), with only small increases in pressure

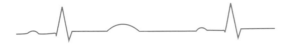

Neck vein pulsations

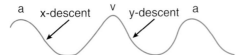

Hepatic vein Doppler

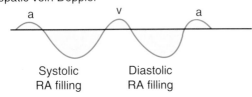

Pulmonary vein Doppler

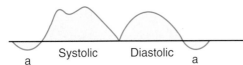

■ **FIGURE 7–5.** Schematic diagram of right atrial (hepatic vein) and left atrial (pulmonary vein) filling patterns and the close correspondence with the pattern of jugular venous pulsations. Pulmonary and hepatic vein patterns appear "opposite" in direction, because the direction of flow in the hepatic vein using a transthoracic subcostal view is away from the transducer (into the right atrium), while the direction of flow from a transthoracic apical view of the pulmonary vein is toward the transducer (into the left atrium).

following atrial (*a* wave) and ventricular (*v* wave) contraction. *Right atrial filling* is characterized by

■ a small reversal of flow following atrial contraction (*a* wave),
■ a systolic phase (which is effectively "diastole" for the atrium) when blood flows from the superior and inferior vena cava into the atrium,
■ a small reversal of flow at end-systole (*v* wave), and
■ a diastolic filling phase when the atrium serves as a conduit for flow from the systemic venous return to the right ventricle.

These filling phases are reflected in the patterns of jugular venous pulsation familiar to the clinician: the *a* wave following atrial contraction, the *x* descent corresponding to atrial systolic filling, the *v* wave with ventricular contraction, and the *y* descent corresponding to atrial diastolic filling. Disease processes affect the jugular venous pulsations and the Doppler pattern of right atrial filling in similar ways.

Left atrial filling from the pulmonary veins also is characterized by

■ a small reversal of flow following atrial contraction (*a* wave),
■ a systolic filling phase,
■ a blunting of flow or brief reversal at end-systole, and
■ a diastolic filling phase.

In normal individuals, the systolic and diastolic filling phases are approximately equal in volume. Normal left atrial pressure is low (5 to 10 mm Hg), corresponding to the normal left ventricular end-diastolic pressure, with slight increases in pressure following atrial (*a* wave) and ventricular (*v* wave) contraction.

Normal Respiratory Changes

The patterns of right and left ventricular diastolic filling show normal respiratory variation. With inspiration, negative intrapleural pressure results in an increase in systemic venous return into the thorax and, thus, into the right atrium. This increased right atrial volume and pressure results in a transient increase in right ventricular diastolic filling volumes and velocities, with a normal magnitude of increase of up to 20% compared with end-expiratory values.

Left atrium filling does *not* increase with inspiration, since pulmonary venous return is entirely intrathoracic and thus not affected significantly by respiratory changes in intrathoracic pressure. In fact, left atrial and, consequently, left ventricular diastolic filling is slightly higher at end-expiration than during inspiration. The mechanism of the observation remains controversial. Some postulate a delay in transit of the increased right ventricular filling to the left side of the heart. Others suggest a decrease in left atrial filling during inspiration due to an increased volume (or "pooling") in the pulmonary venous bed. Less likely, in normal individuals, is impaired left ventricular diastolic filling due to an increase in right ventricular diastolic volume within a fixed-volume pericardium. This last mechanism may become important in patients with pericardial disease (constriction, tamponade) and may partly account for the exaggerated respiratory changes in right ventricular and left ventricular diastolic filling seen in these conditions.

Causes of Diastolic Dysfunction

While diastolic dysfunction can be seen with a wide range of cardiac disorders, there are four basic mechanisms of disease (Table 7–1) that lead to diastolic dysfunction:

TABLE 7-1
Causes of Diastolic Dysfunction

Primary myocardial disease	Dilated cardiomyopathy
	Restrictive cardiomyopathy
	Hypertrophic cardiomyopathy
Secondary hypertrophy	Hypertension
	Aortic stenosis
	Aortic or mitral regurgitation
	Congenital heart disease
Coronary artery disease	Ischemia
	Infarction
Extrinsic constraint	Pericardial tamponade
	Pericardial constriction

- Primary myocardial disease
- Secondary left ventricular hypertrophy
- Coronary artery disease
- Extrinsic constraint

TWO-DIMENSIONAL/ M-MODE EVALUATION

Evaluation of ventricular chamber dimensions and wall thickness is an integral part of the echocardiographic evaluation of diastolic function. In a patient with clinical heart failure, the findings of increased wall thickness with a nondilated chamber and normal systolic function suggest that diastolic dysfunction may be the etiology of "heart failure." Of course, this finding is neither sensitive nor specific for the diagnosis of diastolic dysfunction. Diastolic dysfunction can be present concurrently with systolic dysfunction (e.g., in dilated cardiomyopathy) and may be absent despite ventricular hypertrophy in some situations, such as physiologic hypertrophy in an athlete. On M-mode echocardiography, early studies suggested that the degree and rate of motion of the posterior left ventricular wall might provide a useful measure of diastolic function. In practical terms, the magnitude of these changes is too small to be measured reliably. Other findings on two-dimensional (2D) or M-mode echocardiography that raise the question of diastolic dysfunction include pericardial thickening (as in constrictive pericarditis), the pattern of ventricular septal motion with respiration (especially with tamponade physiology), and dilation of the inferior vena cava and hepatic veins (consistent with elevated right atrial pressures). Tissue characterization of the myocardium using ultrasound techniques may prove to be useful in evaluation of patients with suspected diastolic dysfunction, but

further studies are needed. Thus, direct evaluation of ventricular diastolic function by 2D or M-mode techniques is limited. Instead, attention has focused on the utility of Doppler echocardiography for evaluation of diastolic function.

DOPPLER EVALUATION OF LEFT VENTRICULAR FILLING

Description of Left Ventricular Filling by Doppler Echo

Doppler recordings of left ventricular diastolic filling velocities correspond closely with ventricular filling parameters measured by other techniques (Table 7-2). The normal Doppler ventricular inflow pattern is characterized by a brief interval between aortic valve closure and the onset of ventricular filling (the isovolumic

TABLE 7-2
Doppler Measures of Left Ventricular Diastolic Filling

Left Ventricular Inflow Velocities

Early diastolic filling velocity (E)*
Filling velocity after atrial contraction (A)*
Ratio of E/A*

Intervals

Isovolumic relaxation time (IVRT)*
Deceleration time (DT)*
Atrial filling period $(A_{dur},$ at annulus)*

Acceleration/Deceleration

Time from mitral valve opening to E velocity
Maximal acceleration
Early diastolic deceleration slope

Filling Rates/Volumes

Peak rapid filling rate
Peak atrial filling rate
Stroke volume
Fractional filling rates (first third)

Doppler Myocardial Tissue Velocities

Early diastolic myocardial tissue velocity (E_m)*
Diatolic myocardial tissue velocity after atrial contraction (A_m)*
Ratio of E_m/A_m*

Color M-Mode Doppler

Propagation velocity

Mitral Regurgitant Jet Signal

Rate of decline in LV pressure in early diastole $(-dP/dt)$

*Components of standard examination for diastolic dysfunction.

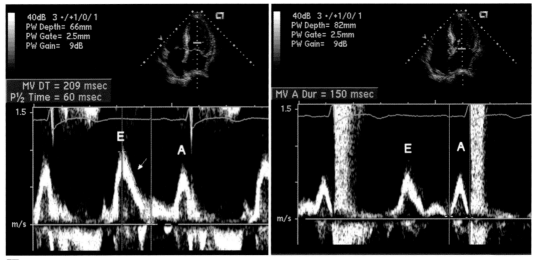

FIGURE 7–6. Normal pattern of left ventricular diastolic filling recorded with pulsed Doppler in an apical four-chamber view at the mitral leaflet tips (*left*) and at the mitral annulus level (*right*). The recording at the mitral tips level is used to measure *E* velocity, *A* velocity, and the deceleration time. The annular flow signal is used for measurement of atrial flow duration. If transmitral stroke volume is calculated, the annular flow signal is used for the velocity time integral.

relaxation time). Immediately following mitral valve opening, there is rapid acceleration of blood flow from the left atrium to the ventricle with an early peak filling velocity of 0.6 to 0.8 m/s occurring 90 to 110 ms after the onset of flow in young, healthy individuals. This early maximum filling velocity (*E* velocity) occurs simultaneously with the maximum pressure gradient between the atrium and ventricle. After this maximum velocity, flow decelerates rapidly (i.e., with a steep slope) in normal individuals with a normal deceleration slope of 4.3 to 6.7 m/s². Deceleration time, defined as the interval from the *E* peak to where a line following the deceleration slope intersects with the zero baseline, ranges from about 140 to 200 ms. Early diastolic filling is followed by a variable period of minimal flow (diastasis), depending on the total duration of diastole. With atrial contraction, left atrial pressure again exceeds ventricular pressure, resulting in a second velocity peak (late diastolic or atrial velocity), which typically ranges from 0.19 to 0.35 m/s in young, normal individuals (Fig. 7–6).

Quantitative Ventricular Filling Velocity and Time Interval Measurements

Quantitative measurements that can be made from the Doppler velocity curve include (Fig. 7–7):

1. *Maximum velocities*: The *E* velocity, the *A* velocity, and their ratio (*E/A* ratio)

2. *Velocity-time integrals*: Total, early diastolic, atrial contribution, first third or half of diastole, and their ratios
3. *Time intervals*: The isovolumic relaxation time, the total duration of diastole, the deceleration time, and the atrial filling period
4. *Measures of acceleration and deceleration*: The time from onset of flow to the *E* velocity, the

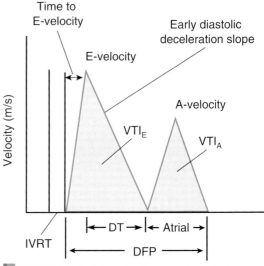

FIGURE 7–7. Schematic diagram of quantitative measurements that can be made from the Doppler left ventricular filling curve.

maximum rate of rise in velocity, and the slope of early diastolic deceleration

Volumetric Flow Rates

To convert the Doppler ventricular inflow *velocity curve* to a *volume curve*, the cross-sectional area of flow must be taken into account. As described in Chapter 2, volumetric flow rates can be calculated as the product of velocity and cross-sectional area in regions where flow is laminar with a spatially symmetric flow pattern. Thus, the instantaneous volume flow rate across the mitral valve can be calculated as instantaneous velocity times the flow cross-sectional area (CSA). Similarly, transmitral stroke volume (SV) can be determined from the integral of the flow velocity curve (VTI) over the diastolic filling period:

$$SV_{transmitral} = VTI \times CSA$$

The standard approach to determining the cross-sectional area of flow across the mitral valve is to calculate the cross-sectional area of flow at the mitral annulus level. Motion of the mitral leaflets is a passive process, with the degree of motion reflecting flow across the valve (in the absence of mitral stenosis). Although there is some tapering of the flow area from the annulus to the leaflet tips, the more rigid mitral annulus is a preferable site for flow measurement rather than the flexible, mobile leaflets. Even though the shape of the mitral annulus is complex in three dimensions, area often is calculated as an ellipse, based on diameter measurements in apical four-chamber and parasternal long-axis views. The even simpler assumption of a circular geometry, using the parasternal long axis diameter, also is a reasonable approximation in most clinical situations (Fig. 7–8).

Combining Doppler left ventricular inflow velocity data with the cross-sectional area of the mitral annulus, additional filling parameters that can be calculated include:

1. *Peak filling rates*: Peak rapid filling rate, atrial peak filling rate, and their ratio
2. *Stroke volume*
3. *Fractional filling rates*: For example, first third filling fraction or the ratio of early to late filling

For each of these parameters, the filling rate is calculated by multiplying the appropriate velocity or velocity-time integral by cross-sectional area. For example, peak rapid filling rate (PRFR) is

$$PRFR \ (mL/s) = E \ velocity \ (cm/s) \times CSA \ (cm^2)$$

Of course, volume flow measurements are accurate only when velocities and diameters are

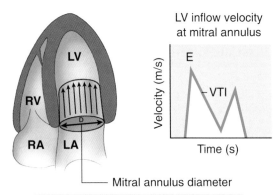

LV inflow velocity at mitral annulus

$$CSA = \pi \ (D/2)^2$$
$$Transmittal \ SV = CSA \times VTI$$
$$Peak \ filling \ rate = E\text{-velocity} \times CSA$$

FIGURE 7–8. Calculation of volumetric flow rates across the mitral annulus. Mitral annular diameter can be measured from both apical four-chamber and parasternal long-axis views to calculate an elliptical cross-sectional area. If a circular cross-sectional area is used as an approximation, the parasternal long-axis annular diameter is used in the calculations.

measured at the same anatomic location, for example, at the annulus level.

Doppler Data Recording

Left ventricular inflow can be recorded in nearly all patients from an apical approach in either a four- or two-chamber view (Table 7–3). This window allows parallel alignment between the ultrasound beam and the direction of left ventricular filling. On transesophageal echocardiography, left ventricular inflow can be recorded from a high esophageal position, taking care to align the Doppler beam parallel to the inflow stream (Fig. 7–9). In some patients, a transgastric apical view also may allow recording of left ventricular inflow, although caution is needed to avoid foreshortening of the ventricle and a nonparallel intercept angle (with resultant underestimation of velocities) from this window.

Inflow velocities should be recorded using pulsed Doppler with the 2 to 3 mm sample volume positioned first at the mitral leaflet tips (for evaluation of diastolic function) and then at the mitral annulus level (for measurement of volume flow rates and the duration of atrial filling) (see Fig. 7–6). With the beam aligned parallel to the flow stream, the 2- to 3-mm sample volume is moved slowly along the length of the ultrasound beam to identify the site of maximal velocity, usually at the mitral leaflet tip level. The velocity range is

TABLE 7–3

Selected Normal Parameters of Diastolic Function

Velocities	
E/A ratio	1.32 ± 0.42
Deceleration slope	5.0 ± 1.4 m/s²
Intervals	
IVRT	63 ± 11 ms
Deceleration time	150–200 ms
$A_{dur}-a_{dur}$	<20 ms
Derived Measures	
Tau	33 ± 6 ms
$-dP/dt$	2048 ± 335 mm Hg/s
Filling Rates	
Peak filling rate	288 ± 66 mL/s
Peak filling rate normalized to	
LV-EDV	2.9 ± 1.0 s⁻¹
Atrial filling rate	229 ± 83 mL/s
Ratio of early to atrial FV1	1.71 ± 0.43
Myocardial Doppler Velocities	
E_m	10.3 ± 2.0 cm/s
A_m	5.8 ± 1.6 cm/s
Ratio of E_m/A_m	2.1 ± 0.9

Data from: Tebbe et al: Clin Cardiol 3:19, 1980; Shapiro, McKenna: Br Heart J 51:637, 1984; Pearson et al: Am Heart J 113:1417, 1987; Snider R et al: Am J Cardiol 56:921, 1985; Garcia-Fernandez et al: Eur Heart J 20:496, 1999.

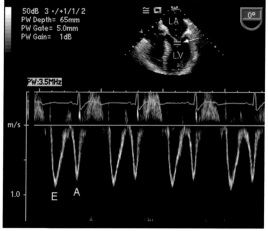

■ **FIGURE 7–9.** Transesophageal recording of left ventricular filling. Flow is directed away from the transducer from this approach.

adjusted to maximize the display of the velocity of interest and avoid signal aliasing. The sweep speed for the spectral display is maximized (100 cm/s) and wall filters are reduced (as allowed by signal quality) so that the velocities approach the baseline, allowing accurate time interval measurements. Flows are recorded at end-expiration during normal breathing. Standard clinical measurements of left ventricular inflow include

- early diastolic filling velocity (E),
- atrial filling velocity (A),
- deceleration time (DT) all at the leaflet tips, and
- atrial filling duration (A_{dur}) at the mitral annulus.

TISSUE DOPPLER MYOCARDIAL IMAGING

As the left ventricle fills in diastole, the myocardial walls expand, or move outward, and this motion can be recorded using pulsed Doppler with the velocity scale, gain and wall filters adjusted to display the velocity of the movement of the myocardium, rather than the intracavity blood flow velocities. The diastolic velocities of the left ventricular myocardium are less dependent on preload than transmitral flow velocities and thus are useful adjunct to filling velocities in evaluation of diastolic function. The pattern of myocardial motion is similar, but inverted and lower in velocity, compared to transmitral flow velocities (Fig 7–10). When myocardial tissue velocities are recorded near the mitral annulus from an apical approach, there is a brief early diastolic velocity peak away from the transducer, corresponding to early diastolic relaxation, with a velocity between 0.10 to 0.14 cm/s, which is termed the *early myocardial velocity* (E_m). Following atrial contraction, a second velocity peak away from the apex is seen (A_m) with a normal ratio of $E_m/A_m > 1.0$. A reduced E_m/A_m indicates impaired relaxation. The pattern of E_m/A_m also helps distinguish normal left ventricular filling from the pseudo-normalized pattern seen in patients with moderate to severe diastolic dysfunction.

Myocardial tissue Doppler signals are recorded using pulsed Doppler in an apical four-chamber view with a small sample volume (2 to 3 mm in length) positioned in the myocardium of the basal ventricular wall, about 1 cm from the mitral annulus. Signals may be recorded from the basal septum or basal lateral wall, although signals tend to be more reproducible from the septum. The velocity scale is decreased to show a range of only about 0.2 m/s, gain is turned to very low levels,

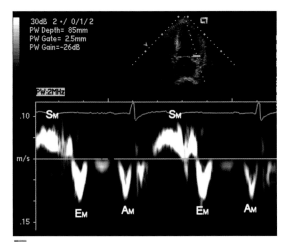

■ **FIGURE 7-10.** Myocardial tissue Doppler recording in a young normal patient with the early myocardial velocity (E_m) greater than the atrial velocity (A_m). The systolic velocity toward the transducer is termed S_m. Note that the velocity scale has a maximum of only 0.15 m/s, compared to 1.5 m/s for left ventricular inflow in Figure 7-6 in the same patient.

and wall filters are reduced to obtain a well-defined signal with clear E_m and A_m peaks. Some instruments have a tissue Doppler setting that automatically makes these adjustments to the pulsed Doppler modality. Recordings are made at end-expiration during normal quiet respiration. Standard clinical measurements from the myocardial tissue Doppler include

■ early diastolic filling velocity (E_m), and
■ filling velocity after atrial contraction (A_m).

ISOVOLUMIC RELAXATION TIME

The isovolumic relaxation time (IVRT) is simply the time interval between aortic valve closure and mitral valve opening. A normal isovolumic relaxation time is approximately 80 to 100 msec, but the normal range varies with age and heart rate. Impaired relaxation is associated with a prolonged IVRT whereas decreased compliance and elevated filling pressures are associated with a shortened IVRT. Thus, this measurement is useful in determining the severity of diastolic dysfunction, particularly in serial studies of patients on medical therapy or with disease progression.

The isovolumic relaxation time is measured from an apical four-chamber view angulated anteriorly to show the outflow tract and aortic valve. Using pulsed Doppler, a 3- to 5-mm sample volume is positioned midway between the aortic and mitral valves to obtain a clear signal showing both aortic outflow and mitral inflow, optimally

with a defined aortic valve closing click. After adjusting gain and decreasing the wall filters, the IVRT is measured as the time interval in milliseconds from the middle of the aortic closure click to the onset of mitral flow (Fig. 7-11).

LEFT ATRIAL FILLING

Doppler Assessment

Left atrial filling is evaluated by Doppler recordings of pulmonary vein flow either from a transesophageal or a transthoracic approach. Again, the Doppler pattern of velocities parallels the normal filling curves, with inflow into the left atrium occurring in two phases, systolic and diastolic. In addition, there is flow deceleration following ventricular contraction and a small reversal of flow after atrial contraction (Fig. 7-12). On transesophageal recordings, the systolic inflow pattern is biphasic in most patients, with an early systolic peak related to atrial relaxation and a second late systolic peak related to displacement of the mitral annulus toward the left ventricular apex. Respiratory variation in flow may be seen in left-heart filling patterns (atrial and ventricular) but is less prominent than the variation seen in right-heart filling *and* is directionally opposite: left-heart filling diminishes slightly with inspiration. Both the pulmonary veins and the left atrium are intrathoracic in their entirety, so negative intrathoracic pressure does not result in a pressure gradient between them. Instead, atrial filling may diminish during inspiration as blood "pools" briefly in the expanded pulmonary veins, which then empty during expiration.

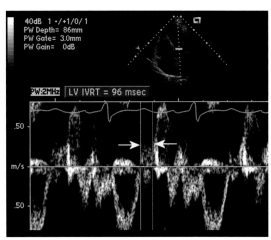

■ **FIGURE 7-11.** The isovolumic relaxation time (IVRT) is measured from aortic valve closure and the onset of mitral flow (*arrows*) and measures 96 ms in this example.

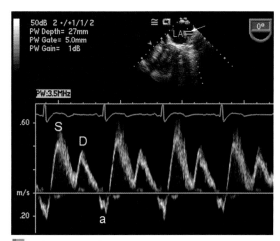

FIGURE 7–12. Normal pattern of left atrial inflow recorded in the left superior pulmonary vein from a transesophageal approach.

Doppler Data Recording

From a transesophageal approach, left atrial inflow patterns can be easily recorded in each of the four pulmonary veins in the transverse plane. Careful positioning and angulation are needed to ensure that the pulsed Doppler sample volume is located in the pulmonary vein itself rather than in the adjacent left atrium. A sample volume size of 5 mm typically is used with wall filters lowered to show the low-velocity components associated with atrial and ventricular contraction. The flow pattern varies somewhat with distance from the pulmonary vein orifice. A distance approximately 1 cm from the orifice provides optimal signal strength with the most consistent inflow pattern.

The left superior pulmonary vein is most easily visualized adjacent to the left atrial appendage, and is directed somewhat anteriorly. The left inferior pulmonary vein can be visualized by advancing the transducer a short distance to see the inflow pattern from this horizontally directed vein. The right pulmonary veins can be imaged by turning the transducer medially to identify the superior right pulmonary vein (again anteriorly directed) and advancing the probe slightly to image the horizontally positioned right inferior pulmonary vein.

From a transthoracic approach, recording pulmonary venous flow patterns is more challenging. Most echocardiographers use the apical four-chamber view, which allows a parallel alignment between the right superior pulmonary vein flow stream and the ultrasound beam. Signal strength may be a limiting factor at this depth of interro-

gation (typically about 14 cm), so careful attention to sample volume position, wall filters, and gain settings is needed to optimize the velocity data. Sample volume positioning may be facilitated by the use of color flow imaging to identify the flow stream from the pulmonary vein into the left atrium. Again, the sample volume should be positioned *in* the pulmonary vein 1 to 2 cm from the orifice. Of note, the biphasic pattern of systolic inflow and atrial reversal may be more difficult to demonstrate on transthoracic compared with transesophageal imaging due to a lower signal-to-noise ratio (Fig. 7–13). In addition, the flow pattern in the left upper pulmonary vein (on transesophageal echocardiography) shows a more laminar flow pattern than the right upper pulmonary vein (on transesophageal or transthoracic echocardiography). Alternate transthoracic windows that may allow recording of pulmonary vein flow in some individuals include subcostal and parasternal short-axis views at the aortic valve level or suprasternal notch views of the left atrium and pulmonary veins. However, intercept angle tends to be suboptimal from these windows. Standard clinical measures of pulmonary venous inflow include

■ peak systolic velocity (PV_S),
■ peak diastolic velocity (PV_D),
■ peak atrial reversal velocity (PV_a), and
■ duration of pulmonary vein atrial reversal (a_{dur}).

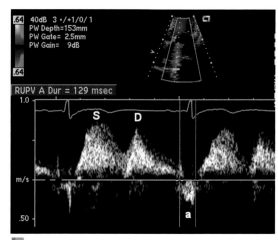

FIGURE 7–13. Normal pattern of left atrial inflow recorded in the right superior pulmonary vein from a transthoracic apical four-chamber view using color flow imaging to aid in positioning the sample volume approximately 1 to 2 cm into the vein. Note the systolic (S) and diastolic (D) filling phases with a slight flow reversal following atrial contraction (*a*).

COLOR DOPPLER M-MODE PROPAGATION VELOCITY

Color Doppler M-mode recordings of left ventricular inflow from an apical approach can be used to measure the propagation velocity as blood moves from the annulus to the apex. The flow propagation velocity is decreased with restrictive ventricular filling and increased with constrictive pericarditis.

Color M-mode propagation velocity is recorded from an apical four chamber view using color flow imaging to place a color M-mode cursor parallel to mitral inflow in the center of the flow stream (Fig. 7–14). Using a narrow sector, minimum depth needed to include the annulus and apex, and an aliasing velocity of 0.5 to 0.7 m/s, the color M-mode signal is recorded at a fast sweep speed (100 to 200 mm/s). With normal diastolic function, the blood flows quickly from the annulus toward the apex resulting in a near vertical M-mode color pattern. The slope of the line along the edge of the color Doppler M-mode in early diastole is termed the *propagation velocity*, with a normal value >50 cm/s. With decreased relaxation, the movement of blood from the annulus to apex is slower so that the slope of color M-mode is prolonged. Accurate recording and measurement of the propagation velocity requires considerable expertise and is not used in all laboratories.

MITRAL REGURGITANT JET

The rate of decline in velocity of the mitral regurgitant jet at end-systole reflects the rate of decrease in left ventricular pressure in early diastole (Fig.

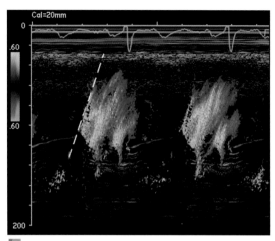

■ FIGURE 7–14. Color Doppler M-mode propagation velocity (*dashed line*) recorded with the color Doppler M-mode cursor positioned in the center of the mitral annulus in an apical four-chamber view. The slope of the Doppler flow as it moves from the annulus (*bottom of scale*) to the apex (*top of the scale*) reflects the rate of left ventricular relaxation.

7–15). This allows measurement of the negative dP/dt from the end-systolic segment of the mitral regurgitant jet, analogous to measurement of positive dP/dt from the initial segment of the jet (see Chapter 6). Unfortunately, the mitral regurgitant jet velocity is also affected by left atrial pressure, which may be elevated with mitral regurgitation independent of abnormalities in diastolic function. In addition, reproducibility of this measurement is suboptimal due to poor signal strength in some patients and measurement of a

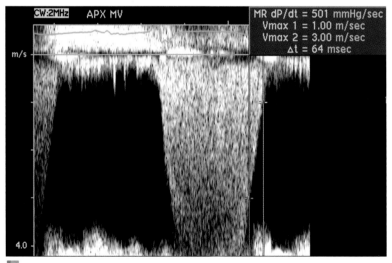

■ FIGURE 7–15. Measurement of −*dP/dt* from the deceleration curve of the mitral regurgitant jet signal.

short interval so that it has not been widely accepted as a standard method for evaluation of diastolic dysfunction.

FACTORS THAT AFFECT DOPPLER EVALUATION OF LEFT VENTRICULAR DIASTOLIC FUNCTION

Normal Variations

Evaluation of left ventricular diastolic function is confounded by the normal variation in ventricular filling related to

- respiration,
- heart rate,
- age, and
- PR interval.

There is normal slight variation (<20%) in left ventricular inflow velocities with respiration. At higher heart rates, diastole is shorter–particularly the period of diastasis–so that the *A* velocity more closely succeeds the *E* velocity. When overlap of these two velocity curves occurs, the *A* velocity, in effect, is "added" to the *E*-velocity curve, resulting in a higher *A* velocity and lower *E/A* ratio (Fig. 7–16). Similarly, a longer PR interval results in an *A* velocity earlier in diastole that may become superimposed on the *E*-velocity curve. At very high heart rates (short diastolic filling periods), the *E*- and *A*-velocity curves become merged into a single *E/A* velocity. Evaluation of a patient with complete heart block but intact atrial contraction often demonstrates this nicely, with the location of the *A* velocity relative to the *E* velocity affecting its magnitude accordingly (Fig. 7–17).

In children and young adults, the majority of ventricular filling occurs in early diastole, with a prominent *E* velocity and only a small contribution to ventricular filling due to atrial contraction (20% of total left ventricular volume). With age, the *E* velocity diminishes, and the atrial contribution becomes more prominent, with equalization of *E* and *A* velocities at approximately age 60

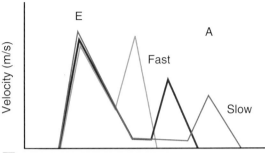

**LV Inflow
Effect of Heart Rate**

▌ FIGURE 7–16. Schematic diagram showing the overlap or "summation" of *A* velocity with *E* velocity that occurs with higher heart rates.

years and reversal of the *E/A* ratio after that age in normal individuals. Early diastolic deceleration time also is progressively prolonged and there is a slight increase in isovolumic relaxation time with age (Table 7–4, Fig. 7–18). Presumably, the mechanism of the changes in left ventricular filling patterns with age is a gradual reduction in the rate of early diastolic relaxation.

Left atrial filling is affected by many of the same variables that affect left ventricular diastolic filling. Higher heart rates result in merging of the systolic and diastolic phases of left atrial filling, while lower heart rates result in clearer separation between them. Changes in left atrial inflow with aging have been described, including a reduction in the diastolic filling phase, a compensatory increase in the systolic filling phase, and a more prominent atrial reversal in subjects older than age 50 (see Fig. 7–18).

Physiologic Factors

Several physiologic variables other than left ventricular diastolic function that also affect the pattern of *left ventricular diastolic filling* include

- preload,
- volume flow rate (e.g., mitral regurgitation),

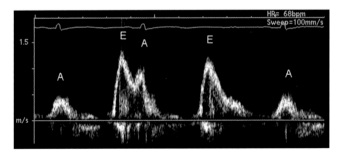

▌ FIGURE 7–17. Left ventricular filling in a patient with an atrial arrhythmia showing the effect of a shorter diastolic interval on the *E/A* pattern.

TABLE 7-4

Effect of Aging on Parameters of Left Ventricular Diastolic Filling in Normal Subjects

Parameter	Age 21-49yr* Mean (95% CI)	Age >50yr* Mean (95% CI)	Age >70yr† Mean (95% CI)
E velocity (m/s)	0.72 (0.44–1.00)	0.62 (0.34–0.90)	0.44 (0.25–0.76)
A velocity (m/s)	0.40 (0.20–0.60)	0.59 (0.31–0.87)	59 (0.38–0.84)
E/A ratio	1.9 (0.7–3.1)	1.1 (0.5–1.7)	0.8 (0.5–1.2)
Deceleration time (ms)	179 (139–219)	210 (138–282)	140 (90–230)
IVRT (ms)	76 (54–98)	90 (56–124)	

*Data from Cohen GI, Pietrolungo JF, Thomas JD, Klein AL: A practical guide to assessment of ventricular diastolic function using Doppler echocardiography. J Am Coll Cardiol 27:1753–1760, 1996. Normal reference values were derived from 61 subjects aged 21 to 49 years and 56 subjects older than 50 years.
†Data from Sagie A, Benjamin EJ, Galdersisi M, et al: Reference values for Doppler indexes of left ventricular diastolic filling in the elderly. J Am Soc Echocardiogr 6:570–576, 1993. Reference values were derived from 114 healthy elderly subjects in the Framingham Heart Study.
CI, confidence interval; IVRT, isovolumic relaxation time.

■ LV systolic function, and
■ atrial contractile function.

While it is clear that Doppler velocity recordings accurately represent left ventricular filling patterns, it should be emphasized again that left ventricular *filling* is not equivalent to left ventricular *diastolic function*.

Left atrial pressure, *preload*, dramatically affects the pattern of left ventricular filling (Fig. 7–19). Increased preload results in an increase in the *E* velocity, a shortened IVRT, and steeper deceleration slope of early diastolic filling. As the left ventricle fills rapidly in early diastole, left ventricular diastolic pressure rises, so atrial contraction results in only a small pressure gradient between the left atrium and the left ventricle and a small *A* velocity. Examples of elevated preload include volume infusion or an elevated left atrial pressure due to elevation of left ventricular end-diastolic pressure.

Mitral regurgitation also results in an increase in *E* velocity both via the mechanism of an elevated left atrial pressure and because of the increased volume flow rate across the mitral valve. Again, the *A* velocity tends to be reduced (Fig. 7–20).

Situations with a reduced left atrial pressure have a reduced *E* velocity due to a smaller gradient between the left atrium and left ventricle at mitral valve opening. Thus, hypovolemia or use of a venodilator (such as nitroglycerin) results in a decrease in the *E* velocity. Reduced preload is unlikely to affect atrial contraction, so the *A*-velocity peak is either unaffected or enhanced

LV Inflow
Effect of Age

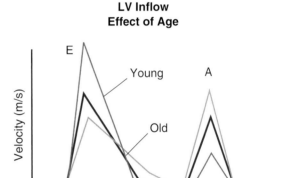

LV Inflow (Pulmonary Venous Flow)
Effect of Age

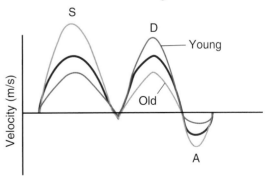

■ **FIGURE 7–18.** Schematic diagram showing the changes in left ventricular (*top*) and left atrial inflow and pulmonary venous flow (*bottom*) patterns that occur with age. The typical pattern seen in younger (age, 50 years) subjects (*solid lines*) is compared with middle-aged (*dotted lines*) and older (age, 70 years) subjects (*dashed lines*).

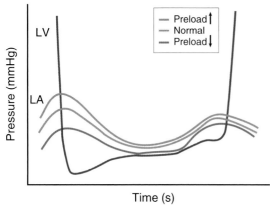

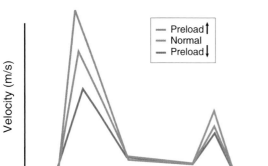

FIGURE 7–19. Effect of preload on left ventricular filling pattern. With increased preload, an increased pressure gradient from the left atrium to the left ventricle at the time of mitral valve opening results in a higher *E* velocity. The *A* velocity remains the same or is reduced if a high end-diastolic pressure results in a smaller left atrial to left ventricular pressure gradient following atrial contraction. The opposite changes occur with decreased preload.

if left ventricular diastolic pressure remains low at the time of atrial contraction.

Left ventricular systolic function affects the pattern of diastolic filling in that, for a given diastolic pressure-volume curve, an increased

end-systolic volume results in a shift to a steeper portion of the pressure-volume curve. Diastolic filling then occurs with a greater increase in pressure for a given increase in volume. This results in an increased *E* velocity and reduced *A* velocity, similar to the pattern seen with decreased compliance due to a shift to a different diastolic pressure-volume curve (see Fig. 7–4).

Atrial contractile function, although not always recognized clinically, can affect the pattern of left ventricular diastolic filling. This is obvious in the case of atrial fibrillation, when no atrial contribution to ventricular filling is seen (Fig. 7–21), or with atrial flutter, when small "flutter" waves in the inflow velocity pattern may be noted, but is less obvious in sinus rhythm with ineffective atrial contraction, which may result in a small *A* velocity.

Pulmonary venous flow patterns also are affected by physiologic factors other than diastolic function with the *systolic filling phase* most affected by

■ left atrial size,
■ left atrial pressure,
■ left atrial compliance, and
■ atrial contractile function.

The velocity and duration of the *atrial reversal* is affected by

■ left atrial contraction,
■ left atrial compliance, and
■ cardiac rhythm.

Despite the potential influence of all these factors on the pattern of left ventricular diastolic filling, the Doppler velocity data still can provide useful information on diastolic dysfunction if carefully interpreted.

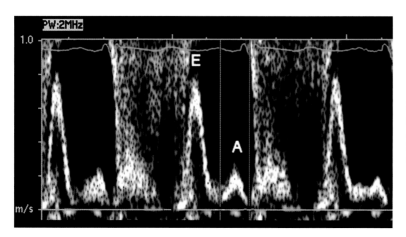

FIGURE 7–20. Left ventricular inflow in a patient with severe mitral regurgitation showing a high *E* velocity due to increased volume flow across the mitral valve and an increased left atrial pressure.

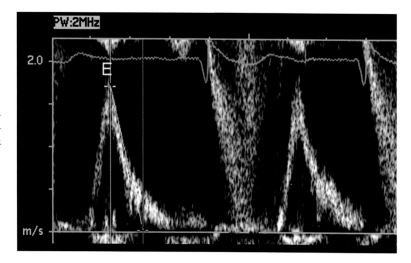

FIGURE 7–21. Left ventricular inflow in a patient with atrial fibrillation shows a single velocity peak and no *A* velocity.

Left Ventricular Relaxation

Mild diastolic dysfunction is characterized by impaired ventricular relaxation with a classic pattern of impaired early diastolic filling and an increased atrial contribution to total left ventricular filling (Fig. 7–22). *Impaired relaxation* (see Fig. 7–3) is associated with

- a reduced E velocity,
- a lengthened IVRT,
- a prolonged early diastolic deceleration time,
- an E/A ratio <1, and
- an E_m/A_m ratio <1.

If left ventricular relaxation is impaired but filling pressures are not elevated, the pulmonary venous pattern is normal with

- a systolic greater than diastolic phase, and
- a normal atrial reversal duration and velocity.

If impaired relaxation is accompanied by elevated filling pressures, the left ventricular inflow pattern continues to show an E/A ratio <1 with a prolonged deceleration time and a myocardial tissue Doppler $E_m/A_m < 1$. However, the IVRT now is in the normal range and the pulmonary venous atrial reversal is prolonged in duration and increased in velocity. This pattern is consistent with mild-to-moderate diastolic dysfunction.

Left Ventricular Compliance

Abnormal ventricular compliance results in rapid early diastolic filling following mitral valve opening with a short IVRT and acceleration time. As the ventricle fills, left ventricular diastolic pressure rises rapidly due to a stiff ventricle with decreased compliance, so a high E velocity is followed by a steep deceleration slope (Fig. 7–23).

The atrial contribution to filling is relatively small, because filling is now occurring on the steep portion of the pressure-volume relationship (see Fig. 7–4). In addition, LV-EDP typically is elevated so there is only a small left atrial to ventricular pressure gradient following atrial contraction.

With reduced left ventricular compliance, the myocardial tissue Doppler shows a reduced E_m/A_m ratio. The pulmonary venous flow pattern in patients with reduced compliance shows diastolic flow greater than systolic flow. Atrial reversal is prominent as well, with an increased velocity and duration of atrial flow, since a high left ventricular diastolic pressure reduces late diastolic left ventricular filling so that atrial contraction results in reversal of flow in the pulmonary veins. Specifically, an atrial reversal velocity > 0.35 m/s and an atrial reversal duration 20 ms greater than the duration of the forward atrial flow across the mitral annulus, are consistent with reduced compliance and an elevated left ventricular end-diastolic pressure.

In summary, *reduced compliance* is associated with

- increased E velocity and E/A ratio,
- low E_m/A_m velocities with an E_m/A_m ratio >1,
- short IVRT,
- decreased deceleration time,
- pulmonary venous diastolic greater than systolic flow, and
- increased velocity and prolonged duration of pulmonary vein atrial reversal.

Diastolic Filling Pressures

Accurate noninvasive assessment of left atrial pressure or of LV-EDP would be of great clinical

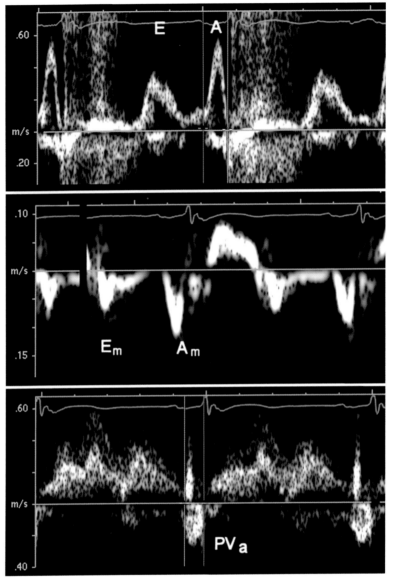

■ **FIGURE 7–22.** Evaluation of left ventricular diastolic filling in a patient with left ventricular hypertrophy and decreased relaxation. The mitral inflow at the leaflet tips (*top*) shows an $E/A < 1$ and a prolonged deceleration time. The myocardial tissue Doppler (*center*) confirms impaired relaxation with an $E_m/A_m < 1$ indicating the mitral flow pattern is not related to loading conditions. The pulmonary venous inflow (*bottom*) shows relatively equal systolic and diastolic components and a normal atrial reversal velocity and duration (*PVa*), consistent with normal left ventricular filling pressures. These findings indicate mild diastolic dysfunction.

utility but has been an elusive goal. Several promising approaches to this problem have been proposed (Table 7–5), but it is not yet clear if any of these methods provides the precision and accuracy needed for sequential evaluation in a critically ill patient. In this situation, invasive measurement of the PAWP serves as a surrogates for left ventricular filling pressure. On the other hand, the data are convincing that Doppler parameters allow identification of patients with elevated filling pressure, even when an exact numerical value cannot be provided.

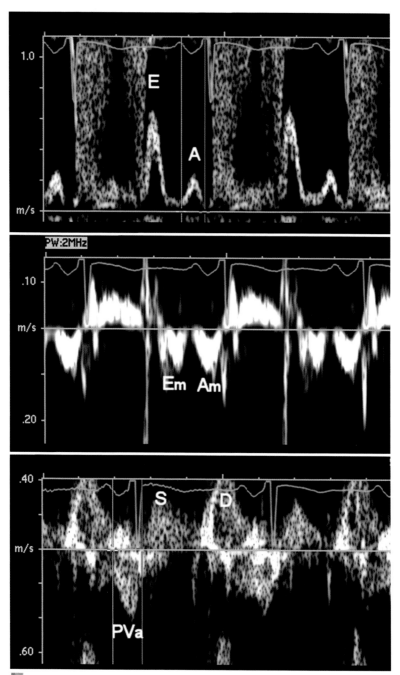

■ **FIGURE 7–23.** Evaluation of left ventricular diastolic filling in a patient with impaired compliance and an elevated left ventricular end-diastolic pressure. The mitral inflow at the leaflet tips (*top*) shows an $E/A > 1$ and a short deceleration time. The myocardial tissue Doppler (*center*) shows about equal E_m and A_m velocities consistent with decreased compliance. The pulmonary venous inflow (*bottom*) shows relatively a larger diastolic than systolic component and an increased atrial reversal (*PVa*) velocity (approximately 0.40 m/s) and duration, consistent with elevated left ventricular filling pressures. These findings are consistent with severe diastolic dysfunction.

TABLE 7-5
Validation of Doppler Measures of Diastolic Function

Reference Standard	Echo Parameter	r	Breakpoints	Sensitivity	Specificity	Reference
Radionuclide filling rates	E/A	0.76	Doppler E/A correlated with radionuclide early to atrial filling ratio			Spirito et al, 1986
Radionuclide filling rates	% atrial contribution	0.83	Relative filling rates, but not peak filling rates, were correlated			Pearson et al, 1988
PAWP	E/A	0.72	$E/A > 1.1$ predicts PAWP > 12 mm Hg			Appleton et al, 1993
PAWP	DT	−0.90	DT ≤ 120 ms predicts PAWP ≥ 20 mm Hg	100%	99%	Giannuzzi et al, 1994
PAWP	E/E_m	0.87	PCWP = 1.24 [E/Ea] + 1.9 mm Hg			Nagueh et al, 1997
LV-EDP	E/A		$E/A > 2.0$ associated with LVEDP > 20 mm Hg	100%	100%	Channer et al, 1986
LV-EDP	A/E ratio of velocity integrals	0.98				Stork et al, 1989
LV-EDP	a_{dur}		$a_{dur} > 0.35$ m/s predicts LV-EDP > 15 mm Hg			Nishimura et al, 1990
LV-EDP	a_{dur}		$a_{dur} > A_{dur}$ predicts LV-EDP > 15 mm Hg	85%	79%	Rossvold et al, 1993
LV-EDP	a_{dur}		$a_{dur} > A_{dur}$ + 20 msec predicts LV-EDP > 12 mm Hg	71%	95%	Appleton et al, 1993
LV-EDP	DT of E-velocity A_{dur}/a_{dur}	−0.74 −0.70	DT < 140 ms predicts LVEDP ≥ 20 mm Hg A_{dur}/a_{dur} ≤ 0.9 predicts LVEDP ≥ 20 mm Hg	90% 90%	99% 90%	Cecconi et al, 1996
LV-EDP	Change in A-velocity during Valsalva	0.85	↓ A wave by 21 ± 15 cm/s with LVEDP < 15 mm Hg ↑ A wave by 18 ± 13 cm/s with LVEDP > 25 mm Hg			Schwammenthal et al, 2000
Mean LVDP	E/E_m	0.64	E/E_m < 8 predicts normal LVDP E/E_m > 15 predicts mean LVDP > 15 mm Hg		86%	Ommen et al, 2000
LAP	$PV_S/(PV_S + PV_D)$	−0.88	$PV_S/(PV_S + PV_D)$ < 55% indicates LAP ≥ 15 mm Hg	91%	87%	Kuecherer et al, 1990
LAP	PV_S/PV_D	0.94				Hoit et al, 1992
LAP	DT of E velocity	0.73	DT < 180 ms predicts LAP ≥ 20 mm Hg	100%	100%	Nishimura et al, 1996
LAP	DT of PV_D	−0.92	DT of PV_D < 175 ms predicts LAP > 17 mm Hg	100%	94%	Kinnaird et al, 2001

Date from Spirito P et al: J Am Coll Cardiol 7:518–526, 1986; Pearson AC et al: Am J Cardiol 61:446–454, 1988; Appleton CP et al: J Am Coll Cardiol 22:1972–1982, 1993; Giannuzzi P et al: J Am Coll Cardiol 23:1630–1637, 1994; Nagueh SF et al: J Am Coll Cardiol 15:1527–1533, 1997; Channer KS et al: Lancet 1 (8488):1005–1007, 1986; Stork TV et al: Am J Cardiol 64:655–660, 1989; Nishimura RA et al: Circulation 8:1488–1497, 1990; Rossvold O et al: J Am Coll Cardiol 21:1687, 1993; Appleton CP et al: J Am Coll Cardiol 22:1972–1982, 1993; Cecconi M et al: J Am Soc Echocardiogr 9:241–250, 1996; Schwammenthal E et al: Am J Cardiol 86:169–174, 2000; Ommen SR et al: Circulation 102:1788–1794, 2000; Kuecherer HF et al: Circulation 82:1127–1139, 1990; Hoit BD et al: Circulation 86:651–659, 1992; Nishimura RA et al: J Am Coll Cardiol 28:1226–1233, 1996; Kinnaird TD et al: J Am Coll Cardiol 37:2025–2030, 2001.

Doppler parameters that indicate an elevated left ventricular filling pressure include a

- pulmonary vein atrial reversal velocity (PV$_a$) > 0.35 m/s,
- pulmonary atrial reversal duration (A$_{dur}$) at least 20 ms > transmitral atrial flow duration (A$_{dur}$),
- pulmonary venous sytolic flow < diastolic flow (S < D),
- deceleration time of the pulmonary venous diastolic flow phase < 175 ms,
- ratio of the early to atrial transmitral velocity (E/A ratio) > 2,
- E-velocity deceleration time < 140 ms, and
- ratio of transmitral E velocity to the myocardial tissue E$_m$ velocity (E/E$_m$) > 15.

In clinical practice, several of these variables are considered in examination of patients with suspected diastolic dysfunction.

In the specific case of patients with aortic regurgitation, the end-diastolic velocity of the aortic regurgitant velocity curve, recorded with continuous-wave Doppler, can be used to calculate the end-diastolic pressure gradient between the aorta and left ventricle using the Bernoulli equation. This pressure gradient then is subtracted from diastolic blood pressure to obtain LV-EDP. For example, if the end-diastolic aortic regurgitant velocity is 3.9 m/s, then the aortic to left ventricular gradient is $4(3.9)^2$ or 61 mmHg. With a diastolic blood pressure of 72 mmHg, LV-EDP would be (72 − 61) = 11 mmHg. While conceptually sound, this approach is limited by the need for a recordable aortic regurgitant jet, dependence on an accurate cuff diastolic blood pressure measurement, and derivation of a small number (LV-EDP) from two larger numbers, so that small errors in either measured variable lead to large errors in the calculated result.

CLINICAL UTILITY

Clinical Assessment of Left Ventricular Diastolic Function

In the clinical setting, evaluation of diastolic ventricular function is complicated by the coexistence of more than one of the factors that affect diastolic filling (Table 7–6). For example, patients with reduced compliance often have an elevated preload. Thus, an elderly patient with reduced compliance may have a pattern of left ventricular filling similar to a younger patient with normal diastolic function (a pattern referred to as *pseudo-normalization*). A patient with impaired relaxation may have coexisting mitral regurgitation, which obscures the changes in LV filling due to diagnostic dysfunction. As these examples illustrate, sorting out the relative contribution of diastolic dysfunction from other physiologic parameters can be difficult in an individual patient.

Furthermore, the factors that affect diastolic filling are not independent. A change in one physiologic parameter (such as left atrial pressure) may affect other parameters (such as atrial compliance and left ventricular contractility). The interdependence of these physiologic parameters complicates not only our ability to evaluate individual patients but also our understanding of the physiology of diastolic filling. From a practical point of view, the combination of myocardial tissue velocity and the pattern of pulmonary venous inflow, in conjunction with left ventricular filling parameters allows more precise delineation of the type and severity of diastolic dysfunction.

Thus, the patient with a "pseudo-normal" pattern of left ventricular inflow will be correctly classified as having reduced compliance based on an $E_m/A_m < 1$ on myocardial tissue Doppler (Fig. 7–24). In addition, the pulmonary venous flow

---

TABLE 7–6					
Classification of Diastolic Dysfunction					
	Normal	**Mild**	**Mild-Moderate**	**Moderate**	**Severe**
Pathophysiology		↓ Relaxation	↓ Relaxation and ↑ LV-EDP	↓ Relaxation, ↓ Compliance, and ↑ LV-EDP	↓ Relaxation, ↓↓ Compliance, and ↑↑ LV-EDP
E/A ratio	1–2	<1	<1	1.0–2.0	>2.0
E$_m$/A$_m$ ratio	1–2	<1	<1	<1	>1
IVRT (msec)	50–100	>100	Normal	↓	↓
DT (msec)	150–200	>200	>200	150–200	<150
PV$_S$/PV$_D$	≥1	PV$_S$ > PV$_D$	PV$_S$ > PV$_D$	PV$_S$ < PV$_D$	PV$_S$ << PV$_D$
PV$_a$ (m/s)	<0.35	<0.35	≥0.35	≥0.35	≥0.35
a$_{dur}$ − A$_{dur}$ (msec)	<20	<20	≥20	≥20	≥20 ms

Based on the Canadian Consensus Guidelines (Rakowki et al: J Am Soc Echocadiogr 9:736–760, 1996; and Yamada et al: J Am Soc Echocardiogr 15:1238–1244, 2002), with modification to include tissue Doppler data; and Redfield: JAMA 289:194–202, 2003.

pattern shows a prominent diastolic phase with an increased velocity and duration of atrial flow reversal, confirming the diagnosis of moderate diastolic dysfunction.

The optimal examination for diastolic dysfunction continues to evolve as new methods are proposed and then either validated in larger studies or abandoned as better techniques become available. Each laboratory needs to develop a protocol for when and how to evaluate diastolic function. My recommendation is that detailed evaluation of diastolic dysfunction be performed in patients referred for evaluation of heart failure symptoms, including dyspnea, and in those with evidence for

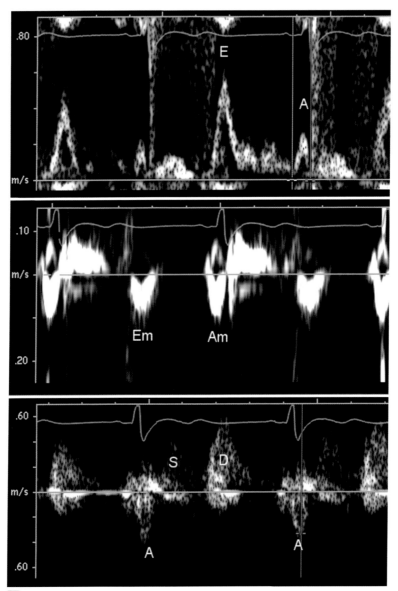

FIGURE 7–24. Evaluation of left ventricular diastolic filling in a patient with a pseudo-normal pattern of left ventricular inflow with an $E/A > 1$ and relatively normal deceleration time (*top*). This pattern is distinguished from normal by the myocardial tissue Doppler (*center*), which shows $E_m < A_m$ velocities and the pulmonary venous inflow pattern (*bottom*). There is a relatively a larger diastolic than systolic component and an atrial reversal (*PVa*) velocity at the upper limits of normal (approximately 0.35 m/s) with a duration slightly longer than the mitral A duration, suggestive of elevated left ventricular filling pressures. These findings are consistent with moderate diastolic dysfunction.

any of the conditions listed in Table 7–1 based on clinical or echocardiographic criteria.

The Canadian Consensus Guidelines for Evaluation of Diastolic Dysfunction provide a useful frame of reference (Table 7–6) for classification from mild to severe based on a limited number of parameters (Figs. 7–25 and 7–26). The recommendations of that document have been modified in this table to replace evaluation of ventricular inflow with Valsalva with the E_m/A_m ratio, because the E_m/A_m ratio likely is more reproducible than changes with the Valsalva maneuver. These guidelines will evolve with increased understanding of the evaluation of diastolic dysfunction.

Myocardial Disease

A variety of diastolic filling patterns can be seen in patients with dilated cardiomyopathy (see Chapter 9) and differences in diastolic function may explain differences in clinical symptoms between patients with similar degrees of systolic dysfunction. When systolic dysfunction is present, the elevated end-systolic volume results in a shift along the pressure-volume curve to a steeper segment. This means that for a given diastolic pressure-volume relationship, compliance is reduced at higher left ventricular volumes. Thus, the expected pattern of diastolic filling in dilated cardiomyopathy is that of reduced compliance: a high E velocity, rapid deceleration slope, low A velocity, and an E/A ratio >1. Keeping in mind that E velocity and E/A ratio usually decrease with age, the finding of a "normal" left ventricular filling pattern in a patient older than 50 years should raise the question of abnormal ventricular compliance.

In cardiac amyloidosis, a specific example of restrictive cardiomyopathy, the patterns of left ventricular diastolic filling and the change in these patterns during the disease course are particularly instructive. With amyloid infiltration of the myocardium, the first change is impaired relaxation, resulting in the classic pattern of mild diastolic dysfunction with a reduced E velocity and increased A velocity (panel A of Figs. 7–25 and 7–26). As the disease progresses, compliance also becomes abnormal, with moderate diastolic dysfunction resulting in a shift from $E/A < 1$ to an $E/A > 1$, with all the other findings of reduced compliance. This "pseudo-normalized" pattern can be distinguished from normal (if the patient is seen at only one point in the disease course) by the pattern of pulmonary venous inflow, which shows a diastolic component greater than the systolic component with an enhanced atrial reversal. The myocardial tissue Doppler signal will show an $E_m/A_m < 1$ (panel C, Figs. 7–25 and 7–26). To

some extent, this description oversimplifies the changes seen in amyloid heart disease, since concurrent changes in left ventricular systolic function, the degree of mitral regurgitation, and left atrial filling pressures also occur, all of which affect the pattern of left ventricular diastolic filling. However, it does serve as a useful framework for understanding the complex changes that occur with diastolic dysfunction.

Patients with hypertrophic cardiomyopathy often have a pattern of left ventricular diastolic filling consistent with impaired relaxation. Some studies have suggested that Doppler evaluation of left ventricular diastolic filling can be used to assess the effects of medical therapy (e.g., beta blockers or calcium channel blockers) on diastolic function in this disease.

Left Ventricular Hypertrophy

The "classic" pattern of mild left ventricular diastolic dysfunction is seen with left ventricular hypertrophy due to hypertension or to valvular aortic stenosis. The predominant abnormality is impaired relaxation, resulting in a pattern of reduced early diastolic filling and an enhanced atrial contribution to filling. The Doppler velocity curve typically shows a prolonged IVRT, reduced acceleration to a reduced E velocity, prolonged early diastolic deceleration slope, an increased A velocity, and an E/A ratio <1. When left ventricular systolic dysfunction supervenes, the elevated LV-EDP and elevated left atrial pressure may result in "pseudo-normalization" of this pattern with an enhanced E velocity (related to a higher mitral valve opening gradient) and reduced A velocity (due to the elevated left ventricular end-diastolic pressure). Coexisting mitral regurgitation also can lead to a "paradoxical" higher E velocity despite impaired ventricular relaxation.

Ischemic Cardiac Disease

In patients with coronary artery disease and no prior myocardial infarction, induction of ischemia results in diastolic dysfunction prior to systolic dysfunction (see Chapter 8). Diastolic filling curves with ischemia induced by balloon inflation during percutaneous transluminal angioplasty show rapid onset of a reduced E velocity, with resolution of these changes as ischemia is relieved. In acute myocardial infarction, a pattern of delayed relaxation is seen acutely. At follow-up, one of several patterns of left ventricular filling may be observed. With successful reperfusion and little myocardial damage, left ventricular diastolic filling returns to normal. With an infarction but preserved left ventricular systolic function, the pattern of impaired relaxation often persists. With

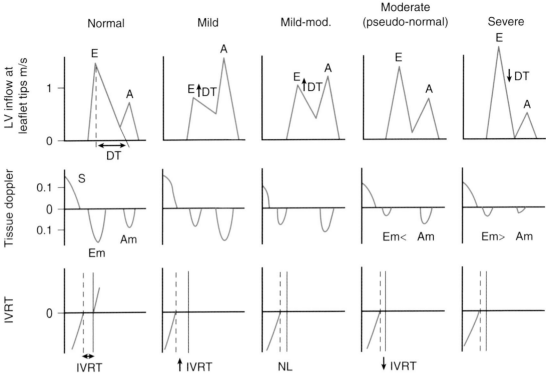

FIGURE 7–25. Diagram of the changes in diastolic parameters with diastolic function ranging from normal to severely impaired, corresponding to the classification in Table 7–6. Left ventricular inflow at the mitral leaflet tips (*top*), tissue Doppler velocities at the base of the septum adjacent to the mitral annulus (*middle*), and the isovolumetric relaxation time (IVRT, *bottom*) are shown. Abbreviations as in other tables and figures.

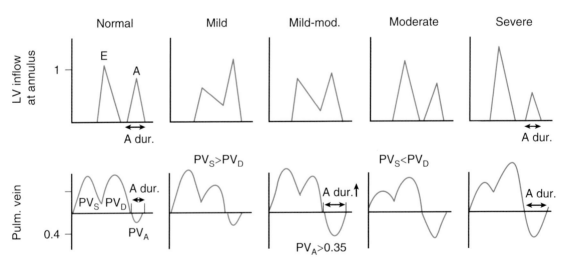

FIGURE 7–26. Evaluation of left atrial pressure is based on the pattern of left ventricular filling recorded at the mitral annulus (*top*) and pulmonary vein flow (*bottom*). With elevated left atrial pressures, the mitral deceleration time (DT) shortens and the velocity and duration of the atrial reversal in the pulmonary veins increase, with an $PV_A > 0.35$ m/s and at least 20 ms longer in duration than the transmitral *A*-duration indicating elevated filling pressures. With diastolic dysfunction, the diastolic phase of pulmonary venous flow exceeds the systolic phase of flow.

a large infarction and significant left ventricular systolic dysfunction, the "pseudo-normalized" pattern of a high E velocity and low A velocity due to a combination of reduced compliance, a high LV-EDP, and a shift along the diastolic pressure volume curve (increased end-systolic volume) can be seen. Thus, an apparent "normal" pattern of left ventricular filling late after myocardial infarction may be due to normal left ventricular diastolic and systolic function or to impaired diastolic and systolic function. As for cardiomyopathy patients, these two groups can be distinguished by a higher E/A ratio, shorter IVRT, and steeper deceleration slope than normal and by the pattern of myocardial tissue Doppler and pulmonary venous flow.

Pericardial Disease

With both pericardial tamponade and pericardial constriction, cardiac filling is impaired by pericardial "extrinsic constraint" and there is marked reciprocal respiratory variation the left and right ventricular filling. In the case of tamponade physiology, filling is impaired in both early and late diastole. With constrictive pericarditis, early diastolic filling tends to be normal, with marked impairment of filling late in diastole when the heart has expanded to the maximum allowed by the fibrotic pericardial encasement. Both these conditions are discussed in more detail in Chapter 10.

RIGHT VENTRICULAR DIASTOLIC FUNCTION

Right Ventricular Filling

The pattern of right ventricular diastolic filling is similar to left ventricular diastolic filling except that maximal velocities are lower (because the tricuspid annulus is larger) and the diastolic filling period is slightly shorter. Although few studies have addressed right ventricular diastolic filling, the same measurements described for left ventricular diastolic filling are applicable.

Doppler Data Recording

On transthoracic echocardiography, right ventricular inflow can be recorded from the parasternal right ventricular inflow view or from the apical four-chamber view (Fig. 7–27). Pulsed Doppler is used with the same technical considerations as apply to recording left ventricular inflow velocities. Evaluation of respiratory variation on inflow velocities is complicated by the respiratory motion of the heart, so care must be taken to ensure a parallel intercept angle between the ultrasound beam and inflow stream throughout the respira-

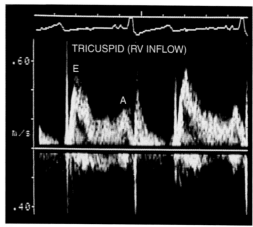

FIGURE 7–27. Doppler right ventricular inflow shows an E velocity and A velocity similar to left ventricular inflow.

tory cycle. This can be accomplished in most patients by using a window where 2D echo shows little respiratory variation in the image plane itself or in the Doppler beam orientation relative to the 2D image.

Physiologic Factors That Affect Right Ventricular Filling

Right ventricular filling appears to be affected by all the same physiologic parameters that affect left ventricular filling, although less attention has been directed toward right ventricular inflow patterns. Again, the major differences between right ventricular and left ventricular filling are (1) timing, (2) reciprocal respiratory variation (as described earlier), and (3) absolute velocities, which are lower for right ventricular inflow because the tricuspid annulus is larger than the mitral annulus.

Right Atrial Filling

Doppler velocity curves of right atrial filling can be recorded in the superior vena cava (from a suprasternal notch approach) or the central hepatic vein (from a subcostal approach), since these central veins empty directly into the right atrium without intervening venous valves. The pattern of right atrial filling recorded by Doppler parallels the jugular venous pressure curves seen clinically (Fig. 7–28). However, the Doppler data represent a more reliable approach, since evaluation of jugular venous patterns is difficult in some patients due to body habitus and interpretation is subjective (with no recorded data).

Again, right atrial filling patterns show respiratory variation in normal individuals with augmentation of right atrial inflow during inspiration, as is seen in the right ventricular inflow pattern. A plausible explanation for these observations is

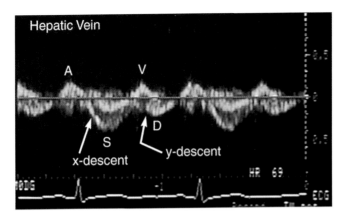

FIGURE 7–28. Normal pattern of right atrial inflow recorded in the central hepatic vein from a subcostal approach. Again, systolic (S) and diastolic (D) antegrade filling with slight flow reversal following atrial (A) contraction is seen.

that the negative intrathoracic pressure with voluntary inspiration (but not with mechanical ventilation) results in an extrathoracic to intrathoracic pressure gradient from the great veins into the right atrium, leading to increased blood flow into the right side of the heart. Right atrial pressure can be estimated by echocardiographic evaluation (from the subcostal window) of the inferior vena cava (IVC) as it enters the right atrium as discussed in Chapter 6 (see Table 6–6).

Right atrial filling is most often evaluated from the subcostal window. After the long-axis view of the inferior vena cava is obtained, the transducer is rotated and angulated to depict the central hepatic vein, which tends to be directed toward the transducer in this view, allowing a parallel intercept angle between the pulsed Doppler beam and hepatic vein flow. Hepatic vein flow is assumed to be representative of inferior vena caval flow, because both enter the right atrium without intervening venous valves. Direct study of inferior vena caval flow is limited by a nearly perpendicular intercept angle.

Right atrial inflow also can be recorded in the superior vena cava from the suprasternal notch window. From the standard aortic arch view, the transducer is angulated toward the patient's right to visualize the superior vena cava adjacent and slightly anterior to the ascending aorta. The pulsed Doppler sample volume is positioned in the superior vena cava, with adjustment of transducer angle and sample volume depth to obtain a well-defined velocity curve. As for other inflow patterns, wall filters are minimized (as allowed by signal-to-noise ratio) to demonstrate the low-velocity flows associated with atrial filling.

From both the superior vena cava and hepatic vein recordings, it is important to distinguish respiratory variation in the Doppler curves due to respiratory variation in the angle between the ultrasound beam and blood flow direction from

true variations in atrial filling volumes. The hepatic vein is small, so several positions often need to be tried to find one that maintains the sample volume in the hepatic vein throughout the respiratory cycle.

The physiologic factors that affect left atrial filling also affect right atrial filling, although (as for ventricular filling) less attention has been focused on physiologic parameters affecting the right side of the heart. Respiratory variation in right atrial filling typically is much more prominent than the respiratory variation seen in left atrial filling.

ALTERNATE APPROACHES TO EVALUATION OF DIASTOLIC DYSFUNCTION

Despite the numerous potential shortcomings of Doppler echocardiographic evaluation of diastolic filling, it has great promise as a repeatable, non-invasive, widely available method for evaluation of diastolic function. Techniques used in the research laboratory (time constant of relaxation, pressure-volume curves, etc.) rarely are applicable to clinical patient treatment. The other available clinical modalities for evaluation of diastolic function include

■ direct intracardiac pressure measurements,
■ contrast angiographic filling curves based on frame-by-frame volume calculations, and
■ radionuclide high-resolution time-activity curves.

SUGGESTED READING

Reviews

1. Smith, MD: Left ventricular diastolic function: Clinical utility of Doppler echocardiography. In: Otto CM (ed): The Practice of Clinical Echocardiography, 2nd ed. Philadelphia: WB Saunders, 2002, pp 113–140.

Advanced discussion of the principles and applications of Doppler evaluation of diastolic function in clinical practice. Includes tables of normal values, case examples, literature review, and 167 references.

2. Gibson DG, Francis DP: Clinical assessment of left ventricular diastolic function. Heart 89:231–238, 2003.

    Review of the physiology of diastole with clear definitions and discussion of relaxation, ventricular filling, and pressure gradients. The effects of asynchronous relaxation (or incoordination of ventricular function) on diastolic filling and the isovolumic relaxation time are emphasized. In addition, the use of Doppler parameters to evaluate patterns of left ventricular diastolic filling and estimate filling pressures is reviewed.

3. Zaqvi TZ: Diastolic function assessment incorporating new techniques in Doppler echocardiography. Rev Cardiovasc Med 4:81–99, 2003.

    Review of Doppler evaluation of diastolic dysfunction with excellent illustrations, appendices on details of the methodology and pitfalls for each parameter, and 133 references. Discussion of utility of Doppler evaluation of diastolic function in clinical practice.

4. Zile MR, Brutsaert DL: New concepts in diastolic dysfunction and diastolic heart failure: Part I: Diagnosis, prognosis, and measurements of diastolic function. Circulation 105:1387–1393, 2002.

    Review of the physiology, clinical presentation and prognosis of diastolic dysfunction with a summary of the Doppler parameters used in clinical practice.

Consensus Guidelines

5. Rakowski H, Appleton C, Chan KL, et al: Canadian consensus recommendations for the measurement and reporting of diastolic dysfunction by echocardiography. J Am Soc Echocardiogr 9:736–760, 1996.

    Consensus document that first reviews the physiologic basis for Doppler measures of diastolic dysfunction and then summarizes recommended measurements and proposes classification on a scale from mild to severe dysfunction as summarized in Table 7–6. The use of Doppler myocardial velocity data (E_m and A_m) is not addressed in this document but has been added to the figures and tables in this chapter.

Prevalence of Diastolic Dysfunction

6. Yamada H, Goh PP, Sun JP, et al: Prevalence of left ventricular diastolic dysfunction by Doppler echocardiography: Clinical application of the Canadian Consensus guidelines. J Am Soc Echocardiogr 15:1238–1244, 2002.

    In a series of 520 consecutive patients, diastolic dysfunction was present in 56% and was classified as mild in 19%, mild-to-moderate in 2%, moderate in 22%, and severe in 12% using the Canadian Consensus classification. In the 99 patients with clinical evidence of heart failure, diastolic dysfunction was the primary etiology in 38% with most patients having underling hypertensive or coronary heart disease.

7. Redfield MM, Jacobsen SJ, Burnett Jr JC, et al: Burden of systolic and diastolic ventricular dysfunction in the community: Appreciating the scope of the heart failure epidemic. JAMA 1289:194–202, 2003.

    In a cross-sectional survey of 2042 adults over age 45, the prevalence of heart failure was 2.2%. However, 44% of these patients had an ejection fraction > 50% suggesting diastolic dys-

function as the cause of clinical symptoms. The approach to classification of diastolic dysfunction based on mitral inflow, response to Valsalva maneuver, Doppler tissue imaging, and pulmonary venous flow is summarized.

Validation of Doppler Parameters

8. Spirito P, Maron BJ, Bonow RO: Noninvasive assessment of left ventricular diastolic function: Comparative analysis of Doppler echocardiographic and radionuclide angiographic techniques. J Am Coll Cardiol 7:518–526, 1986.

    Comparison of Doppler and radionuclide angiographic evaluation of diastolic filling in 12 normal subjects and 25 patients with cardiac disease. Good correlations were noted between Doppler and radionuclide measures of the ratio of early to late diastolic filling (r = 0.76), the time interval from end-systole to end of early rapid filling (r = 0.83), and the slope of the early flow velocity peak versus peak filling rate (r = 0.79).

9. Rokey R, Kuo LC, Zoghbi WA, et al: Determination of parameters of left ventricular diastolic filling with pulsed Doppler echocardiography: Comparison with cineangiography. Circulation 71:543–550, 1985.

    Comparison of Doppler and cineangiographic measures of left ventricular diastolic filling in 30 patients showed that the Doppler curve resembles the first derivative of the angiographic volume curve. Doppler and angiographic peak filling rate (r = 0.87) and normalized peak filling rate (r = 0.83) correlated well.

10. Nishimura RA, Schwartz RS, Tajik AJ, Holmes DR: Noninvasive measurement of rate of left ventricular relaxation by Doppler echocardiography: Validation with simultaneous cardiac catheterization. Circulation 88:146–155, 1993.

    The time constant of left ventricular relaxation (tau) can be calculated from the Doppler mitral regurgitant velocity signal using a semilogarithmic method with a zero asymptote, after conversion of velocities to pressures, using the Bernoulli equation. However, this approach requires knowledge of left atrial pressure and has only limited accuracy for detection of changes in tau in an individual patient.

11. Chen C, Rodriguez L, Lethor JP, et al: Continuous wave Doppler echocardiography for noninvasive assessment of left ventricular dP/dt and relaxation time constant from mitral regurgitant spectra in patients. J Am Coll Cardiol 23:970–976, 1994.

    In 12 patients with mitral regurgitation, Doppler-derived measures correlated well with invasive data for maximum +dP/dt (r = 0.91), maximum –dP/dt (r = 0.89), and tau (r = 0.93).

12. Berk MR, Xie G, Kwan OL, et al: Reduction of left ventricular preload by lower body negative pressure alters Doppler transmitral filling patterns. J Am Coll Cardiol 16:1387–1392, 1990.

    To avoid confounding effects of pharmacologic intervention, preload was reduced by lower body negative pressure. Decreased preload resulted in a reduced E velocity, no change in A velocity, a reduced E/A ratio, and a reduction in mean acceleration and deceleration with a corresponding prolongation of the pressure half-time.

13. Thomas JD, Choong CYP, Flachskampf FA, Weyman AE: Analysis of the early transmitral Doppler velocity curve: Effect of primary physiologic changes and compensatory preload adjustment. J Am Coll Cardiol 16:644–655, 1990.

    Elegant description of early diastolic filling with mathematical explanations (for the mathematically inclined) and clear diagrams showing the effects of changes in each parameter (for the rest of us).

14. Kuecherer HF, Muhiudeen IA, Kusumoto FM, et al: Estimation of mean left atrial pressure from transesophageal pulsed Doppler echocardiography of pulmonary venous flow. Circulation 82:1127–1139, 1990.

    In 47 patients undergoing cardiovascular surgery, the systolic fraction of pulmonary venous inflow correlated with mean left atrial pressure (r = −0.88). A systolic fraction < 55% had a sensitivity of 91% and a specificity of 87% for detection of a left atrial pressure ≥ 15 mm Hg.

15. Pozzoli M, Capamolla S, Pinna G, et al: Doppler echocardiography reliably predicts pulmonary artery wedge pressure in patients with chronic heart failure with and without mitral regurgitation. J Am Coll Cardiol 27:883–893, 1996.

    Simultaneous right heart catheterization and Doppler studies were performed in 231 patients with chronic heart failure. Pulmonary wedge pressure correlated most closely with the deceleration rate of early mitral filling and the systolic fraction of pulmonary venous flow. Regression equations for noninvasive calculation of pulmonary wedge pressure are proposed.

16. Hofmann T, Keck A, van Ingen G, et al: Simultaneous measurement of pulmonary venous flow by intravascular catheter Doppler velocimetry and transesophageal Doppler echocardiography: Relation to left atrial pressure and left atrial and ventricular function. J Am Coll Cardiol 26:239–249, 1995.

    In 32 patients undergoing open heart surgery, simultaneous measurement of left atrial pressure, pulmonary venous flow velocity by Doppler catheter, and transesophageal recording of pulmonary venous flow demonstrate close agreement between Doppler catheter and velocity data. Left atrium pressure correlated with the ratio of systolic to diastolic peak velocity, the systolic velocity-time integral, the time to maximal flow velocity, and the ratio of systolic to diastolic flow duration.

17. Nishimura RA, Appleton CP, Redfield MM, et al: Noninvasive Doppler echocardiographic evaluation of left ventricular filling pressures in patients with cardiomyopathies: A simultaneous Doppler echocardiographic and cardiac catheterization study. J Am Coll Cardiol 28:1226–1233, 1996.

    In patients with systolic left ventricular dysfunction, left atrial pressure correlated directly with the E/A ratio, and inversely with the early diastolic deceleration time. In contrast, correlation was poor in patients with hypertrophic cardiomyopathy due to multiple other factors affecting diastolic filling in these patients.

18. Kircher BJ, Himelman RB, Schiller NB: Noninvasive estimation of right atrial pressure from the inspiratory collapse of the inferior vena cava. Am J Cardiol 66:493–496, 1990.

    The inferior vena cava size and respiratory motion are related to right atrial pressure such that a 50% respiratory collapse in inferior vena cava diameter has a sensitivity of 87% and specificity of 82% for detection of a right atrial pressure < 10 mm Hg.

19. Takatsuji H, Mikami T, Urasawa K, et al: A new approach for evaluation of left ventricular diastolic function: Spatial and temporal analysis of left ventricular filling flow propagation by color M-mode Doppler echocardiography. J Am Coll Cardiol 27:365–371, 1996.

    Propagation velocity on a color M-mode of left ventricular filling from an apical approach was defined as the distance/time ratio between the mitral orifice and the point where velocity decreased to 70% of its initial value. Compared to micromanometer pressure data, propagation velocity correlated with the time constant of relaxation (tau) and with peak −dP/dt in a series of 40 patients.

20. Ommen SR, Nishimura RA, Appleton CP, et al: Clinical utility of Doppler echocardiography and tissue Doppler imaging in the estimation of left ventricular filling pressures: A comparative simultaneous Doppler-catheterization study. Circulation 102:1788–1794, 2000.

    Simultaneous catheter pressures and Doppler data were recorded in 100 consecutive patients undergoing cardiac catheterization. Isolated parameters of left ventricular filling correlated with mean left ventricular diastolic pressure only in patients with an ejection fraction < 50%. The best Doppler predictor of mean LV diastolic pressure was the ratio of the early mitral inflow velocity (E) to the early diastolic velocity of the mitral annulus (E_m). A stepwise approach to evaluation of diastolic function, using multiple parameters, is recommended.

21. Schwammenthal E, Popescu BA, Popescu AC, et al: Noninvasive assessment of left ventricular end-diastolic pressure by the response of the transmitral a-wave velocity to a standarized Valsalva maneuver. Am J Cardiol 86:169–174, 2000.

    Recording left ventricular inflow during the Valsalva maneuver allows unmasking of elevated filling pressures when the E/A ratio is < 1.0. The change in the A velocity during Valsalva correlates closely (r = 0.87) with left ventricular end-diastolic pressure, regardless of resting E/A ratio, with an increase in A velocity ≥ 9 cm/s during Valsalva indicating an LV end-diastolic pressure > 25 mm Hg.

22. Kinnaird TD, Thompson CR, Munt BI: The deceleration time of pulmonary venous diastolic flow is more accurate than the pulmonary artery occlusion pressure in predicting left atrial pressure. J Am Coll Cardiol 37:2025–2030, 2001.

    In 93 patients undergoing cardiac surgery, directly measured left atrial pressure was compared to transesophageal Doppler measures of left ventricular and left atrial filling. The best predictor of left atrial pressure was the deceleration time of the pulmonary vein diastolic flow curve (r = −0.92), which was identified in the first set of patients and then validated in a second group. The deceleration time was measured as the time interval from peak diastolic flow to a point on the baseline extrapolated from the slope of the deceleration curve. A pulmonary venous diastolic deceleration time < 175 ms was 100% sensitive and 94% specific for a left atrial pressure > 17 mm Hg.

Clinical Outcomes

23. Pinamonti B, Zecchin M, Di Leanarda A, et al: Persistence of restrictive left ventricular filling pattern in dilated cardiomyopathy: An ominous prognostic sign. J Am Coll Cardiol 29:604–612, 1997.

    In 110 patients with dilated cardiomyopathy, a restrictive pattern of ventricular filling at baseline, with persistence of this pattern at a 3-month follow-up study, was predictive of high mortality and cardiac transplantation rates.

24. Poulsen SH, Jensen SE, Moller JE, Egstrup K: Prognostic value of left ventricular diastolic function and association with heart rate variability after a first acute myocardial infarction. Heart 86:376–380, 2001.

    In 64 consecutive patients with first myocardial infarction, multivariate predictors of cardiac death and readmission for heart failure were ejection fraction and an E velocity deceleration time ≤ 140 ms.

25. Gerdts E, Bjornstad H, Toft S, et al: Impact of diastolic Doppler indices on exercise capacity in hypertensive patients with electrocardiographic left ventricular hypertrophy (a LIFE substudy). J Hypertens 20:1223–1229, 2002.

   In 60 hypertensive patients, multivariate predictors of peak exercise load included male gender, a higher resting E/A ratio, a greater decreased in IVRT with exercise and a higher exercise heart rate. These findings emphasize the importance of diastolic function in clinical manifestations of disease.

26. Wang M, Yip GW, Wang AY, et al: Peak early diastolic mitral annulus velocity by tissue Doppler imaging adds independent and incremental prognostic value. J Am Coll Cardiol 41:820–826, 2003.

   In 353 patients with known cardiac disease and 165 normal subjects, diastolic function was evaluated by echocardiography. The strongest predictors of cardiac death were the early diastolic tissue Doppler mitral annulus velocity (E_m) and left atrial size. E_m provided incremental value in prediction of clinical outcome compared to other Doppler measures of diastolic function.

The Echo Exam *Diastolic Dysfunction*

Parameter	Physiologic Descriptor
Relaxation	$-dP/dt$ or tau
Compliance	dV/dt
Filling pressure	LV-EDP or LAP or PAW

EDP, end-diastolic pressure; LAP, left atrial pressure; PAWP, pulmonary artery wedge pressure.

Echo Exam

Left ventricular (LV) inflow at mitral leaflet tips
   E = Early diastolic filling velocity (m/s)
   A = Filling velocity after atrial contraction (m/s)
   DT = Deceleration time (msec)*

LV inflow at mitral annulus
   A_{dur} = duration of atrial filling velocity in msec

Myocardial tissue Doppler at base of septum
   E_m = Early diastolic filling velocity (m/s)
   A_m = Filling velocity after atrial contraction (m/s)

Isovolumic relaxation time
   IVRT = isovolumic relaxation time (msec)

Pulmonary venous inflow
   PV_S = peak systolic velocity
   PV_D = peak diastolic velocity
   PV_a = peak atrial reversal velocity
   a_{dur} = pulmonary vein atrial reversal duration

*DT, time interval from peak velocity to baseline, extrapolated from slope of diastolic deceleration curve.

Example

A 62-year-old man with amyloidosis has an echocardiogram that shows a symmetric increase in wall thickness with an ejection fraction of 52%. The following parameters of diastolic function are recorded.

E velocity	1.1 m/s
A velocity	0.6 m/s
Deceleration time (DT)	160 ms
A_{dur}	130 ms
E_m/A_m ratio	<1
IVRT	40 ms
PV_S /PV_D	<1
PV_a	0.4 m/s
a_{dur}	155

The E/A ratio is >1 but the E_m/A_m ratio is less than 1, indicating a pattern of pseudonormalization suggestive of moderate diastolic dysfunction with decreased compliance. Moderate diastolic dysfunction is confirmed by the short IVRT and relatively short deceleration time.

There also is evidence of elevated filling pressures with a PV_a>0.35 m/s and with the duration of pulmonary vein atrial flow minus the duration of atrial flow at the mitral annulus >20 ms.

Quantitation of Diastolic Function

Parameter	Modality	View	Recording	Measurements
LV inflow at leaflet tips	Pulsed Doppler	A4C with 2–3 mm sample volume positioned at mitral leaflet tips	Parallel to flow Normal expiration Low wall filters	*E* and *A* peak velocities DT along outer edge of spectral envelope using linear slope from peak to baseline
LV inflow at annulus	Pulsed Doppler	A4C with 2 mm sample volume at mitral annulus	Parallel to flow, normal expiration, low wall filters	A_{dur}
Myocardial tissue Doppler	Pulsed Doppler	A4C with 2–3 mm sample volume placed within basal segment of septal wall	Very low gain settings Low wall filters	E_m and E_m/A_m
IVRT	Pulsed Doppler	Anteriorly angulated A4C with 3–5 mm sample volume midway between aortic and mitral valves	Clear aortic closing click and clear onset of transmitral flow, low wall filters	IVRT as time interval from middle of aortic closure click to onset of mitral flow
Pulmonary venous inflow	Pulsed Doppler (color to guide location)	Right superior pulmonary vein in A4C view using color flow to depict flow	2 mm sample volume 1–2 cm into pulmonary vein	PV_a, a_{dur}, and relative ratio of S/D

Classification of Diastolic Dysfunction

Pathophysiology	Normal	Mild ↓ Relaxation	Mild-Moderate ↓ Relaxation and ↑ LV-EDP	Moderate ↓ Relaxation, ↓ Compliance, and ↑ LV-EDP	Severe ↓ Relaxation ↓↓ Compliance, and ↑↑ LV-EDP
E/A ratio	1–2	<1	<1	1.0–2.0	>2.0
E_m/A_m ratio	1–2	<1	<1	<1	>1
IVRT (ms)	50–100	>100	Normal	↓	↓
DT (ms)	150–200	>200	>200	150–200	<150
PV_S/PV_D	≥1	$PV_S > PV_D$	$PV_S > PV_D$	$PV_S < PV_D$	$PV_S \ll PV_D$
PV_a (m/s)	<0.35	<0.35	≥0.35	≥0.35	≥0.35
$a_{dur} - A_{dur}$ (ms)	<20	<20	≥20	≥20	≥20 ms

Based on the Canadian Consensus Guidelines (Rakowki et al: J Am Soc Echocadiogr 9:736–760, 1996; and Yamada et al: J Am Soc Echocardiogr 15:1238–1244, 2002), with modification to include tissue Doppler data; and Redfield: JAMA 289:194–202, 2003.

ISCHEMIC CARDIAC DISEASE

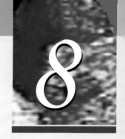

8

G iven the high prevalence of coronary artery disease, evaluation of patients with suspected or documented ischemic disease is one of the most common indications for echocardiography. Echocardiographic evaluation focuses on the functional outcome of coronary artery disease—specifically systolic wall thickening and endocardial motion—rather than on direct imaging of the coronary arteries. While the proximal left main and right coronary arteries often can be identified, even on transthoracic images, tomographic imaging techniques currently do not provide the detailed knowledge of distal vessel anatomy or the location and severity of coronary artery narrowings that is needed for patient management. Coronary angiography remains the procedure of choice for direct assessment of coronary artery anatomy.

However, echocardiography offers detailed functional assessment of segmental and global left ventricular systolic function both at rest and after interventions to induce ischemia. In many cases, this functional assessment provides critical data for patient management. For example, stress echocardiography is a reliable approach for the initial diagnosis of coronary artery disease, especially in patients with a nondiagnostic stress electrocardiogram (ECG). Another example is the use of echocardiography in the emergency department for early diagnosis of acute myocardial infarction in patients with equivocal electrocardiograms. In addition, the central role of echocardiography in evaluation for complications of acute myocardial infarction has long been recognized. Finally, echocardiography often provides important prognostic data in patients with coronary artery disease.

BASIC PRINCIPLES

Relationship between Coronary Artery Anatomy and Segmental Wall Motion

While coronary anatomy varies to some degree from patient to patient, the overall pattern of coronary artery branching is relatively uniform (Fig. 8–1). The left main coronary artery arises from the superior aspect of the left coronary sinus of

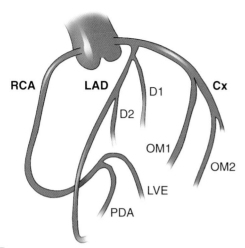

FIGURE 8–1. Schematic drawing of coronary artery anatomy showing the left anterior descending (LAD) artery with diagonal (D1 and D2) branches, the circumflex artery (Cx) with obtuse marginal branches (OM1 and OM2), and the right coronary artery (RCA) giving rise to the posterior descending artery (PDA) and left ventricular extension (LVE) branch.

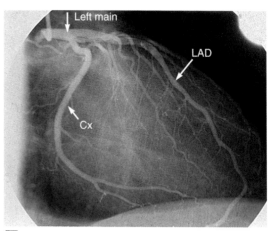

FIGURE 8–2. Normal left coronary artery in a right anterior oblique projection showing the left anterior descending (LAD) and circumflex (Cx) coronary arteries.

Valsalva and divides into (1) the left anterior descending artery, which extends via the interventricular groove down the anterior wall to (and sometimes around) the left ventricular apex; and (2) the circumflex artery, which continues laterally in the atrioventricular groove. The right coronary artery arises from the superior aspect of the right coronary sinus of Valsalva and extends inferomedially following the atrioventricular groove. Approximately 80% of patients have a *right-dominant* coronary circulation; the right coronary artery gives rise to the posterior descending artery, which lies in the inferior interventricular groove supplying both the inferior aspect of the ventricular septum and the inferior free wall (Figs. 8–2 and 8–3). In approximately 20% of patients, the coronary circulation is *left dominant*; the circumflex artery gives rise to the posterior descending artery.

The posterior left ventricular wall may be supplied by extension branches from the right coronary artery or by obtuse marginal branches of the circumflex arteries. The lateral wall is supplied by obtuse marginal branches of the circumflex artery. The left anterior descending artery supplies the anterior portion of the interventricular septum via septal perforating branches and the anterior wall via diagonal branches. There is marked individual variability in the blood supply to the left ventricular apex. In some cases, the left anterior descending artery extends around the apex to supply the apical segment of the inferior wall. In

other cases, the posterior descending artery extends around the apex to supply the apical segment of the anterior wall. More commonly, the blood supply to the apex arises from both the left anterior descending and the posterior descending coronary arteries.

Segmental wall motion abnormalities seen by echocardiography correspond closely with the coronary artery blood supply to the myocardium. A standardized nomenclature for tomographic imaging of the heart allows consistency of terms, correlations between different imaging techniques and a known relationship of each segment to coronary anatomy. The standardized terminology for tomographic planes is short axis, vertical long axis (equivalent to echocardiographic two-chamber

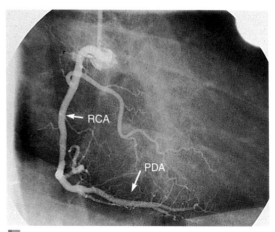

FIGURE 8–3. Normal right coronary anatomy with the posterior descending artery (PDA) seen in a right anterior oblique projection.

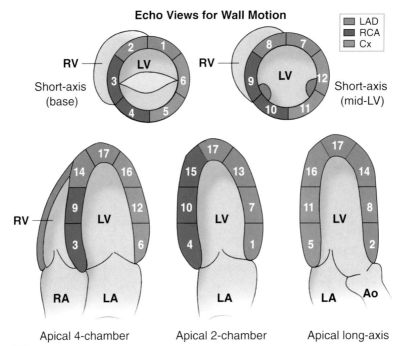

FIGURE 8–4. Echocardiographic views for wall motion evaluation. In the short-axis view, at the base and midventricular levels, the left ventricle is divided into the anterior (*1, 7*), anterior septal (*2, 8*), inferior septal (*3, 9*), inferior (*4, 10*), inferolateral (*5, 11*), and anterolateral (*6, 12*) segments. In the apical region, there are four segments: anterior (*13*), septal (*14*), inferior (*15*), and lateral (*16*) plus the tip of the apex (*17*). The territory of the left anterior descending artery is indicated in blue, the right coronary artery in red, and the left circumflex coronary artery in yellow.

plane), and horizontal long axis (equivalent to echocardiographic four-chamber plane). An additional plane provided by echocardiography is the echo long-axis view (which includes the aortic valve).

From base to apex, the left ventricle is divided into three segments—basal, mid-cavity, and apical—to correspond to proximal, middle, and apical lesions of the coronary arteries (Fig. 8–4). In a short-axis view, both at the basal (mitral valve) and mid-cavity (or papillary muscle) levels, the ventricle is divided clockwise, beginning with the interventricular groove, into six segments: the anterior wall, the anterolateral wall, the inferolateral (or posterior) wall, the inferior wall, the inferior septal, and the anterior septal walls. The apical region is divided into four segments because of the normal tapering of the ventricle toward the apex: anterior, lateral, inferior, and septal, with an additional segment for the tip of the apex. This results in 17 myocardial segments. The location of wall motion abnormalities can be reported descriptively, using a series of drawings showing different echocardiographic views, using a target diagram with the apex in the center and

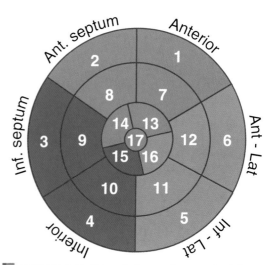

FIGURE 8–5. "Target" diagram for reporting left ventricular segmental wall motion with the apex in the center of the circle and the base around the circumference. Segment numbers and coronary artery territories correspond to those shown in Figure 8–4.

the base around the circumference (Fig. 8–5), or using more quantitative display formats.

The segmental wall motion abnormalities seen with ischemia or infarction correspond to the coronary anatomy as follows:

1. Left anterior descending artery disease results in wall motion abnormalities of the anterior septum, anterior free wall, and apex. Depending on the degree to which diagonal branches supply the lateral wall, abnormalities may be seen for the anterolateral wall as well. If the left anterior descending artery extends around the apex, apical segments of the inferior and inferolateral walls may be affected. The location of the lesion along the length of the coronary artery affects the pattern of wall motion. A lesion in the distal third of the vessel affects only the apex; a lesion in the midsegment of the vessel affects the midcavity and apical segments, while a proximal lesion affects the entire wall including the basal segments.
2. Circumflex artery disease affects wall motion of the anterolateral and posterolateral left ventricular walls. Again, the extent of segmental wall motion is related to the exact coronary anatomy in an individual patient. Echocardiography is particularly helpful in patients with circumflex disease because this myocardial region often is "silent" electrocardiographically and is not well seen on a single-plane right anterior oblique left ventricular angiogram.
3. Posterior descending artery disease results in abnormal wall motion in the inferior septum, inferior free wall, and inferolateral (posterior) left ventricular segments. If the posterior descending artery is a short vessel, the apex will not be affected, while extensive wall motion abnormalities of the apex may be seen if the posterior descending artery extends to supply the ventricular apex.

Other patterns of abnormal wall motion are seen with lesions of the branches of the three major coronary arteries. For example, isolated disease in a diagonal branch of the left anterior descending artery results in a discrete wall motion abnormality in the portion of the anterolateral wall supplied by that vessel. Proximal right coronary artery disease can result in ischemia or infarction of the right ventricular free wall.

Collateral vessels and previous bypass surgery also affect the pattern of wall motion. If a myocardial segment has a balanced oxygen demand/supply ratio, wall motion will be normal whether blood flow is supplied antegrade by the native vessel, by collateral vessels, or by a bypass graft.

Echocardiographic Views for Evaluation of Left Ventricular Wall Motion

Transthoracic Imaging

Regional systolic function for each segment of the left ventricle can be assessed on transthoracic imaging by combining data from multiple image planes. Standard views for evaluation of wall motion are

- short-axis (base, mid-LV, and apex) view,
- four-chamber view,
- two-chamber view, and
- long-axis view.

In the parasternal long-axis view, the basal and midventricular segments of the anterior septum and posterior left ventricular walls are seen. In the parasternal short-axis view, circumferential images of the left ventricle at the base and midventricular levels are obtained. Note that if the transducer is angulated toward the apex from a fixed parasternal position, progressively more apical segments of the posterior wall are imaged while the *same* segment of the septum is included in the ultrasound image plane. A more parallel alignment between image planes may be obtained by moving the transducer apically to obtain short-axis midcavity and (sometimes) apical views of the left ventricle (Fig. 8–6). In either case, evaluation of wall motion from other windows is helpful for avoiding misdiagnosis related to an oblique image plane. The apical segments rarely are adequately depicted from the parasternal window.

From the apical window, evaluation of left ventricular wall motion is performed in four-chamber, two-chamber, and long-axis views. Detailed evaluation of the extent of abnormal myocardium is possible by slow rotation of the image plane between the standard views. In the four-chamber view, the inferior septum and anterolateral wall are seen. Anterior angulation to include the aortic valve allows visualization of portions of the anterior septum. In the two-chamber view, the anterior and inferior free walls are seen. Endocardial and epicardial definition of the anterior wall may be difficult due to attenuation by adjacent overlying lung tissue. This problem can be alleviated by careful patient positioning and imaging during held respiration. In the apical long-axis view, the anterior septum and inferolateral (posterior) wall are seen (analogous to the parasternal long-axis view).

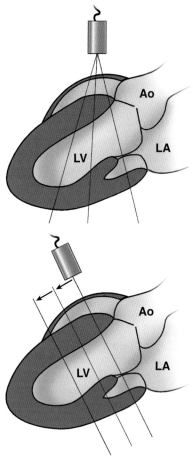

nearest the transducer and the anterior and anterolateral walls are most distal (Fig. 8–7).

Real-time volumetric imaging from an apical approach avoids many of these limtiations. Simultaneous apical views at set angles of rotation or multiple parallel short-axis views can be generated from the three-dimensional (3D) volume set, allowing rapid evaluation of wall motion in multiple myocardial segments on the same cardiac cycles. A limitation of apical volumetric scans is that the endocardium is imaged using the lateral, rather than axial, resolution of the ultrasound beam, which may limit identification of endocardial borders for quantitative analysis (see Chapter 4).

FIGURE 8–6. Angulation of the transducer from a fixed parasternal position results in short-axis views that intersect similar segments of the septum but progressively more apical segments of the posterior wall. By moving the transducer apically, more parallel image planes can be obtained.

Note that while these three apical image planes are approximately 60° to each other, there is some individual variation in their exact relationship. In addition, variation in coronary anatomy between individuals results in variable patterns of abnormal wall motion. Care is needed in positioning the transducer at the apex to avoid foreshortening of the ventricle from this approach. Integration of data from parasternal and apical approaches, taking into account image quality in each view, allows assessment of each myocardial segment in at least two views.

Finally, evaluation from a subcostal approach may be helpful. In the subcostal four-chamber view, the inferior septum and anterolateral wall are imaged. In the subcostal short-axis view, the inferior and inferolateral (posterior) walls are

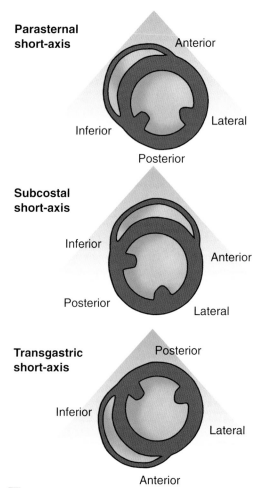

FIGURE 8–7. The wall segments seen in the short-axis view from transthoracic parasternal and subcostal, and transesophageal transgastric approach are shown. Correct identification of wall segments is facilitated by noting the position of the septum and the papillary muscles.

Transesophageal Imaging

When transthoracic images are inadequate or in certain monitoring situations (e.g., intraoperative monitoring of left ventricular function), regional left ventricular function can be evaluated from a transesophageal approach. From the high left atrial position, a four-chamber view of the left ventricle is obtained (in the 0° plane of the transesophageal echocardiographic probe) showing the inferior septum and lateral wall. Rotating the image plane to approximately 60° provides a two-chamber view with demonstration of the anterior and inferior walls, while further rotation to approximately 120° results in a long-axis view with imaging of the anterior septum and inferolateral (posterior) wall. Again, the exact degree of rotation to obtain these views varies slightly from patient to patient. In addition, transducer position and angulation may require adjustment as the image plane is rotated using anatomic landmarks to ensure optimal images with inclusion of the apical segments. Even with optimal technique, these views may be foreshortened; that is, the apparent apex represents an oblique plane through the anterolateral wall, while the true left ventricular apex is not seen.

From the transgastric position the transverse image plane provides short-axis views of the left ventricle at the base (mitral valve) and midcavity (papillary muscle) level. Rotation of the image plane at this position provides a two-chamber view, although the apex may be foreshortened. Further advancement of the probe may allow acquisition of an "apical" four-chamber view (in the 0° plane) by flexing the probe tip. However, the ventricle may be foreshortened and the true apex missed if the left ventricular apex does not lie on the diaphragm without intervening lung tissue in a position accessible from the transgastric approach.

Transesophageal imaging of left ventricular wall motion is indicated

- for intraoperative assessment of global and segmental left ventricular function, and
- in critically ill patients when transthoracic views are inadequate.

Sequence of Events in Ischemia

Irreversible myocardial damage (e.g., infarction) results in wall motion abnormalities that are present at rest. With an acute infarction, wall thickness is normal, but systolic wall thickening and endocardial motion are reduced or absent. An old myocardial infarction is characterized by thinning and increased echogenicity of the affected segments due to scarring and fibrosis, in addition to abnormal motion and absent wall thickening.

In contrast, ischemia is a reversible imbalance in the myocardial oxygen demand/supply ratio. Even with substantial coronary artery narrowing, blood flow is adequate for myocardial oxygen demands at rest. However, when the narrowing exceeds approximately 70% of the luminal cross-sectional area, blood flow becomes inadequate to meet increased myocardial oxygen demands with exercise, pharmacologic interventions, or mental stress, resulting in ischemia. When oxygen demand returns to baseline, blood flow again is adequate, ischemia resolves, and wall motion returns to normal. Thus, wall motion *at rest* is normal in patients with coronary artery disease if there has been no previous myocardial infarction.

The sequence of changes as a region of myocardium becomes ischemic is as follows (Fig. 8–8). The first detectable changes associated with heterogeneity of flow to the left ventricle are biochemical followed by a significant perfusion defect (detectable by radionuclide techniques). Next, regional myocardial dysfunction, characterized by both abnormal diastolic relaxation and compliance and impaired systolic wall thickening and endocardial motion, occurs in rapid succession (within a few cardiac cycles). Ischemic ST-segment depression on electrocardiography and clinical angina are relatively late manifestations of ischemia and are not seen consistently. Echocardiography, by detecting abnormal regional wall motion, provides a useful noninvasive method for evaluating ischemia that should be more sensitive than electrocardiography given this sequence of events. Echocardiography differs from radionuclide techniques in that the functional consequences of ischemia, rather than the pattern of myocardial perfusion, are assessed.

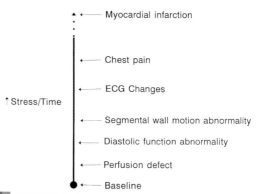

FIGURE 8–8. Schematic diagram of the sequence of events in myocardial ischemia.

Evaluation of Global and Regional Ventricular Function in Coronary Artery Disease

Global left ventricular systolic function can be evaluated either qualitatively or quantitatively in patients with coronary artery disease using the approaches described in Chapter 6. Because the pattern of left ventricular dysfunction typically is *not* uniform, it is important that qualitative evaluation is based on multiple tomographic views. If quantitative methods are applied, approaches that incorporate endocardial borders from at least two tomographic planes are most appropriate. In patients with coronary artery disease, the left ventricular ejection fraction is essential clinical data because it is a crucial variable in clinical decision making concerning surgical intervention.

Segmental (or regional) left ventricular systolic function most often is evaluated using a semiquantitative scoring system. The endocardial motion for each defined myocardial segment is described as normal, hypokinetic, akinetic, or dyskinetic, with a score from 1 to 4 corresponding to these descriptive terms. Hyperkinesis also may be scored (Table 8–1). Some clinicians prefer to subclassify the degree of hypokinesis as mild, moderate, or severe, but such a subclassification often has significant interobserver and intraobserver variability. An overall wall motion score index can be derived by dividing the sum of scores for each segment by the number of segments evaluated:

Wall motion score index =

Sum of individual segment scores/

Number of segments visualized

Several more sophisticated approaches to quantiation of wall motion have been proposed. Most of these represent modifications of angiographic techniques, such as the centerline method for quantitative wall motion analysis. Quantitiative evaultion of wall motion by echocardiography requires

■ identification and tracing of the endocardium at end-diastole and end-systole,
■ evaluation of wall motion in multiple tomographic views,
■ knowledge of the degree of variability of normal wall motion, and
■ correction for the effects of left ventricular translation, rotation, and torsion.

As automated edge-detection programs become faster and are validated for echocardiographic data, quantitative analysis of segmental function will become more feasible in the clinical setting. Approaches that incorporate 3D reconstruction of the left ventricle improve data acquisition times and may dimish the effects of cardiac motion that potentially result in imaging different regions of myocardium in systole versus diastole for a given tomographic plane. Although wall thickening may be a more sensitive method for evaluation of regional ventricular function, most current approaches continue to rely on endocardial motion.

MYOCARDIAL ISCHEMIA

Basic Principles

Because echocardiographic wall motion at rest is normal in a patient with significant coronary artery disease and no prior myocardial infarction, imaging *during ischemia* is needed for diagnosis. Inducing ischemia during echocardiographic imaging is referred to as *stress echocardiography*. Ischemia can be induced by increasing myocardial oxygen demand either with exercise or by pharmacologic interventions (Table 8–2).

Stress Echocardiography

Exercise Echocardiography

Exercise echocardiography typically is performed using standard exercise-test protocols. Supine or upright bicycle exercise protocols have the advantage that echocardiographic

TABLE 8–1		
Qualitative Scale for Assessment of Segmental Wall Motion on Echocardiography		
Score*	Wall Motion	Definition
1	Normal	Normal endocardial inward motion and wall thickening in systole
2	Hypokinesis	Reduced endocardial motion and wall thickening in systole
3	Akinesis	Absence of inward endocardial motion or wall thickening in systole
4	Dyskinesis	Outward motion or "bulging" of the segment in systole, usually associated with thin, scarred myocardium

*A score of 0 may be used for hyperkinesis, defined as increased endocardial inward motion and wall thickening in systole.

TABLE 8–2

Stress Echocardiography

Type of Stress	Advantages	Disadvantages
Treadmill exercise	Widely available High workload	Imaging post-ETT only
Upright bicycle	Imaging during exercise	Imaging may be technically difficult Lower workload
Supine bicycle	Imaging during exercise	Lower workload Supine position affects exercise physiology
Dobutamine	Continuous imaging Does not require physically active patient	Potential adverse effects of dobutamine Lower level of stress achieved
Dipyridamole	Continuous imaging Does not require physically active patient	Potential adverse effects of dipyridamole Induction of relative flow inequality rather than ischemia per se

ETT, exercise treadmill testing.

imaging can be performed during exercise at each progressive level of exertion, including maximal exercise. Treadmill exercise protocols have the advantage that a higher total workload can be achieved but the disadvantage that imaging can only be performed after exercise. Wall motion abnormalities that resolve very rapidly after exercise may be missed.

Resting images are acquired in digital cine-loop format for standard views of the left ventricle. Standard exercise protocols are used with monitoring of the 12-lead ECG, blood pressure, and symptoms by a qualified medical professional during and following the exercise protocol. The risks of exercise echocardiography are the risks of the exercise test itself. Either during maximal exercise (supine or sitting bicycle) or immediately after exercise (treadmill), digital cine-loop image acquisition is repeated. Typically, four or more sequential cycles are recorded digitally, and the examiner subsequently chooses the best image for comparison with the baseline views (Fig. 8–9). This allows elimination of poor quality images due to respiratory motion. Next, the rest and exercise cine-loop digital images are displayed side by side so that endocardial motion and wall thickening for each myocardial region can be compared. A systematic approach, comparing each segment in turn, is needed for detection of subtle abnormalities (Fig. 8–10).

Interpretation of an exercise stress echocardiogram includes incorporation of data on the maximum workload achieved (exercise duration), the heart rate and blood pressure response to exercise, the presence of arrhythmias, and clinical symptoms, as well as evaluation of the echocardiographic images.

Dobutamine Stress Echocardiography

EVALUATION FOR ISCHEMIA. Pharmacologic stress testing with intravenous dobutamine is based on the increased heart rate and contractility induced by this potent beta agonist. Typically, infusions are started at a low dose (5 mg/kg/min) and increased incrementally every 3 to 5 minutes with a calibrated infusion pump until the maximum dose (30 to 40 mg/kg/min) or an endpoint has been reached. Atropine is added, if needed, to achieve an appropriate increase in heart rate with a typical goal of 85% of the patient's maximum predicted heart rate. To minimize the likelihood of significant adverse effects and to optimize the quality of the data obtained, a dobutamine stress echocardiography examination requires a well-defined study protocol performed in the appropriate clinical setting.

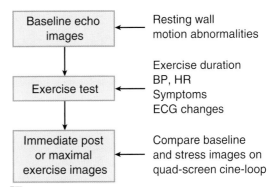

FIGURE 8–9. Flowchart of an exercise echocardiography protocol. BP, blood pressure; HR, heart rate; ECG, electrocardiogram.

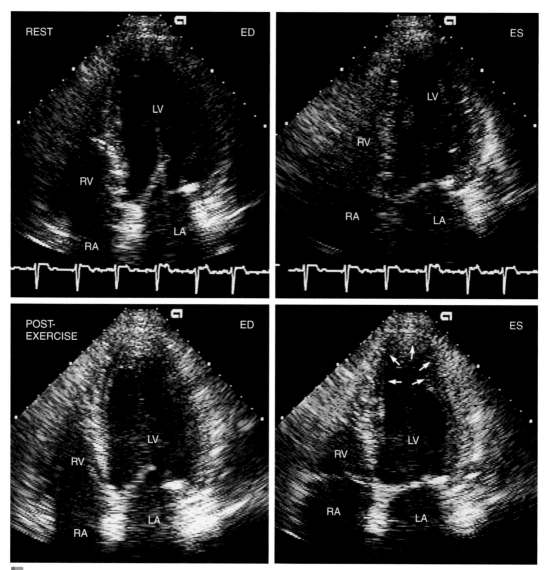

■ **FIGURE 8–10.** Frames from an abnormal exercise echo study showing the development of apical akinesis *(arrows)* with exercise. End-diastolic (ED) images are shown on the left, end-systolic (ES) on the right, with rest images on the top and exercise images on the bottom. The patient was found to have a severe proximal left anterior descending artery stenosis on coronary angiography.

Patient monitoring during dobutamine stress echocardiography includes

■ periodic blood pressure measurement (usually every 2 to 3 minutes),
■ continuous ECG rhythm monitoring, and
■ careful observation for clinical symptoms or signs.

Appropriate equipment, medications, and trained personnel should be immediately available in the event of an adverse effect, including a cardiac defibrillator, emergency cardiac medications, intravenous esmolol (a beta blocker that counter-acts the effects of dobutamine), and a qualified physician.

After an intravenous line for administration of the dobutamine has been placed, the patient is positioned in a left lateral decubitus position on an echo-stretcher with an apical cutout to allow optimal image acquisition throughout the study protocol. Initially, the intravenous line is filled only with saline solution while resting data are obtained. Data collection at baseline, after 3 minutes at each dosage level, and during recovery includes heart rate, blood pressure, symptoms, a 12-lead ECG, and echocardiographic images (Fig.

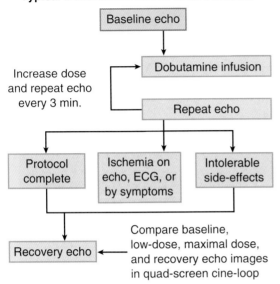

Typical Dobutamine Stress Echo Protocol

FIGURE 8-11. Flowchart of dobutamine stress echo protocol.

8-11). Standard views include parasternal short-axis images at the base and mid-cavity levels and apical four-chamber, two-chamber, and long-axis images with digital image acquisition in each view. Some centers also record Doppler left ventricular filling and ejection velocities at each stage of the stress protocol.

Endpoints for stopping the test are

- reaching the maximum protocol dose,
- patient discomfort,
- a definite wall motion abnormality involving two or more adjacent segments,
- ST-segment elevation on ECG,
- reaching 85% of maximum predicted heart rate for age,
- a systolic blood pressure > 200 or < 100 mm Hg *or* a diastolic blood pressure > 120 mm Hg, or
- significant ventricular arrhythmias.

Although complications are uncommon when appropriate precautions are observed, reported adverse effects include anxiety, tremulousness, palpitations, arrhythmias, paresthesias, and chest pain. Note that because the purpose of the test is to induce ischemia, some patients will have either echocardiographic changes or ECG evidence of ischemia and may experience angina. However, the frequency of angina may be less than that with standard ECG stress testing because the protocol can be stopped as soon as wall motion abnormalities are seen (which often is before angina occurs). Hypotension occurs in up to 10% of patients because of peripheral β_2-receptor–

mediated vasodilation but, unlike hypotension with exercise testing, is *not* a predictor of severe coronary disease or a worse prognosis. Contraindications to dobutamine stress echocardiography include unstable angina, uncontrolled hypertension, or sensitivity to dobutamine.

The echocardiographic images are interpreted after reformatting the digital images so that each quadrant of the screen shows a single view at rest (upper left), low-dose (upper right), maximal dose (lower left), and recovery phase (lower right). For each myocardial segment, wall motion is compared on these images in a systematic fashion. Since wall thickening and endocardial motion normally increase with dobutamine, an abnormal test is defined as the observation of hypokinesis or akinesis in a region that had normal wall motion at rest (Figs. 8–12 and 8–13).

EVALUATION FOR MYOCARDIAL VIABILITY. In addition to detection of ischemic myocardium, dobutamine stress echocardiography has been proposed as a method to evaluate for myocardial viability in regions that are "stunned" or "hibernating." For example, after treatment of myocardial infarction with thrombolytic therapy, the extent of residual viable myocardium in the area at risk may be unclear early after the event because of myocardial "stunning." Alternatively, a patient with chronic coronary artery disease may have hypokinesis or akinesis at baseline due to "hibernating" myocardium, which may recover with revascularization. In both these settings, echocardiographic imaging during low-dose (5 to 10 mg/kg/min) dobutamine infusion has been reported to show improved wall thickening and endocardial motion in viable segments of the myocardium. Of course, at higher dobutamine doses, worsening of regional function may occur due to induction of ischemia. This pattern of initial improvement at low dose, with subsequent worsening of myocardial function at higher dobutamine doses, is referred to as a biphasic response.

Other Stress Modalities

Dipyridamole has been proposed for echocardiographic stress testing by some investigators based on the differential pattern of coronary blood flow induced by this agent: increased blood flow in normal coronary arteries with a *relative* decrease in blood flow in diseased vessels. Overall success with this approach has been higher with perfusion imaging (e.g., thallium) because the difference in blood flow between regions supplied by normal versus abnormal coronary arteries can be seen on the radionuclide images. Results with echocardiographic imaging have been less consistent, since actual ischemia (not just a relative difference in

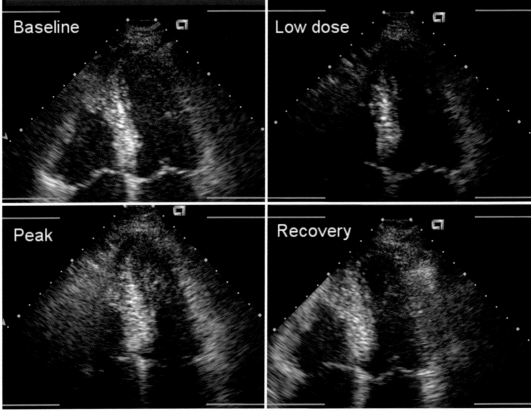

■ **FIGURE 8–12.** Normal dobutamine stress echocardiography showing the standard display format for the apical four-chamber view at end-systole at baseline (*upper left*), low-dose (5 mg/kg/min) dobutamine (*upper right*), high-dose (40 mg/kg/min) dobutamine (*lower left*), and recovery images (*lower right*). Note the marked decrease in end-systolic cavity area from baseline to peak dose images. This format is also used for the apical two-chamber, long-axis, and parasternal short-axis views.

blood flow) is needed to induce a wall motion abnormality.

Limitations/Technical Aspects

Stress echocardiography has a high sensitivity and specificity for diagnosis of significant coronary artery disease (Tables 8–3 and 8–4). In addition, it allows reliable definition of the anatomic location and extent of ischemic myocardium. However, stress echocardiography does have potential technical and physiologic limitations:

■ Endocardial definition
■ Cardiac and respiratory motion
■ Inadequate stress or workload
■ Abnormal resting left ventricular function

Assessment of endocardial wall motion and wall thickening requires adequate delineation of the endocardium for each myocardial segment. Careful attention to patient positioning, transducer orientation, and image processing parame-

ters can improve image quality, but definition of certain segments, particularly the anterior wall, may be difficult in some individuals due to adjacent lung tissue. Some centers use contrast agents that opacify the left ventricle after intravenous administration to enhance detection of regional wall motion abnormalities when endocardial definition is suboptimal even with harmonic imaging (Fig. 8–14).

Exercise and postexercise imaging can be limited by respiratory interference due to a rapid respiratory rate. Digital acquisition in cine-loop format of several cycles, followed by selection of the best images, is necessary for correct interpretation. The possible effects of cardiac translation and rotation, both between systole and diastole and between baseline and stress, should be considered in comparisons of wall motion. The interpretation of a stress echocardiographic study includes a description of image quality as an indicator of the reliability of these results. Suboptimal images should be interpreted with caution.

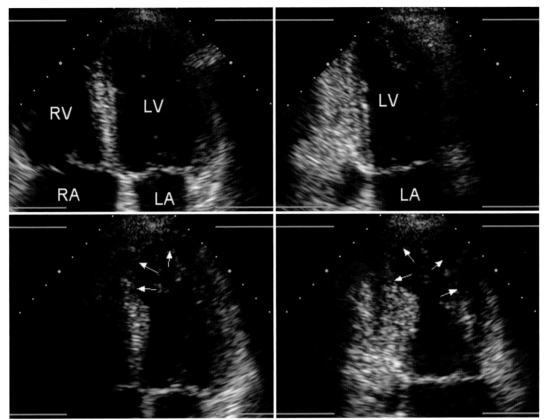

■ **FIGURE 8–13.** Example of an abnormal dobutamine stress echocardiographic study with baseline images (*top*) at end-systole in an apical four-chamber view (*left*) and apical two-chamber view (*right*), and the peak dose (40 mg/kg/min dobutamine plus 0.5 mg atropine) end-systolic images on the bottom. The apical segments of the septum, anterior, and inferior walls became akinetic at peak dobutamine dose (*arrows*), indicating significant coronary artery disease in the left anterior descending artery distribution.

TABLE 8–3				
Selected Studies on the Diagnostic Accuracy of Exercise Echocardiography Compared with Coronary Angiography*				
First Author/Year	**N**	**Percentage with Documented CAD**	**Sensitivity (%)**	**Specificity (%)**
Limacher/1984	73	–	91	88
Armstrong/1987	123	82	87	86
Ryan/1988	64	47	78	100
Sawada/1989	57 (women)	49	86	86
Crouse/1991	228	77	97	64
Marwick/1992	179	64	84	86
Quinones/1992	112	77	74	88

CAD, coronary artery disease.
*In all studies, significant coronary artery disease was defined as a 50% stenosis in an epicardial vessel.
Data from Limacher et al: Circulation 67:1211–1218, 1984; Armstrong et al: J Am Coll Cardiol 10:531–538, 1987; Ryan et al: 11:993–999, 1988; Sawada, et al: 14:1440–1447, 1989; Crouse et al: Am J Cardiol 67:1213–1218, 1991; Marwick et al: J Am Coll Cardiol 19:74–81, 1992; Quinones et al: Circulation 85:1026–1031, 1992.

TABLE 8-4

Selected Studies on Diagnostic Accuracy of Dobutamine Stress Echocardiography Compared with Coronary Angiography

First Author/Year	Source of Subjects	N	Percentage with Documented CAD	Percentage Stenosis Considered Significant	Sensitivity (%)	Specificity (%)
Berthe/1986	Post-AMI	30	100	50	85	88
Cohen/1991	Chest pain	70	27	70	86	95
Sawada/1991	Coronary angio	103	44	50	89	85
Mazeika/1992	Coronary angio	50	26	70	78	93
Martin/1992	Coronary angio	40	35	50	76	60
Segar/1992	Coronary angio	85	–	50	95	82
Marcovitz/1992	Coronary angio	141	21	50	96	66
Marwick/1993	Coronary angio	217	65	50	72	83

CAD, coronary artery disease; AMI, acute myocardial infarction; angio, angiography.
Data from Berthe et al: Am J Cardiol 58:1167–1172, 1986; Cohen et al: Am J Cardiol 67:1311–1318, 1991; Sawada et al: Circulation 83:1602–1614, 1991; Mazeika et al: J Am Coll Cardiol 19:1203–1211, 1992; Martin et al: Annals Int Med 116:190–196, 1992; Segar et al: J Am Coll Cardiol 19:1197–1202, 1992; Marcovitz et al: Am J Cardiol 69:1269–1273, 1992; Marwick et al: J Am Coll Cardiol 22:159–167, 1993.

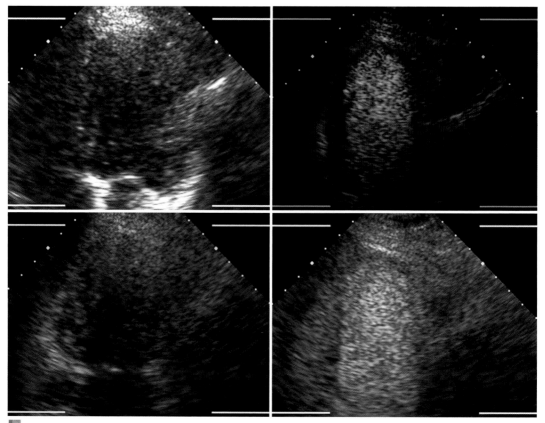

▪ **FIGURE 8–14.** This patient has suboptimal endocardial defintion even with harmonic imaging and careful patient positioning as shown in the apical four-chamber (*top*) and two-chamber (*bottom*) views on the left. After intravenous injection of galactose contrast, opacification of the left ventricular chamber is seen (*right*) with clear definition of the endocardial border, allowing evaluation of regional and global systolic function.

Potential physiologic limitations are related to the fact that abnormal wall motion occurs only *during* ischemia. First, if the "stress" used does *not* induce ischemia, no wall motion abnormality will be seen even if significant coronary disease is present. For example, a patient with limited exercise duration due to hip pain may not achieve a level of exertion that results in ischemia. Similarly, a pharmacologic "stress" that does not induce ischemia will not induce a wall motion abnormality. Second, the duration of ischemia is important. If ischemia has resolved by the time imaging is performed, the wall motion abnormality will not be detected. This is of particular concern with treadmill exercise, since echocardiographic imaging is performed after exertion, although this possible limitation may be offset by the higher maximum workload achieved prior to the recovery period compared with bicycle exercise protocols.

Stress echocardiography in patients with abnormal global or regional function at rest is more difficult to interpret than in subjects with normal resting left ventricular systolic function. The presence of a segmental motion abnormality at rest implies that coronary artery disease, with prior myocardial infarction, is present. With stress imaging, new wall motion abnormalities in regions remote from the site of resting abnormal wall motion indicate additional areas of ischemia. Evaluation of areas adjacent to the resting wall motion abnormality may be problematic due to a potential tethering effect by the abnormal region.

In patients with global systolic dysfunction at rest—which may be due to end-stage ischemic disease, cardiomyopathy, or chronic valvular disease—stress echocardiography is much less specific for the diagnosis of coronary disease. Differentiation of end-stage ischemic disease from a primary cardiomyopathy is discussed under the section on myocardial infarction below. Stress echocardiography also may be helpful in some patients with cardiomyopathy or valvular disease, depending on the specific clinical question.

Alternate Approaches

Exercise Electrocardiography

Exercise ECG remains a standard test for evaluation of patients with suspected or known coronary artery disease. Even though it has a lower sensitivity and specificity for diagnosis of coronary disease compared with imaging techniques, it continues to provide important prognostic data at a low cost in many patients. Imaging techniques most often are needed in subgroups with high false-positive (e.g., women with chest pain) or

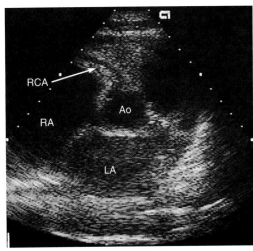

FIGURE 8–15. Right coronary artery (RCA) seen on a transthoracic parasternal short-axis view.

false-negative rates on stress ECG and in patients with an abnormal resting ECG that obscures exercise-induced ischemic changes.

Direct Echocardiographic Imaging of the Coronary Arteries

The origins of the right and left coronary arteries often can be identified on transthoracic imaging (Fig. 8–15). On transesophageal imaging, the proximal left coronary can be followed to its bifurcation into left anterior descending and circumflex arteries (Figs. 8–16 and 8–17), and often

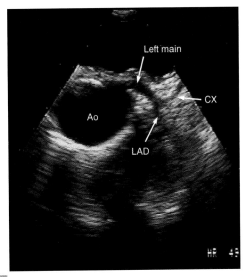

FIGURE 8–16. Left main coronary artery on transesophageal imaging showing its bifurcation into left anterior descending (LAD) and circumflex (Cx) arteries.

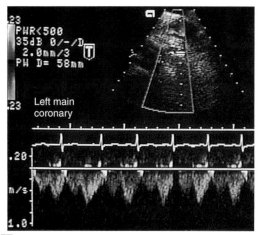

FIGURE 8–17. Doppler recording of coronary artery blood flow in the left main coronary artery from a transesophageal approach showing predominant diastolic flow.

these branches can be imaged for a portion of their length, as can the right coronary artery. However, clinical decision making usually requires detailed knowledge of the entire extent of the coronary anatomy. Tomographic imaging is a suboptimal method for evaluation of the relatively small coronary vessels that move with the epicardial surface of the heart.

Radionuclide Techniques/ Positron Emission Tomography

Radionuclide perfusion imaging techniques with thallium or sestamibi immediately after exercise and at rest after redistribution are well-validated methods for evaluation of coronary artery disease patients (Fig. 8–18). These techniques also can be performed using dipyridamole to induce heterogeneity in blood flow or with dobutamine to induce ischemia. Compared with stress echocardiography, radionuclide techniques have the advantage that image quality is less dependent on each patient's body habitus, although attenuation due to breast tissue may be a problem in women. Disadvantages of radionuclide techniques include a higher cost, it is less easily performed at the bedside, and it uses ionizing radiation (albeit a low dose). Technical factors are important with both techniques, and data quality at a particular institution depends in part on experience.

Positron emission tomography combines physiologic and anatomic data and theoretically allows assessment of myocardial metabolism and perfusion. This technique is not widely available clinically, although research applications are considerable.

Coronary Angiography

Coronary angiography remains the standard of reference for evaluation of coronary artery disease. Cinefluoroscopic films of coronary anatomy in multiple views allow detailed assessment of both proximal and distal coronary anatomy.

Clinical Utility

Diagnosis of Coronary Artery Disease

Stress echocardiography is used for the diagnosis of significant coronary artery disease. The accuracy of stress echocardiography is highly dependent on image quality, specifically endocardial definition, with most investigators reporting success rates for obtaining diagnostic images after treadmill exercise of 85% to 100%. The success rate for image acquisition and the quality of the images obtained tend to be greater with supine exercise (in which the patient can be positioned optimally) and with pharmacologic stress (which has the added advantage of little increase in respiratory interference).

Compared with coronary angiography, with significant disease defined as 50% narrowing of an epicardial coronary artery, exercise echocardiography has an overall sensitivity of 74% to 97% and a specificity of 64% to 100% for diagnosing the presence of coronary artery disease (see Table 8–4). Sensitivity is highest for multivessel disease (>90%) and lowest for single-vessel disease (60% to 80%) in these studies. In comparison, exercise electrocardiography had a much lower sensitivity at 51% to 63% and specificity at 62% to 74%, while exercise thallium-201 perfusion imaging tended to have an accuracy similar to echocardiography, with a sensitivity of 61% to 94% and a specificity of 81%.

Extent and Location of Ischemic Areas

When image quality is adequate, stress echocardiography also allows accurate evaluation of the location and extent of the area of ischemic myocardium. By integrating data from multiple views, a reasonable estimate of the location of significant coronary lesions can be made. Echocardiographic estimates of which and how many coronary arteries are affected correlate well with angiographic findings.

Prognostic Implications

The relationship between stress echocardiographic results and clinical outcome has been evaluated in several studies (Fig. 8–19). Exercise echocardiography in patients after myocardial

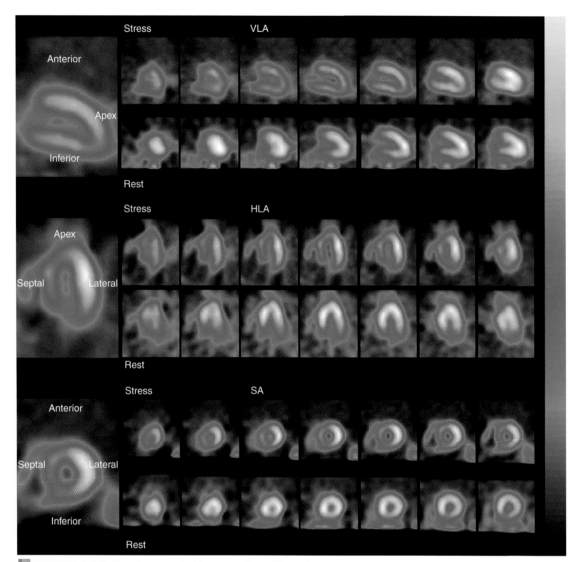

■ **FIGURE 8-18.** Exercise stress dual-isotope radionuclide study; resting images were acquired with 201-thallium and exercise images with Tc-Sestamibi. Three views are shown. *Top:* The vertical long-axis (VLA) images from the septum to lateral wall are shown with the stress images on the top and the rest images on the bottom. *Middle:* Horizontal long-axis (HLA) images are shown from posterior to anterior. *Bottom:* Short-axis (SA) images from apex to base are displayed. On the exercise images, there is an inferior wall perfusion defect starting in the apical slice on the short-axis view and extending to the midcavity and basal slices. On the rest images, there is complete redistribution consistent with ischemia without previous infarction in the inferior wall. (Courtesy of James H. Caldwell, Jr., MD.)

infarction predicts subsequent cardiac events with a positive predictive value of 63% to 80% and a negative predictive value of 78% to 95%. In patients with suspected coronary artery disease, the presence of an inducible wall motion abnormality predicts cardiac events (myocardial infarction, revascularization, death) over the subsequent 12 months with a sensitivity of 45% (positive predictive value of only 34%) but a specificity of 86% (negative predictive value of 91%). In patients undergoing noncardiac vascular surgery, dobutamine stress echocardiography is 100% sensitive and 69% specific for prediction of perioperative unstable angina, myocardial infarction, or death. In another study, the risk of postoperative events was 0% in those with a low-risk dobutamine stress study, 9% in those with an intermediate risk study, and 43% in those with a high-risk study.

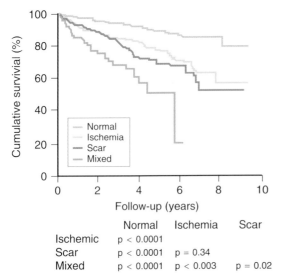

	Normal	Ischemia	Scar
Ischemic	p < 0.0001		
Scar	p < 0.0001	p = 0.34	
Mixed	p < 0.0001	p = 0.003	p = 0.02

FIGURE 8–19. Kaplan-Meier survival for cardiac mortality based on results of dobutamine stress echocardiography in 3156 patients with known or suspected coronary artery disease. (From Marwick TH, et al: Prediction of mortality using dobutamine echocardiography. J Am Coll Cardiol 37:754–760, 2001. Used with permission.)

MYOCARDIAL INFARCTION

Basic Principles

Myocardial infarction is irreversible injury to the myocardium due to prolonged ischemia, usually secondary to acute thrombotic occlusion of an epicardial coronary artery at the site of an atherosclerotic plaque. Initially, the affected myocardium becomes akinetic, with normal wall thickness. Over time (4 to 6 weeks), the involved myocardial segments show thinning of the wall and increased echogenicity. A transmural infarction (>50% of wall thickness pathologically, Q waves on ECG clinically) results in a definite area of akinesis and wall thinning. A nontransmural infarction (<50% wall thickness pathologically, no Q waves on ECG) may result in a lesser degree of wall thinning and in hypokinesis rather than akinesis.

Because ischemic myocardium also is akinetic in a patient with chest pain, echocardiography cannot distinguish acute infarction from ongoing ischemia. Furthermore, with prolonged ischemia or with successful reperfusion therapy for acute myocardial infarction, a phenomenon called *stunned myocardium* may be seen, where the wall motion abnormality persists for 24 to 72 hours even though irreversible damage has not occurred. Some investigators also propose that prolonged persistence of wall motion abnormali-

ties that can be reversed by reperfusion can occur—termed *hibernating myocardium.* Echocardiographic imaging cannot distinguish between these conditions since it shows the regional myocardial function at the time imaging is performed. The converse of this principle also should be kept in mind. Normal wall motion implies that there is no ischemia *at the time* the images were acquired. Thus, normal wall motion *between* episodes of chest pain does not exclude a diagnosis of unstable angina.

Echocardiographic Imaging

The myocardial segments affected and the echocardiographic views for assessment of myocardial infarction are the same as described for myocardial ischemia.

An occlusion of the left anterior descending artery results in akinesis of the anterior septum, anterior free wall, and apex (Fig. 8–20). Imaging in parasternal long- and short-axis views and in apical views demonstrates these segmental wall motion abnormalities. In the acute setting (Fig. 8–21), the unaffected walls may be hyperkinetic. Overall left ventricular systolic function typically is moderately depressed with an average ejection fraction of $41\% \pm 11\%$ after an unreperfused anterior myocardial infarction due to a proximal left anterior descending artery occlusion.

Occlusion of the posterior descending artery results in an inferior myocardial infarction with akinesis of the inferior septum, the inferior free wall, and (to a variable extent) the inferolateral (posterior wall) (Fig. 8–22). Parasternal and apical views again are used. The subcostal approach may be particularly helpful in patients with poor image quality from parasternal and apical windows. Typically, overall left ventricular systolic function is only mildly depressed, with an average postinfarction ejection fraction of $53\% \pm 10\%$ after an unreperfused inferior infarction. With inferior infarction, the echocardiographer also should evaluate for possible concurrent right ventricular infarction.

Occlusion of the circumflex artery, resulting in a lateral myocardial infarction, is less common and often is electrocardiographically "silent." Akinesis of the anterolateral and posterolateral walls is seen, with a mild to moderately depressed ejection fraction depending on the extent of myocardium supplied by the circumflex artery in that individual.

Note that these "classic" patterns of wall motion abnormalities will vary with individual variation in coronary anatomy and the location of the occlusion along the length of the coronary

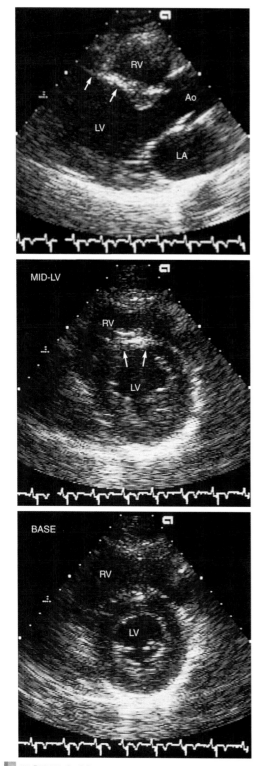

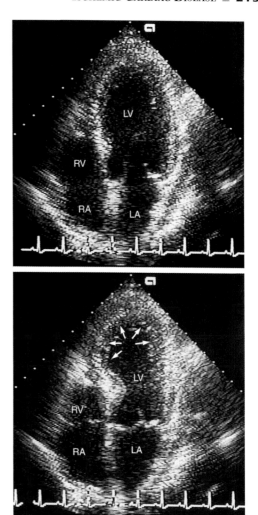

FIGURE 8–21. Acute anterior myocardial infarction seen in an apical four-chamber view in diastole (*top*) and systole (*bottom*). The apical septum is akinetic (*arrows*), although the myocardium is not yet thinned and scarred.

FIGURE 8–20. Old anterior myocardial infarction with thinning and increased echogenicity of the distal septum (*arrows*) seen in the parasternal long-axis view (*top*) and short-axis views at the mid–left ventricular level (*middle*). With this mid–left anterior descending artery occlusion, the basal septum (*bottom*) is normal.

artery. Also, these patterns will be altered by the use of reperfusion therapy.

In acute myocardial infarction, diastolic function, as well as systolic function, is abnormal. Acutely, early diastolic relaxation is impaired, with a reduced E velocity on the left ventricular inflow curve. With successful reperfusion, this pattern of diastolic filling tends to normalize over the subsequent 1 to 2 weeks. With large infarctions that are not reperfused, the E velocity also increases after infarction; however, in this situation, this change in inflow velocity reflects an increased left ventricular end-diastolic pressure rather than "normalization" of the left ventricular filling pattern. In patients with moderate to severely reduced systolic function, the E/A ratio correlates positively with left ventricular end-

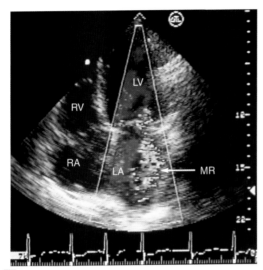

FIGURE 8-22. Mitral regurgitation due to papillary muscle dysfunction after inferior myocardial infarction.

diastolic and left atrial pressures (i.e., a higher E/A ratio indicates a higher left ventricular end-diastolic pressure) due to the overriding effect of left atrial pressure on the early diastolic filling velocity. It is most helpful to interpret patterns of left ventricular diastolic filling in an individual patient over time with side-by-side comparisons of the echocardiographic findings and integration with other clinical data (see Chapter 7).

Limitations/Alternate Approaches

As for other applications of echocardiography, image quality can be a limiting factor in patients with poor ultrasound tissue penetration. However, with optimal patient positioning, an experienced sonographer, and a state-of-the-art instrument, diagnostic images can be obtained in nearly all patients.

The standard approach to the diagnosis of acute myocardial infarction includes two of the following three findings:

■ A typical clinical presentation
■ Diagnostic ECG changes
■ A consistent pattern of elevation in serum cardiac enzyme levels

When typical findings of acute myocardial infarction are present, the diagnosis rarely is in doubt. Unfortunately, many patients have an atypical clinical presentation, and ECG changes may be nondiagnostic

Radionuclide imaging for acute myocardial infarction is based on the principle of detection of areas of hypoperfusion. The finding of a normal radionuclide perfusion pattern in patients pre-

senting with chest pain has a high specificity for the absence of acute myocardial infarction. Sensitivity for acute infarction is lower since an old infarction cannot be distinguished from an acute infarction with this approach.

Coronary angiography, of course, remains the standard of reference for identification of an occluded coronary artery. Concurrent left ventriculography can identify wall motion abnormalities using a right anterior oblique view, showing the anterior wall, apex, and inferior wall in silhouette (Fig. 8-23), and a left anterior oblique view to evaluate the lateral wall (which is superimposed on the ventricular chamber in the right anterior oblique view). The current standard of care for acute myocardial infarction often includes percutaneous coronary revascularization, so many of these patients go directly to the catheterization laboratory at the time of presentation.

Clinical Utility

Diagnosis of Acute Myocardial Infarction in the Emergency Department

In a patient presenting to the emergency department with chest pain and a nondiagnostic ECG,

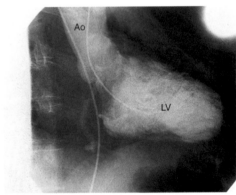

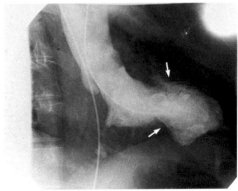

FIGURE 8-23. Left ventricular angiography with diastolic (*top*) and systolic (*bottom*) frames showing an akinetic apex (*between arrows*) due to myocardial infarction.

echocardiographic assessment of global and segmental wall motion can be helpful in clinical decision making. The presence of a segmental wall motion abnormality indicates that coronary artery disease is present—an acute infarction, ischemia, or an old infarction. Associated hyperkinesis of uninvolved segments suggests an acute event. Many emergency departments now use small portable ("hand-held") ultrasound devices for this indication.

The presence of a new wall motion abnormality may justify prompt coronary angiography for a possible acute coronary intervention. Global left ventricular systolic dysfunction also is an important prognostic sign, indicating significant cardiac disease and the need for further evaluation. Normal wall motion *during pain* is consistent with a very low likelihood of acute myocardial infarction, so it may be possible to send the patient to a non–coronary care unit bed depending on the clinical setting. However, normal wall motion once pain has resolved is less diagnostic, because unstable angina may be present with wall motion abnormalities seen only *during* episodes of ischemia.

Some clinical centers now use exercise echocardiography in the early evaluation of patients presenting with chest pain to allow triage to further inpatient versus outpatient evaluation. Patients with a diagnostic ECG, history of coronary disease, or unstable hemodynamics receive prompt standard treatment. In the remainder, after exclusion of myocardial infarction by serial enzyme level measurement, stress testing is performed to identify those with coronary artery disease. Other centers use radionuclide imaging techniques in the chest pain evaluation unit (see Suggested Readings 20 and 21).

Evaluation of Interventional Therapy for Acute Myocardial Infarction

In a patient with a definite myocardial infarction by clinical and ECG criteria, echocardiography allows assessment of the location and extent of "myocardium at risk." Once reperfusion therapy has been initiated, echocardiography can be used to assess its effects, although the several-day time lag between successful reperfusion and normalization of wall motion ("stunned" myocardium) makes this evaluation most meaningful before hospital discharge or at outpatient follow-up. However, echocardiography can be helpful in identification of recurrent ischemia in patients with recurrent chest pain by identification of wall motion abnormalities in regions that previously were normal. At long-term follow-up after myocardial infarction, echocardiography allows assessment of global ventricular function and long-term ventricular dilation due to "infarct expansion."

Complications of Myocardial Infarction

Echocardiography is the procedure of choice for initial evaluation of the post–myocardial infarction patient with a new systolic murmur with a differential diagnosis of

■ mitral regurgitation,
■ ventricular septal defect, or
■ ventricular rupture with pseudoaneurysm formation.

Most commonly, the etiology of the murmur is *mitral regurgitation* due to either papillary muscle dysfunction, abnormal wall motion of the segment underlying a papillary muscle, or papillary muscle rupture. The presence and severity of mitral regurgitation are evaluated using Doppler techniques (see Chapter 12), and the etiology is inferred from two-dimensional (2D) imaging. Partial or complete rupture of the papillary muscle is a catastrophic complication that can be recognized as a flail leaflet with an attached mass (the papillary muscle head) that prolapses into the left atrium in systole (Fig. 8–24). Transesophageal imaging is indicated when this diagnosis is suspected unless the diagnosis is clear on transthoracic images.

Another cause of a new systolic murmur after myocardial infarction is a *ventricular septal defect* due to necrosis and rupture of a focal area of the interventricular septum (Figs. 8–25 and 8–26). Identification of the rupture site may be difficult with 2D imaging, especially since this complication tends to occur with *small* infarcts so that the wall motion abnormality may be subtle. Evaluation with Doppler ultrasound establishes the diagnosis, with a high-velocity left-to-right systolic jet recorded with continuous-wave Doppler ultrasound and systolic turbulence on the right ventricular side of the septum recorded with conventional pulsed Doppler or color flow imaging.

When *ventricular rupture* occurs in the free wall of the left ventricle (instead of in the septum), mortality is extremely high due to extravasation of blood into the pericardial space and acute pericardial tamponade. However, some patients have a temporary respite due to containment of the rupture by pericardial adhesions or by thrombosis at the rupture site. In these patients, echocardiography may establish the diagnosis, prompting

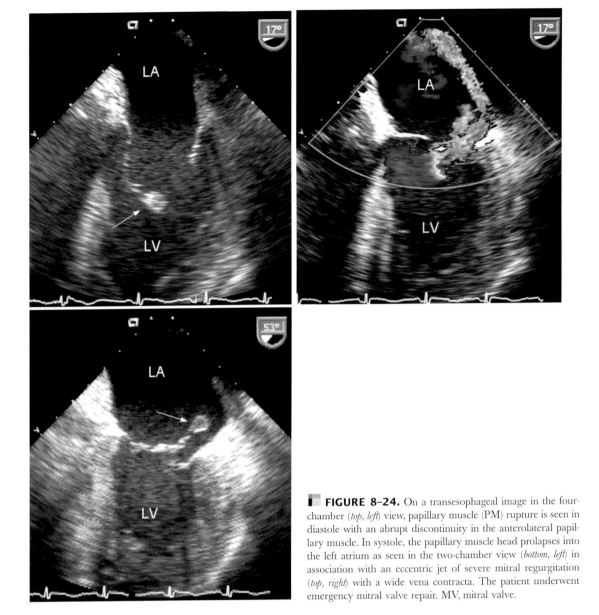

FIGURE 8-24. On a transesophageal image in the four-chamber (*top, left*) view, papillary muscle (PM) rupture is seen in diastole with an abrupt discontinuity in the anterolateral papillary muscle. In systole, the papillary muscle head prolapses into the left atrium as seen in the two-chamber view (*bottom, left*) in association with an eccentric jet of severe mitral regurgitation (*top, right*) with a wide vena contracta. The patient underwent emergency mitral valve repair. MV, mitral valve.

emergency surgery (Fig. 8-27). Echocardiographic clues of ventricular rupture (in the appropriate clinical setting) include a diffuse or localized pericardial effusion and a discrete segmental wall motion abnormality. Occasionally, the site of rupture can be demonstrated on 2D imaging, and rarely, flow from the ventricle into the pericardial space can be demonstrated with Doppler techniques.

A chronic, contained ventricular rupture is called a *pseudoaneurysm* (Figs. 8-28 and 8-29). A left ventricular pseudoaneurysm has a wall composed of pericardium (no myocardial fibers). Characteristic features are

- an abrupt transition from normal myocardium to the aneurysm,
- an acute angle between the normal myocardium and aneurysm,
- a narrow "neck" at the site of rupture,
- a ratio of the "neck" diameter to the maximum diameter <0.5, and
- partial filling of the aneuysm with thrombus.

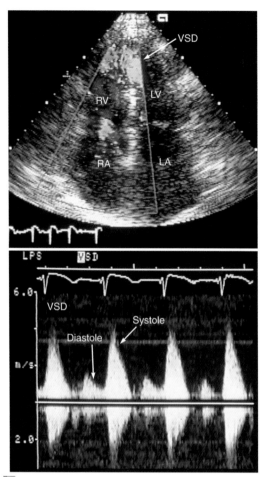

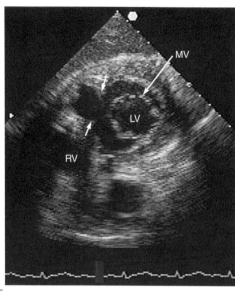

■ FIGURE 8–27. Transgastric short-axis image showing acute left ventricular rupture after myocardial infarction. There in an abrupt discontinuity in the left ventricular wall (*arrows*) with flow in and out of a thrombus-lined section of the pericardium. Rapid diagnosis allowed surgical intervention in this patient.

■ FIGURE 8–25. Color flow image showing left-to-right flow across an apical ventricular septal defect (VSD) after myocardial infarction (*top*). Continuous-wave Doppler (*bottom*) shows high-velocity left-to-right flow in systole with lower-velocity left-to-right flow in diastole across the defect.

■ FIGURE 8–26. Postmyocardial infarction ventricular septal defect (VSD) seen on left ventriculography in a left anterior oblique image plane. There is rapid appearance of contrast in the right ventricle (RV) after injection into the left ventricle (LV).

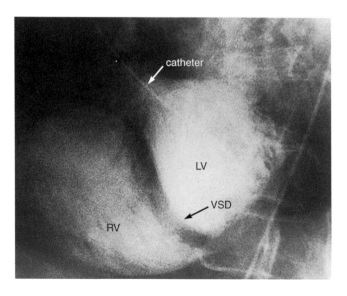

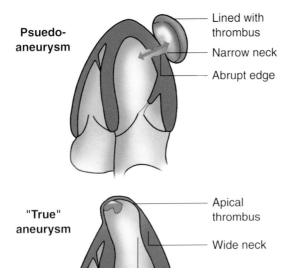

FIGURE 8–28. Schematic diagram of a pseudo-aneurysm versus a true aneurysm

Often, flow in and out of the pseudoaneurysm is seen, and clinically, a corresponding apical murmur may be appreciated on auscultation. While long-term survival has been described occasionally in patients with a pseudoaneurysm, correct echocardiographic diagnosis is essential. Surgical repair usually is recommended given a high likelihood of spontaneous rupture.

Other complications of acute myocardial infarction include

■ pericardial effusion,
■ right ventricular infarction,
■ LV aneurysm, or
■ LV thrombus.

A *pericardial effusion* also can be seen after myocardial infarction as a nonspecific response to transmural infarction. This effusion may be asymptomatic or may be associated with clinical symptoms (chest pain) and signs (ECG changes) of acute pericarditis. While usually benign, tamponade physiology can occur.

Another complication of acute myocardial infarction for which echocardiography is the diagnostic procedure of choice is *right ventricular infarction*. Clinical diagnosis requires a high level of suspicion. Other clinical tests, such as ST-segment elevation in right-sided ECG leads, are not as sensitive or specific as echocardiography. Right ventricular infarction most often is associated with an inferior left ventricular infarct. Echocardiographic findings include right ventricular hypokinesis or akinesis with variable degrees of right ventricular dilation. This diagnosis significantly changes the clinical management of these patients (i.e., low cardiac output is treated with volume infusions rather than with afterload reduction or inotropic agents).

Longer-term complications of acute myocardial infarction include aneurysm formation, left ventricular thrombi, and the sequelae of the irreversible decrease in left ventricular systolic function. A *left ventricular aneurysm* is defined echocardiographically as a dyskinetic region with a diastolic contour abnormality (Fig. 8–30). Apical

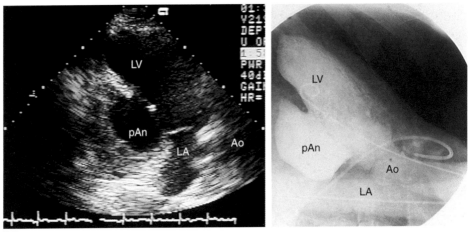

FIGURE 8–29. Apical long-axis view showing a chronic basal aneurysm filled with thrombus with a narrow neck (*left*) consistent with a pseudoaneurysm (pAn). Angiography (oriented to match the apical long-axis view) shows a similar appearance (*right*).

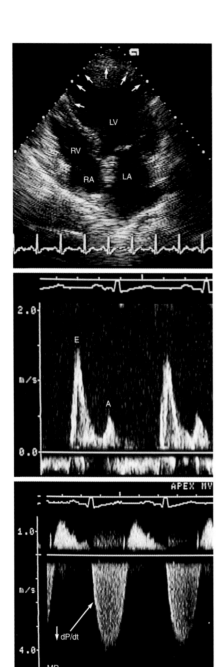

obtuse angle between the aneurysm and body of the left ventricle. The ratio of the diameter of the junction between the aneurysm and the remainder of the left ventricle to the maximum aneurysm diameter is >0.5.

Left ventricular thrombi form in regions of stasis of blood flow, such as in an apical aneurysm or overlying an area of akinesis in other regions of the left ventricle. Evidence of severely reduced overall ventricular function, an aneurysm, an akinetic area, and the appearance of a spontaneous contrast effect in the left ventricle all increase the likelihood of left ventricular thrombus formation. Only rarely (as in hypereosinophilic syndrome) do ventricular thrombi occur in the absence of an underlying wall motion abnormality.

A thrombus is identified as an area of increased echogenicity within the ventricular chamber, distinct from the endocardium. Often, the thrombus protrudes into the chamber with a convex contour, but laminated thrombus with a concave contour following the endocardial curve also can be seen. Care is needed to distinguish a thrombus from prominent apical trabeculation with a false tendon or "web" traversing the apex of the left ventricular chamber.

Diagnosis of apical thrombi is enhanced by using a 5-MHz transducer (improved near-field resolution), sliding the transducer medially from the apical window, and then angulating posteriorly to obtain a short-axis view of the apex. These procedures allow clear definition of the apical endocardium in most individuals. However, if images are suboptimal, appropriate interpretation should indicate that a thrombus "cannot be excluded," especially if the patient is at high risk of left ventricular thrombus formation. Note that transesophageal imaging is rarely helpful for this diagnosis because the apex often cannot be visualized and is in the far field of the image plane.

FIGURE 8–30. Apical dilation and systolic dyskinesis (*top*) consistent with an apical aneurysm. The pattern of left ventricular inflow (*middle*) shows a prominent *E* velocity consistent with an elevated left ventricular end-diastolic pressure. The mitral regurgitant velocity curve in this patient (*bottom*) shows a reduced *dP/dt*.

END-STAGE ISCHEMIC CARDIAC DISEASE

Differentiation from Other Causes of Left Ventricular Systolic Dysfunction

The diagnosis of coronary artery disease is clear in patients with definite segmental wall motion abnormalities that correspond to the distribution of coronary blood flow (Table 8–5). In end-stage ischemic disease, repeated transmural and subendocardial infarctions result in a diffuse pattern of abnormal wall thickening and endocardial

aneurysms are most common, but inferobasal aneurysms also may be seen. Note that a "true" left ventricular aneurysm, unlike a "false" or pseudoaneurysm, is lined by (thinned) myocardium. There is a smooth transition from normal myocardium to the thinned area with an

TABLE 8–5

Differentiation of Left Ventricular Systolic Dysfunction Due to End-Stage Ischemic Disease from Dilated Cardiomyopathy or Chronic Valvular Disease

Findings	End-Stage Ischemic Disease	Dilated Cardiomyopathy	Chronic Valvular Disease
Left-ventricular ejection fraction	Moderate-severely depressed	Moderate-severely depressed	Moderate-severely depressed
Segmental wall motion abnormalities	May be present	Absent	Absent
Right ventricular systolic function	Normal	Decreased	Variable
Pulmonary artery pressures	Elevated	Elevated	Elevated
Valve leaflets	Normal	Normal	Abnormal
Mitral regurgitation	Moderate	Moderate	Moderate-severe
Aortic regurgitation	Not significant	Not significant	Moderate-severe

motion. Thus, when global systolic dysfunction is present, it may be difficult to differentiate between end-stage ischemic disease and systolic dysfunction due to long-standing valvular disease or a dilated cardiomyopathy (Fig. 8–31).

Echocardiographic Approach

Several features of the echocardiographic examination help in this differentiation. The segmental pattern of left ventricular wall motion is examined carefully in each tomographic plane. While patients with a dilated cardiomyopathy may have a somewhat asymmetric pattern of wall motion with relative preservation at the ventricular base, definite areas of akinesis or wall thinning suggest ischemic disease. The degree of reduction in overall ventricular function (ejection fraction) is important in patient management but does not assist in determining the etiology of disease.

Right ventricular size and systolic function are normal in patients with ischemic disease unless there has been a previous right ventricular infarction. Dilated cardiomyopathy occasionally affects the two ventricles in differing degrees but most often results in a symmetric pattern of right and left ventricular dilation and reduced systolic function.

Mitral valve regurgitation typically accompanies both dilated cardiomyopathy and end-stage ischemic disease due to one of several mechanisms, including mitral annular dilation, reduced papillary muscle function, or malalignment of the papillary muscles. Left ventricular dilation and systolic dysfunction *due to* chronic mitral regurgitation, in contrast to mitral regurgitation due to ventricular dilation and dysfunction, usually are associated with anatomic abnormalities of the

mitral leaflets themselves (e.g., myxomatous or rheumatic disease).

Pulmonary artery pressures are elevated to variable degrees in patients with left ventricular dysfunction of any etiology, due to chronic elevation in left ventricular end-diastolic pressure. Pulmonary pressures can be estimated from the tricuspid regurgitant jet velocity or from the pulmonary artery systolic velocity curve as described in Chapter 6. Mild degrees of tricuspid valve regurgitation are common in ischemic disease, but moderate or severe regurgitation usually is a response to chronic pulmonary hypertension or chronic right ventricular dilation and systolic dysfunction.

Note that aortic regurgitation is *not* a consequence of left ventricular dilation or systolic dysfunction. Left ventricular dilation typically does not result in an increase in the diameter of the aortic annulus or adjacent outflow tract. The finding of moderate or severe aortic regurgitation implies primary valvular disease or aortic root dilation.

Left ventricular thrombi may be present with severe left ventricular dysfunction of any etiology. The observation of reduced systolic function should prompt a search for apical thrombi, but this finding does not help in the differential diagnosis.

Limitations/Alternate Approaches

If a diagnosis of end-stage ischemic disease versus a primary cardiomyopathy would alter patient management, coronary angiography may be needed for a definitive diagnosis, to document the exact site and severity of coronary lesions, and to assess the distal vessel anatomy.

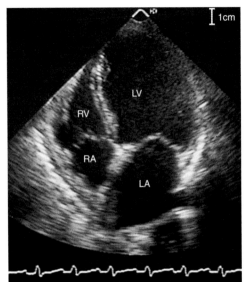

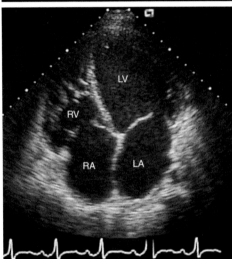

■ **FIGURE 8–31.** End-stage ischemic heart disease (*top*) and a dilated cardiomyopathy (*bottom*) often appear similar on 2D echocardiography. Note that the patient with ischemic disease has normal right ventricular size and systolic function.

SUGGESTED READING

General

1. Armstrong VF, Pellikka PA, Ryan T, et al: Stress echocardiography: Recommendations for performance and interpretation of stress echocardiography. J Am Soc Echocardiogr 11:97–104, 1998.

   This position paper from the American Society of Echocardiography summarizes the optimal methods of performing pharmacologic and stress echocardiography. Details include the imaging technique, required equipment, personnel, and analysis techniques. Contraindications, accuracy, and prognostic implications also are summarized.

2. Cerqueira MD, Weissman NJ, Dilsizian V, et al: Standardized myocardial segmentation and nomenclature for tomographic imaging of the heart. American Heart Asso-

ciation Writing Group on Myocardial Segmentation and Registration for Cardiac Imaging. Circulation 105: 538–542, 2002.

   Standards for defining cardiac image orientation and myocardial segments that can be used by all imaging modalities to enhance correlation between different approaches. The standard reference for cardiac displays is defined as the long axis of the left ventricle. The names used for image planes are short axis (90° to long axis), vertical long axis (apical two-chamber plane), and horizontal long axis (four-chamber plane). Myocardial segments are defined at the basal and mid-ventricular level as (clockwise from the anterior septal insertion) as anterior, anterolateral, inferolateral, inferior, inferoseptal, and anteroseptal. There are four apical segments (anterior, septal, inferior, and lateral).

Exercise Echocardiography

3. Marcovitz PA: Exercise echocardiography: Stress testing in the initial diagnosis of coronary artery disease and in patients with prior revascularization or myocardial infarction. In: Otto CM (ed): The Practice of Clinical Echocardiography, 2nd ed. Philadelphia: WB Saunders, 2002, pp 275–300.

   The clinical application of exercise echocardiography is discussed in detail including necessary equipment and personnel, interpretation of stress images, a comparison of treadmill versus bicycle exercise testing, and the relative advantages and disadvantages of exercise echocardiography compared to other diagnostic approaches. Topics include the utility of exercise echocardiography for detection of coronary artery disease, and evaluation after revascularization or acute myocardial infarction. The value of exercise echocardiography for detection of coronary artery disease in women (sensitivity 86% to 88%, specificity 84% to 86%) is emphasized; 143 references.

4. Olmos LI, Dakik J, Gordon R, et al: Long-term prognostic value of exercise echocardiography compared with exercise ^{201}Tl, ECG, and clinical variables in patients evaluated for coronary artery disease. Circulation 98: 2679–2686, 1998.

   In 225 patients undergoing exercise echocardiographic and nuclear stress tests, cardiac events at a mean follow-up of 3.7 years were predicted by induction of ischemia on echocardiography (odds ratio 4.1, 95% confidence interval 1.32 to 12.79) or a perfusion defect on [201]thallium (odds ratio 4.93, 95% confidence interval 1.72 to 14.08). The authors conclude that echocardiographic and radionuclide stress studies provide comparable prognostic data.

5. Marwick TH, Mehta R, Arheart K, Lauer MS: Use of exercise echocardiography for prognostic evaluation of patients with known or suspected coronary artery disease. J Am Coll Cardiol 30:83–90, 1997.

   In 463 patients undergoing exercise echocardiography, ischemia was defined as an exercise-induced new or worsened wall motion abnormality on 2D echocardiography. Multivariate predictors of cardiac events or revascularization at 44 ± 11 months were the percent age-predicted maximal heart rate and ischemia (relative risk 5.06, 95% confidence interval [CI] 3.09 to 8.29, P < .0001). Echocardiographic data provided incremental predictive value compared to clinical and exercise data alone.

6. Heupler S, Mehta R, Lobo A, et al: Prognostic implications of exercise echocardiography in women with known or suspected coronary artery disease. J Am Coll Cardiol 30:414–420, 1997.

In 508 women undergoing stress echocardiography, there was no evidence of ischemia in 81%, 13% had an new or worsened wall motion abnormality with exercise, and 6% had evidence of old myocardial infarction. At follow-up (41 ± 10 months), 7% had cardiac events including 17 cardiac deaths and 19 patients with myocardial infarction or revascularization for progressive symptoms. Independent predictors of outcome were known coronary artery disease and echocardiographic ischemia (odd ratio 4.3, 95% CI 2.1 to 8.7, $P < .0001$).

7. Kafka HF, Leach AJ, Fitzgibbon GM: Exercise echocardiography after coronary artery bypass surgery: Correlation with coronary angiography. J Am Coll Cardiol 25:1019–1023, 1994.

A total of 213 exercise echocardiographic studies were performed in 182 patients 2 weeks to 21 years after coronary artery bypass grafting for suspected recurrent ischemia. Compared to coronary angiography, exercise echocardiography had a positive predictive value of 71% for vascular compromise in one vascular territory and 98% for ischemic involving more than one coronary artery distribution. False negative results were most likely with ischemia isolated to the posterolateral region of the left ventricle.

Dobutamine Stress Echocardiography

8. Marwick TH: Stress echocardiography with non-exercise techniques: Principles, protocols, interpretation, and clinical applications. In Otto CM (ed): The Practice of Clinical Echocardiography, 2nd ed. Philadelphia: WB Saunders, 2002, pp 301–339.

Concise summary of the principles, technical aspects, and clinical utility of pharmacologic stress echocardiography. Comprehensive tables summarize clinical studies evaluating the sensitivity and specificity of dobutamine stress, vasodilator stress, and atrial pacing stress echocardiography; 286 references.

9. Mertes H, Sawada SG, Ryan T, et al: Symptoms, adverse effects, and complications associated with dobutamine stress echocardiography: Experience in 1118 patients. Circulation 88:15–19, 1993.

Complications of dobutamine stress echocardiography that required termination of the test protocol included noncardiac symptoms (nausea, anxiety, headache, tremor, urgency) in 3%, and angina pectoris in 19.3% (which was relieved by sublingual nitroglycerin or a short-acting beta blocker in all cases). Arrhythmias included premature ventricular contractions in 15%, premature atrial contractions in 8%, and nonsustained ventricular tachycardia in 40 (3.5%) patients. There were no deaths, myocardial infarctions, or episodes of sustained ventricular tachycardia.

10. Geleijnse ML, Fioretti PM, Roelandt JR: Methodology, feasibility, safety and diagnostic accuracy of dobutamine stress echocardiography. J Am Coll Cardiol 30:595–606, 1997.

This review summarizes the data from 2246 patients having dobutamine stress echocardiography at 28 different centers. The risk of ventricular fibrillation or myocardial infarction was 1/2000 and there were no reported deaths. Dobutamine stress echocardiography was nondiagnostic in about 5% due to poor image quality and in 10% due to submaximal stress. In the remainder, the overall sensitivity was 80% with a specificity of 84% for detection of coronary artery disease. Sensitivity was higher for three-vessel (92%) compared to two-vessel (86%) or one-vessel (74%) disease and was lowest for circumflex artery disease.

11. Poldermans D, Arnese M, Fioretti PM, et al: Sustained prognostic value of dobutamine stress echocardiography for late cardiac events after major noncardiac vascular surgery. Circulation 95:53–58, 1997.

The risk of cardiac events after major noncardiac vascular surgery (mean follow-up 19 ± 11 months) is increased in those with extensive (risk 6.5 times higher) or limited inducible ischemia (risk 2.9 times higher) on preoperative dobutamine stress echocardiography compared to those with no wall motion abnormalities. Risk also is increased (3.8 times) in those with a resting wall motion abnormality on echocardiography. (See accompanying editorial by Bach and Eagle on pages 8 to 10 in the same issue of Circulation.)

12. Bates JR, Sawada SG, Segar DS, et al: Evaluation using dobutamine stress echocardiography in patients with insulin-dependent diabetes mellitus before kidney and/or pancreas transplantation. Am J Cardiol 77:175–179, 1996.

An abnormal dobutamine stress echocardiographic study was associated with a cardiac event rate of 45% compared to an event rate of only 6% in those with a normal study (mean follow-up 1.1 ± 0.7 years).

13. Ahmad M, Zie T, McCulloch M, et al: Real-time three-dimensional dobutamine stress echocardiography in assessment of ischemia: Comparison with two-dimensional dobutamine stress echocardiography. J Am Coll Cardiol 37:1303–1309, 2001.

Real time simultaneous acquisition of multiple views of the left ventricle is as accurate as 2D imaging for detection of wall motion abnormalities and provides unique views of the left ventricle, as well as shorter scanning times.

14. Das MK, Pellikka PA, Mahoney DW, et al: Assessment of cardiac risk before nonvascular surgery: dobutamine stress echocardiography in 530 patients. J Am Coll Cardiol 35:1647–1653, 2000.

Inducible ischemia on dobutamine stress echocardiography had a sensitivity of 100% and specificity of 63% for prediction of perioperative cardiac death (1 patient) or nonfatal myocardial infarction (31 patients). Patients with ischemia evident at <60% of maximum predicted heart rate had a risk of perioperative events of 43% compared to a risk of only 9% in those with ischemia evident at a heart rate >60% of maximum predicted.

15. Marwick TH, Case C, Sawada S, et al: Prediction of mortality using dobutamine echocardiography. J Am Coll Cardiol 37:754–760, 2001.

Cardiac mortality after a normal dobutamine stress echocardiogram was 1% per year for the first 4 years of follow-up. Echocardiographic evidence of ischemia was an independent predictor of outcome with a 4-year survival (cardiac death) of about 80% for those with inducible ischemia and 60% for those with both ischemia and evidence of akinesis or dyskinesis at rest.

16. Sicari R, Pasanisi E, Venneri L, et al. for the Echo Persantine International Cooperative (EPIC) Study Group and the Echo Dobutamine International Cooperative (EDIC) Study Group: Stress echo results predict mortality: A large-scale multicenter prospective international study. J Am Coll Cardiol 41:589–595, 2003.

In 7333 patients undergoing pharmacologic stress echocardiography, followed for a mean of 2.6 years, there was evidence for ischemia in 35%. Cardiac events (sudden death and fatal myocardial infarction) occurred in 2.1% of the study group with a Kaplan

Meier survival of 92% for those with a normal stress test, compared to 71% for those with ischemia.

Myocardial Infarction

17. Wang S, Fleischmann KE: Role of echocardiography in evaluating patients presenting to the emergency room with acute chest pain: Diagnosis, triage treatment decisions, outcomes. In: Otto CM (ed): The Practice of Clinical Echocardiography, 2nd ed. Philadelphia: WB Saunders, 2002, pp 235–250.

    Review of the potential utility of echocardiography for triage, risk stratification, and detection of other causes of chest pain in patients with suspected myocardial infarction. The concept of a chest pain center and cost-effectiveness of various approaches are discussed; 71 references

18. Mohler ER 3rd, Ryan T, Segar DS, et al: Clinical utility of troponin T levels and echocardiography in the emergency department. Am Heart J 135:253–260, 1998.

    The combination of cardiac troponin T levels and a new wall motion abnormality on echocardiography performed in the emergency department had a positive predictive value of 84% and a negative predictive value of 90% for adverse cardiac events in 100 patients admitted for chest discomfort.

19. Fleischmann KE, Goldman L, Robiolio PA, et al: Echocardiographic correlates of survival in patients with chest pain. J Am Coll Cardiol 23:1390–1396, 1994.

    In 513 presenting to the emergency department with chest pain, 92% were admitted to the hospital, 48% had ischemic changes on ECG, 46% had a history of coronary artery disease, and 21% suffered an acute myocardial infarction. At 28½-month follow-up 20% had died (57% cardiovascular) with echocardiographic predictors of overall mortality, and death from cardiovascular causes being severe left ventricular systolic dysfunction and moderate or severe mitral regurgitation (even when adjusted for clinical and ECG variables).

20. Kontos MC, Arrowood JA, Paulsen WH, Nixon JV: Early echocardiography can predict cardiac events in emergency department patients with chest pain. Ann Emerg Med 31:550–557, 1998.

    Echocardiography performed within 4 hours of presentation for chest pain in 260 patients had a higher sensitivity (91%) than ECG (40%) for prediction of cardiac events (myocardial infarction or revascularization). Specificity of echocardiography (75%) was lower than ECG (94%), most likely related to the definition of an abnormal echocardiogram as a regional wall motion abnormality or an ejection fraction <40%.

21. Bholasingh R, Cornel JH, Kamp O, et al: Prognostic value of predischarge dobutamine stress echocardiography in chest pain patients with a negative cardiac troponin T. J Am Coll Cardiol 41:596–602, 2003.

    In 377 patients with chest pain but a nondiagnostic ECG and negative troponin, cardiovascular events (death, myocardial infarction, unstable angina, or revascularization) occurred in 8/26 (31%) with an abnormal and 14/351 (4%) of patients with a normal dobutamine stress echo at a mean follow-up of 6 months.

Myocardial Viability

22. Lualdi JC, Douglas PS: Echocardiography for the assessment of myocardial viability. J Am Soc Echocardiogr 10:772–781, 1997.

    Excellent review on the use of low-dose dobutamine stress echocardiography for assessment of myocardial viability. Other methods for assessing viability also are discussed.

23. Zoghbi WA: Evaluation of myocardial viability with contrast echocardiography. Am J Cardiol 90(Suppl 10A): 65J–71J, 2002.

    Review of the use of myocardial contrast echocardiography to evaluate myocardial perfusion and microvascular integrity.

24. Arnese M, Corvel JH, Salustri A, et al: Prediction of improvement of regional left ventricular function after surgical revascularization: A comparison of low dose dobutamine echocardiography with 201 Tl single-photon emission computed tomography. Circulation 91: 2748–2752, 1995.

    The sensitivity of wall motion with low-dose dobutamine for prediction of recovery of function after revascularization was 74% compared to 89% for 201-thallium poststress reinjection scintigraphy. However, the specificity of low dose dobutamine was 95% compared to 48% for 201-thallium SPECT imaging suggesting that the nuclear technique overestimates the probability of postoperative recovery.

Complications of Acute Myocardial Infarction

25. Foster E, Tseng ZH: Echocardiography in the coronary care unit: Management of acute myocardial infarction, detection of complications, and prognostic implications. In: Otto CM (ed): The Practice of Clinical Echocardiography, 2nd ed. Philadelphia: WB Saunders, 2002, pp 251–275.

    This chapter summarizes the pathophysiologic correlates of the echocardiographic findings in acute myocardial infarction, the role of echocardiography in patient management, and the utility of echocardiography for detecting complications of acute myocardial infarction. 241 references.

26. Oliva PB, Hammill SC, Edwards WD: Cardiac rupture, a clinically predictable complication of acute myocardial infarction: Report of 70 cases with clinicopathologic correlations. J Am Coll Cardiol 22:720–726, 1993.

    Cardiac rupture should be suspected after myocardial infarction in the setting of pericarditis, repetitive emesis, restlessness, and agitation, or if there is a deviation from the expected pattern of T-wave evolution on ECG. Prompt echocardiography can establish the diagnosis of cardiac rupture, allowing rapid intervention.

27. Visser CA, Kan G, Meltzer RS, et al: Incidence, timing, and prognostic value of left ventricular aneurysm formation after myocardial infarction: A prospective, serial echocardiographic study in 158 patients. Am J Cardiol 57:729–732, 1986.

    Left ventricular aneurysm formation was seen within 3 months in 22% of patients with nonreperfused myocardial infarctions—29 of 90 (32%) anterior and 6 of 68 (9%) posterior infarctions.

28. Asinger RW, Mikell FL, Elsperger J, Hodges M: Incidence of left ventricular thrombosis after acute transmural myocardial infarction. N Engl J Med 305:297–302, 1981.

    In the prethrombolytic era, the incidence of apical thrombus detectable by 2D echocardiography was 0 of 35 inferior infarctions and 12 of 35 (34%) anterior infarctions. Thrombi occurred only in areas of akinesis or dyskinesis.

29. Kinch JW, Ryan TJ: Right ventricular infarction. N Engl J Med 330:1211–1217, 1994.

A concise and well-written review of the clinical presentation, diagnosis, and management of right ventricular infarction. The echocardiographic approach is emphasized and compared with ECG and hemodynamic and radionuclide findings; 78 references.

30. Catherwood E, Mintz GS, Kotler MN, et al: Two-dimensional echocardiographic recognition of left ventricular pseudoaneurysm. Circulation 62:294–303, 1980.

Characteristic echocardiographic findings in left ventricular pseudoaneurysm are presented.

31. Gatewood RP Jr, Nanda NC: Differentiation of left ventricular pseudoaneurysm with two-dimensional echocardiography. Am J Cardiol 46:869–878, 1980.

Characteristic echocardiographic findings in left ventricular pseudoaneurysm are presented.

Clinical Outcome after Myocardial Infarction

32. Greco CA, Salustri A, Seccareccia F, et al: Prognostic value of dobutamine echocardiography early after uncomplicated acute myocardial infarction: A comparison with exercise electrocardiography. J Am Coll Cardiol 29:261–267, 1997.

An abnormal predischarge dobutamine stress echocardiographic study after myocardial infarction was associated with a relative risk of 5.5 (95% CI 1.14 to 23.16) for cardiac death and myocardial infarction at follow-up (mean 17 ± 13 months). Dobutamine stress echocardiography was an independent predictor of outcome on multivariate analysis when other clinical and exercise variables were included in the analysis.

33. Sicari R, Picano E, Landi P, et al: Prognostic value of dobutamine-atropine stress echocardiography early after acute myocardial infarction. J Am Coll Cardiol 29:254–260, 1997.

Dobutamine atropine stress echocardiography was performed an average of 12 days after myocardial infarction in 778 patients. Evidence of myocardial viability in regions with abnormal resting wall motion was associated with unstable angina over a follow-up interval of 9 ± 7 months, whereas inducible ischemia was predictive of cardiac-related death.

34. Senior R, Swimburn JM: Incremental value of myocardial contrast echocardiography for the prediction of recovery of function in dobutamine nonresponsive myocardium early after acute myocardial infarction. Am J Cardiol 91:397–402, 2003.

Dobutamine echocardiography and intravenous myocardial contrast echocardiography in 96 patients an average of 4.6 days after myocardial infarction showed that independent predictors of recovery of function included both dobutamine and myocardial contrast data.

35. Balcells E, Powers ER, Lepper W, et al: Detection of myocardial viability by contrast echocardiography in acute infarction predicts recovery of resting function and contractile reserve. J Am Coll Cardiol 41:827–833, 2003.

Myocardial contrast perfusion predicted recovery of contractile function after revascularziation in 30 patients with myocardial infarction.

36. Lancellotti P, Hoffer EP, Pierard LA: Detection and clinical usefulness of a biphasic response during exercise echocardiography early after myocardial infarction. J Am Coll Cardiol 41:1142–1147, 2003.

In 114 patients undergoing stress echocardiography and quantitative coronary angiography after first myocardial infarction, echocardiographic evidence of ischemia in the infarct region predicted infarct-related artery stenosis with a sensitivity of 75% and a specificity of 76%. A biphasic response predicted recovery of function after reperfusion.

The Echo Exam *Ischemic Cardiac Disease*

Myocardial Ischemia

Stress echo modalities
   Treadmill exercise
   Supine bicycle
   Dobutamine
Digital cine-loop views
   Short axis mid-cavity
   Apical 4-chamber
   Apical 2-chamber
   Apical long-axis
Interpretation
   Exercise duration
   Heart rate and blood pressure
   Symptoms
   Wall motion at rest and with stress
   EF at rest and with stress
Utility
   Diagnosis of coronary artery disease
   Severity of disease
     Nnumber of vessels involved
     Extent of myocardium at risk
   Overall LV systolic function
   Diastolic LV function
   Clinical prognosis

Acute Myocardial Infarction

Detection of wall motion abnormalities
Evaluation of recurrent chest pain
Assessment of the response to reperfusion
Complications of acute myocardial infarction
   LV systolic dysfunction
   LV thrombus
   Aneurysm formation
   Acute mitral regurgitation
   Ventricular septal defect
   LV rupture (pseudoaneurysm)
   Pericardial effusion

LV Pseudoaneurysm

Abrupt transition from normal myocardium to aneurysm
Acute angle between myocardium and aneurysm
Narrow neck
Ratio of neck diameter to aneurysm diameter <0.5
May be lined with thrombus

End-Stage Ischemic Disease

LV systolic dysfunction
   Deceased ejection fraction
   Decreased dP/dt
   Regional pattern may be seen
RV systolic dysfunction
   May be present if RV infarction or if pulmonary
     pressures elevated
Mitral regurgitation (MR)
   Diverse mechanisms of ischemic MR
     LV dilation and systolic dysfunction
     Regional wall motion abnormality
     Papillary muscle dysfunction or rupture
   Quantitate severity (see Chapter 12)
LV aneurysm and thrombus formation

Stress Echocardiography

Parameter	Modality	View	Recording	Interpretation
Resting regional wall motion	2D	PSAX mid-cavity level Apical 4-chamber Apical 2-chamber Apical long-axis	Depth that includes only LV, optimize endocardial definition, use contrast if needed	Select optimal image from series of digital cine loops
Stress regional wall motion	2D	PSAX mid-cavity level Apical 4-chamber Apical 2-chamber Apical long-axis	Same depth as baseline, optimize endocardial definition, use contrast if needed	Compare optimal baseline and stress images in same views
Clinical and hemodynamic data		Symptoms Heart rate and rhythm Blood pressure	Continuous during exam, report values at each stage of stress	Maximal workload affects accuracy of echo results for detection of ischemia
LV systolic function	2D Doppler	Ejection fraction *dP/dt*	See section on systolic function for details	

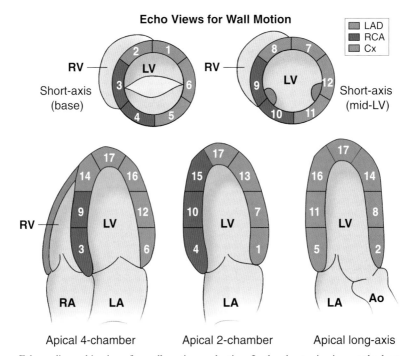

Echocardiographic views for wall motion evaluation. In the short-axis view, at the base and midventricular levels, the left ventricle is divided into the anterior (*1, 7*), anterior septal (*2, 8*), inferior septal (*3, 9*), inferior (*4, 10*), inferolateral (*5, 11*), and anterolateral (*6, 12*) segments. In the apical region, there are four segments: anterior (*13*), septal (*14*), inferior (*15*), and lateral (*16*) plus the tip of the apex (*17*). The territory of the left anterior descending artery is indicated in blue, the right coronary artery in red, and the left circumflex coronary artery in yellow.

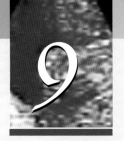

CARDIOMYOPATHIES, HYPERTENSIVE AND PULMONARY HEART DISEASE

Cardiomyopathy is defined as a primary disease of the myocardium, excluding myocardial dysfunction due to ischemia or chronic valvular disease. There are several possible approaches to classification of cardiomyopathies, such as etiology or anatomy, but a physiologic classification is most useful clinically. The three basic physiologic categories of cardiomyopathy are

- dilated,
- hypertrophic, and
- restrictive.

The disease process in an individual patient may correspond closely with one of these physiologic categories; however, overlap between these categories (particularly between dilated and restrictive) can occur. Echocardiographic evaluation focuses on confirming the diagnosis and type of cardiomyopathy present and on defining the physiologic consequences of the disease process in that individual.

While hypertensive and pulmonary heart disease, strictly speaking, are not cardiomyopathies, they are included in this chapter because their clinical and echocardiographic presentation may mimic a cardiomyopathy. In addition, evaluation of the post–cardiac-transplant patient is included.

DILATED CARDIOMYOPATHY

Basic Principles

Dilated cardiomyopathy is characterized by four-chamber enlargement with impaired systolic function of both ventricles. The list of possible etiologies is long and includes postviral, toxins (e.g., alcohol), parasitic diseases (e.g., Chagas' disease), peripartum, and idiopathic (Table 9–1). The physiology of dilated cardiomyopathy is characterized predominantly by

■ impaired left ventricular contractility,
■ reduced cardiac output, and
■ elevated left ventricular end-diastolic pressure.

Clinically, patients most often present with heart failure, with initial complaints ranging from symptoms of pulmonary or systemic venous congestion to symptoms of low forward cardiac output. Coexisting mitral regurgitation frequently is present secondary to left ventricular and mitral annular dilation. In addition, pulmonary hypertension develops in most patients in response to the chronic elevation in left atrial pressure. Left ventricular diastolic dysfunction often coexists with

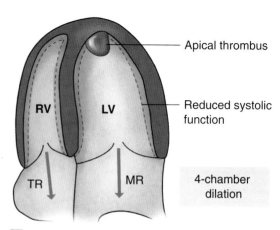

■ **FIGURE 9–1.** Schematic diagram of the key features of dilated cardiomyopathy in an apical four-chamber view. All four chambers are enlarged with reduced left and right ventricular (LV and RV) systolic function. *Dashed lines* indicate the limited extent of endocardial motion between end-diastole and end-systole. An apical thrombus is present. Secondary mitral and tricuspid regurgitation are indicated by the *arrows* (LA, left atrium; RA, right atrium).

systolic dysfunction but typically is not the predominant feature of this disease.

Echocardiographic Approach

Echocardiographic imaging from standard windows allows evaluation of the size and function of all four cardiac chambers with particular attention to the two ventricles (Figs. 9–1 and 9–2):

■ Left ventricular systolic function
  ■ Qualitative global and regional function
  ■ Quantitative end-diastolic and end-systolic dimensions or volumes
  ■ Ejection fraction
■ Right ventricular systolic function
  ■ Qualitative size and systolic function
  ■ Pulmonary artery systolic pressure

In addition to two-dimensional (2D) imaging, other signs of poor left ventricular systolic function include:

■ M-mode
  ■ Increased mitral E-point to septal separation (EPSS)
  ■ Reduced anteroposterior aortic root motion
  ■ Delayed mitral valve closure
■ Doppler
  ■ Reduced aortic ejection velocity
  ■ Reduced dP/dt
  ■ Associated mitral regurgitation
  ■ Diastolic dysfunction

TABLE 9–1
Examples of Potential Causes of Dilated Cardiomyopathy
Idiopathic
Toxins (alcohol, medications, cobalt, snake bites)
Metabolic (thiamine deficiency, acromegaly)
Peripartum
Infections (Chagas' disease, postviral)
Systemic diseases (e.g., immune-mediated injury)
Inherited disorders (Duchenne's muscular dystrophy, sickle cell anemia)

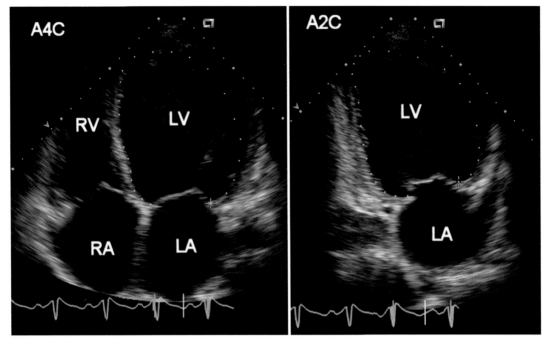

FIGURE 9–2. Echocardiographic images in a patient with dilated cardiomyopathy. In the apical four-chamber view (*left*), dilation of all four cardiac chambers is seen. In the apical two-chamber view (*right*), the left ventricle and atrium are seen. In real time, right and left ventricular systolic functions are severely reduced.

The increased EPSS is due to a combination of left ventricular dilation and reduced mitral leaflet motion due to low transmitral flow rates. Reduced anteroposterior aortic root motion reflects reduced left atrial filling and emptying (Fig. 9–3). The Doppler findings of a reduced aortic ejection velocity and velocity-time integral indicate a reduced stroke volume, although compensatory mechanisms (including left ventricular dilation) result in a normal stroke volume at rest

in many individuals. A slow rate of rise in velocity of the mitral regurgitant jet indicates a reduced rate of increase in left ventricular pressure in early systole (dP/dt). Associated atrioventricular valve regurgitation can be assessed with Doppler techniques (see Chapter 12) and often is moderate in severity (Fig. 9–4). Pulmonary pressures usually are elevated and can be estimated from the velocity in the tricuspid regurgitant jet, as described in Chapter 6.

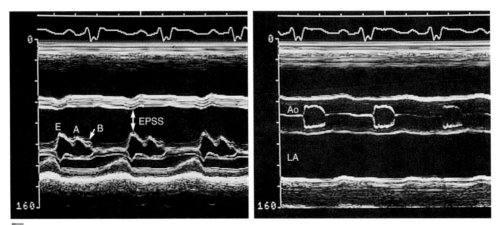

FIGURE 9–3. M-mode findings in dilated cardiomyopathy. There is increased mitral *E*-point septal separation (EPSS) and a "B-bump" (*left*) and decreased aortic root motion with early closure of the aortic valve (*right*).

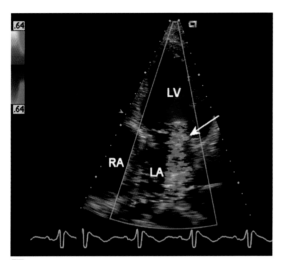

FIGURE 9–4. Color Doppler imaging of a central mitral regurgitant jet in an apical four-chamber view in a patient with dilated cardiomyopathy. The mitral valve leaflets are normal with functional mitral regurgitation due to ventricular dilation and abnormal alignment of the papillary muscles.

The pattern of left ventricular diastolic filling can be evaluated with Doppler recordings of left ventricular inflow. Early in the disease course, a reduced E velocity and increased A velocity consistent with impaired early diastolic relaxation may be observed. However, once left ventricular function has deteriorated significantly, the pattern changes to that of an increased E velocity and reduced A velocity. In this situation, the high ratio of E to A velocity most likely indicates a high left atrial pressure (increased gradient from left atrium to left ventricle at mitral valve opening) and a high

left ventricular end-diastolic pressure (reduced A velocity) (Fig. 9–5). This pattern of mitral inflow, often termed *pseudonormalization*, can be distinguished from a normal inflow pattern by the pulmonary venous inflow signal, which shows an increased atrial reversal velocity signal and an increased ratio of antegrade diastolic to systolic flow and by the pattern of mitral annular motion on Doppler tissue imaging, which shows a decreased E_m velocity. An echocardiographic finding that correlates with an elevated end-diastolic pressure is the M-mode finding of a delayed rate of mitral valve closure, termed a *B-bump* or *AC-shoulder* (see Fig. 9–3).

When significant left ventricular systolic dysfunction is present (ejection fraction <35%), a careful search for apical left ventricular thrombus is indicated (Fig. 9–6). Details on the technical aspects of identifying a left ventricular thrombus are given in Chapter 8.

Limitations/Technical Considerations

Echocardiography rarely can establish the etiology of a dilated cardiomyopathy, even though it is instrumental both in confirming the presence of ventricular dysfunction and in providing prognostic data. The echocardiographic appearance of a dilated cardiomyopathy is fairly uniform despite a wide range of disease processes. One exception is Chagas' heart disease; these patients typically have a left ventricular apical aneurysm with minimal involvement of the ventricular septum. In patients with endomyocardial fibrosis due to Chagas' disease, there is apical obliteration with a small ventricular chamber, atrial enlargement, and atrioventricular valve regurgitation. While

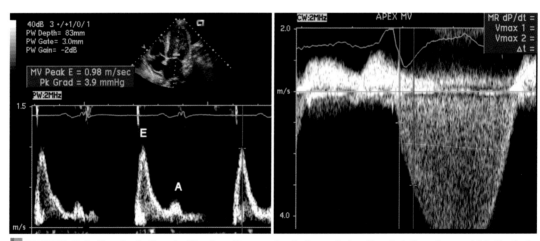

FIGURE 9–5. Doppler findings in dilated cardiomyopathy. Left ventricular diastolic inflow shows a high E velocity and low A velocity suggestive of "pseudo-normalization" due to an elevated end-diastolic pressure (*left*). The mitral regurgitant jet shows a slow rate of rise in velocity consistent with a reduced dP/dt (*right*).

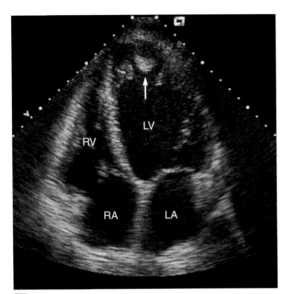

■ **FIGURE 9–6.** Left ventricular apical thrombus (*arrow*) in an apical four-chamber view in a patient with dilated cardiomyopathy.

Chagas' disease is rare in North America and Europe, it is endemic in South and Central America and may be diagnosed in immigrants from those areas. Recognition of the echocardiographic features of this disease may prompt the correct diagnosis in a nonendemic area.

In most patients with dilated cardiomyopathy, an exact etiology cannot be identified, even when all diagnostic modalities are used. The most useful additional data are a careful patient history to uncover possible precipitating factors. An endomyocardial biopsy is rarely diagnostic except when an infiltrative process (e.g., amyloid, sarcoid, hemochromatosis) is present. Findings of "myocarditis" are nonspecific and usually do not change the therapeutic approach.

Clinical Utility

Echocardiographic evaluation is indicated at the initial presentation of a patient with symptoms consistent with dilated cardiomyopathy. If an echocardiogram performed in a patient with a suspected dilated cardiomyopathy shows no significant impairment of left ventricular systolic dysfunction, a careful search is needed for other causes of heart failure symptoms such as

■ coronary artery disease,
■ valvular disease,
■ hypertensive heart disease,
■ pericardial disease, and
■ pulmonary heart disease.

Whenever the clinical presentation suggests heart failure, a comprehensive examination of systolic and diastolic function is needed, even when the core echocardiographic examination does not show obvious evidence of dysfunction. If the echocardiogram is consistent with the clinical diagnosis of dilated cardiomyopathy, detailed information on ventricular function, chamber sizes, associated valvular disease, and pulmonary artery pressures is obtained.

Periodic echocardiography is essential for optimal care of patients with dilated cadiomyopathy. The detailed assessment available by echocardiography aids in appropriate tailoring of medical therapy. In addition, repeat echocardiograms are needed for any change in clinical status that suggests an interval change in ventricular function. A severe decrease in ventricular systolic function may prompt consideration of cardiac transplantation.

In the intensive care unit, echocardiographic evaluation can be helpful in patients with dilated cardiomyopathy to assess left ventricular function, pulmonary artery pressures, the degree of coexisting mitral regurgitation, and to estimate left ventricular filling pressure. Evaluation of an individual patient's response to afterload reduction therapy can be performed by repeat ejection fraction measurements or by sequential noninvasive measurements of pulmonary pressures and cardiac output (see Chapter 6 and Fig. 9–7).

Alternate Approaches

If measurement of pulmonary vascular resistance is needed (e.g., in a heart transplant candidate), cardiac catheterization is indicated. Although echocardiographic measures of pulmonary pressure are accurate, calculation of pulmonary vascular resistance currently is not reliable enough for clinical decision making although promising methods are in development (see Suggested Reading in Chapter 6).

HYPERTROPHIC CARDIOMYOPATHY

Basic Principles

Hypertrophic cardiomyopathy is an autosomal dominant inherited disease of the myocardium (with variable penetrance) related to abnormalities in the β-myosin heavy-chain gene. Predominant anatomic features of this disease (Fig. 9–8) are

■ asymmetric hypertrophy of the left ventricle,
■ normal ventricular systolic function,
■ impaired diastolic left ventricular function, and
■ subaortic dynamic obstruction in some individuals.

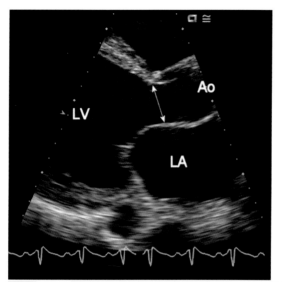

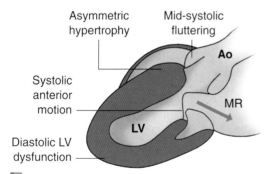

FIGURE 9-7. Calculation of stroke volume in a patient with dilated cardiomyopathy is based on measurement of LV outflow tract diameter from a parasternal long-axis view (*top*) for calculation of a circular cross-sectional area (CSA$_{LVOT}$) and the left ventricular outflow tract velocity-time integral (VTI$_{LVOT}$) is recorded just proximal to the aortic valve from an apical approach using a pulsed Doppler sample volume length of 5 to 10 mm (*bottom*). Stroke volume (SV) is calculated as VTI × CSA. Cardiac output is stroke volume times heart rate. Calculation of stroke volume in this patient is complicated by mechanical alternans related to severe systolic dysfunction with marked variation in the outflow velocity (*arrows*) on alternating beats despite normal sinus rhythm.

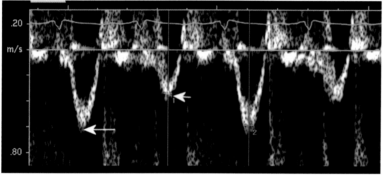

FIGURE 9-8. Schematic diagram of the typical features of hypertrophic cardiomyopathy in a parasternal long-axis view. There is midsystolic closure and coarse fluttering of the aortic valve leaflets, asymmetric septal hypertrophy with sparing of the basal posterior wall, normal left ventricular systolic function with impaired diastolic function, dynamic outflow tract obstruction with systolic anterior motion of the mitral valve leaflets, and mitral regurgitation.

Other important clinical features of this disease are a high risk of sudden death (especially during exertion); symptoms of angina, exercise intolerance, and syncope; and a systolic murmur on cardiac auscultation.

The *pattern* of left ventricular hypertrophy in patients with hypertrophic cardiomyopathy can be quite variable, ranging from "classic" septal hypertrophy to isolated apical hypertrophy (Fig. 9-9). In addition, the *degree* of myocardial thickening is quite variable, even within a family. Hypertrophy may be confined to the anterior segment of the ventricular septum (type I) or may involve the anterior and posterior segments of the septum (type II) with sparing of the lateral, posterior, and inferior walls. Some patients have extensive ventricular hypertrophy with normal wall thickness seen only in the basal segment of the posterior wall (type III). An unusual pattern of hypertrophy is apical hypertrophic cardiomyopathy (type IV), which is of particular note to the echocardiographer because it can be missed if the marked displacement of the apical endocardium is not recognized. Clinically, the clue to an apical

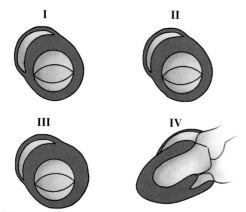

I   II

III   IV

■ FIGURE 9–9. Schematic diagram of patterns of ventricular hypertrophy in hypertrophic cardiomyopathy in a parasternal basal short-axis view. Type I = hypertrophy confined to anterior septum; type II = anterior and posterior septum involved; type III = extensive hypertrophy sparing only the basal posterior wall; type IV = apical hypertrophy (in a long-axis schematic view).

pattern of hypertrophy is inverted precordial T waves on the electrocardiogram. The common feature of all these hypertrophy patterns is normal thickness (or "sparing") of the basal posterior left ventricular wall. In the parasternal long- and short-axis views, this region is seen at the base (between the papillary muscle and mitral annulus) posterior to the mitral valve leaflets.

In patients with subaortic obstruction, apposition of the anterior leaflet of the mitral valve against the hypertrophied ventricular septum is seen in systole. This obstruction is dynamic rather than fixed, both in the sense that it occurs only in mid to late systole and in the sense that the presence and severity of obstruction can be altered by loading conditions. These features contrast with the relatively fixed obstruction of aortic valve stenosis, which persists from the onset to the end of ejection and in which the severity of the stenosis is relatively insensitive to changes in loading conditions. Dynamic outflow obstruction in hypertrophic cardiomyopathy typically has a pattern of onset in midsystole, with the maximum left ventricular to aortic pressure gradient occurring in late systole (Figs. 9–10 and 9–11). Controversy persists regarding the mechanism of dynamic obstruction and the lack of a clear relationship between clinical status and hemodynamic findings. Of note, late systolic obstruction occurs after the majority of the stroke volume has been ejected, thus minimally affecting forward stroke volume in most patients.

Obstruction can be diminished by maneuvers that increase ventricular volume, an increase in preload or a decrease in contractility, or by maneuvers that increase afterload. Conversely, the degree of obstruction is increased by

- a reduction in preload,
- an increase in contractility, or
- a decrease in afterload.

All these conditions are similar in that they reduce left ventricular volume. Some patients with no or minimal evidence of outflow obstruction at rest develop obstruction with maneuvers performed during the physical examination or with echocardiography. Clinically useful maneuvers include examination during a postpremature contraction beat (increased contractility), with Valsalva maneuver (decreased preload), or after inhalation of amyl nitrate (decreased afterload and preload). All of these maneuvers lead to an increase in the degree of dynamic obstruction with a louder murmur and an increased Doppler velocity. Dynamic outflow obstruction usually is associated with mitral regurgitation, since the systolic anterior motion of the leaflets in systole disrupts normal coaptation. A posteriorly directed mitral regurgitant jet of mild to moderate severity originates at the malcoapted segment of the leaflets (Fig. 9–12).

Left ventricular systolic function typically is normal in patients with hypertrophic cardiomyopathy. However, left ventricular diastolic function is abnormal, accounting for many of the heart failure symptoms in patients with hypertrophic cardiomyopathy. The thickened myocardium exhibits impaired relaxation and decreased compliance.

Echocardiographic Approach

Left Ventricular Asymmetric Hypertrophy

Evaluation of the pattern and extent of left ventricular hypertrophy is made from multiple tomographic views. In the parasternal long-axis view, particular attention is focused on the posterobasal wall between the papillary muscle and the mitral annulus. Although the wall in this region is not thickened in patients with hypertrophic cardiomyopathy, it is thickened in patients with concentric hypertrophy due to other etiologies (e.g., hypertension, restrictive cardiomyopathy). Two-dimensional guided M-mode tracings provide the best endocardial definition for measurement of septal and posterior wall thickness, although 2D measurements can be used when image quality is adequate. Two-dimensional imaging in both long- and short-axis views is used to ensure that the M-mode beam is perpendicular to the left ventricu-

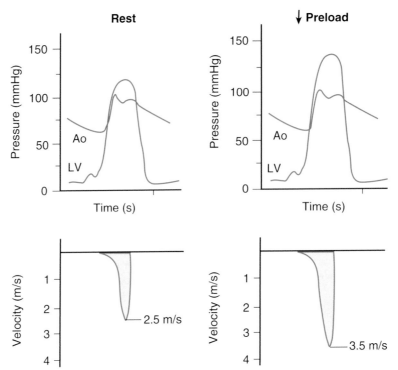

FIGURE 9–10. Schematic diagrams of the pressure gradient and velocity curve in dynamic outflow obstruction due to hypertrophic cardiomyopathy. At rest, a small gradient is present only in late systole between the left ventricle (LV) and aorta (Ao). The continuous-wave Doppler curve shows a late-peaking velocity of 2.5 m/s, with the origin of this velocity being the subaortic region. With alterations in loading conditions (decreased preload), the degree of obstruction increases dramatically. A late peaking, high-velocity (3.5 m/s) Doppler curve now is obtained.

lar walls and to avoid inclusion of right ventricular trabeculation in the septal wall thickness.

The parasternal long-axis view also offers the best opportunity to define the exact relationship between the pattern of septal hypertrophy and the outflow tract (Fig. 9–13). This is important when a surgical approach, such as myotomy-myectomy, is being considered, because surgical visualization usually is retrograde across the aortic valve, allowing only limited direct inspection of the septal endocardium and little information on the extent of septal thickening or the degree of septal curvature. The extent and pattern of hypertrophy also is important if percutaneous catheter ablation is being considered. Parasternal short-axis views from base to apex allow assessment of the latero-medial extent of the hypertrophic process.

Some degree of bulging of the septum into the left ventricular outflow tract, often called a septal "knuckle," is seen in normal older individuals. This apparent septal prominence most likely is due to increased tortuosity of the aorta resulting in a more acute angle between the basal septum

and aortic root. There is no evidence that this septal contour pattern is inherited or associated with clinical events so that these patients should not be considered to have hypertrophic cardiomyopathy.

Apical views again allow visualization of the pattern and extent of hypertrophy. Diagnosis of apical hypertrophy can be difficult, since endocardial definition may be poor and the endocardial surface (which may be located up to one third the distance from the apical epicardium to the base) may be missed if image quality is suboptimal (Fig. 9–14). In some cases, the epicardium may be mistaken for the apical endocardium. A careful examination, when the referring physician has alerted the echocardiographer to this possible diagnosis, avoids this potential pitfall. Color or pulsed Doppler examination is helpful in demonstrating the absence of blood flow in the "apical" region, which is occupied by the hypertrophied myocardium. If needed, echo contrast can be used to better define the endocardial border.

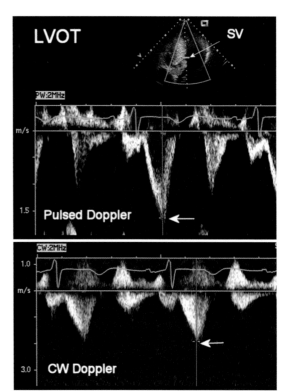

FIGURE 9–11. In a patient with hypertrophic cardiomyopathy, pulsed Doppler examination from the apex with the sample volume (SV) moved progressively toward the aortic valve, demonstrates a subaortic late-peaking systolic velocity curve. Continuous-wave Doppler in a patient confirms the typical late-peaking systolic velocity curve due to dynamic outflow tract obstruction, which is mild in this patient with a maximum velocity of only 1.8 m/s at rest.

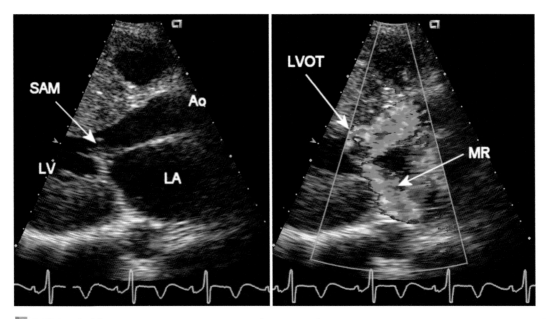

FIGURE 9–12. Parasternal long-axis 2D image (*left*) and color flow image (*right*) showing systolic anterior motion of the mitral leaflets (SAM), and mitral regurgitation (MR) in a patient with hypertrophic cardiomyopathy. The posteriorly directed MR jet originates from the malcoapted segment of the mitral leaflets in association with systolic anterior motion. Turbulence in the LV outflow tract (LVOT) is seen due to subaortic dynamic obstruction

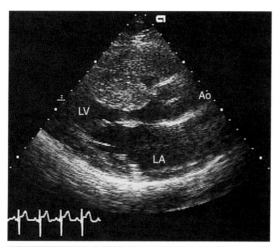

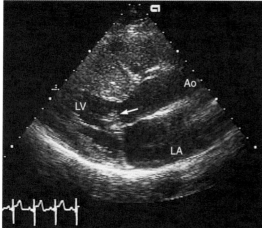

FIGURE 9-13. Two-dimensional images of hypertrophic cardiomyopathy in a parasternal long-axis view at end-diastole (*top*) and end-systole (*bottom*). Systolic anterior motion of the mitral valve is seen (*arrow*).

Qualitative and quantitative evaluation of left ventricular systolic function is performed using standard approaches (see Chapter 6).

Left Ventricular Diastolic Function

Left ventricular diastolic function is evaluated using Doppler recordings of

■ left ventricular inflow across the mitral valve,
■ left atrial inflow in the pulmonary vein,
■ myocardial Doppler tissue velocity, and
■ isovolumic relaxation time.

Parameters of diastolic function are evaluated as described in Chapter 7. Typical changes in patients with hypertrophic cardiomyopathy include a prolonged isovolumic relaxation time, reduced *E* velocity, enhanced *A* velocity, and increased duration and velocity of the pulmonary

vein a-reversal. These findings are consistent with impaired diastolic relaxation and an elevated left ventricular end-diastolic pressure. However, there is marked patient variability depending on the severity of diastolic dysfunction in each patient. Seqential studies may show changes after medical or surgical therapy that are consistent with improved diastolic filling.

Dynamic Outflow Tract Obstruction

In a subset of patients with hypertrophic cardiomyopathy, subaortic obstruction is present, characterized by

■ systolic anterior motion of the mitral leaflet,
■ mid-systolic closure of the aortic valve,
■ late peaking high velocity flow in the outflow tract, and
■ variability in the severity of obstruction with certain maneuvers:
 ■ post-PVC beats
 ■ amyl nitrate inhalation
 ■ exercise

IMAGING. In a patient with dynamic left ventricular outflow tract obstruction, long-axis images show the classic finding of systolic anterior motion of the mitral valve with apposition of the mitral leaflet and septum in mid- to late systole. M-mode recordings may be helpful in that with pathologic systolic anterior motion, the rate of anterior leaflet motion is more rapid than the anterior motion of the posterior wall in systole (Fig. 9–15). A "contact lesion" on the ventricular septum at the site of mitral leaflet impingement may be seen in some patients.

Short-axis views also show the systolic anterior motion of the mitral valve leaflets. Frame-by-frame analysis shows the cross-sectional area of the outflow tract throughout systole.

Apical 2D views are helpful for demonstrating the abnormal mitral leaflet motion, especially the apical long-axis and the anteriorly angulated four-chamber views. Note that the degree of systolic anterior motion may not be uniform from medial to lateral across the mitral leaflets, so imaging in multiple planes with slight adjustments in transducer angulation may be needed to demonstrate the presence and extent of dynamic outflow obstruction.

The aortic valve shows normal leaflet opening in early systole, followed by midsystolic abrupt partial closure with coarse fluttering of the aortic valve leaflets in late systole due to late systolic dynamic outflow obstruction. Again, these rapid leaflet movements are best documented on M-mode recordings. The aortic leaflets themselves may be sclerotic because of the long-term effect of

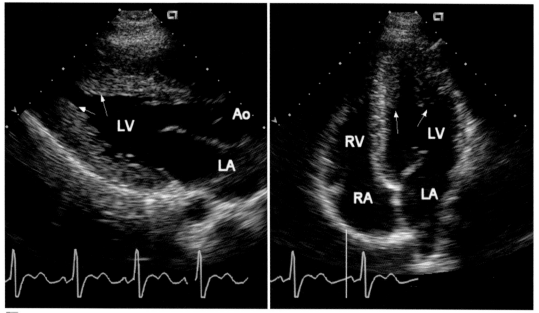

■ FIGURE 9-14. Apical hypertrophic cardiomyopathy with marked thickening of the apical segments (*arrows*) in a parasternal long-axis (*left*) and apical four-chamber view (*right*).

a turbulent jet as a result of subaortic obstruction, and some degree of coexisting aortic regurgitation may be noted.

DOPPLER EVALUATION. Doppler studies provide a more direct evaluation of the presence, location, and degree of dynamic subaortic obstruction than do imaging techniques. With conventional pulsed or color flow imaging, the site of obstruction is identified based on the location of the poststenotic turbulence. Both parasternal and apical long-axis views are useful for this examination.

Using pulsed Doppler from an apical approach, the sample volume is slowly moved from the apex progressively toward the base, recording the velocity curve at each step. Proximal to the outflow obstruction, velocities are normal. At the site of obstruction, the velocity increases abruptly to a velocity reflecting the degree of obstruction (as stated in the Bernoulli equation). This approach, using stepwise evaluation with pulsed Doppler ultrasound, is advantageous in that intracavity gradients due to apical hypertrophy or apposition of the papillary muscle with the

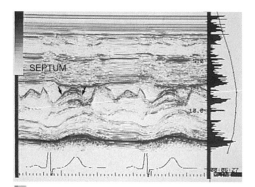
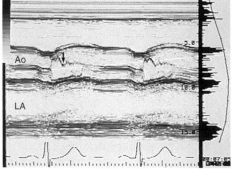

■ FIGURE 9-15. M-mode at the mitral valve level (*left*) in a patient with dynamic outflow obstruction due to hypertrophic cardiomyopathy showing the classic septal hypertrophy and systolic anterior motion (SAM) of the mitral leaflets (*arrows*). An M-mode view at the aortic valve level (*right*) shows midsystolic closure of the aortic valve (*arrow*) followed by coarse fluttering of the leaflets.

septum will be recognized and not mistaken for subaortic dynamic obstruction (Fig. 9–16).

Continuous-wave Doppler from an apical approach typically shows a late-peaking high-velocity systolic jet in patients with dynamic left ventricular outflow tract obstruction. The shape of this curve is distinctive, corresponding to the temporal course of the left ventricular to aortic pressure gradient (see Fig. 9–10). Again, because continuous-wave Doppler measures velocities along the entire length of the ultrasound beam, other techniques are needed to confirm the depth of origin of the signal. In patients with hypertensive heart disease or hypovolemia, the combination of left ventricular hypertrophy and hyperdynamic systolic function may result in a similar late-peaking high-velocity systolic waveform. However, in these patients the site of obstruction is not subaortic; it is closer to the apex, at the midventricular level.

PROVOCATIVE MANEUVERS. When features suggestive of hypertrophic cardiomyopathy are present and there is no evidence for outflow obstruction at rest, maneuvers to "provoke" outflow obstruction may be performed to make a definite diagnosis or to relate the patient's symptoms to the echocardiographic findings. When only a modest degree of obstruction is seen at rest, interventions to increase the degree of obstruction may be performed for similar reasons.

A spontaneous premature ventricular contraction (PVC) results in an increased degree of obstruction on the post-PVC beat due to increased left ventricular contractility. Alternatively, the strain phase of the Valsalva maneuver increases obstruction by decreasing preload (smaller left ventricular cavity size) but is difficult to perform simultaneously with echocardiography due to changes in cardiac position and lung interference as the patient performs the maneuver.

A simple and reasonably safe method to provoke dynamic outflow obstruction in the echocardiography laboratory is amyl nitrate inhalation under direct physician supervision. This medication results in a brief decrease in preload (venodilation) and decrease in afterload (arterial dilation), both of which increase the degree of obstruction. A moderate degree of tachycardia may occur, but the duration of action of this inhaled medication is brief. The sonographer records the continuous-wave Doppler signal in the left ventricular outflow tract before, during, and after administration of amyl nitrate by the physician to document the effects of the medication on the degree of outflow obstruction. Attention is needed to maintain a parallel intercept angle between the ultrasound beam and the high-

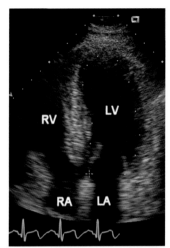

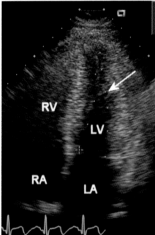

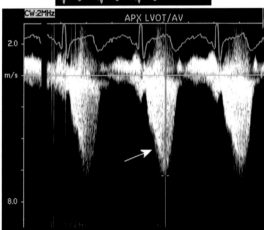

▌ FIGURE 9–16. Example of a concentrically hypertrophied hyperdynamic left ventricle in diastole (*top*) with mid-cavity obliteration at end-systole (*middle*) resulting in a late-peaking high-velocity outflow tract Doppler curve (*bottom*). This patient was anemic and febrile at the time of this examination. Hypertensive hyperdynamic mid-cavity obstruction must be distinguished from the dynamic subaortic obstruction seen in hypertrophic cardiomyopathy.

velocity jet, particularly with respect to the phase of the respiratory cycle. The physician monitors heart rate, rhythm, symptoms, and blood pressure. Care is needed to ensure that only the patient (and not the other individuals in the room) are exposed to the medication.

Exercise echocardiography also may be helpful in patients with hypertrophic cardiomyopathy. Continuous-wave Doppler outflow velocity recordings are made at rest and immediately postexercise to assess for inducible outflow obstruction.

Mitral Valve Abnormalities

The mitral valve is anatomically and functionally abnormal in the majority of patients with hypertrophic cardiomyopathy. Functionally, mitral regurgitation results from systolic anterior motion of the leaflets into the outflow tract leading to late systolic failure of coaptation and a consequent posteriorly directed regurgitant jet. However, anatomic abnormalities are present as well. Both autopsy and echocardiographic studies demonstrate that the mitral leaflets have an increased surface area and a longer length (particularly the anterior leaflet) compared to normal subjects. In addition, the degree of coaptation is excessive, and the coaptation plane is displaced posteriorly. About 10% of patients have anomalous papillary muscle anatomy with direct insertion of the papillary muscle into the leaflet.

Limitations/Technical Considerations

As discussed previously, it is important to distinguish hypertrophic cardiomyopathy with dynamic subaortic obstruction associated with systolic anterior motion of the mitral leaflet from a concentrically hypertrophied ventricle due to other disease processes (such as hypertension). In some situations, the hypertrophied ventricle may be hyperdynamic, with midcavity obliteration resulting in an intracavity gradient. The distinction between hypertrophic cardiomyopathy and a hyperdynamic concentrically hypertrophied ventricle can be made by careful attention to the 2D images (sparing of the basal posterior wall in hypertrophic cardiomyopathy) and M-mode findings (characteristic aortic and mitral valve motion) and by evaluation of the depth of origin of the high-velocity jet using conventional pulsed, high pulse repetition frequency (HPRF), and color Doppler techniques. The patient's clinical and family history also are important for making this distinction.

Another difficult problem is separating the degree of outflow obstruction due to dynamic subaortic obstruction from that due to valvular aortic stenosis in the rare patient with both conditions. In the presence of serial stenoses, an accurate measure of the pressure drop across each narrowing may not be possible, since the simplified Bernoulli equation applies to a single stenosis. However, HPRF Doppler may allow examination of velocities at each site, indicating the relative contribution of each site to the total degree of obstruction to ventricular outflow. Occasionally, a patient with valvular aortic stenosis and a hypertrophied ventricle will demonstrate dynamic subaortic obstruction only after aortic valve replacement. Some of these patients have hypertrophic cardiomyopathy that is "unmasked" by the afterload reduction of valve replacement. Others have a hyperdynamic ventricle with a midcavity pressure gradient that may resolve as the degree of left ventricular hypertrophy decreases postoperatively.

Clinical Utility

Diagnosis and Screening

Echocardiography is the procedure of choice for accurate diagnosis of hypertrophic cardiomyopathy. Since this is an inherited disorder, screening with echocardiography is indicated for all first-degree relatives of the affected individual. This diagnosis significantly changes clinical management even in asymptomatic individuals, given the high risk of sudden death with exertion, and has important implications for genetic counseling.

Evaluation of Medical Therapy

In patients with a definite diagnosis of hypertrophic cardiomyopathy, Doppler findings can be used to assess the impact of medical therapy. Specifically, the pattern of left ventricular diastolic filling after institution of therapy to improve diastolic function (such as beta blockers or calcium channel blockers) may show an improvement in early diastolic filling. The degree of dynamic outflow obstruction also may show improvement on medical therapy.

Monitoring of Percutaneous Septal Ablation

Echocardiography plays an important role in patient selection for catheter septal ablation procedures and for monitoring the procedure in the catheterization laboratory. In the catheterization laboratory, baseline and postprocedure Doppler data are used in conjunction with invasive hemodynamics to assess the reduction in outflow obstruction (Fig. 9–17). After the procedure, sequential echocardiographic studies may show continued improvement in the extent of outflow obstruction due to healing and fibrosis of the

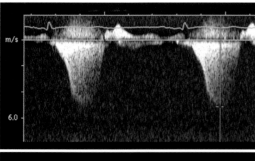

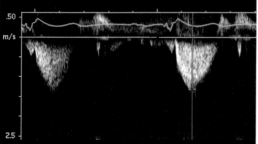

FIGURE 9–17. In a patient with obstructive hypertrophic cardiomyopathy undergoing a catheter septal ablation procedure, transthoracic echocardiography in the catheterization laboratory demonstrates severe obstruction at baseline with a late peaking outflow tract velocity of 5 m/s (*top*). After the septal ablation, the maximum velocity was 1.4 m/s (*bottom*).

infarcted septal myocardium. In the patient being considered for percutaneous or surgical treatment for hypertrophic cardiomyopathy, knowledge of the extent, distribution, and curvature of septal hypertrophy determines the location and size of the muscle segment to be removed or ablated. With the catheter positioned in a septal coronary branch, contrast is injected during echocardiographic imaging to show the specific location and extent of the area perfused by that vessel before delivery of the ablation agent (Fig. 9–18).

Surgical Therapy

Intraoperative monitoring of myotomy-myectomy allows evaluation of the adequacy of the procedure in relieving outflow tract obstruction. Transesophageal imaging may provide adequate images of the myectomy site; however, epicardial imaging often is preferable since the septum is located anteriorly relative to the esophagus. Doppler evaluation for residual obstruction postbypass should be performed under hemodynamic conditions as similar as possible to the baseline state, because the degree of obstruction is influenced by loading conditions. Color flow imaging is helpful in excluding residual obstruction but when the

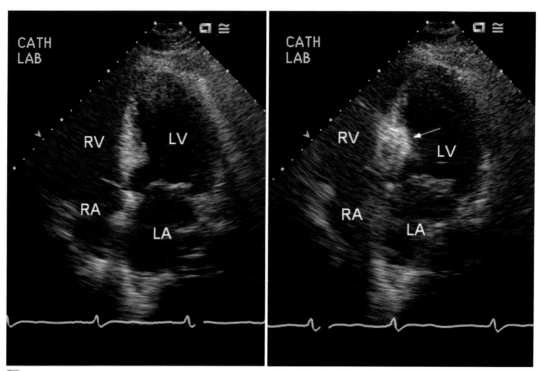

FIGURE 9–18. In a patient with obstructive hypertrophic cardiomyopathy undergoing catheter septal ablation, an apical four-chamber view recorded in the cardiac catheterization laboratory (Cath Lab) with the patient supine, the baseline image on the *left* shows septal hypertrophy. The image on the *right* shows contrast in the septum (*arrow*) defining the area perfused by the septal branch that will be injected with the ablation agent.

subaortic flow pattern remains abnormal, quantitative Doppler velocity data are needed. Careful examination for a postoperative ventricular septal defect also should be performed.

It may be difficult to obtain an accurate continuous-wave Doppler recording of the degree of outflow obstruction in the operating room because the transesophageal approach rarely provides a transgastric apical view from which the beam can be aligned parallel to the jet. An epicardial apical position may not be obtainable with a median sternotomy because the transducer often is too large to fit under the ribs at the apex. Placement of a sterile transducer on the ascending aorta with inferior angulation toward the outflow tract may allow a parallel intercept angle in some patients.

Alternate Approaches

Usually, echocardiography provides all the data needed for clinical management of a patient with suspected or diagnosed hypertrophic cardiomyopathy. Alternate tomographic imaging techniques can provide data on the anatomic pattern of hypertrophy but do not allow evaluation of abnormal diastolic filling or the presence and degree of dynamic outflow tract obstruction.

When the echocardiographic findings and clinical presentation are discrepant, cardiac catheterization may be helpful. First, evaluation of coronary anatomy may be indicated, since coexisting epicardial coronary artery disease may explain some symptoms in a patient with hypertrophic cardiomyopathy. Second, recordings of left ventricular and aortic pressures at rest and after provocative maneuvers to increase or decrease dynamic outflow obstruction and with slow "pullback" across the outflow tract and aortic valve allow more detailed hemodynamic evaluation. This is particularly helpful in the patient with sequential stenoses in the subaortic region and at the aortic valve level.

In the operating room, direct left ventricular and aortic pressure measurements after myectomy may be helpful if residual obstruction is suspected.

RESTRICTIVE CARDIOMYOPATHY

Basic Principles

Restrictive cardiomyopathy is characterized by normal left ventricular systolic function with impaired diastolic function due to a stiff, hypertrophied left ventricle. Heart failure symptoms are due to the resultant elevation in left ventricular end-diastolic pressure and the inability to increase cardiac output with exercise due to impaired diastolic filling. Note that heart failure—defined as the inability to maintain a normal cardiac output or maintenance of a normal cardiac output only with an elevated left ventricular end-diastolic pressure—can occur with normal systolic function. In many patients with restrictive cardiomyopathy, right-sided failure predominates initially with symptoms of peripheral edema and ascites.

As the disease process progresses, an individual patient may progress from an anatomic/hemodynamic pattern consistent with restrictive cardiomyopathy to a pattern showing some features of dilated cardiomyopathy, ending with a picture indistinguishable from dilated cardiomyopathy.

Compared with dilated cardiomyopathy, restrictive cardiomyopathy is an uncommon diagnosis. Examples of the etiology of restrictive cardiomyopathy include

■ infiltrative processes:
  ■ amyloidosis,
  ■ hemochromatosis,
  ■ glycogen storage disease,
■ inflammatory diseases:
  ■ sarcoidosis,
  ■ hypereosinophilic syndrome.

An unusual cause of restrictive cardiomyopathy is the hypereosinophilic syndrome. This systemic disease is characterized by hypereosinophilia with involvement of the lungs, bone marrow, brain, and heart. Cardiac involvement is typical and exhibits unique echocardiographic features. In this syndrome, left ventricular thrombus formation occurs in the absence of an underlying wall motion abnormality (particularly in the apex), resulting in gradual apical "obliteration" (as seen on angiography) or filling in of the apex with an echogenic mass (on echocardiography). Thrombus formation also occurs under the posterior mitral valve leaflet, leading to adherence of the posterior leaflet to the endocardium and significant mitral regurgitation.

Echocardiographic Approach

Typical echocardiographic features (Figs. 9–19 and 9–20) in the untreated patient with restrictive cardiomyopathy include

■ nondilated, thick-walled left ventricle,
■ normal LV systolic function,
■ abnormal LV diastolic function,
■ right ventricular free wall thickening,
■ bi-atrial enlargement,
■ moderate pulmonary hypertension, and
■ elevated right atrial pressure (dilated inferior vena cava).

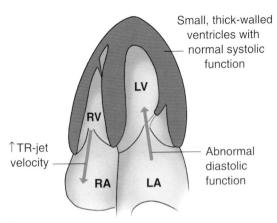

FIGURE 9–19. Schematic diagram of the typical features of restrictive cardiomyopathy, which include a thick-walled, small left ventricle (LV) with impaired diastolic function, left and right atrial enlargement (LA, RA), and signs of secondary pulmonary hypertension, including paradoxical septal motion and a high-velocity tricuspid regurgitant (TR) jet.

The pattern of left ventricular diastolic filling parallels the abnormalities in left ventricular diastolic function in this disease. However, interpretation is complicated both by the numerous confounding factors that affect left ventricular diastolic filling (see Chapter 7) and by temporal changes in diastolic filling as the disease progresses in an individual patient. Early in the disease course, impaired diastolic relaxation of the left ventricle results in impaired early diastolic filling. The Doppler left ventricular inflow curve shows a reduced E velocity, increased A velocity, prolonged isovolumic relaxation time, and decreased early diastolic deceleration slope. The myocardial tissue Doppler signal shows a reduced E_m and increased A_m velocity (Fig. 9–21). The pulmonary vein flow curve shows a reduced diastolic filling phase and normal systolic filling phase, resulting in a decreased ratio of systolic to diastolic pulmonary venous flow.

As the disease progresses, left atrial pressure rises, resulting in an increased pressure gradient from the left atrium to left ventricle at mitral valve opening. Along with reduced diastolic compliance of the left ventricle, this increased mitral opening pressure leads to an increased E velocity and a rapid deceleration slope. The A velocity is reduced due to a combination of increased left ventricular end-diastolic pressure and reduced atrial contractile function (Fig. 9–22). Thus the pattern of diastolic filling in established restrictive cardiomyopathy (which may coincide with the initial clinical presentation) is similar to the "big

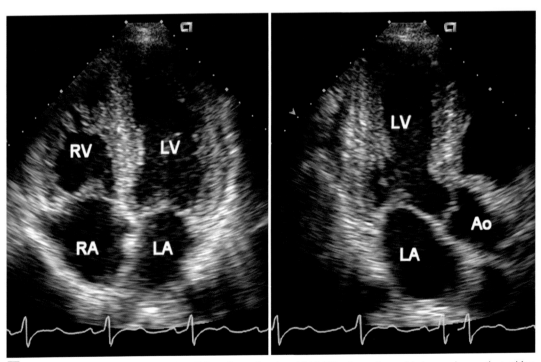

FIGURE 9–20. Apical four-chamber (*left*) and two-chamber (*right*) 2D echocardiographic images in a patient with a restrictive cardiomyopathy due to amyloidosis. There is biventricular hypertrophy, biatrial enlargement, and both systolic and diastolic dysfunction of the left ventricle. Mild, diffuse valve thickening also is present.

Early

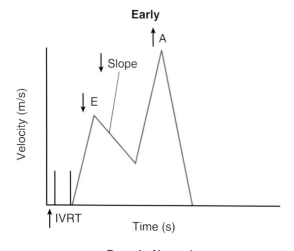

Pseudo-Normal

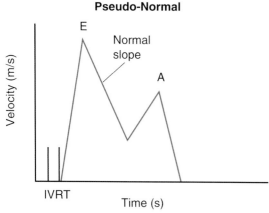

Late

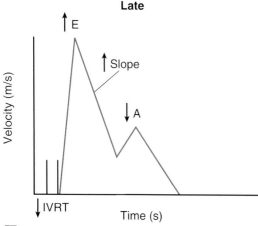

FIGURE 9–21. Schematic diagrams of left ventricular diastolic filling in restrictive cardiomyopathy. Early in the disease course, ventricular relaxation abnormalities predominate, and the E velocity and early deceleration slope are reduced while the isovolumic relaxation time and A velocity are increased. Pseudo-normalization occurs as left ventricular end-diastolic pressure rises, resulting in relatively normal E and A velocities. With advanced (late) disease, ventricular compliance decreases, resulting in a high E velocity, steep deceleration slope, short isovolumic relaxation time, and reduced A velocity.

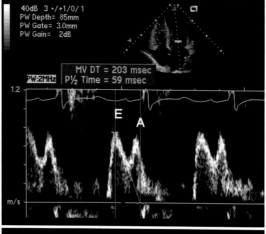

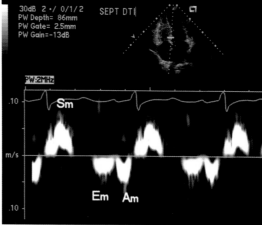

FIGURE 9–22. Left ventricular diastolic filling in a patient with a restrictive cardiomyopathy shows pseudonormalization with an E velocity slightly greater than the A velocity (*top*). This pattern is distinguished from normal by the tissue Doppler myocardial velocity (*bottom*) showing reduced early motion (E_m), compared to the motion after atrial contraction (A_m). Same patient as Fig. 9–20.

E, little A" pattern seen in normal young individuals. However, this "pseudo-normal" pattern of LV filling can be distinguished from normal by

■ the rapid early diastolic deceleration time (LV inflow);
■ a reduced E_m velocity (annular tissue velocity);
■ an increased PV_a velocity and duration; and
■ the patient's age, clinical presentation, and other associated echocardiographic findings.

With a pseudo-normal left ventricular inflow pattern, the myocardial tissue velocity shows a marked reduction in the E_m velocity with the ratio of the transmitral E velocity to the E_m velocity corresponding to the elevation in left ventricular end-diastolic pressure. In addition, pulmonary venous inflow in diastole is normal or increased as blood flows in a conduit from the pulmonary veins to left ventricle while systolic filling is decreased. When atrial contraction occurs, the increased resistance to left ventricular filling results in an increase in the velocity and duration of the atrial flow reversal in the lower resistance pulmonary veins (Fig. 9–23). Thus pulmonary venous flow shows an increased diastolic phase, reduced systolic phase, and prominent *a*-wave flow reversal. This is in contrast to the normal pattern of nearly equal systolic and diastolic pulmonary venous inflow curves (Fig. 9–24) and a small *a* wave.

Examination of right atrial filling by recording hepatic vein (or superior vena cava) flow patterns also can be helpful. These patterns correspond to the physical findings of the neck vein pulsations

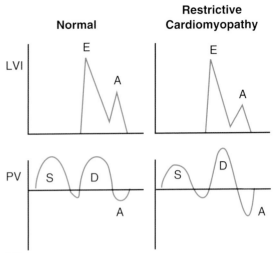

FIGURE 9–24. Schematic diagrams of left ventricular inflow (LVI) and pulmonary vein (PV) Doppler flow patterns with normal diastolic function and in restrictive cardiomyopathy. Although the inflow patterns are similar superficially, the "pseudo-normal" pattern has a steeper deceleration slope and lower *A* velocity. The pulmonary vein flow shows increased diastolic filling and a prominent *A* reversal compared with the normal pattern.

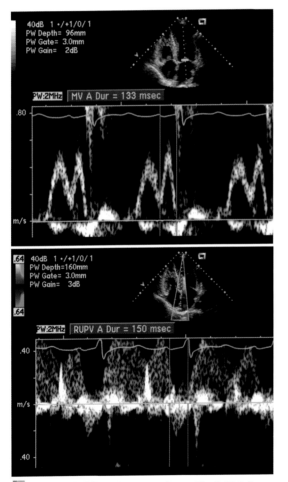

FIGURE 9–23. In the same patient as Fig. 9–22, left ventricular inflow recorded with the sample volume at the mitral annulus (*top*) is used to measure the *A*-wave duration (133 ms), which then is compared to the a-reversal duration (150 ms) in the pulmonary vein (*bottom*). The *A* duration < PV$_a$ duration is consistent with an elevated LV end-diastolic pressure.

seen in patients with restrictive cardiomyopathy. Using this analogy, the hepatic vein flow pattern typically shows a prominent reverse flow phase with atrial contraction (*a* wave) followed by a rapid filling curve in systole (*x* descent). The diastolic phase of right atrial filling is blunted corresponding to a diminished *v* wave and *y* descent. These findings correspond to the pattern of right atrial pressure recordings at catheterization; the x descent represents the "dip," and the blunted systolic filling phase represents the "plateau" of the dip-and-plateau pattern.

Late in the disease course, a restrictive pattern of left ventricular filling is seen with an increased *E* velocity and reduced *A* velocity, steep early diastolic deceleration slope and reduced isovolumic relaxation time.

Limitations/Technical Considerations

Differentiation of restrictive cardiomyopathy from constrictive pericarditis is problematic. Both have a similar clinical presentation, and both are characterized by preserved left ventricular systolic function with impaired diastolic filling. Features that distinguish these two conditions include the patterns of atrial and ventricular diastolic filling, the presence or absence of pericardial thickening, and the degree of associated pulmonary hypertension. However, no single feature is diagnostic of either condition (see Table 10–2).

Attention to technical details is necessary in recording Doppler atrial and ventricular filling patterns, particularly their relationship to the phase of respiration. Respiratory variation is assessed most reliably using a respirometer to mark the onsets of inspiration and expiration. Before recording Doppler signals, 2D and color flow imaging is used to convince the sonographer that there is no significant respiratory variation in the angle between the ultrasound beam and the direction of blood flow because respiratory changes in intercept angle could result in apparent changes in velocity even under constant-flow conditions due to the erroneous assumption that cosine θ remains 1 in the Doppler equation. Once a constant intercept angle is ascertained, recordings of left ventricular diastolic inflow are made with the sample volume positioned at the mitral leaflet tips.

Recording right atrial filling patterns is straightforward using a subcostal approach with the pulsed Doppler sample volume positioned in the central hepatic vein. This vein connects directly to the inferior vena cava and right atrium, with no intervening venous valve, and conveniently lies parallel to the direction of the ultrasound beam from the subcostal window.

Left atrial filling is more technically challenging to record due to signal attenuation at the depth of the pulmonary veins from an apical approach. Other transthoracic acoustic windows rarely allow interrogation of pulmonary vein flow at a near-parallel intercept angle. A transesophageal approach is helpful if recordings of pulmonary vein flow are inadequate on transthoracic interrogation and are needed for patient management.

Tissue Doppler myocardial velocity should be recorded in a four-chamber apical approach with a small sample volume (2 mm) positioned at the myocardium adjacent to the medial mitral annulus. Gain setting and wall filters should be low (50 to 100 Hz) with the velocity scale expanded to optimally display the phasic waveform.

Clinical Utility

In a patient with symptoms of heart failure, a diagnosis of restrictive cardiomyopathy may not have been suspected on clinical grounds. In some cases, echocardiographic findings may provide the first clues pointing toward this diagnostic possibility. In a patient with known restrictive cardiomyopathy, echocardiography can be used to follow disease progression. A meticulous examination with careful attention to technical details and with integration of 2D, Doppler, and clinical data may allow differentiation of restrictive cardiomyopathy from constrictive pericarditis.

Alternate Approaches

Diagnostic evaluation of the patient with probable restrictive cardiomyopathy may include cardiac catheterization with measurement of intracardiac pressures at rest and with volume loading, endomyocardial biopsy, and chest computed tomographic imaging (to detect pericardial calcification or thickening). In some cases, constrictive pericarditis may remain a diagnostic possibility despite the results of these tests. The diagnosis of constrictive pericarditis is critical, since it can be treated by removal of the adherent pericardial layers. In patients in whom there is a high level of suspicion but nondiagnostic test results, thoracotomy may be indicated to confirm (and treat) or exclude a diagnosis of pericardial constriction.

HYPERTENSIVE HEART DISEASE

Basic Principles

Hypertensive heart disease is an end-organ consequence of systemic hypertension. Chronic systemic pressure overload results in left ventricular hypertrophy to maintain normal wall stress. Initially, diastolic function is impaired, while systolic function remains normal. With long-standing hypertension, systolic dysfunction and ventricular dilation can occur. Typical echocardiographic findings (Fig. 9–25) associated with chronic hypertension include

■ left ventricular hypertrophy,
■ diastolic dysfunction,

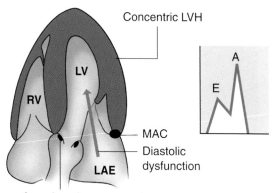

▌ FIGURE 9–25. Schematic diagram of hypertensive heart disease in an anteriorly angulated apical four-chamber view. Note concentric ventricular hypertrophy (LVH), mitral annular calcification (MAC), left atrial enlargement (LAE), aortic (Ao) vlave sclerosis, aortic root dilation, and impaired early diastolic relaxation ($E < A$).

- aortic root dilation,
- aortic valve sclerosis,
- mitral annular calcification,
- left atrial enlargement, and
- atrial fibrillation.

Echocardiographic Approach

Ventricular Hypertrophy

Standard imaging views demonstrate concentric left ventricular hypertrophy with increased wall thickness and a nondilated chamber (Fig. 9–26). In contrast to hypertrophic cardiomyopathy, the pattern of hypertrophy is symmetric, including involvement of the basal posterior wall. M-mode recordings confirm an increased end-diastolic wall thickness (>11 mm). Left ventricular mass can be estimated from M-mode data, assuming hypertrophy is symmetric, but preferably is calculated from 2D data (see Chapter 6).

Diastolic Function

Left ventricular diastolic function is characterized by impaired early diastolic relaxation (Fig. 9–27). This results in a prolonged isovolumic relaxation time (IVRT), reduced E velocity, reduced E/A ratio, and prolonged deceleration slope. Interestingly, in individuals with physiologic hypertrophy (due to physical conditioning), diastolic dysfunction is not seen even when increased wall thickness is present. In pathologic hypertrophy (due to hypertension), diastolic dysfunction often is the first evidence of end-organ damage, usually antedating clear evidence of anatomic hypertrophy.

Systolic Function

Typically, systolic function is preserved early in the disease course. Segmental wall motion abnormalities are not seen unless coexisting coronary artery disease is present. With a small, hypertrophied, normally functioning left ventricular chamber, midcavity obliteration at end-systole may be seen with an associated Doppler velocity curve showing a brief, late-systolic high-velocity signal. The duration of this intracavity gradient is briefer than that seen with hypertrophic cardiomyopathy, the level of obstruction is midventricular rather than subaortic, and systolic anterior motion of the mitral leaflets is not seen. Midcavity obliteration is exacerbated by hypovolemia or increased contractility.

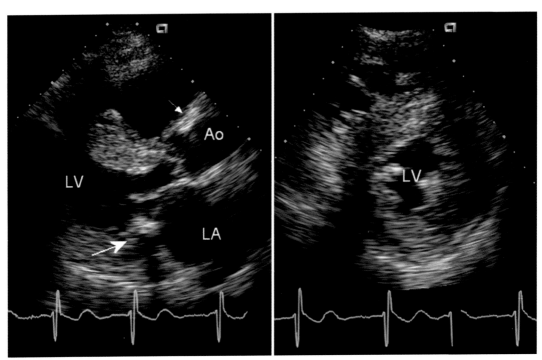

FIGURE 9–26. Parasternal long-axis (*left*) and short-axis (*right*) views with the typical echocardiographic findings in hypertensive heart disease with concentric left ventricular hypertrophy, mitral annular calcification with shadowing (*large arrow*), aortic valve sclerosis, and increased echogenicity of the ascending aorta (*small arrow*).

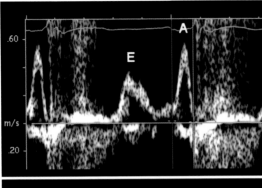

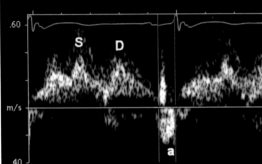

■ **FIGURE 9–27.** Left ventricular inflow (*top*) and pulmonary venous flow (*bottom*) in a patient with hypertension and concentric hypertrophy. Mild diastolic dysfunction is present with impaired relaxation as evidenced by the *E/A* ratio < 1 and the prolonged deceleration time. However, left ventricular end-diastolic pressure is normal with a low velocity and short duration of the pulmonary vein atrial reversal (*a*).

Other Echocardiographic Findings

Aortic root dilation often is present in hypertensive patients and is associated with increased tortuosity of the ascending aorta, arch, and descending aorta. Increased irregular echogenicity of the aortic walls, representing atherosclerosis, also may be noted. In uncomplicated hypertension, the aortic annulus itself is not dilated. The aortic valve leaflets usually show sclerotic changes and associated mild aortic regurgitation. Mitral annular calcification frequently is present in patients with chronic hypertension and is one cause of mild-to-moderate mitral regurgitation in these patients. Left atrial enlargement is due to a combination of a chronically elevated left ventricular end-diastolic pressure and mitral regurgitation.

Limitations/Technical Considerations

Left ventricular mass determinations are dependent on optimal image quality with clear definition of endocardial and epicardial surfaces and on correct endocardial border tracing at end-diastole

and end-systole. It remains controversial whether 2D or M-mode mass calculations are optimal, especially given cost considerations in large patient populations. Differentiation of hypertensive heart disease from hypertrophic or restrictive heart disease is based on the pattern of hypertrophy, associated echocardiographic findings, and integration of the echocardiographic and clinical data.

Clinical Utility

Diagnosis and Prognosis

Left ventricular mass, measured by echocardiography, is a strong predictor of clinical outcome in patients with hypertension. In subjects with borderline hypertension, increased left ventricular mass identifies a subgroup of patients with a poor prognosis without medical therapy. In patients with definite hypertension, the degree of left ventricular hypertrophy reflects the chronic elevation of systemic pressure, in theory serving as an index of the temporally averaged blood pressure over long periods. Thus, left ventricular mass may be a more accurate method for assessing the severity of hypertension than occasional blood pressure recordings in the physician's office or even 24-hour recordings of blood pressure.

Choices of Medical Therapy

Some hypertension clinics tailor medical therapy in individual patients based on noninvasive Doppler echo evaluation of hemodynamics. Because blood pressure equals cardiac output times systemic vascular resistance, hypertension can be due to elevation of either one or both of the components of this equation. To assess hemodynamics noninvasively in hypertensive patients, cardiac output is measured using Doppler recordings of ascending aortic flow and 2D aortic diameter measurements (see Chapter 6). Systemic vascular resistance then is calculated from the cuff blood pressure and Doppler cardiac output. Appropriate medications are chosen based on the specific hemodynamics in each patient.

Efficacy of Medical Therapy

Determination of left ventricular mass also is useful in assessing the long-term effect of medical therapy. Again, rather than measuring blood pressure at rare intervals in the disease course, the chronic end-organ effects of hypertension on the left ventricle are measured. It seems plausible that effective antihypertensive therapy should reverse end-organ changes; specifically, it should result in regression of left ventricular hypertrophy.

Evaluation of Heart Failure Symptoms

In a patient with chronic hypertension, heart failure symptoms may be due to diastolic or systolic left ventricular dysfunction, superimposed coronary artery disease, or superimposed valvular disease. Early in the disease course, pathologic hypertrophy is associated with impaired early diastolic filling. Impaired ventricular filling leads to elevated left atrial pressures and pulmonary venous hypertension, resulting in dyspnea. Diagnosis of diastolic dysfunction with preserved systolic function can be made by echocardiography and has important clinical implications, since the therapy for heart failure symptoms is quite different for diastolic versus systolic dysfunction.

An extreme form of preserved systolic function with left ventricular hypertrophy and heart failure symptoms has been observed in hypertensive patients and has been termed *hypertensive hypertrophic cardiomyopathy*. This condition is characterized by normal to hyperdynamic systolic function, concentric hypertrophy, diastolic dysfunction, and a midventricular late systolic gradient due to cavity obliteration. Strictly speaking, this combination of findings is not a "cardiomyopathy" but simply represents severe end-organ damage due to hypertension. However, awareness of this specific clinical picture results in consideration of this diagnosis in patients in whom hypertrophic or restrictive cardiomyopathy otherwise might be suspected.

With long-standing hypertension, impairment of left ventricular contractility can occur, even in the absence of coexisting coronary artery disease. Physiologically, elevated afterload (as in valvular aortic stenosis) is the proximate cause of systolic dysfunction. However, systolic function may not improve even with aggressive antihypertensive therapy when systolic dysfunction is long-standing, suggesting that irreversible changes in ventricular contractility have occurred. End-stage hypertensive heart disease has an echocardiographic appearance similar to that of end-stage dilated cardiomyopathy.

Alternate Approaches

The need for routine echocardiographic evaluation of patients with hypertension is controversial. Medical management based on intermittent office blood pressure measurements remains standard practice at most medical centers. When needed, estimates of the chronicity of blood pressure elevation can be obtained by 24-hour blood pressure monitors or evaluation of other end-organ damage (e.g., renal function, retinal examination). While electrocardiographic estimates of left ventricular hypertrophy are less accurate and precise than echocardiographic measurements, there is a substantial cost differential between these diagnostic tests.

EVALUATION OF THE POST–CARDIAC-TRANSPLANT PATIENT

Basic Principles

Echocardiographic evaluation of the post–cardiac-transplant patient typically is directed toward one of three goals: (1) assessment of cardiac anatomy and physiology prompted by a specific clinical problem, (2) the elusive goal of noninvasive diagnosis of early rejection of the transplanted heart, or (3) diagnosis of posttransplant coronary artery disease.

Clinical problems encountered in the post–cardiac-transplant patient include:

1. Pericardial effusion, particularly early postoperatively
2. Right ventricular systolic dysfunction due to inadequate myocardial preservation at the time of transplantation, persistently elevated pulmonary vascular resistance, or transplant rejection
3. Left ventricular systolic dysfunction due to inadequate myocardial preservation, acute rejection early after transplantation, or superimposed coronary artery disease at a longer interval after transplantation

Primary valvular disease, of course, is uncommon due to screening of donor hearts before transplantation. However, mitral or tricuspid regurgitation secondary to ventricular dysfunction and annular dilation may be seen. Diastolic dysfunction is an early marker of rejection.

Echocardiographic Approach

Normal Findings after Cardiac Transplantation

Typically, right and left ventricular size, wall thickness, and systolic function are normal in the absence of perioperative complications or rejection. However, abnormal septal motion is the norm with anterior motion of the septum in systole with a slight decrease in the extent of systolic thickening of the septal myocardium. Valvular anatomy and function are normal, with small amounts of mitral, tricuspid, and pulmonic regurgitation present at a prevalence similar to that in normal individuals. The suture lines in the aorta and pulmonary artery may be difficult to appreciate, depending on the distance of the suture lines from the valve planes and the type of surgical procedure. A small pericardial effusion is seen early in the postoperative period but rarely persists beyond a few weeks. Pulmonary artery pressures may show some degree of persistent elevation as calculated from the velocity in the tricuspid regurgitant jet and estimates of right atrial pressure.

If the surgical approach included anastomoses of the normal and donor atrium, a normal echocardiogram after cardiac transplantation will show bi-atrial enlargement (Fig. 9–28) with a variably prominent ridge between the donor and recipient portions of both right and left atrium. The atrial suture line should not be mistaken for an abnormal atrial mass (Fig. 9–29). When transplantation is performed with anastomosis of the superior and inferior vena cava for the right atrium and a cuff of tissue with the pulmonary veins for the left atrium, there is little atrial enlargement and suture lines may not be evident.

Evaluation of Abnormal Findings

The echocardiographic approach to the posttransplant patient with suspected cardiac dysfunction is similar to that in any patient, with the proviso that the expected findings after transplantation (such as the atrial suture line) are recognized. Pericardial effusions often are loculated due to postoperative pericardial adhesions, so careful examination in multiple tomographic planes from parasternal, apical, and subcostal windows is essential when this diagnosis is suspected.

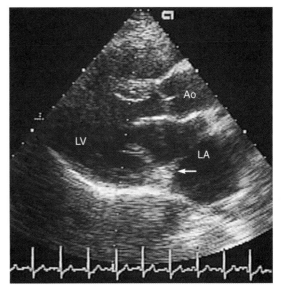

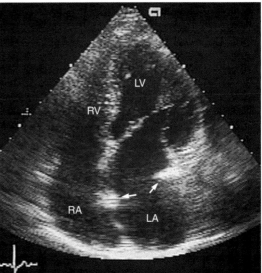

FIGURE 9–29. Parasternal long-axis (*top*) and apical four-chamber view (*bottom*) in a posttransplant patient showing bi-atrial enlargement with a prominent suture line (*arrows*).

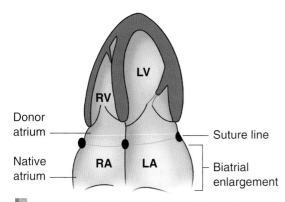

FIGURE 9–28. Schematic diagram of the posttransplant heart. Note the suture line between the donor and native atria resulting in an appearance of biatrial enlargement. Right and left ventricular size and systolic function are normal. With the more recent surgical techniques, an atrial suture line is not present.

Transplant Rejection

With acute rejection, echocardiography shows increased left ventricular mass, decreased systolic function, and an increase in the echogenicity of the myocardium. In addition, a new or increasingly pericardial effusion may accompany acute rejection.

With mild or early rejection, 2D echocardiographic changes are subtle and are not accurate or reproducible enough to allow adjustment of immunosuppressive medications in individual patients. Instead, proposed echocardiographic approaches to diagnosis of early rejection have focused on measures of diastolic function, specifically measures of early diastolic relaxation. The Doppler changes in acute rejection include

- decreased pressure half-time (increased early diastolic deceleration slope),
- decreased isovolumetric relaxation time, and
- increased E velocity.

Using the patient as his or her own baseline, a significant change, defined as >20% for E velocity and >15% for pressure half-time or isovolumic relaxation time, is consistent with rejection. Some transplant centers have found these measures clinically useful but most centers continue to rely on endomyocardial biopsy. More refined approaches to ultrasonic tissue characterization appear promising, since they may detect interstitial edema early in the course of rejection.

Transplant Coronary Artery Disease

As survival after cardiac transplantation has improved, increasing numbers of patients are seen with posttransplant coronary artery disease. Transplant coronary disease differs from typical atherosclerosis in that both epicardial vessels and the microvasculature are diffusely involved and the disease course often is accelerated. Echocardiographic exercise stress testing has a higher prevalence of false-negative results due to the diffuse disease process masking regional wall motion abnormalities. Dobutamine stress echocardiography is more accurate in this patient population and now is routine at many transplant centers. However, coronary angiography may be needed for a definitive diagnosis, often with concurrent intravascular ultrasound examination of the coronary arteries.

Limitations/Technical Considerations/Alternate Approaches

The standard method for evaluation of transplant rejection remains transvenous endomyocardial biopsy. Some centers use echocardiographic (rather than fluoroscopic) guidance for this procedure. Because echocardiographic images are tomographic, any segment of the biotome shaft going through the image plane will appear to be the "tip." Thus, it is crucial to identify the open forceps of the biotome for correct identification of the biopsy site. A subcostal window often is most practical, since, with the patient supine, clear views of the right ventricle and septum are obtained, and the sonographer is clear of the sterile field (usually the right internal jugular vein approach is used). In some cases, the apical view also may be helpful.

PULMONARY HEART DISEASE

Chronic versus Acute Pulmonary Disease

Chronic pulmonary hypertension, whether due to intrinsic lung disease, recurrent pulmonary emboli, or primary pulmonary hypertension, results in a group of clinical signs and symptoms termed *cor pulmonale*. The underlying pathophysiology of this clinical syndrome is chronic pressure overload of the right ventricle as it ejects into a high-resistance pulmonary vascular bed. Initially, compensatory hypertrophy of the right ventricle occurs with preserved systolic function. Over time, right ventricular contractility deteriorates, and right ventricular dilation, moderate to severe tricuspid regurgitation, and consequent right atrial enlargement are seen (Fig. 9–30).

Acute pulmonary embolism also can affect right-sided heart function due to the sudden onset of elevated pulmonary vascular resistance. Echocardiographic evaluation may be helpful in assessing pulmonary artery pressures and right ventricular function in patients with either chronic or acute pulmonary hypertension.

Echocardiographic Approach

Pulmonary Pressures

Standard approaches for noninvasive evaluation of pulmonary artery pressures (PAP), as described in Chapter 6, are applicable to the patient with

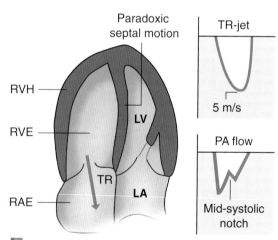

FIGURE 9–30. Schematic diagram of the key features of pulmonary heart disease. Right ventricular hypertrophy (RVH) and enlargement (RVE) are seen with paradoxic septal motion. Secondary tricuspid regurgitation (TR) and right atrial enlargement (RAE) are common. Elevated pulmonary artery pressures will be reflected in the high-velocity tricuspid regurgitant jet velocity and midsystolic notching in the pulmonary artery velocity curve.

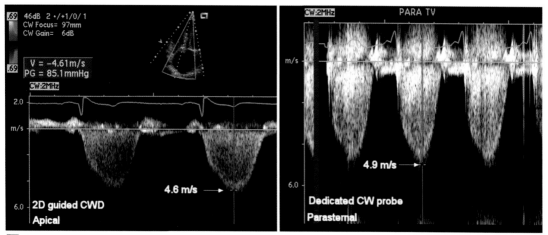

FIGURE 9–31. Tricuspid regurgitant jet in a patient with primary pulmonary hypertension. Using 2D and color guided continuous wave (CW) Doppler from the apex, a clear signal is obtained, although signal strength is low, with a maximum jet of only 4.6 m/s. The use of a dedicated CW probe (*right*) provides a stronger signal and a higher jet velocity is obtained from a parasternal window. The maximum velocity of 4.9 m/s indicates a right ventricular to right atrial pressure difference of 96 mm Hg. Right atrial pressure was elevated at 10 mm Hg, so estimated pulmonary artery systolic pressure is 106 mm Hg. Note the faint linear spread of the signal at peak of the curve (see third beat in *right panel*). This faint signal is due to the transit time effect and care is needed to avoid including these signals in the velocity measurement.

suspected or known pulmonary hypertension. The most reliable approach is to record the maximum tricuspid regurgitant jet velocity (V_{TR}) for calculation of the right ventricular to right atrial systolic pressure difference (Fig. 9–31). Care is needed to interrogate the tricuspid regurgitant jet from multiple acoustic windows (apical, parasternal) with careful transducer angulation to obtain a parallel intercept angle between the ultrasound beam and jet. Right atrial pressure (RAP) is estimated from the size and respiratory variation in the inferior vena cava. Then pulmonary artery systolic pressure (in the absence of pulmonic stenosis) is calculated as

$$PAP = 4(V_{TR})^2 + RAP$$

Diastolic pulmonary artery pressure can be estimated from the velocities in the pulmonic regurgitant Doppler curve (see Chapter 6).

Indirect signs of pulmonary hypertension often are seen on echocardiography that indicate the presence, but not the exact severity, of pulmonary hypertension. An M-mode recording through the pulmonic valve shows a reduced *a*-wave and midsystolic closure of the valve. This pattern has a reasonably high specificity (>90%) for detecting pulmonary hypertension but a low sensitivity (30% to 60%). This motion pattern is paralleled by the Doppler velocity curve, which shows an abrupt midsystolic deceleration of flow (Fig. 9–32). Signs of right ventricular pressure overload, including abnormal ventricular septal

motion, may be valuable clues suggesting the presence of pulmonary hypertension.

Right Ventricular Pressure Overload

The response of the right ventricle to chronic pressure overload is hypertrophy and dilation (Fig. 9–33). The increase in thickness of the right ventricular free wall is best seen on the subcostal view. Ventricular septal motion is abnormal or "paradoxical" with anterior motion of the septum during systole both on M-mode and 2D imaging. A rational explanation for this pattern of septal motion is based on the concept that the septum

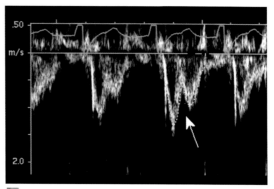

FIGURE 9–32. Pulmonary artery velocity curve showing midsystolic notching (*arrow*) due to severe pulmonary hypertension.

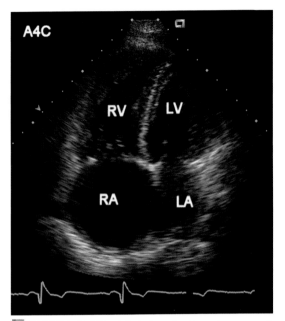

FIGURE 9–33. Apical four-chamber view at end-diastole in a patient with cor pulmonale. There is right ventricular enlargement, right ventricular hypertrophy, paradoxical septal motion, and reduced systolic function of the right ventricle.

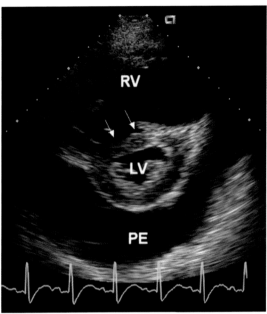

FIGURE 9–34. Parasternal short-axis view in a patient with pulmonary hypertension and a pericardial effusion (PE) shows severe right ventricular enlargement with flattening of the ventricular septum in diastole.

moves toward the center of mass of the heart during systole. With right ventricular hypertrophy, the center of mass is shifted anteriorly, so the septum moves toward the center of the right ventricle instead of the normal pattern of motion toward the center of the left ventricle. On 2D imaging, the curvature of the septum is reversed in both systole and in early to middiastole. In contrast, right ventricular volume overload is characterized by diastolic flattening of the septum in late diastole with a normal curvature in systole, due to increased volume flow into the right ventricle (compared with the left ventricle) in diastole but normal ventricular pressures in systole (Fig. 9–34).

With long-standing or acute pulmonary hypertension, right ventricular systolic dysfunction can occur, with secondary dilation serving as a compensatory mechanism to maintain forward stroke volume. However, right ventricular dilation leads to tricuspid regurgitation due to annular dilation and malalignment of the papillary muscles. This superimposed volume overload results in further right ventricular dilation and more tricuspid regurgitation. Right atrial dilation is due to both pressure (v wave) and volume (tricuspid regurgitation) overload of the right atrium.

Secondary Tricuspid Regurgitation

Tricuspid regurgitation secondary to pulmonary hypertension and/or right ventricular systolic dysfunction can be evaluated with color Doppler flow imaging from parasternal, apical, and subcostal views. Severe regurgitation results in systolic flow reversal in the inferior vena cava and hepatic veins. Careful attention to tricuspid valve anatomy is needed to ensure that other etiologies of tricuspid regurgitation (e.g., vegetation, rheumatic, carcinoid, Ebstein's anomaly) are not present.

The intensity of the continuous-wave Doppler tricuspid regurgitant jet relates to the severity of regurgitation, but the velocity relates to the right ventricular to right atrial pressure difference. With acute tricuspid regurgitation, a rapid falloff in velocity in late systole may be seen consistent with a right atrial v wave.

Limitations/Technical Considerations

The major limitation of echocardiography in evaluation of cor pulmonale is poor ultrasound tissue penetration resulting in poor image quality and low Doppler signal strength. Hyperexpanded lungs obscure the standard acoustic windows in many patients with chronic lung disease. However, adequate image quality may be obtained with current instruments in nearly all patients.

Assessment of the severity of pulmonary hypertension depends on obtaining a parallel intercept angle between the ultrasound beam and tricuspid regurgitant jet. Underestimation of pulmonary artery pressures should be considered in all patients, especially when Doppler signal strength is suboptimal or when the Doppler data and clinical setting are discrepant. The absence of a recordable tricuspid regurgitant jet does not indicate normal pulmonary pressures. In this situation, the echocardiographer should indicate that the data are inadequate and alternate diagnostic approaches should be considered. Overestimation of pulmonary pressures from the tricuspid regurgitant signal can be avoided by measuring the outer edge of the dark spectral envelope, but avoiding the slight spectral broadening at peak velocity that results from the transit time effect (see Fig. 9–31).

Clinical Utility

In the patient with chronic lung disease and right heart failure, echocardiography allows confirmation of a clinical diagnosis of cor pulmonale, assessment of the degree of pulmonary hypertension, and evaluation of right ventricular size and systolic dysfunction.

In patients with primary pulmonary hypertension, echocardiography is essential to exclude other causes of pulmonary hypertension, such as an atrial septal defect or mitral regurgitation. In addition, noninvasive measurement of pulmonary pressure now is routinely used for evaluating changes in pulmonary pressures with medical therapy.

In the patient with an acute pulmonary embolus, imaging may show a residual thrombus originating from or in transit through (from a deep vein thrombosis) the right side of the heart. Transesophageal imaging can demonstrate thrombus in the main, right, or left pulmonary artery. However, the sensitivity of echocardiography for diagnosis of pulmonary embolism based on demonstrating a thrombus is low because the thrombus is lodged more distally in the pulmonary vasculature in most cases. In addition, adequate visualization of the pulmonary artery bifurcation is not possible in all patients due to interposition of the air-filled trachea and bronchi. Indirect signs of pulmonary embolism include

- elevated pulmonary artery pressures,
- evidence of acute right ventricular pressure overload,
- right ventricular dilation and dysfunction, and
- tricuspid regurgitation.

Similar findings may be seen in patients with chronic recurrent pulmonary emboli. The possibility of pulmonary embolism should be strongly considered in patients with these findings even when a different working clinical diagnosis or "reason for echo" was entertained. Often patients in whom pulmonary embolism is subsequently diagnosed are initially referred for nonspecific indications including "chest pain," "dyspnea," or "heart failure."

Alternate Approaches

Cardiac catheterization allows direct measurement of right ventricular and pulmonary artery pressures and calculation of pulmonary vascular resistance. Right ventricular size and systolic function can be evaluated by angiography.

Clinically, the standard approach for diagnosis of pulmonary embolism is a radionuclide lung ventilation-perfusion scan or rapid computed tomography. These data often are combined with a radionuclide or vascular diagnostic evaluation for deep venous thrombus. In some cases, pulmonary angiography is needed with injection of contrast material directly into the main pulmonary artery.

SUGGESTED READING

Dilated Cardiomyopathy

1. Lewis JF: Doppler and two-dimensional echocardiographic evaluation in acute and long-term management of the heart failure patient. In: Otto CM (ed): The Practice of Clinical Echocardiography, 2nd ed. Philadelphia: WB Saunders, 2002, pp 571–587.

   Summary of the echocardiographic findings and the clinical implications of the echocardiographic data in terms of further diagnostic evaluation, therapy, and long-term prognosis.

2. Waller BF: Pathology of the cardiomyopathies. J Am Soc Echocardiogr 1:4–19, 1988.

   Review of the pathology and pathophysiology of cardiomyopathies. Excellent illustrations.

3. Acquatella H, Schiller NB: Echocardiographic recognition of Chagas' disease and endomyocardial fibrosis. J Am Soc Echocardiogr 1:60–68, 1988.

   Review of the echocardiographic findings in Chagas' disease.

4. Lapu-Bula R, Robert A, DeKock M, et al: Risk stratification in patients with dilated cardiomyopathy: Contribution of Doppler-derived left ventricular filling. Am J Cardiol 82:779–785, 1998.

   In 197 consecutive patients with dilated cardiomyopathy, multivariate predictors of outcome (death or cardiac transplantation) were New York Heart Association functional class, left ventricular ejection fraction, E/A ratio, and systolic blood pressure. These data emphasize the importance of diastolic dysfunction in predicting clinical outcome in heart failure patients.

5. Juilliere Y, Barbier G, Feldmann L, et al: Additional predictive value of both left and right ventricular ejection fraction on long-term survival in idiopathic dilated cardiomyopathy. Eur Heart J 18:276–280, 1997.

Multivariate analysis identified only left and right ventricular ejection fractions as predictors of clinical outcome (death or heart transplantation) in 62 consecutive patients with dilated cardiomyopathy followed for 2.2 ± 1.3 years. This finding emphasizes the importance of right ventricular function in patients with dilated cardiomyopathy.

6. Wong M, Johnson G, Shabetai R, et al: Echocardiographic variables as prognostic indicators and therapeutic monitors in chronic congestive heart failure: Veterans Affairs Cooperative Studies V-HeFT I and II. Circulation 87(Suppl VI):65–70, 1993.

Echocardiographic variables including E-point septal separation, systolic left ventricular interval dimension, and the ratio of ventricular radius to wall thickness were shown to be predictors of mortality in patients with congestive heart failure in a large randomized trial (V-HeFT).

7. Faris R, Coats AJ, Henein MY: Echocardiography derived variables predict outcome in patients with nonischemic dilated cardiomyopathy with or without a restrictive filling pattern. Am Heart J 144:343–350, 2002.

A restrictive left ventricular filling pattern was present in 58% of a retrospective cohort including 337 patients with dilated cardiomyopathy. A restrictive filling pattern was a strong predictor of mortality with an adjusted hazard ratio of 3.2 (95% CI 1.8 to 5.7).

8. Aikawa K, Sheehan FH, Otto CM, et al: The severity of functional mitral regurgitation depends on the shape of the mitral apparatus: A three-dimensional echo analysis. J Heart Valve Dis 11:627–636, 2002.

Quantitative 3D echocardiography was used to evaluate the anatomy of the mitral valve and left ventricle in 13 patients with functional mitral regurgitation (MR) in association with dilated cardiomyopathy. The mechanism of functional MR in dilated cardiomyopathy appears to be related to outward displacement of the anterior papillary muscle with widening of the central chordal angle, apical displacement of the coaptation point, and annular dilation.

9. Kwan J, Shiota T, Agler DA, et al: Geometric differences of the mitral apparatus between ischemic and dilated cardiomyopathy with significant mitral regurgitation: Real-time three-dimensional echocardiographic study. Circulation 107:1135–1140, 2003.

Real time 3D echocardiography was used to study 26 patients with ischemic mitral regurgitation, 18 dilated cardiomyopathy patients with mitral regurgitation, and 8 control subjects. Asymmetrical distortion of the angle between the annular plane and valve leaflets was seen with ischemic mitral regurgitation compared to symmetric changes in patients with dilated cardiomyopathy.

Hypertrophic Cardiomyopathy

10. Woo A, Wigle ED, Rakowski H: Echocardiography in the evaluation and management of patients with hypertrophic cardiomyopathy. In: Otto CM (ed): The Practice of Clinical Echocardiography, 2nd ed. Philadelphia: WB Saunders, 2002, pp 588–612.

This chapter details the echocardiographic findings in hypertrophic cardiomyopathy and correlates the echocardiographic data with clinical, genetic, and pathophysiologic aspects of the disease process.

11. Maron BJ: Hypertrophic cardiomyopathy: A systematic review. JAMA 287:1308–1320, 2002.

Review of the epidemiology, clinical course, and management of hypertrophic cardiomyopathy.

12. Solomon SD, Wolff S, Watkins H, et al: Left ventricular hypertrophy and morphology in familial hypertrophic cardiomyopathy associated with mutations of the beta-myosin heavy chain gene. J Am Coll Cardiol 22:498–505, 1993.

Two-dimensional echocardiograms were compared in 39 genetically affected and 30 unaffected family members. The spectrum of abnormal findings in genetically affected individuals was broad, with a maximal left ventricular wall thickness ranging from 11 to 40 (mean 24) mm. In the affected group, 62% had systolic anterior motion of the mitral leaflet, 79% had reversed septal curvature, and 77% had a septal/free wall ratio >1.3.

13. Schwammenthal E, Nakatani S, He S, et al: Mechanism of mitral regurgitation in hypertrophic cardiomyopathy, mismatch of posterior to anterior leaflet length and mobility. Circulation 98:856–865, 1998.

These authors propose that the mechanism of mitral regurgitation in patients with hypertrophic cardiomyopathy and systolic anterior motion of the valve is inadequate mobility and coaptation of the posterior leaflet.

14. Hagueh SR, Ommen SR, Lakkis NM, et al: Comparison of ethanol septal reduction therapy with surgical myectomy for the treatment of hypertrophic obstructive cardiomyopathy. J Am Coll Cardiol 38:1701–1706, 2001.

Outcomes with surgical myotomy-myectomy and with alcohol septal ablation were similar when patients from two institutions were compared. The use of contrast echocardiography to guide the percutaneous septal ablation appears to reduce the incidence of complete heart block requiring pacemaker implantation.

15. Firoozi S, Elliott PM, Sharma S, et al: Septal myotomy-myectomy and transccoronary septal alcohol ablation in hypertrophic obstructive cardiomyopathy: A comparison of clinical, haemodynamic and exercise outcomes. Eur Heart J 23:1617–1624, 2002.

In a comparison of 20 patients treated with septal ablation and 24 patients undergoing surgical myectomy for symptoms refractory to medical therapy, although the reduction in outflow gradient with similar with both approaches (from about 85–90 mm Hg to 15–20 mm Hg), myectomy was associated with a greater improvement in exercise tolerance.

16. Ho CY, Sweitzer NK, McDonough B, et al: Assessment of diastolic function with Doppler tissue imaging to predict genotype in preclinical hypertrophic cardiomyopathy. Circulation 105:2992–2297, 2002.

A myocardial tissue Doppler velocity (E$_m$ < 15 cm/s) in combination with an elevated ejection fraction (≥68%) is specific (100%) for detection of genetically affected individuals without other phenotypic evidence for hypertrophic cardiomyopathy. However, the low sensitivity (44%) of E$_m$ and ejection fraction suggest that continued periodic evaluation of individuals with a family history but no overt findings for hypertrophic cardiomyopathy is warranted.

17. Ward RP, Weinert L, Spencer KT, et al: Quantitative diagnosis of apical cardiomyopathy using contrast echocardiography. J Am Soc Echocardiogr 15:316–322, 2002.

Contrast echocardiography improves the accuracy of the echocardiographic diagnosis of apical cardiomyopathy and should be considered in patients with unexplained symmetric precordial T-wave inversion or increased apical uptake on single-photon emission computed tomography, but a nondiagnostic transthoracic echo. A contrast enhanced apical thickness >2.0 cm was seen in those with apical hypertrophic cardiomyopathy.

18. Ommen SR, Park SH, Click RL, et al: Impact of intra-operative transesophageal echocardiography in the surgical management of hypertrophic cardiomyopathy. Am J Cardiol 90:1022–1024, 2002.

    The findings with intraoperative monitoring of surgical myectomy in 256 consecutive patients are reported. In addition to monitoring the procedure, baseline evaluation is important for detection of other structural abnormalities. After the procedure, unexpected severe mitral regurgitation was seen in eight patients and a ventricular septal defect was found in two patients.

Restrictive Cardiomyopathy

19. Thamilarasan M, Klein AL: Restrictive cardiomyopathy: Diagnosis and prognostic implications. In: Otto CM (ed): The Practice of Clinical Echocardiography, 2nd ed. Philadelphia: WB Saunders, 2002, pp 613–638.

    Detailed discussion of the importance of echocardiography in the diagnosis, management, and evaluation of prognosis in patients with restrictive cardiomyopathies.

20. Klein AL, Hatle LK, Taliercio CP, et al: Prognostic significance of Doppler measures of diastolic function in cardiac amyloidosis: A Doppler echocardiography study. Circulation 83:808–816, 1991.

    Left ventricular diastolic filling in cardiac amyloidosis is characterized by reduced early diastolic filling and an enhanced atrial contribution to filling early in the disease course, with progression to rapid early filling and a reduced atrial contribution late in the disease course ("pseudonormalization"). The Doppler pattern of left ventricular diastolic filling was predictive of clinical outcome in 63 consecutive patients. Those with a deceleration time ≤150 ms had a 1-year probability of survival of 49% compared with 76% in those with a deceleration time >150 ms (P < .0001).

21. Palka P, Lange A, Donnellly JE, Nihoyannopoulos P: Differentiation between restrictive cardiomyopathy and constrictive pericarditis by early diastolic Doppler myocardial velocity gradient at the posterior wall. Circulation 102:655–662, 2000.

    Use of tissue Doppler myocardial velocities may help distinguish restrictive cardiomyopathy from constrictive pericarditis. Compared to patients with constrictive pericarditis, those with restrictive cardiomyopathy have lower systolic (S_m) and early diastolic (E_m) velocities. In addition, a positive myocardial velocity is seen during isovolumic relaxation in those with restrictive cardiomyopathy.

22. Rajagopalan N, Garcia MJ, Rodriquez L, et al: Comparison of new Doppler echocardiographic methods to differentiate constrictive pericardial heart disease and restrictive cardiomyopathy. Am J Cardiol 87:86–94, 2001.

    Measures of diastolic function that distinguish constrictive pericarditis from restrictive cardiomyopathy were:

Parameter	Sensitivity	Specificity
Mitral E-velocity respiratory variation ≥ 10%	*84%*	*91%*
Pulmonary vein D velocity respiratory variation ≥ 18%	*79%*	*91%*
Doppler tissue E_m ≥ 8.0 cm/s	*89%*	*100%*
Color M-mode propagation velocity ≥ 100 cm/s	*74%*	*91%*

Hypertensive Heart Disease

23. Gottdiener JS, Diamond JA, Phillips RA: Hypertension: Impact of echocardiographic data on treatment options, prognosis and assessment of therapy. In: Otto CM (ed): The Practice of Clinical Echocardiography, 2nd ed. Philadelphia: WB Saunders, 2002, pp 705–739.

    This chapter reviews approaches to evaluation of left ventricular mass in population-based studies with emphasis on technique reproducibility and cost. The clinical relevance of echocardiography in determining the prognosis and in tailoring medical therapy in the hypertensive patient is discussed.

24. Cuspidi C, Michev L, Severgnini B, et al: Change in cardiovascular risk profile by echocardiography in medium-risk elderly hypertensives. J Hum Hypertens 17:101–106, 2003.

    In 223 elderly (≥65 yr) pateints with a new diagnosis of hypertension, echocardiographic left ventricular hypertrophy (LVH) was present in 56%. The addition of LVH to conventional clinical measures of risk decreasd the classification of patients as medium risk from 56% to 29% and increased the number for high risk from 44% to 56%.

25. Schillaci G, DeSimone G, Reboldi G, et al: Change in cardiovascular risk profile by echocardiography in low- or medium-risk hypertension. J Hypertens 20:1519–1525, 2002.

    In 792 hypertensive adults classified as low or medium risk by clinical criteria, echocardiographic left ventricular hypertrophy was present in 29%, idenfying a higher risk subgroup that would benefit from immediate drug treatment.

26. Ren JF, Pancholy SB, Iskandrian AS, et al: Doppler echocardiographic evaluation of the spectrum of left ventricular diastolic dysfunction in essential hypertension. Am Heart J 127:906–913, 1994.

    In 41 patients with essential hypertension, left ventricular mass was inversely correlated with the normalized peak filling rate (r = −0.89). In patients with concentric hypertrophy, the normalized peak filling rate was decreased despite normal end-diastolic and end-systolic volumes, suggesting that diastolic dysfunction occurs early in the clinical course of hypertensive heart disease and may precede evidence of systolic dysfunction.

27. Karam R, Lever HM, Healy BP: Hypertensive hypertrophic cardiomyopathy or hypertrophic cardiomyopathy with hypertension? A study of 78 patients. J Am Coll Cardiol 13:580–584, 1989.

    These authors emphasize that the clinical and echocardiographic features of elderly hypertensive patients with "hypertensive hypertrophic cardiomyopathy" are similar to those of normotensive patients with hypertrophic cardiomyopathy alone.

Evaluation after Heart Transplantation

28. Valantine HA, Schnittger I: Role of echocardiography in the evaluation of patients after heart transplantation. In: Otto CM (ed): The Practice of Clinical Echocardiography, 2nd ed. Philadelphia: WB Saunders, 2002, pp 658–678.

    An approach to evaluation of the posttransplant patient, in which echocardiographic data are key, is presented. The role of echocardiography in detection of transplant rejection and in diagnosis of transplant coronary artery disease is reviewed.

29. Miller LW, Labovitz AJ, McBride LA, et al: Echocardio-graphically guided endomyocardial biopsy. A 5-year experience. Circulation 78:99–102, 1988.

Description of utility of echocardiography for guiding endomyocardial biopsy in 4700 individual biopsies in 58 patients. Only two complications occurred.

30. Burgess MI, Bhattacharyya A, Ray SG: Echocardiography after cardiac transplanation. J Am Soc Echocardiogr 15:917–925, 2002.

Review of evaluation of the posttransplant patient including detection of rejection, evaluation for coronary artery disease, and echo guidance for endomyocardial biopsy; 73 references.

Pulmonary Heart Disease

31. Wong SP, Otto CM: Echocardiographic findings in acute and chronic pulmonary disease. In: Otto CM (ed): The Practice of Clinical Echocardiography, 2nd ed. Philadelphia: WB Saunders, 2002, pp 739–760.

The technical aspects of noninvasive measurement of pulmonary pressures are reviewed followed by a discussion of the clinical utility of echocardiography in patients with pulmonary disease including acute pulmonary embolism, chronic obstructive pulmonary disease, primary pulmonary hypertension, and evaluation before and after lung transplantation.

32. Hinderliter AL, Willis PW 4th, Long WA, et al, for the PPH Study Group: Frequency and severity of tricuspid regurgitation determined by Doppler echocardiography in primary pulmonary hypertension. Am J Cardiol 91:1033–1037, 2003.

In 78 patients with primary pulmonary hypertension, tricuspid regurgitation was detected in 97% with a velocity of 4.6 ± 0.6 m/s. Tricuspid regurgitation was severe in 37%, moderate in 23%, and mild in 40% of patients with severity related to annular and right ventricular dilation. Severe tricuspid regurgitaiton was associated with an elevated right atrial pressure, depressed cardiac index, and impaired exercise tolerance.

33. Raymond RJ, Hinderliter AL, Willis PW, et al: Echocardiographic predictors of adverse outcomes in primary pulmonary hypertension. J Am Coll Cardiol 39:1214–1219, 2002.

In 81 patients with primary pulmonary hypertension, echocardiographic predictors of death or lung transplantation were pericardial effusion, indexed right atrial area, and paradoxical septal motion.

34. Cotton CL, Gandhi S, Vaitkus PT, et al: Role of echocardiography in detecting portopulmonary hypertension in liver transplant candidates. Liver Transpl 8:1051–1054, 2002.

In patients undergoing evaluation for orthotopic liver transplantation, echocardiographic estimates of pulmonary systolic pressure have a high negative predictive value (92%) for excluding significant portopulmonary hypertension. However, positive predictive value is low (38%) due to overestimation of pulmonary pressures by echocardiography so that right heart catheterization is needed when the echocardiographic pulmonary pressure estimate is >50 mm Hg.

The Echo Exam *Cardiomyopathies, Hypertensive and Pulmonary Heart Disease*

Echo Differential Diagnosis of Heart Failure

Ischemic disease
Valvular disease
Hypertensive heart disease
Cardiomyopathy
   Dilated
   Hypertrophic
   Restrictive

Pericardial disease
   Constriction
   Tamponade
Pulmonary heart disease

Cardiomyopathies: Typical Features

	Dilated	Hypertrophic	Restrictive
LV systolic function	Moderately-severely ↓	Normal	Normal
LV diastolic function	May be abnormal	Abnormal	Abnormal
LV hypertrophy	↑LV mass due to left ventricular dilation with normal wall thickness	Asymmetric LV hypertrophy	Concentric LV hypertrophy
Chamber dilation	All four chambers	Left and right atrial dilation if MR is present	Left and right atrial dilation
Outflow tract obstruction	Absent	Dynamic LV outflow tract obstruction may be present	Absent
Left ventricular end-diastolic pressure	Elevated	Elevated	Elevated
Pulmonary artery pressures	Elevated	Elevated	Elevated

Differentiation of Cause of Increased Wall Thickness

	Hypertensive Heart Disease	Hypertrophic Cardiomyopathy	Restrictive Cardiomyopathy
Left ventricular hypertrophy	+	+	+
Pattern of hypertrophy	Concentric	Asymmetric	Concentric
Clinical history of hypertension	+	Absent	Absent
Outflow obstruction	Midventricular cavity obliteration	Dynamic subaortic obstruction	Absent
RV hypertrophy	Absent	May be present	+
Pulmonary hypertension	Mild	Mild	Moderate
LV systolic function	Normal initially but may be reduced late in disease course	Normal	Normal initially but may be reduced late in disease course
LV diastolic function	Abnormal	Abnormal	Abnormal

+ = present.

257

Echo Approach to the Cardiomyopathies

Modality	Echo Views and Flows	Measurements
Imaging	LV size and systolic function	LV-EDV, LV-ESV Apical biplane EF
	Degree and pattern of LV hypertrophy	LV-mass
	Evidence for dynamic outflow tract obstruction	SAM of the mitral valve Aortic valve midsystolic closure
	RV size and systolic function	
	LA size	
Doppler Echo	Associated valvular regurgitation	Measure vena contracta, quantitate if more than mild
	LV diastolic function	Standard diastolic function evaluation with classification of severity and estimate of LV-EDP
	LV systolic function	dP/dt from MR jet Calculation of cardiac output
	Pulmonary pressures	TR-Jet and IVC for PA systolic pressure Evaluate PR jet for PA diastolic pressure Consider measures of pulmonary resistance
	Color, pulsed, and CW Doppler to quantitate outflow obstruction	Maximum outflow tract gradient

PERICARDIAL DISEASE

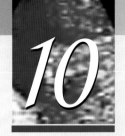

10

PERICARDIAL ANATOMY AND PHYSIOLOGY

The pericardium consists of two serous surfaces surrounding a closed, complex, saclike potential space. The visceral pericardium is continuous with the epicardial surface of the heart. The parietal pericardium is a dense but thin fibrous structure that is apposed to the pleural surfaces laterally and blends with the central tendon of the diaphragm inferiorly. Around the right and left ventricles and the ventricular apex, the pericardial space is a simple ellipsoid structure conforming to the shape of the ventricles. Around the systemic and pulmonary venous inflows and around the great vessels, the parietal and visceral pericardia meet to close the "ends" of the sac—these areas often are referred to as *pericardial reflections*. The pericardial space encloses the right atrium and right atrial appendage anteriorly and laterally, with pericardial reflections around the superior and inferior vena cava near their junction with the right atrium. Superiorly, the pericardium extends a short distance along the great vessels, with a small "pocket" of pericardium surrounding the great arteries posteriorly—the *transverse sinus*. The pericardial space extends lateral to the left atrium, and a blind pocket of the pericardium extends posterior to the left atrium, between the four pulmonary veins—the *oblique sinus* (Fig. 10-1). The pericardial space normally contains a small amount (5 to 10 mL) of fluid that may be detectable with echocardiography.

Anatomically, the pericardium isolates the heart from the rest of the mediastinum and from the lungs and pleural spaces. In addition, it may serve a lubricating function to allow normal rotation and translation of the heart during the cardiac cycle. However, the normal physiologic function of the pericardium is unclear. Some investigators suggest that the pericardium exerts a "restraining" effect on normal cardiac filling, while others argue that the pericardium has no significant hemodynamic function. In either case, the importance of the pericardium becomes clear with disease processes such as inflammation, infection, or malignancy.

PERICARDITIS

Basic Principles

Pericarditis is inflammation of the pericardium, and it can be due to a variety of causes, including bacterial or viral infection, trauma, uremia, and transmural myocardial infarction (Table 10-1).

259

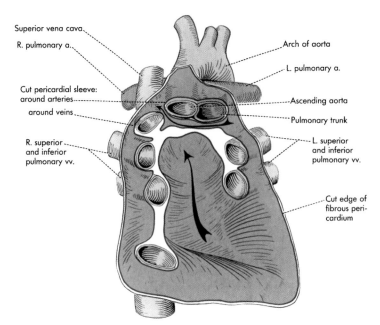

Superior vena cava
R. pulmonary a.
Cut pericardial sleeve: around arteries
around veins
R. superior and inferior pulmonary vv.
Arch of aorta
L. pulmonary a.
Ascending aorta
Pulmonary trunk
L. superior and inferior pulmonary vv.
Cut edge of fibrous pericardium

FIGURE 10–1. The posterior wall of the pericardial sac after the heart has been removed by severing its continuity with the great arteries and veins and by cutting the two pericardial sleeves that surround the arteries and veins. The parietal serous pericardium is dark gray; the fibrous pericardium is white; the horizontal arrow is in the transverse sinus; the vertical arrow is in the oblique sinus of the pericardium. (Reprinted with permission from Rosse C, Goddum-Rosse P: Hollinshead's Textbook of Anatomy, 5th ed. Philadelphia: Lippincott-Raven, 1997.)

Clinically, the diagnosis of pericarditis is based on the characteristic triad of

■ chest pain,
■ electrocardiographic changes including ST elevation, and
■ the presence of a pericardial rub on auscultation.

TABLE 10–1

Differential Diagnosis of Pericardial Effusion/Pericarditis

I. Infections
   A. Postviral pericarditis
   B. Bacterial
   C. Tuberculosis
II. Malignant
   A. Metastatic disease (e.g., lymphoma, melanoma)
   B. Direct extension (lung carcinoma, breast carcinoma)
   C. Primary cardiac malignancy
III. "Inflammatory"
   A. Post-myocardial infarction (Dressler's syndrome)
   B. Uremia
   C. Collagen-vascular disease
   D. Postcardiac surgery
IV. Intracardiac-pericardial communications
   A. Blunt or penetrating chest trauma
   B. Postcatheter procedures (electrophysiology studies, percutaneous coronary intervention, valvuloplasty)
   C. Left ventricular rupture post-myocardial infarction

While it is probable that most patients with pericarditis have a pericardial effusion at some point in the disease course, a pericardial effusion is not a necessary criterion for diagnosis of pericarditis. Interestingly, there is no correlation between the size of the pericardial effusion and the presence or absence of a pericardial "rub" on physical examination.

Echocardiographic Approach

In a patient with suspected pericarditis, the echocardiogram may show a pericardial effusion of any size or pericardial thickening with or without an effusion, or it may be entirely normal. A pericardial effusion is recognized as an echolucent space around the heart, as described in detail in the following sections (Fig. 10–2).

Pericardial thickening is evidenced by increased echogenicity of the pericardial reflection on two-dimensional (2D) imaging and as multiple par-allel reflections posterior to the left ventricle on M-mode recordings (Fig. 10–3). However, because the pericardium typically is the most echogenic structure in the image, it can be difficult to distinguish normal from thickened pericardium.

A careful echocardiographic examination from several windows is needed when pericarditis is suspected, since effusion or thickening can be localized and may be seen in only certain tomographic views. If a pericardial effusion is present, the possibility of tamponade physiology should be considered. If pericardial thickening is present, examination for evidence of constrictive physiology should be considered (see following sections).

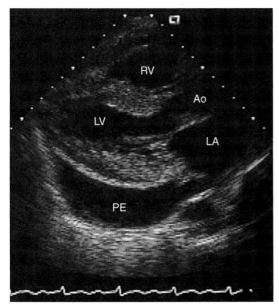

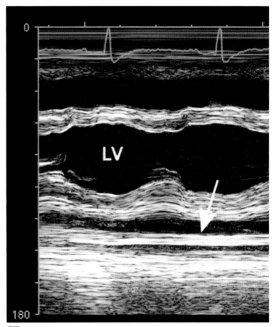

FIGURE 10-3. Pericardial thickening on M-mode echocardiography appears as multiple parallel dense echos *(arrow)* posterior to the left ventricular epicardium. This patient also has a small pericardial effusion, seen on M-mode as an echo-free space between the flat pericardium and moving posterior wall.

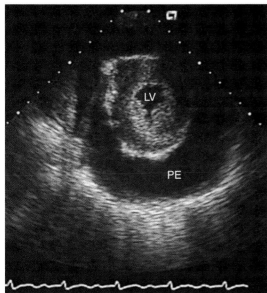

FIGURE 10-2. Parasternal long- and short-axis views of a large posterior pericardial effusion (PE).

Clinical Utility

Pericarditis is a clinical diagnosis that cannot be made independently by echocardiography. The goal of the echocardiographic examination is to evaluate for pericardial effusion or thickening.

PERICARDIAL EFFUSION

Basic Principles and Tamponade Physiology

A variety of disease processes can result in a pericardial effusion with a differential diagnosis similar to that for pericarditis (see Table 10-1). The physiologic consequences of fluid in the pericardial space depend both on the volume and rate of fluid accumulation. A slowly expanding pericardial effusion can become quite large (>1000 mL) with little increase in pericardial pressure, whereas rapid accumulation of even a small volume of fluid (50 to 100 mL) can lead to a marked increase in pericardial pressure (Fig. 10-4).

Tamponade physiology occurs when the pressure in the pericardium exceeds the pressure in the cardiac chambers, resulting in impaired cardiac filling. As pericardial pressure increases, filling of each cardiac chamber is sequentially impaired, with lower-pressure chambers (atria) affected before higher-pressure chambers (ventricles). The compressive effect of the pericardial fluid is seen most clearly in the phase of the cardiac cycle when pressure is lowest in that chamber—systole for the atrium, diastole for the ventricles. Filling pressures become elevated as a compensatory mechanism to maintain cardiac output. In fully developed tamponade, diastolic pressures in all four cardiac chambers are equal (and elevated) due to exposure of the entire heart to the elevated pericardial pressure.

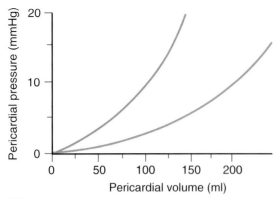

FIGURE 10–4. Schematic graph of pericardial pressure versus pericardial volume for an acute effusion (*blue line,* with a steep pressure-volume relationship) and for a chronic effusion (*yellow line,* where large volumes may lead to only mild pressure elevation).

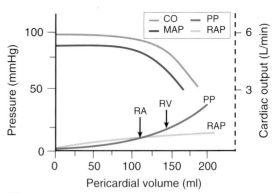

FIGURE 10–5. Schematic graph showing the relationship between pericardial pressure (PP), right atrial pressure (RAP), mean arterial pressure (MAP), and cardiac output (CO). Note that when pericardial pressure exceeds right atrial (RA) pressure, blood pressure and cardiac output fall. When right ventricular (RV) pressure is exceeded (*at the arrow*), cardiac output and mean arterial pressure fall further.

Clinically, tamponade physiology is manifested as low cardiac output symptoms, hypotension, and tachycardia. Jugular venous pressure is elevated and pulsus paradoxus (an inspiratory decline >10 mm Hg in systemic blood pressure) is present on physical examination. The clinical finding of pulsus paradoxus is closely related to the echo findings of reciprocal respiratory changes in right and left ventricular filling and emptying (Fig. 10–5).

Echocardiographic Approach to Diagnosis of Pericardial Effusion

Diffuse Effusion

A pericardial effusion is recognized on 2D echocardiography as an echolucent space adjacent to the cardiac structures. In the absence of prior pericardial disease or surgery, pericardial effusions usually are diffuse and symmetric with clear separation between the parietal and visceral pericardium (Fig. 10–6). A relatively echogenic area anteriorly, in the absence of a posterior effusion, most likely represents a normal pericardial fat pad. M-mode recordings are helpful, especially with a small effusion, showing the flat posterior pericardial echo reflection and the moving epicardial echo with separation between the two in both systole and diastole.

In patients with recurrent or long-standing pericardial disease, fibrinous stranding within the fluid and on the epicardial surface of the heart may be seen (Fig. 10–7). When a malignant effusion is suspected, it is difficult to distinguish this nonspecific finding from metastatic disease. Features suggesting the latter include a nodular appearance, evidence of extension into the myocardium, and the appropriate clinical setting.

The size of the pericardial effusion is considered to be small when the separation between parietal and visceral pericardium is less than 0.5 cm, moderate when it is 0.5 to 2 cm, and large when it is greater than 2 cm. More quantitative measures of the size of the pericardial effusion rarely are needed in the clinical setting.

Loculated Effusion

In the postoperative patient or the patient with recurrent pericardial disease, a *loculated* pericardial effusion can occur. In this situation, the effusion is localized by adhesions to a small area of the pericardial space or consists of several separate areas of pericardial effusion, separated by adhesions. Recognition of a loculated effusion is especially important because hemodynamic compromise can occur with even a small, strategically located fluid collection. In addition, drainage of a loculated effusion may not be possible from a percutaneous approach (Fig. 10–8).

Distinguishing from Pleural Fluid

To reliably exclude the possibility of a loculated pericardial effusion, echocardiographic evaluation requires a careful examination from multiple acoustic windows. The parasternal approach demonstrates the extent of the fluid collection at the base of the heart in both long- and short-axis views. Note that pericardial fluid may be seen posterior to the left atrium (in the oblique sinus), as well as posterior to the left ventricle. Care should be taken that the coronary sinus or descending thoracic aorta is not mistaken for pericardial fluid. In fact, these structures can help in distinguishing pericardial from pleural fluid, since

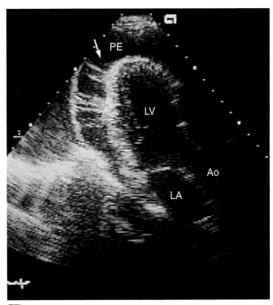

FIGURE 10–7. Fibrinous stranding with adhesions between the visceral and parietal pericardia in a chronic effusion seen on an apical long-axis view.

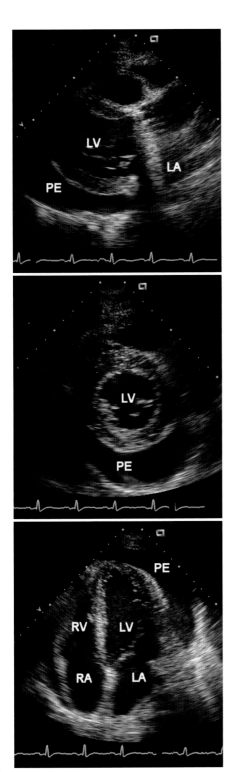

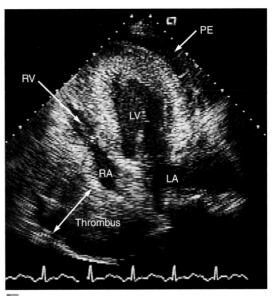

FIGURE 10–8. Apical four-chamber view showing a localized pericardial thrombus *(arrows)* compressing the right ventricle and atrium, leading to tamponade physiology in this postoperative patient.

FIGURE 10–6. Pericardial effusion seen from an parasternal long-axis view *(top)*, short-axis view *(middle)*, and apical four-chamber view *(bottom)* in a patient early after mecahnical aortic valve replacement. Note the shadowing and reverberations from the valve in the parasternal long-axis view.

a left pleural effusion will extend posterolateral to the descending aorta, whereas a pericardial effusion will track anterior to the descending aorta (Fig. 10–9). When a large left pleural effusion is present, sometimes cardiac images can be obtained with the transducer on the patient's back (Fig. 10–10).

In the apical views, the lateral, medial, and apical extent of the effusion can be appreciated. In the apical four-chamber view, an isolated echo-free space superior to the right atrium most likely represents pleural fluid. The subcostal view demonstrates fluid between the diaphragm and right ventricle and is particularly helpful in echo-guided pericardiocentesis (Fig 10–11). The sensitivity and specificity of echocardiography for detection of a pericardial effusion are very high.

Echocardiographic Approach to Pericardial Tamponade

When cardiac tamponade occurs with a diffuse moderate to large pericardial effusion (Fig. 10–12), the associated physiologic changes are evident on echocardiographic and Doppler examination, including

- right atrial systolic collapse,
- right ventricular (RV) diastolic collapse,
- reciprocal respiratory changes in RV and left ventricular (LV) volumes,
- reciprocal respiratory changes in RV and LV filling, and
- inferior vena cava plethora.

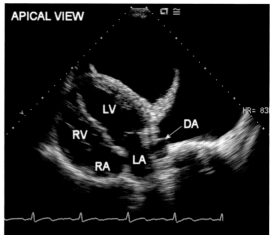
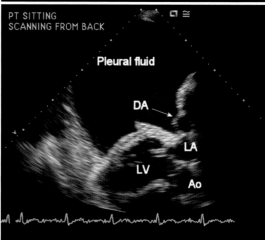

FIGURE 10–10. In a view with the transducer moved laterally from the apical position *(top)* a large left pleural effusion is seen. This can be distinguished from pericardial fluid by the position of the descending aorta (DA), the presence of compressed lung, and identification of both layers of the pericardium adjacent to the myocardium. Images also were obtained with the transducer on the patient's back *(bottom)*, demonstrating the relationship bewteen the pleural fluid and the descending aorta.

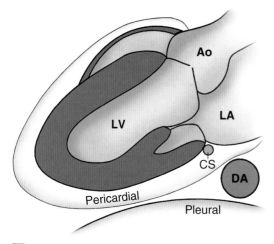

FIGURE 10–9. Schematic diagram of the relationship between a pericardial effusion and the descending aorta (DA) compared with a left pleural effusion. Pericardial fluid tracks posterior to the left atrium (LA) in the oblique sinus of the pericardium, anterior to the descending aorta.

Right Atrial Systolic Collapse

When intrapericardial pressure exceeds right atrial systolic pressure (lowest point of the atrial pressure curve), inversion or collapse of the right atrial free wall occurs. Because the right atrial free wall is a thin, flexible structure, brief right atrial wall inversion can occur in the absence of tamponade physiology. However, the longer the duration of right atrial inversion relative to the cycle length, the greater is the likelihood of cardiac tamponade. Inversion for greater than one third of systole has a sensitivity of 94% and a specificity of 100% for the diagnosis of tamponade. Careful

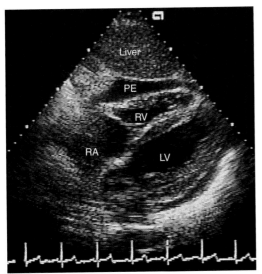

FIGURE 10–11. Pericardial effusion seen from a subcostal view.

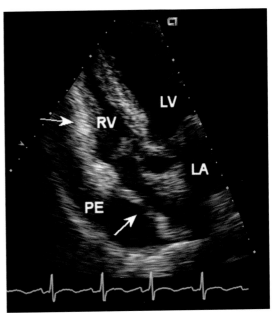

FIGURE 10–13. Apical four-chamber view showing systolic collapse on the right atrial free wall *arrow)* in a patient with clinical tamponade physiology. PE, pericardial effusion.

frame-by-frame 2D-image analysis is needed for this evaluation (Fig. 10–13).

Right Ventricular Diastolic Collapse

RV diastolic collapse occurs when intrapericardial pressure exceeds RV diastolic pressure *and* when the RV free wall is normal in thickness and compliance. The presence of RV hypertrophy or infiltrative diseases of the myocardium may allow

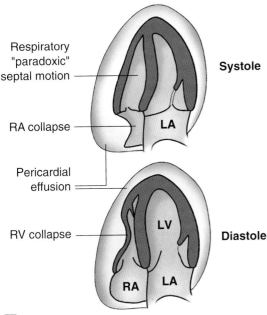

FIGURE 10–12. Schematic diagram of 2D echo findings with tamponade physiology.

development of a pressure gradient between the pericardial space and RV chamber without inversion of the normal contour of the free wall. Right ventricular diastolic collapse is best appreciated in the parasternal long-axis view or from a subcostal window. If the timing of right ventricular wall motion is not clear on 2D imaging, an M-mode recording through the right ventricular free wall is helpful. The presence of RV diastolic collapse is somewhat less sensitive (60% to 90%) but more specific (85% to 100%) than brief right atrial systolic collapse for diagnosing tamponade physiology (Fig. 10–14).

Reciprocal Changes in Ventricular Volumes

Reciprocal respiratory variation in RV and LV volumes may be seen on 2D imaging when tamponade is present. In the apical four-chamber view, an increase in RV volume with inspiration (shift in septal motion toward the left ventricle in diastole and toward the right ventricle in systole) and a decrease during expiration (normalization of septal motion) can be appreciated. This pattern of motion corresponds to the physical finding of pulsus paradoxus. The proposed explanation for this observation is that total pericardial volume (heart chambers plus pericardial fluid) is fixed in tamponade so that as intrathoracic pressure becomes more negative during inspiration, enhanced RV filling limits LV diastolic filling. This pattern reverses during expiration.

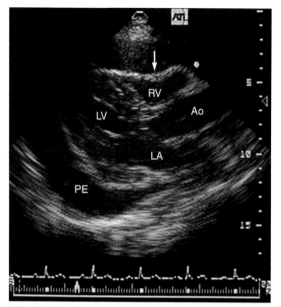

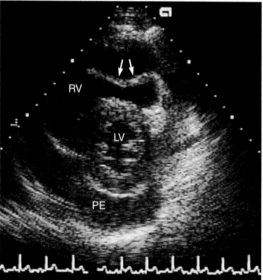

■ **FIGURE 10–14.** Parasternal long-axis *(above)* and short-axis *(below)* views showing right ventricular diastolic collapse *(arrows)*.

Respiratory Variation in Diastolic Filling

Doppler recordings of RV and LV diastolic filling in patients with tamponade physiology show a similar pattern. With inspiration, the RV early diastolic filling velocity is augmented, while LV diastolic filling diminishes (Figs. 10–15 and 10–16). In addition, the flow velocity integral in the pulmonary artery increases with inspiration, while the aortic flow velocity integral decreases. In the acutely ill patient, these changes can be difficult to demonstrate in part due to respiratory changes in the intercept angle between the

Doppler beam and the flow of interest causing artifactual apparent velocity changes. Differentiating the normal respiratory variation in diastolic filling from the excessive variation (>25%) seen in tamponade may be subtle in borderline cases. Tamponade physiology is not an all-or-none phenomenon; a patient may exhibit varying degrees of hemodynamic impairment as the degree of pericardial compression (pericardial pressure) increases.

Plethora of the Inferior Vena Cava

Inferior vena cava plethora, a dilated inferior vena cava with less than 50% inspiratory reduction in diameter near the inferior vena cava–right atrium junction, also has been proposed as a sensitive (97%), albeit nonspecific (40%), indicator of tamponade physiology. This simple finding reflects the elevated right atrial pressure seen in tamponade.

Limitations/Alternate Approaches

Echocardiography is very sensitive for the diagnosis of pericardial effusion, even when loculated, if care is taken to examine the heart in multiple tomographic planes from multiple acoustic windows. Loculated effusions can be difficult to assess in certain locations, particularly if localized to the atrial region, because the effusion itself may be mistaken for a normal cardiac chamber.

The etiology of the pericardial effusion is not always evident on echocardiographic examination. Irregular pericardial or epicardial masses in a patient with a known malignancy certainly raise the possibility of a malignant effusion, but this appearance can be mimicked by fibrinous organization of a long-standing pericardial effusion. Masses adjacent to the cardiac structures (in the mediastinum) resulting in pericardial effusion can be missed with echocardiography. Wide-view tomographic imaging procedures, such as computed tomography (CT) or magnetic resonance imaging (MRI), are helpful in these cases.

Obviously, whether a pericardial effusion is infected or inflammatory in etiology cannot be determined with echocardiography. Depending on the associated clinical findings in each case, diagnostic pericardiocentesis and/or pericardial biopsy may be indicated to establish the correct diagnosis.

With pericardial effusion due to cardiac rupture, either as a consequence of myocardial infarction or trauma, the site of rupture itself rarely can be detected, so a high level of suspicion is needed when this diagnosis is a possibility. In some cases, the site of left ventricular rupture is "contained" by pericardial adhesions, resulting in

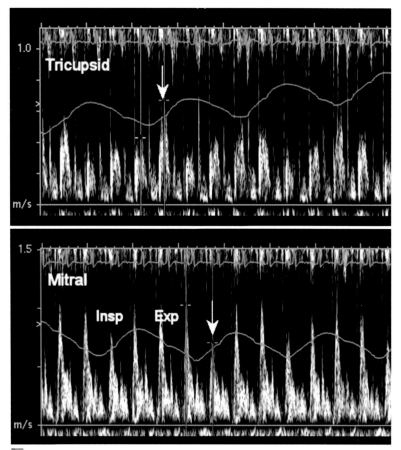

■ **FIGURE 10–15.** Doppler recording of left ventricular inflow with superimposed respirometer tracing in a patient with tamponade showing increased triscupid flow and decreased mitral *(arrows)* on the first beat after inspiration, reflecting the reciprocal respiratory changes in right and left ventricular diastolic filling.

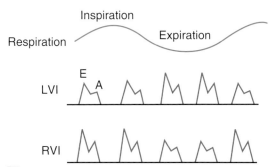

■ **FIGURE 10–16.** Schematic diagram of left and right ventricular diastolic inflow (RVI and LVI) Doppler curves with tamponade physiology showing enhanced right ventricular (and reduced left ventricular) diastolic filling with inspiration and a reversal of this pattern during expiration.

formation of a pseudoaneurysm. A *pseudoaneurysm* is defined as a saccular structure communicating with the ventricle with walls composed of pericardium. In contrast, the walls of a "true" aneurysm are composed of thinned, scarred myocardium (see Chapter 8).

Clinical Utility

Diagnosis of Pericardial Effusion

Echocardiography is the procedure of choice for diagnosis of pericardial effusion. When transthoracic images are inadequate, as occasionally occurs (especially in postoperative patients), transesophageal imaging, or an alternate tomographic imaging procedure (MRI, CT) may be needed. Echocardiography can be helpful in establishing a diagnosis of pericardial tamponade but requires integration with other clinical data.

In evaluating a patient for cardiac tamponade, it is essential to remember that tamponade is a clinical and hemodynamic diagnosis. Furthermore, varying degrees of tamponade physiology may be seen. The most important finding on echocardiography in a patient with suspected pericardial tamponade is whether a pericardial effusion is present. The absence of a pericardial effusion *excludes* the diagnosis, again taking care that a loculated effusion is not missed. Only rarely does tamponade physiology result from other mediastinal contents under pressure (i.e., air due to barotrauma or a compressive mass). Conversely, in a patient with convincing clinical evidence for tamponade, the presence of a moderate to large pericardial effusion on echocardiography *confirms* the diagnosis; further evaluation with Doppler is not not needed and may delay appropriate intervention.

In intermediate cases, either when the clinical diagnosis has not been considered or when the clinical evidence is equivocal, 2D findings of chamber collapse and inferior vena cava plethora and Doppler findings showing marked respiratory variation in right and left ventricular filling may be helpful, in conjunction with the clinical data. Another diagnostic test that is helpful in making

this diagnosis is right-sided heart catheterization showing a depressed cardiac output and equalization of right atrial, right ventricular diastolic, and pulmonary artery wedge pressures.

Echo-Guided Pericardiocentesis

The success rate without complications of percutaneous needle pericardiocentesis can be enhanced by using echocardiographic guidance. With the patient in the position planned for the procedure, the optimal transcutaneous approach is identified based on the location of the effusion, the distance from the chest wall to the pericardium, and the absence of intervening structures. The transducer angle and pericardial depth are noted, and the transducer position is marked prior to prepping the site for the procedure. After the procedure, the residual amount of pericardial fluid is assessed using standard tomographic views (Fig. 10–17). If monitoring during the procedure is needed, an acoustic window that allows visualization of the effusion but does not compromise the sterile field is identified. (Alternatively, a sterile sleeve is used for the transducer.) Note that with *tomographic* imaging it is difficult to

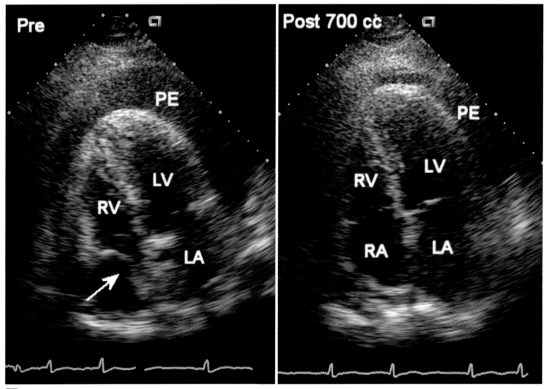

■ **FIGURE 10–17.** Apical four-chamber view recorded in the catheterization laboratory immediately pre- and post-pericardicentesis with removal of 700 mL of fluid. On the pre-pericardicentesis image *(left)* a large pericardial effusion (PE), small ventricular chamber, and right atrial collapse *(arrow)* are seen. The post-pericardicentesis image *(right)* shows a reduction in size of the effusion, an increase in right and left ventricular volumes and a normal contour of the right atrial wall.

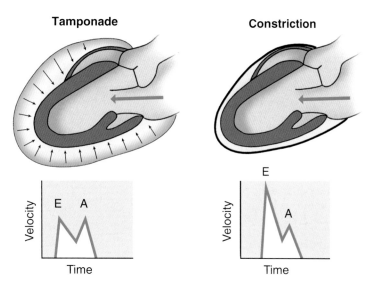

Tamponade

Constriction

FIGURE 10–18. Schematic diagram of pericardial tamponade compared with pericardial constriction. With tamponade, diastolic filling is impaired in both early and late diastole due to the elevated pericardial pressures "compressing" the heart. With constriction, early diastolic filling is rapid but ends abruptly when the volume limits of the rigid pericardial space are reached.

identify the *tip* of the needle, since any segment of the needle passing through the image plane may appear to be the tip. Scanning in both superoinferior and lateromedial directions during imaging helps minimize this source of error. Confirmation that the needle tip is in the pericardial space can be made by injecting a *small* amount of agitated sterile saline solution through the needle to achieve an echo-contrast effect.

PERICARDIAL CONSTRICTION

Basic Principles

In constrictive pericarditis, the visceral and parietal layers of the pericardium are adherent, thickened, and fibrotic, resulting in impairment of diastolic ventricular filling. Pericardial constriction can occur after repeated episodes of pericarditis, after cardiac surgery, after radiation therapy, and from a variety of other causes. The diagnosis often is delayed because clinical symptoms are nonspecific–fatigue and malaise due to low cardiac output–and physical findings either are subtle (elevated jugular venous pressure, distant heart sounds) or occur only late in the disease course (ascites and peripheral edema).

The physiology of constrictive pericarditis is characterized by impaired diastolic cardiac filling due to the abnormal pericardium surrounding the cardiac structures, acting like a rigid "box" (Fig. 10–18). Early diastolic filling is rapid, with an abrupt cessation of ventricular filling as diastolic

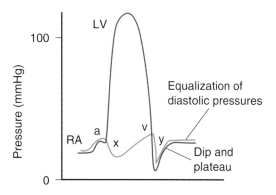

Constrictive Pericarditis

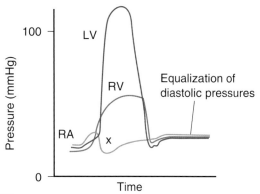

Pericardial Tamponade

FIGURE 10–19. Typical pressure tracings in tamponade and constriction.

pressure increases—when the "box" is "full." Pressure tracings (Fig. 10–19) typically show

- a brief, rapid fall of ventricular pressure in early diastole, followed by
- a high early diastolic pressure plateau (*dip-plateau* or *square-root sign*),
- a rapid descent of right atrial pressure with the onset of ventricular filling (*y* descent),
- only modest elevation of RV and pulmonary artery systolic pressures,
- a RV diastolic pressure plateau that is a third or more of systolic pressure, and
- equalization of diastolic pressures in the RV and LV even after volume loading.

Echocardiographic Approach

Imaging

Typically, left ventricular wall thickness, internal dimensions, and systolic function are normal in the patient with constrictive pericarditis. Left atrial enlargement is seen due to chronic left atrial pressure elevation. Pericardial thickening may be evident on 2D imaging as increased echogenicity in the region of the pericardium (Fig. 10–20). Careful examination from several acoustic windows is needed because the spatial distribution of pericardial thickening may be asymmetric. From the parasternal approach, an M-mode recording shows multiple dense echos, posterior to the LV epicardium, moving parallel with each

other. These echos persist even at a low-gain setting. High time resolution M-mode recordings also may demonstrate an abrupt posterior motion of the ventricular septum in early diastole, with flat motion in middle diastole and abrupt anterior motion following atrial contraction (Fig. 10–21). This pattern of motion appears to be due to initial rapid RV diastolic filling, followed by equalization of filling of right and left ventricles as the "plateau" phase of the pressure curve is reached, and increased RV filling after atrial contraction. The left ventricular posterior wall endocardium shows little posterior motion during diastole (<2 mm from early to late diastole) due to the impairment of diastolic filling resulting in a "flat" pattern of diastolic posterior wall motion. On subcostal views, the inferior vena cava and hepatic veins are dilated, reflecting the elevated right atrial pressure.

Doppler Examination

The Doppler findings in constrictive pericarditis reflect the abnormal hemodynamics in this condition (Fig. 10–22), including

- characteristic patterns of right and left atrial filling,
- respiratory variation in LV and RV filling, and
- respiratory variation in the isovolumic relaxation time (IVRT).

Pulsed Doppler recordings of hepatic vein flow (from a subcostal approach) measure right atrial filling and show a prominent *a* wave and a deep *y* descent (Fig. 10–23) and a marked increase in flow velocities with inspiration. Similarly, pulsed Doppler recordings of pulmonary vein flow

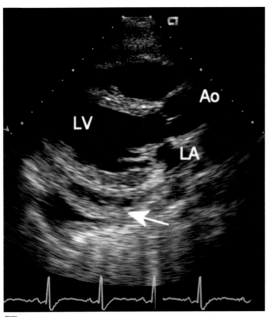

■ **FIGURE 10–20.** Constrictive pericarditis from a parasternal long-axis view with both thickened pericardium (*arrow*) and a small effusion.

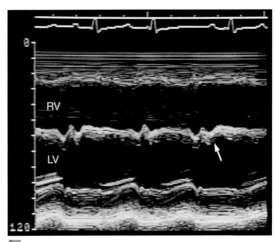

■ **FIGURE 10–21.** M-mode in constrictive pericarditis showing rapid anterior motion of the septum (*arrow*) with atrial contraction before the QRS on the ECG.

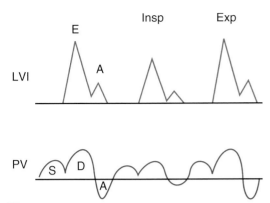

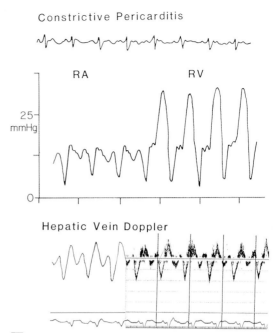

FIGURE 10–22. Schematic diagram of the Doppler flow patterns in constrictive pericarditis. Left ventricular inflow shows reduced early diastolic filling with inspiration, while the pulmonary vein shows a prominent *a* wave and blunting of the systolic filling phase.

(transthoracic apical four-chamber view or transesophageal approach) indicate left atrial filling and again show a prominent *a* wave, prominent *y* descent, a prominent diastolic filling phase, and blunting of the systolic phase of atrial filling.

Both RV and LV diastolic filling show a high *E* velocity due to rapid early diastolic filling occurring simultaneously with the initial high atrial to ventricular pressure difference during the brief early diastolic "dip" in ventricular pressure. As LV pressure increases, filling abruptly ceases, reflected in a short deceleration time of the *E*-velocity curve. Little ventricular filling occurs in late diastole due to the elevated LV diastolic pressure (the "plateau") and the constrictive effect of the thickened pericardium. Doppler recordings of ventric-

FIGURE 10–23. Pressure tracing and hepatic vein flow in a patient with constrictive pericarditis. Note the prominent *a* wave, flat diastolic segment, and prominent *y* descent, all consistent with the "square-root sign" or dip and plateau in the pressure tracings.

ular inflow thus show a very small *A*-velocity following atrial contraction.

Marked reciprocal respiratory variations in RV and LV diastolic inflow velocities are seen due to the differing effects of changes in intrapleural pressure on filling of the two ventricles (Fig 10–24). With inspiration, intrapleural pressure becomes

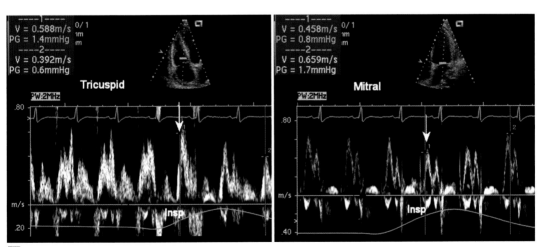

FIGURE 10–24. Respiratory variation in right and left ventricular diastolic filling in a pateint with constrictive pericarditis. There in an increase in tricuspid and decrease in mitral flow velocities on the first beat after inspiration *(arrows)* with the decrease greater than 25% compared to the maximum velocities.

more negative, resulting in augmentation of RV diastolic filling and inflow velocity. LV filling velocities *decrease* with inspiration and *increase* with expiration. Similar directional changes occur in normal individuals, with the respiratory changes being more marked (variation >25%) with constrictive pericarditis.

The LV isovolumic relaxation time–measured from the aortic closure to the mitral opening click on Doppler recordings–increases by a mean of 20% with inspiration in patients with constrictive pericarditis.

Comparison of Pericardial Tamponade, Constrictive Pericarditis, and Restrictive Cardiomyopathy

Although the hemodynamics of pericardial tamponade and pericardial constriction have some similarities, differentiating between these two diagnoses usually is straightforward based on the presence or absence of a pericardial effusion (Table 10–2). Differentiating constrictive pericarditis from a restrictive cardiomyopathy is more difficult. Both are characterized by clinical signs and symptoms of elevated venous pressure and low cardiac output, and both show a normal-sized LV chamber with normal systolic function on 2D echocardiography. Pericardial thickening may be difficult to appreciate, and other 2D and M-mode findings may not reliably differentiate between these two diagnoses. A difference (>25%) in maximum E velocity from expiration to inspiration has been suggested as a useful method for distinguishing constrictive pericarditis from restrictive cardiomyopathy. These characteristic Doppler findings may favor one clinical diagnosis over another and, in conjunction with other clinical data, may be definitive in some cases. However, Doppler data are far from accurate due to overlap between groups in the Doppler findings and due to differing hemodynamics in patients with restrictive cardiomyopathy depending on disease stage (see Chapter 9). One of the most helpful findings on Doppler examination is estimation of pulmonary artery systolic pressure from the tricuspid regurgitant jet velocity. Patients with restrictive cardiomyopathy typically have moderate-to-severe pulmonary hypertension, while those with constrictive pericarditis have only mild elevations in pulmonary pressures.

TABLE 10–2

Comparison of Pericardial Tamponade, Constriction, and Restrictive Cardiomyopathy

	Pericardial Tamponade	Constrictive Pericarditis	Restrictive Cardiomyopathy
Hemodynamics			
Right atrial pressure	↑	↑	↑
RV/LV filling pressures	↑, RV = LV	↑, RV = LV	↑, LV > RV
Pulmonary artery pressures	Normal	Mild elevation (35–40 mm Hg systolic)	Moderate-severe elevation (≥60 mm Hg systolic)
RV diastolic pressure plateau		>⅓ peak RV pressure	<⅓ peak RV pressure
Radionuclide diastolic filling		Rapid early filling, impaired late filling	Impaired early filling
2D Echo	Moderate-large PE	Pericardial thickening without effusion	Left ventricular hypertrophy Normal systolic function
Doppler Echo	Reciprocal respiratory changes in RV and LV filling Inferior vena cava plethora	$E > a$ on LV inflow Prominent y descent in hepatic vein Pulmonary venous flow = prominent a wave, reduced systolic phase Respiratory variation in IVRT and in E velocity	(1) Early in disease $e < A$ on LV inflow (2) Late in disease $E > a$ (3) Constant IVRT (4) Absence of significant respiratory variation
Other diagnostic tests	Therapeutic/diagnostic pericardiocentesis	CT or MRI for pericardial thickening	Endomyocardial biopsy

CT, computed tomography; IVRT, isovolumic relaxation time; LV, left ventricle; MRI, magnetic resonance imaging; PE, pericardial effusion; RV, right ventricular.

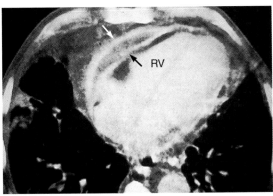 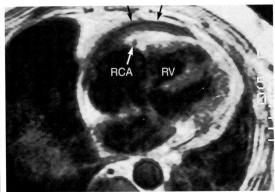

▌ FIGURE 10–25. In a patient with tuberculous constrictive pericarditis, chest CT *(left)* shows thickening of visceral and parietal pericardial layers surrounding consolidated caseous material as alternating bands of light and dark anterior to the right ventricle *(arrows)*. In a second patient with constrictive pericarditis, the chest MRI *(right)* shows pericardial thickening as a low signal band *(dark area)* anterior to the right ventricle *(arrow)*. Epicardial fat is high signal *(white)* with the right coronary artery (RCA) indicated.

Limitations/Alternate Approaches

When the diagnosis of constrictive pericarditis is in question, several alternate approaches may be helpful. Chest fluoroscopy shows calcification of the pericardium in approximately 50% of cases of constrictive pericarditis. Either chest CT or MRI scanning is more definitive for detection of pericardial thickening, especially when it is asymmetric (Fig. 10–25). Evaluation of early diastolic ventricular filling on frame-by-frame angiography or by radionuclide techniques also has been proposed as a method to distinguish constrictive pericarditis from restrictive cardiomyopathy. Endomyocardial biopsy occasionally will confirm a diagnosis of restrictive cardiomyopathy due to an infiltrative process.

Right- and left-sided heart catheterization with recording of intracardiac pressures and waveforms, including simultaneous recording of RV and LV diastolic pressures after volume loading, remains the standard of reference for diagnosis of constrictive pericarditis. However, even with this technique, some cases will be missed, so exploratory thoracotomy may be needed to make a definitive diagnosis. If present, pericardial constriction then can be relieved by surgical removal of the pericardium.

Clinical Utility

The diagnosis of pericardial constriction remains a problem, with no single diagnostic feature on echocardiographic or Doppler examination. However, the conjunction of several findings in a patient in whom the level of clinical suspicion is high increases the likelihood of this diagnosis and may be definitive in some cases. Conversely, the echo and Doppler findings may provide the first clues for this diagnosis in a patient in whom it was not previously considered, for example, a patient presenting with ascites and no cardiac history.

SUGGESTED READING
Pericardial Effusion

1. Markiewicz W, Brik A, Brook G, et al: Pericardial rub in pericardial effusion: Lack of correlation with amount of fluid. Chest 77:643–646, 1980.

   In 76 patients with a pericardial effusion, a rub was noted on auscultation in 4 of 13 (30%) with a small effusion, 23 of 40 (58%) with a moderate effusion, and 10 of 23 (43%) patients with a large effusion. These findings suggest that the size of the effusion cannot be predicted from the presence or absence of a rub.

2. Markiewicz W, Monakier I, Brik A, et al: Clinical-echocardiographic correlations in pericardial effusion. Eur Heart J 3:260–266, 1982.

   Of 100 patients with an effusion on echocardiography, 49 had a clinical course consistent with acute pericarditis (idiopathic in 23, postradiation therapy in 7, Dressler's syndrome in 7, purulent in 4, and other in 7). In the 51 patients with chronic pericarditis, the etiology was carcinoma in 20, heart disease in 12, uremia in 7, rheumatoid arthritis in 5, chronic idiopathic pericarditis in 4, and other in 3 patients.

3. Permanyer-Miralda G, Sagrista-Sauleda J, Soler-Soler J: Primary acute pericardial disease: A prospective series of 231 consecutive patients. Am J Cardiol 56:623–630, 1985.

   Of 231 patients with primary acute pericarditis, "therapeutic pericardiocentesis" was performed in 44 for tamponade physiology, while 32 had a "diagnostic" pericardiocentesis for suspected purulent pericarditis. The diagnostic yield was 29% for therapeutic and 6% for diagnostic pericardiocentesis. The overall diagnostic yield of pericardial biopsy was only 22%.

4. Drummond JB, Seward JB, Tsang TS, et al: Outpatient two-dimensional echocardiography-guided pericardiocentesis. J Am Soc Echocardiogr 11:433–435, 1998.

   Discussion of patient selection and the approach to pericardiocentesis using echocardiographic guidance.

Tamponade Physiology

5. Gillam LD, Guyer DE, Gibson TC, et al: Hydrodynamic compression of the right atrium: A new echocardiographic sign of cardiac tamponade. Circulation 68:294–301, 1983.

Right atrial free wall systolic inversion that persists for a third or more of the cycle length had a sensitivity of 94% and specificity of 100% for the diagnosis of tamponade physiology in 127 patients (19 with tamponade).

6. Leimgruber P, Klopfenstein HS, Wann LS, Brooks HL: The hemodynamic derangement associated with right ventricular diastolic collapse in cardiac tamponade: An experimental echocardiographic study. Circulation 68: 612–620, 1983.

In an experimental model, right ventricular diastolic collapse occurred when intrapericardial pressure exceeded right ventricular diastolic pressure and was associated with a 21% reduction in cardiac output (but no change in mean aortic pressure). Of note, right ventricular diastolic collapse did not occur in the presence of right ventricular hypertrophy.

7. Reddy PS, Curtiss EL, Uretsky BF: Spectrum of hemodynamic changes in cardiac tamponade. Am J Cardiol 55:1487–1491, 1990.

The range of hemodynamic compromise that can be seen with tamponade physiology is emphasized in this study of 77 consecutive patients with greater than 150 mL of pericardial fluid. In group I, intrapericardial pressures were less than right atrial and pulmonary artery wedge pressures. In group II, intrapericardial and right atrial pressures had equalized. In group III, intrapericardial, right atrial, and pulmonary artery wedge pressures were equal. All subjects improved after pericardiocentesis, with the greatest improvement seen in group III.

8. Gonzalez MS, Basnight MA, Appleton CP: Experimental cardiac tamponade: A hemodynamic and Doppler echocardiographic reexamination of the relation of right and left heart ejection dynamics to the phase of respiration. J Am Coll Cardiol 18:243–252, 1991.

In this model, there was an inverse relationship between peak left and right ventricular systolic pressures and ejection times, and between pulmonary and aortic flow velocities, when tamponade physiology was present. This suggests that the mechanism of pulsus paradoxus is the reciprocal changes in right and left ventricular filling due to a "fixed" total cardiac volume in tamponade.

9. Gonzalez MS, Basnight MA, Appleton CP: Experimental pericardial effusion: Relation of abnormal respiratory variation in mitral flow velocity to hemodynamics and diastolic right heart collapse. J Am Coll Cardiol 17:239–248, 1991.

Respiratory changes in left ventricular diastolic filling are exaggerated in tamponade, with this variation occurring before equalization of intracardiac pressures and definite right-sided heart collapse. The presence of excessive respiratory variation, but not its magnitude, is predictive of tamponade physiology.

10. Picard MH, Sanfilippo AJ, Newell JB, et al: Quantitative relation between increased intrapericardial pressure and Doppler flow velocities during experimental cardiac tamponade. J Am Coll Cardiol 18:234–242, 1991.

In contrast to Suggested Reading 9, these authors did note a quantitative relationship between the degree of increase in intrapericardial pressure and the percentage change in inflow/outflow patterns with respiration.

11. Chuttani K, Pandian NG, Mohanty PK, et al: Left ventricular diastolic collapse: An echocardiographic sign of regional cardiac tamponade. Circulation 83:1999–2006, 1991.

Loculated effusions, especially after cardiac surgery, can cause compression of individual cardiac chambers leading to tamponade physiology. Conventional signs of tamponade may be absent on echocardiography in these cases.

12. Himelman RB, Kircher B, Rockey DC, Schiller NB: Inferior vena cava plethora with blunted respiratory response: A sensitive echocardiographic sign of cardiac tamponade. J Am Coll Cardiol 12:1470–1477, 1988.

Dilation of the inferior vena cava reflects an elevated right atrial pressure. Plethora of the inferior vena cava had a sensitivity of 97% but a specificity of only 40% for the diagnosis of pericardial tamponade. False-positive results occurred in patients with right ventricular failure, tricuspid regurgitation, and pulmonary hypertension.

13. Eisenberg MJ, Schiller NB: Bayes' theorem and the echocardiographic diagnosis of cardiac tamponade. Am J Cardiol 68:1242–1244, 1991.

Using Bayes' theorem, the predictive values of right ventricular collapse, right atrial collapse, and inferior vena cava plethora for the diagnosis of tamponade were calculated (using published sensitivities and specificities for these variables). When the pretest probability of tamponade is high (>50%), both right atrial and right ventricular collapse have high positive and negative predictive values. With a medium (10%) or low (1%) pretest likelihood, all three variables have a high (>97%) negative predictive value (i.e., tamponade can be excluded if absent) but a low positive predictive value.

Constrictive Pericarditis

14. Schnittger I, Bowden RE, Abrams J, Popp RL: Echocardiography: Pericardial thickening and constrictive pericarditis. Am J Cardiol 42:388–395, 1978.

Description of echocardiographic diagnosis of pericardial thickening and correlation with surgical, autopsy, and catheterization findings.

15. von Bibra H, Schober K, Jenni R, et al: Diagnosis of constrictive pericarditis by pulsed Doppler echocardiography of the hepatic vein. Am J Cardiol 63:483–488, 1989.

In patients with constrictive pericarditis, hepatic vein flow showed abrupt reversal in late systole and mid-diastole, similar to the "W pattern" seen on physical examination of the neck veins. This hepatic vein flow pattern had a sensitivity of 68% and a specificity of 100% for the diagnosis of constrictive pericarditis in 51 patients (13 with constrictive pericarditis, 13 controls, 12 with right ventricular pressure overload, and 12 with right ventricular pressure and volume overload).

16. Hatle LK, Appleton CP, Popp RL: Differentiation of constrictive pericarditis and restrictive cardiomyopathy by Doppler echocardiography. Circulation 79:357–370, 1989.

Patients with constrictive pericarditis showed marked respiratory variation in left and right ventricular inflow velocities and isovolumic relaxation times, while patients with restrictive cardiomyopathy did not have respiratory variation. With constrictive pericarditis, the first beat after inspiration showed a decrease in left ventricular inflow velocity, an increase in right ventricular inflow velocity, and an increase in left ventricular isovolumic relaxation time. These changes resolve after pericardiectomy.

17. Aroney CN, Ruddy RD, Dighero H, et al: Differentiation of restrictive cardiomyopathy from pericardial constric-

tion: Assessment of diastolic function by radionuclide angiography. J Am Coll Cardiol 13:1007–1014, 1989.

Diastolic filling curves were evaluated using radionuclide techniques. In patients with constrictive pericarditis, the rate of early diastolic filling and the time to peak filling rate were increased, while the atrial contribution to left ventricular filling was decreased compared with patients with restrictive cardiomyopathy and normal individuals.

18. Garcia MJ, Rodriquez L, Ares M, et al: Differentiation of constrictive pericarditis from restrictive cardiomyopathy: Assessment of left ventricular diastolic velocities in longitudinal axis by Doppler tissue imaging. J Am Coll Cardiol 27:108–114, 1996.

The peak velocity of longitudinal axis expansion, measured with Doppler tissue imaging, is reduced in patients with restrictive cardiomyopathy due to intrinsic myocardial disease. In contrast, longitudinal axis expansion is normal with constrictive pericarditis, as elastic recoil of the myocardium is not affected by extrinsic pericardial compression.

19. Oh JF, Tajik AJ, Appleton CP, et al: Preload reduction to unmask the characteristic Doppler features of constrictive pericarditis: A new observation. Circulation 95:3799–3800, 1997.

Increased filling pressures can mask the reciprocal changes in right and left ventricular diastolic filling seen in patients with constrictive pericarditis. If this diagnosis is suspected on clinical grounds, repeat recordings of ventricular filling after decreasing filling volumes is warranted (for example, in the sitting rather than supine position).

20. Oki T, Tabata T, Yamada H, et al: Right and left ventricular wall motion velocities as diagnostic indicators of constrictive pericarditis. Am J Cardiol 81:465–470, 1998.

Doppler tissue imaging demonstrates an abrupt outward motion of the ventricular walls immediately after the early diastolic filling velocity in patients with constrictive pericarditis compared to normal subjects. This finding has potential value for diagnosis of constrictive pericarditis.

21. Sun JP, Abdalla IA, Yang XS, et al: Respiratory variation of mitral and pulmonary venous Doppler flow velocities in constrictive pericarditis before and after pericardiectomy. J Am Soc Echocardiogr 14:1119–1126, 2001.

In 30 patients undergoing pericardiectomy for constrictive pericarditis, there was a significant decrease after surgery in respiratory variation in peak mitral E-velocity, and in pulmonary vein systolic and diastolic flow velocities. Persistent symptoms were associated with persistent respiratory variation in left ventricular inflow and pulmonary venous flow velocities.

22. Abdalla IA, Murray RD, Lee JC, et al: Does rapid volume loading during transesophageal echocardiography differentiate constrictive pericarditis from restrictive cardiomyopathy. Echocardiography 19:125–134, 2002.

Rapid intravenous infusion of normal saline during transesophageal echocardiography in patients with suspected diastolic dysfunction was well tolerated and enhanced the respiratory variation in the pulmonary vein diastolic flow curve seen in patients with constrictive pericarditis.

The Echo Exam *Pericardial Disease*

Pericardial Effusion

Views Parasternal
Apical
Subcostal

Distinguish from pleural fluid

Size Small (<0.5 cm)
Moderate (0.5–2.0 cm)
Large (>2.0 cm)

Diffuse vs loculated

Evaluate for tamponade physiology if moderate or large

Constrictive Pericarditis

M-mode/2D

Pericardial thickening
Normal LV size and systolic function
LA enlargement
Flattened diastolic wall motion
Abrupt posterior motion of the ventricular septum in early diastole
Dilated inferior vena cava and hepatic veins

Doppler

Prominent y descent on hepatic vein or superior vena cava flow pattern
LV inflow shows prominent E velocity with a rapid early diastolic deceleration slope and a small or absent A velocity
Increase in LV-IVRT by >20% on first beat after inspiration
Respiratory variations in RV/LV diastolic filling (difference >25%) with inspiratory ↑RV ↓LV filling with inspiration
Pulmonary venous flow shows prominent a wave and blunting of systolic phase

Pericardial Tamponade

Clinical Findings

Low cardiac output
Elevated venous pressures
Pulsus paradoxus
Hypotension

2D-Echo

Moderate-large pericardial effusion
Right atrial systolic collapse (duration greater than a third of systole)
Right ventricular diastolic collapse
Reciprocal respiratory changes in RV and LV volumes
Inferior vena cava plethora

Doppler

Respiratory variation in RV and LV diastolic filling
Increased RV filling on first beat after inspiration
Decreased LV filling on first beat after inspiration

LV Pseudoaneurysm

Abrupt transition from normal myocardium to aneurysm
Acute angle between myocardium and aneurysm
Narrow neck
Ratio of neck diameter to aneurysm diameter <0.5
May be lined with thrombus

VALVULAR STENOSIS

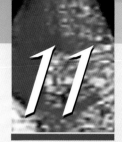

11

BASIC PRINCIPLES

Approach to Evaluation of Valvular Stenosis

Narrowing, or stenosis, of a cardiac valve can be due to a congenitally abnormal valve, a postinflammatory process (e.g., rheumatic), or age-related calcification. As the degree of valve opening decreases, the increasing obstruction to blood flow results in an increased flow velocity and pressure gradient across the valve. In isolated valve stenosis, clinical symptoms typically occur when the valve orifice is reduced to one quarter its normal size. In mixed stenosis and regurgitation, symptoms can occur when each lesion, if isolated, would be considered only moderate in severity.

Secondary changes in patients with valvular stenosis include the response of the specific cardiac chambers affected by pressure overload.

The ventricular response to pressure overload is hypertrophy; the atrial response is dilation. Chronic pressure overload also can lead to irreversible changes in other upstream cardiac chambers and in the pulmonary vascular bed (e.g., in mitral stenosis).

Complete echocardiographic evaluation of the patient with valvular stenosis includes

- diagnostic imaging of the valve to define the etiology of stenosis,
- quantitation of stenosis severity,
- evaluation of coexisting valvular lesions,
- assessment of left ventricular systolic function,
- the response to chronic pressure overload of other upstream cardiac chambers, and the pulmonary vascular bed.

This echocardiographic evaluation then is integrated with pertinent clinical data for a complete evaluation of the patient.

Fluid Dynamics of Valvular Stenosis

High-Velocity Jet

The fluid dynamics of a stenotic valve are characterized by the formation of a laminar, high-velocity jet in the narrowed orifice. The flow profile in cross section at the origin of the jet is relatively blunt (or flat) and remains blunt as the jet reaches its narrowest cross-sectional area in the vena contracta, slightly downstream from the anatomic orifice (Fig. 11–1). Thus the narrowest cross-sectional area of flow (physiologic orifice area) is smaller than the anatomic orifice area. The magnitude of the difference between physiologic and anatomic area depends on orifice geometry and the Reynold's number (a descriptor of the inertial and shear stress properties of the fluid). The ratio of the physiologic to anatomic orifice area is known as the *discharge coefficient.*

The length of the high-velocity jet is dependent on orifice geometry as well and can be vari-

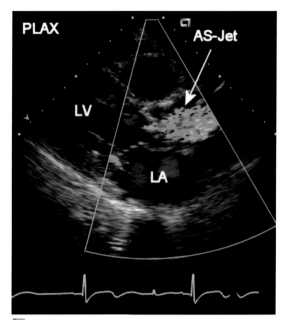

▌ FIGURE 11–2. Color flow imaging in calcific valvular aortic stenosis in a parasternal long-axis view. The post-stenotic flow disturbance identifies the site of obstruction at the valvular level, but the laminar jet is short so that a jet direction is not clearly demonstrated.

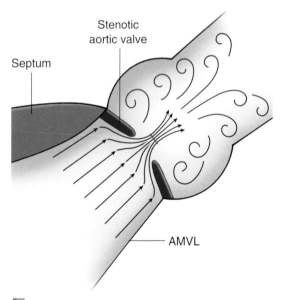

▌ FIGURE 11–1. Schematic illustration of the fluid dynamics of the stenotic aortic valve in systole. The left ventricular outflow tract (LVOT) is bounded by the septum and anterior mitral valve leaflet (AMVL). As LVOT flow accelerates and converges, a relatively flat velocity profile occurs proximal to the stenotic valve, as indicated by the *arrowheads.* Flow accelerates in a spatially small zone adjacent to the valve as blood enters the narrowed orifice. In the stenotic orifice, a high-velocity laminar jet is formed with the narrowest flowstream (vena contracta, indicated by the *dots*) occurring downstream from the orifice. Beyond the jet, flow is disturbed, with blood cells moving in multiple directions and velocities. (Reprinted with permission from Judge KW, Otto CM: Cardiol Clin 8:203, 1990.)

able in the clinical setting with, for example, a very short jet across a deformed, irregular, calcified aortic valve and a longer jet across a smoothly tapering, symmetric, rheumatic mitral valve or a congenitally stenotic semilunar valve (Figs. 11–2 and 11–3).

Relationship between Pressure Gradient and Velocity

The pressure gradient across the stenotic valve is related to the velocity in the jet, according to the unsteady Bernoulli equation:

$$\Delta P = \underbrace{\tfrac{1}{2}\rho(v_2^2 - v_1^2)}_{\substack{\text{Convective} \\ \text{acceleration}}} + \underbrace{\rho(dv/dt)dx}_{\substack{\text{Local} \\ \text{acceleration}}} + \underbrace{R(v)}_{\substack{\text{Viscous} \\ \text{resistance}}}$$

$$(11–1)$$

where ΔP is the pressure gradient across the stenosis (mm Hg), ρ is the mass density of blood (1.06×10^3 kg/m^3), v_2 is velocity in the stenotic jet, v_1 is velocity proximal to the stenosis, $(dv/dt)dx$ is the time-varying velocity at each distance along the flowstream, and R is a constant describing the viscous losses for that fluid and orifice. Historically, Daniel Bernoulli first described this equation in approximately 1738 from studies of steady water flow in rigid tubes. The concepts were later expanded and refined by Euler. Of note, these

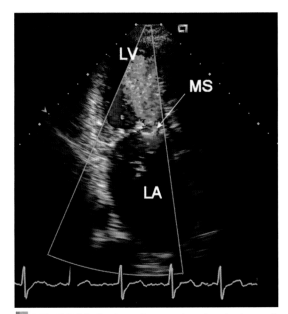

■ **FIGURE 11–3.** Color flow imaging of a mitral stenosis jet in an apical long-axis view. Note the long jet directed toward the LV apex with a well-defined proximal isovelocity surface area on the left atrial side of the valve.

equations may not be strictly applicable to pulsatile blood flow in compliant chambers and vessels, although clinical studies have shown that remarkably accurate pressure-gradient predictions can be made with this approach. This equation was first applied to Doppler data by Holen in 1976 for stenotic mitral valves and by Hatle in 1979 for stenotic aortic valves.

Eliminating the terms for viscous losses and acceleration, substituting known values for the mass density of blood, and adding a conversion factor for measuring velocity in units of meters per second (m/s) and pressure gradient in millimeters of mercury (mm Hg), the Bernoulli equation can be reduced to

$$\Delta P = 4(v_2^2 - v_1^2) \qquad (11\text{-}2)$$

If the proximal velocity is less than 1 m/s, as is commonly the case for stenotic valves, it becomes even smaller when squared [for example, $(0.8)^2 = 0.64$]. Thus the proximal velocity often can be ignored in the clinical setting so that:

$$\Delta P = 4v^2 \qquad (11\text{-}3)$$

This simplified Bernoulli equation allows highly accurate and reproducible calculation of maximum pressure gradients (from maximum velocity) and mean pressure gradients (by integrating the instantaneous pressure difference over the flow period).

Distal Flow Disturbance

Distal to the stenotic jet, the flowstream becomes disorganized with multiple blood flow velocities and directions, although fully developed turbulence, as strictly defined in fluid dynamic terms, may not occur. The distance that this flow disturbance propagates downstream is related to stenosis severity. In addition, the *presence* of a downstream flow disturbance can be extremely useful in defining the exact anatomic site of obstruction, for example, allowing differentiation of subvalvular outflow obstruction (flow disturbance on the ventricular side of the valve) from valvular obstruction (flow disturbance only distal to the valve).

Proximal Flow Patterns

Proximal to a stenotic valve, flow is smooth and organized (laminar) with a normal flow velocity. The spatial flow velocity profile proximal to a stenotic valve depends on valve anatomy, inlet geometry, and the degree of flow acceleration. For example, in calcific aortic stenosis, the acceleration of blood flow by ventricular systole coupled with a tapering outflow tract geometry results in a relatively uniform flow velocity (a "flat" flow profile) across the outflow tract just proximal to the stenotic valve. Immediately adjacent to the valve orifice there is acceleration as flow converges to form the high-velocity jet, but this region of proximal acceleration is spatially small. The flow profile differs slightly for congenital aortic stenosis in that the proximal acceleration region under the domed leaflets in systole is larger than with calcific stenosis. However, proximal flow patterns are similar regardless of disease etiology in that a relatively flat velocity profile is present at the aortic annulus.

In contrast, the flow pattern proximal to the stenotic mitral valve is quite different (Fig. 11–4). Here, the left atrial to left ventricular pressure gradient drives flow passively from the large inlet chamber (the left atrium) abruptly across the stenotic orifice. Proximal flow acceleration is prominent over a large region of the left atrium. The three-dimensional (3D) velocity profile is curved; that is, flow velocities are faster adjacent to and in the center of a line continuous with the jet direction through the narrowed orifice and slower at increasing radial distances from the valve orifice. The proximal velocity profile of an atrioventricular valve thus is hemi-elliptical, unlike the more flattened velocity profile proximal to a stenotic semilunar valve. Any 3D surface area proximal to a narrowed orifice at which all the

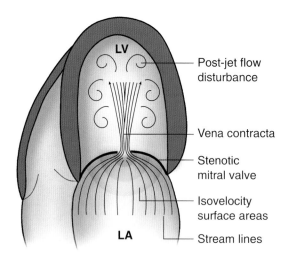

FIGURE 11–4. Schematic diagram of the fluid dynamics of rheumatic mitral stenosis. The stream lines of flow accelerate as they approach the stenotic orifice, with several curved proximal isovelocity surface areas indicated. The mitral stenosis jet is long, with the postjet flow disturbance occurring adjacent and distal to the laminar jet.

blood velocities are equal can be referred to as a *proximal isovelocity surface area* (PISA).

The clinical importance of these flow patterns is that stroke volume can be calculated proximal to a stenotic valve based on knowledge of the cross-sectional area of flow and the spatial mean flow velocity over the period of flow, as described in Chapter 6. This concept applies to the flat flow profile proximal to a stenotic aortic valve (used in the continuity equation), to the proximal flow patterns seen in mitral stenosis, and to the PISAs seen with regurgitant lesions (see Chapter 12).

AORTIC STENOSIS

Diagnostic Imaging of the Aortic Valve

Aortic valve stenosis in adults most often is due to

- calcific aortic stenosis,
- congenital valve disease (bicuspid or unicuspid), or
- rheumatic valve disease.

Calcific Aortic Stenosis

The most common etiology of valvular aortic stenosis in adults is age-related calcification of an anatomically normal trileaflet valve. Calcification occurs slowly over many years and initially presents on two-dimensional (2D) echo as aortic valve "sclerosis"—areas of increased echogenicity,

typically at the base of the valve leaflets, without significant obstruction to left ventricular outflow. Clinically significant obstruction tends to occur from age 70 to 85. When obstruction is present, 2D imaging shows a marked increase in echogenicity of the leaflets consistent with calcific disease and reduced systolic opening. When aortic stenosis is suspected, a systolic leaflet separation of 15 mm or more by 2D or 2D-guided M-mode echocardiography reliably excludes severe obstruction. When the leaflets are abnormal and systolic separation is less than 15 mm, the degree of obstruction may be mild, moderate, or severe, depending on the cross-sectional area of the narrowed orifice. Direct measurement of valve area on short-axis 2D imaging is possible in some patients either with excellent transthoracic images or from a transesophageal approach. However, directly planimetered aortic valve areas should be interpreted with caution due to the complex 3D anatomy of the orifice in calcific degenerative stenosis. It is critical to ensure that the image plane is aligned at the narrowest orifice of the valve, although if the orifice is nonplanar, planimetry of apparent valve area may be misleading. Even when carefully performed, 2D valve area reflects anatomic valve area, whereas Doppler data provide functional valve area (Fig. 11–5).

Bicuspid Aortic Valve

Secondary calcification of a bicuspid aortic valve can be difficult to distinguish from calcification of a trileaflet valve once stenosis becomes severe. Average age at symptom onset is younger for adults with bicuspid valve stenosis, with presentation typically between the ages of 45 and 65.

Earlier in the disease course, a bicuspid valve can be identified on 2D parasternal short-axis views by demonstrating that there are only two open leaflets in systole (Fig. 11–6). Long-axis views show systolic bowing of the leaflets into the aorta, resulting in a "domelike" appearance. M-mode recordings may help in identifying a bicuspid valve if an eccentric closure line is present but can be misleading in terms of the degree of leaflet separation if the M-mode is taken through the base, rather than the tips, of the bowed leaflets. Similarly, planimetry of valve area may be erroneous if the image plane is not aligned with the narrowest point at the leaflet tips.

Typically, the two leaflets are unequal in size, with the anterior (if the leaflet opening is anteroposterior) or rightward (if the leaflet opening is lateromedial) leaflet being larger. Many bicuspid valves have a raphe in the larger leaflet so that the closed valve in diastole appears trileaflet; accurate identification of the number of aortic valve leaflets

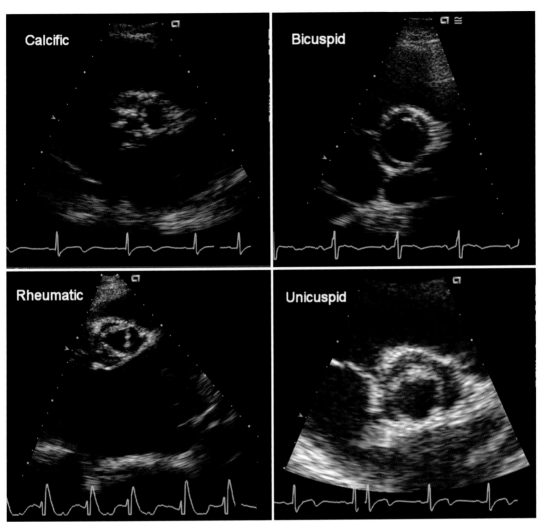

■ FIGURE 11–5. Parasternal mid-systolic short axis views of the four most common causes of valvular aortic stenosis. Calcific aortic stenosis is characterized by calcific masses on the aortic side of the leaflet that result in increased leaflet stiffness without commissural fusion. Calcific shadowing and reverberations limit image quality. In a young patient with a congenital bicuspid valve, the two leaflets (with a raphe in the anterior leaflet) open widely in systole. Later in life, secondary calcific changes are seen that result in stenosis. The diagnostic features of rheumatic stenosis are commissural fusion and mitral valve involvement, with the characteristic triangular aortic valve opening in systole. The unicuspid valve, seen in young adults, has only one point of attachment (at the 6 o'clock position) with a funnel-shaped valve opening. Planimetry of valve area is inaccurate unless the image plane is at the narrowest segment of the doming valve in systole.

can be made only in systole. Doppler interrogation of the aortic valve should be performed whenever a bicuspid valve is suspected to evaluate for stenosis and/or regurgitation.

Rheumatic Aortic Stenosis

Rheumatic valvular disease preferentially involves the mitral valve, so rheumatic aortic stenosis is diagnosed when aortic disease occurs concurrently with rheumatic mitral valve disease. The rheumatic disease process results in commissural fusion of the aortic leaflets, similar to the pathology seen

in rheumatic mitral stenosis. Two-dimensional imaging may show increased echogenicity along the leaflet edges, commissural fusion, and systolic doming of the aortic leaflets. Often, however, the echocardiographic images appear similar to those of calcific aortic stenosis (other than the presence of rheumatic mitral valve disease).

Congenital Aortic Stenosis

Congenital aortic stenosis usually is diagnosed in childhood, but some patients may not become symptomatic until young adulthood or may

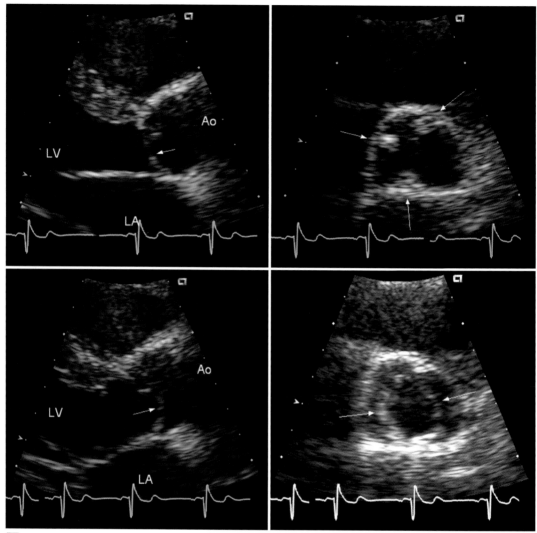

■ **FIGURE 11–6.** Bicuspid aortic valve with diastolic *(top)* and systolic *(bottom)* frames shown in parasternal long-axis *(left)* and short-axis *(right)* views. Note the diastolic sagging and systolic doming of the leaflets in the long-axis view. In short-axis view, only two leaflets are seen to open in systole with the commissures at 4- and 10-o'clock positions.

present with restenosis after surgical valvotomy performed in childhood or adolescence. These patients most often have a unicuspid valve with a single eccentric orifice and prominent systolic doming.

Differential Diagnosis

The differential diagnosis of left ventricular outflow obstruction includes

■ fixed subvalvular obstruction (a subaortic membrane or a muscular subaortic stenosis),
■ dynamic subaortic obstruction (hypertrophic cardiomyopathy), and
■ supravalvular stenosis.

In a patient with a clinical diagnosis of valvular aortic stenosis, the echocardiographic study should demonstrate whether the obstruction is, in fact, valvular or if one of these other diagnoses accounts for the clinical presentation (Fig. 11–7).

A subaortic membrane should be suspected in young adults when the valve anatomy is not clearly stenotic, yet Doppler examination reveals a high transaortic pressure gradient. Since the membrane may be poorly depicted on a transthoracic study, transesophageal imaging should be considered when this diagnosis is suspected (see Fig. 17–3). The spatial orientation of the jet and the shape of the continuous-wave Doppler velocity curve are similar for fixed obstructions,

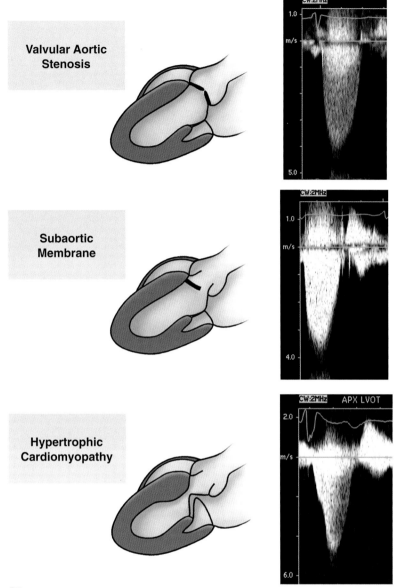

FIGURE 11–7. Examples of the shape of the continuous-wave Doppler velocity curve in valvular aortic stenosis, fixed subvalvular obstruction due to a subaortic membrane, and dynamic obstruction due to hypertrophic cardiomyopathy. Note that the continuous-wave curves for subvalvular and valvular aortic stenosis are similar, although coarse fluttering of the valve with subvalvular obstruction results in a "rough" appearance of the systolic velocity curve. These can be distinguished by 2D and color flow imaging. The shape of the curve with dynamic obstruction is distinctly different with the velocity peaking in late systole.

whether sub-, supra-, or valvular, but careful pulsed Doppler or color flow imaging allows localization of the level of obstruction by detection of the poststenotic flow disturbance.

In dynamic outflow obstruction, the timing and shape of the late-peaking continuous-wave Doppler velocity curve are distinctive. In addition, the degree of obstruction changes dramatically with provocative maneuvers, as detailed in Chapter 9. In the occasional patient with both subvalvular *and* valvular obstruction, high-pulse-repetition-frequency Doppler ultrasound can be helpful in defining the maximum velocities at each site of obstruction.

Quantitation of Stenosis Severity

The severity of valvular aortic stenosis can be determined accurately using equations derived from our understanding of the fluid dynamics of a stenotic valve. Standard evalution of stenosis severity includes

- measurement of maximum aortic jet velocity,
- calculation of maximum and mean transaortic pressure gradients,
- determination of continuity equation valve area, and the
- ratio of outflow tract to aortic jet velocity.

Pressure Gradients

Maximum transaortic pressure gradient (ΔP_{max}) can be calculated from the maximum aortic jet velocity (V_{max}) using the simplified Bernoulli equation (Fig. 11–8):

$$\Delta P_{max} = 4V_{max}^2 \qquad (11\text{–}4)$$

Mean pressure gradient (ΔP_{mean}) can be calculated by digitizing the aortic jet velocity curve (where $v_1, \ldots, v_n$, are instantaneous velocities) and averaging the instantaneous gradients over the systolic ejection period.

$$\Delta P_{mean} = \frac{4v_1^2 + 4v_2^2 + 4v_3^2 + \cdots + 4v_n^2}{n}$$
$$(11\text{–}5)$$

Interestingly, in native aortic valve stenosis, transaortic pressure gradient correlates closely and linearly with maximum transaortic gradient so that mean gradient can be approximated from published regression equations as

$$\Delta P_{mean} = (\Delta P_{max}/1.45) + 2\,\text{mm Hg} \qquad (11\text{–}6)$$

or (from a different study)

$$\Delta P_{mean} = 2.4(V_{max})^2 \qquad (11\text{–}7)$$

Note that these two equations give similar results.

With careful attention to technical details, Doppler-determined pressure gradients are accurate, as has been demonstrated in numerous in vitro and animal models and in clinical studies (Table 11–1). Although Doppler maximum gradients correspond to maximum instantaneous gradients by catheter measurement and Doppler mean gradients correspond to catheter-measured mean gradients, neither Doppler gradient correlates with the peak-to-peak gradient reported at catheterization. In fact, peak aortic and peak left ventricular pressures do not occur simultaneously, so none of the instantaneous velocities recorded with Doppler ultrasound are strictly comparable

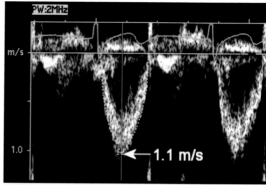

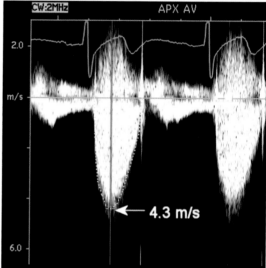

█ FIGURE 11–8. Pulsed Doppler recording of LV outflow tract velocity *(top)* and continuous-wave Doppler recording of an aortic stenosis jet *(bottom)*. The continuous wave Doppler was recorded from an apical approach with a dedicated nonimaging transducer after evaluation from several windows with careful angulation to identify the highest velocity jet. This represents the most parallel intercept angle between the direction of blood flow and the stenotic jet. The maximum pressure gradient is calculated as $\Delta P = 4v^2$, with mean pressure gradient determined by integrating the instantaneous gradients over the systolic ejection period. The velocity ratio is 0.26.

with this clinical measurement. Potential confusion about Doppler pressure gradient data in an individual patient can be avoided by clearly identifying the specific type of gradient measured, for example "maximum instantaneous" or "mean systolic" (Fig. 11–9).

Physiologic changes in pressure gradient should be taken into consideration when comparing nonsimultaneous data recordings and in patient management decisions. Pressure gradients depend on volume flow rate, as well as the degree of valve narrowing, so in an individual patient the

TABLE 11-1					
Selected Studies Validating Doppler Pressure Gradients in Valvular Stenosis (in vivo Simultaneous Data)					
First Author/ Year	**N**	**Study Group/Model**	**R**	**Range (mm Hg)**	**SEE (mm Hg)**
Callahan/1985	120	Supravalvular constriction (canines)	$0.99\ (\Delta P_{max})$ $0.98\ (\Delta P_{mean})$	7–179 N/A	5.2 4.3
Smith/1985	88	Supravalvular constriction (canines)	$0.98\ (\Delta P_{max})$ $0.98\ (\Delta P_{mean})$	5–166 5–116	5.3 3.3
Currie/1985	100	Adults with valvular aortic stenosis	$0.92\ (\Delta P_{max})$ $0.92\ (\Delta P_{mean})$	2–180 0–112	15 10
Smith/1986	33	Adults with valvular aortic stenosis	$0.85\ (\Delta P_{max})$	27–138	N/A
Simpson/1985	24	Adults with valvular aortic stenosis	$0.98\ (\Delta P_{max})$	0–120	N/A
Burwash/1993	98	Chronic valvular aortic stenosis (canines)	$0.95\ (\Delta P_{max})$ $0.91(\Delta P_{mean})$	10–128 5–77	8.4 5.3

Data from Callahan et al: Am J Cardiol 56:989–993, 1985; Smith et al: J Am Coll Cardiol 6:1306–1314, 1985; Currie et al: Circulation 71:1162–1169, 1985; Smith et al: Am Heart J 111:245–252, 1986; Simpson et al: Br Heart J 53:636–639, 1985; Burwash et al: Am J Physiol 265 (Heart Circ Physiol 34):H734–H1743, 1993.

pressure gradient will rise when transaortic stroke volume increases (e.g., anxiety, exercise) and will fall when stroke volume decreases (e.g., sedation, hypovolemia).

The dependence of pressure gradients on volume flow rate can lead to erroneous conclusions about stenosis severity in adult patients with either a chronically elevated or depressed transaortic stroke volume. For example, a patient with coexisting aortic regurgitation will have a high transaortic pressure gradient with only a moderate degree of valve narrowing. Conversely, a patient with left ventricular systolic dysfunction or coexisting mitral regurgitation may have a low transaortic pressure gradient despite severe aortic stenosis. These coexisting conditions are common in adults with valvular aortic stenosis, so determination of the stenotic orifice area is essential for complete evaluation of disease severity.

Continuity Equation Valve Area

Aortic valve area can be calculated based on the principle of continuity of flow. Specifically, the

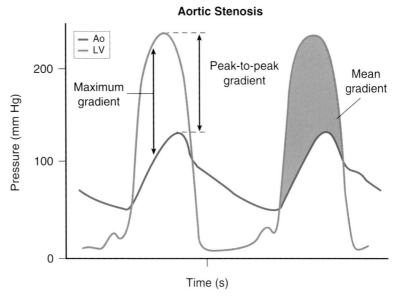

Aortic Stenosis

FIGURE 11-9. Example of left ventricular (LV) and aortic (Ao) pressures measured with fluid-filled catheters in a patient with severe valvular aortic stenosis. Note that the maximum instantaneous gradient is greater than the peak-to-peak gradient. Mean gradient is indicated by the shaded area.

stroke volume (SV) just proximal to the aortic valve (SV_{LVOT}) and that in the stenotic valve orifice (SV_{Ao}) are equal:

$$SV_{LVOT} = SV_{Ao} \qquad (11\text{--}8)$$

If flow is laminar with a spatially flat velocity profile,

$$SV = CSA \times VTI \qquad (11\text{--}9)$$

where CSA is the cross-sectional area of flow (cm²), SV is stroke volume (cm³), and VTI is the velocity-time integral (cm). Because flow both proximal to and in the aortic jet itself is laminar with a reasonably flat velocity profile,

$$CSA_{LVOT} \times VTI_{LVOT} = CSA_{Ao} \times VTI_{Ao} \qquad (11\text{--}10)$$

All the variables in this equation can be measured with 2D or Doppler echo except CSA_{Ao}, which is the stenotic aortic valve area (AVA) itself. Rearranging the equation,

$$AVA = (CSA_{LVOT} \times VTI_{LVOT})/VTI_{Ao} \qquad (11\text{--}11)$$

Thus, the measurements needed to calculate valve area with the continuity equation are (Fig. 11–10):

■ LV outflow tract diameter,
■ LV outflow tract velocity time integral, and
■ aortic jet velocity time integral.

LV outflow tract diameter, measured on a 2D parasternal long-axis midsystolic image, is used to calculate a circular outflow tract cross-sectional area (CSA). The velocity-time integral in the outflow tract is recorded with pulsed Doppler echocardiography from an apical approach. The velocity-time integral in the aortic stenosis jet is recorded with continuous-wave Doppler ultra-

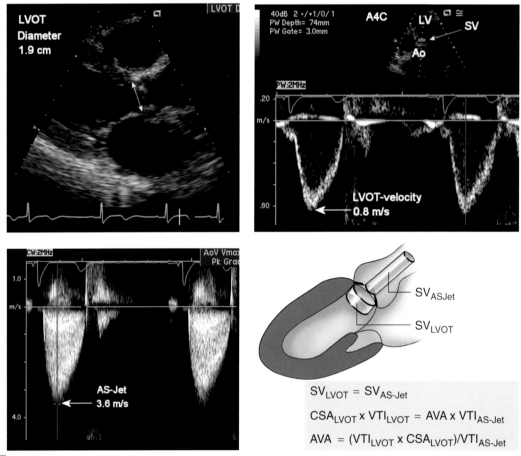

■ **FIGURE 11–10.** Continuity equation aortic valve area (AVA) calculations require measurement of left ventricular outflow tract diameter from a parasternal long-axis view for circular cross-sectional area (CSA) calculation *(above, right)*, pulsed Doppler recording of the left ventricular outflow tract velocity-time integral (VTI) from an apical approach *(above, left)*, and continuous-wave Doppler recording of the aortic stenosis velocity-time integral (VTI AS-jet) from whichever window gives the highest-velocity signal.

sound from the window that yields the highest velocity signal.

For clinical use, the continuity equation can be simplified by substituting maximum velocities (V) for velocity-time integrals. Since the shape and timing of outflow tract and aortic jet velocity curves are similar, their ratios are nearly identical:

$$VTI_{LVOT}/VTI_{Ao} = V_{LVOT}/V_{Ao} \quad (11–12)$$

The simplified continuity equation then is

$$AVA = CSA_{LVOT} \times (V_{LVOT}/V_{Ao}) \quad (11–13)$$

Outflow tract diameter must be measured in each patient for accurate valve area calculations. While the group mean outflow tract diameter is smaller in women than in men and correlates with body size when people of all ages from infancy to adulthood are considered, in the adult population, the relationship between gender or body size (either body surface area, height, or weight) and outflow tract diameter is weak. On the other hand, outflow tract diameter tends to remain constant in a given adult patient over time. Apparent differences in diameter at follow-up visits are more likely to represent measurement error than an actual interval anatomic change. Thus, the ratio of outflow tract velocity to aortic jet velocity can be used to follow disease progression in individual patients.

Velocity Ratio

Although not strictly comparable to valve area, the velocity ratio also may be a useful measure of stenosis severity that, in effect, is "indexed" for body size. Obviously, normal valve area is dependent on body size—infants and children have smaller valve areas than adults and large adults are expected to have larger valve areas than small adults. One way to take the effect of body size into account is to "index" valve area by dividing it by body surface area (BSA):

$$Aortic\ valve\ index = AVA/BSA \quad (11–14)$$

An alternate approach is to define the "normal" valve area for that individual as the cross-sectional area of the outflow tract. Then, the increase in velocity from outflow tract to aortic jet reflects stenosis severity regardless of body size. If

$$"Normal"\ AVA = CSA_{LVOT}$$

and

$$Actual\ AVA \cong "normal"\ AVA \times \frac{V_{LVOT}}{V_{Ao}}$$

then

$$\frac{Actual\ AVA}{"Normal"\ AVA} = \frac{V_{LVOT}}{V_{Ao}} \quad (11–15)$$

A velocity ratio near 1 indicates little obstruction, a velocity ratio of 0.5 indicates a valve area that is one half normal, and a velocity ratio of 0.25 indicates a valve area reduced to one fourth its normal value (see Fig. 11–8).

Technical Considerations and Potential Pitfalls

Continuity equation valve areas have been well validated in comparison with Gorlin formula valve areas calculated from invasive measurements of pressure gradient and cardiac output (Table 11–2). Some of the discrepancies between Doppler echo and invasive measurements of valve area are due to measurement variability for the invasive data and to limitations of the Gorlin formula itself. However, technical considerations in recording the Doppler and 2D echo data and the measurement variability of the noninvasive technique also are important (Table 11–3).

With careful attention to technical details, an experienced laboratory can obtain accurate noninvasive data for calculation of transaortic pressure gradients and valve areas in nearly all adults with valvular aortic stenosis. However, accurate noninvasive quantitation of aortic stenosis severity is a technically demanding procedure, and a significant learning-curve effect is seen in each laboratory for this clinical application. There are several potential pitfalls in the Doppler approach, as detailed below. Each laboratory should confirm the accuracy of its data by comparison with those of an experienced echocardiography laboratory or with other diagnostic tests.

THE AORTIC JET. Owing to the high velocities seen in aortic stenosis (usually 3 to 7 m/s), continuous-wave Doppler ultrasound is needed for accurate measurement of the aortic jet signal. When aortic stenosis is suspected, the examination should include use of a nonimaging, dedicated continuous-wave Doppler transducer. The smaller "footprint" of the dedicated transducer allows optimal positioning and angulation of the ultrasound beam. In addition, a dedicated continuous-wave transducer has a higher signal-to-noise ratio than a combined imaging and Doppler transducer.

In recording the aortic jet velocity signal, a search is made for the highest-frequency shift. This signal then is assumed to represent a near-parallel intercept angle (θ) between the ultrasound beam and the direction of the jet. In this situation,

TABLE 11–2

Selected Studies of Aortic Valve Area Determination

First Author/ Year	Comparison	N	Study Group	R*	Range (cm²)	SEE* (cm²)
Hakki/1981	Simplified vs. original Gorlin formula	60	Aortic stenosis	0.96	0.2–2.0	0.10
Skjaerpe/1985	Cont eq vs. Gorlin	30	Aortic stenosis	0.89	0.4–2.4	0.12
Zoghbi/1986	Cont eq vs. Gorlin	39	Aortic stenosis	0.95	0.4–2.0	0.15
Otto/1986	Cont eq vs. Gorlin	48	Aortic stenosis	0.71	0.2–3.7	0.32
Teirstein/1986	Cont eq vs. Gorlin	30	Aortic stenosis	0.88	0.3–1.6	0.17
Oh/1988	Cont eq vs. Gorlin	100	Aortic stenosis	0.83	0.2–1.8	0.19
Danielson/ 1989	Cont eq vs. Gorlin	100	Aortic stenosis	0.96	0.4–2.0	–
Cannon/1985	Gorlin vs. videotape of valve opening	42	Porcine valves in pulsatile flow model	0.87	0.6–2.5	0.28
	New formula vs. actual orifice area	42	Porcine valves in pulsatile flow model	0.98	0.6–2.5	0.11
Segal/1987	Cont eq vs. actual valve area		In vitro pulsatile flow with orifice plates	0.99	0.05–0.5	0.016
	Gorlin formula vs. actual valve area			0.87		0.047
Cannon/1988	Gorlin vs. known valve area	135	Prosthetic aortic valves	0.39	0.6–2.3	–
Nishimura/ 1988	Cont eq vs. Gorlin	55	Pre-BAV	0.72	0.2–0.9	0.10
			Post-BAV	0.61	0.5–1.3	0.17
Desnoyers/ 1988	Cont eq vs. Gorlin	42	Pre-BAV	0.74	0.3–1.3	–
Tribouilloy/ 1994	TEE vs. cont eq	54	Aortic stenosis	0.96	0.3–2.0	0.11
	TEE vs. Gorlin			0.90		0.12
Cormier/1996	TEE vs. Gorlin	45	Aortic stenosis	0.74	0.5–1.4	–
Kim/1997	TEE vs. Gorlin	81	Aortic stenosis	0.89	0.4–2.0	0.04

*If not stated in the publication, statistics were calculated from the raw data provided in tables. A blank indicates that data for this calculation were not available.

AS, aortic stenosis; BAV, balloon aortic valvuloplasty; Cont eq, continuity equation; Gorlin, Gorlin formula valve area; TEE, Planimetered 2D valve area on transesophageal echocardiography.

Data from Hakki et al: Circulation 63:1050–1055, 1981; Skjaerpe et al: Circulation 72:810–818, 1985; Zoghbi et al: Circulation 73:452–459, 1986; Otto et al: J Am Coll Cardiol 7:509–517, 1986; Teirstein et al: J Am Coll Cardiol 8:1059–1065, 1986; Oh et al: J Am Coll Cardiol 11:1227–1234, 1988; Danielson et al: Am J Cardiol 63:1107–1111, 1989; Cannon et al: Circulation 71:1170–1178, 1985; Segal et al: J Am Coll Cardiol 9:1294–1305, 1987; Cannon et al: Am J Cardiol 62:113–116, 1988; Nishimura et al: Circulation 78:791–799, 1988; Desnoyers et al: Am J Cardiol 62:1078–1084, 1988; Tribouilloy et al: Am Heart J 128:526–532, 1994; Cormier et al: Am J Cardiol 77:882–885, 1996; Kim KS et al: Am J Cardiol 79:436–441, 1997.

TABLE 11-3

Pitfalls in Echocardiographic Evaluation of Aortic Stenosis

Technical

Acoustic access
Intercept angle between aortic stenosis jet and ultrasound
  beam
Outflow tract diameter imaging
Respiratory motion
Learning-curve effect

Interpretation

Identification of flow signal origin (AS vs. MR)
Beat-to-beat variability (AF, PVCs)
Intra- and interobserver measurement variability
Calculation errors

Physiology

Interim changes in heart rate or stroke volume
Dependence of velocity and ΔP on volume flow rate
Progression of AS severity

Standards of Reference

Maximum vs. peak-to-peak ΔP
Continuity vs. Gorlin formula valve areas

cosine θ equals 1 and thus can be ignored in the Doppler equation (see Chapter 1). Any deviation from a parallel intercept angle will result in underestimation of jet velocity. For example, an intercept angle of 30° will result in a measured velocity of 4.3 m/s when the actual velocity is 5 m/s. Underestimation of velocity, which is squared in the Bernoulli equation, results in a large error in calculated pressure gradient. However, intercept angles within 15° of parallel will result in an error in velocity measurement of 5% or less.

The direction of the aortic jet often is eccentric relative to both the plane of the aortic valve and the long axis of the aorta and rarely can be predicted from the 2D images. Occasionally, jet direction can be visualized with color flow imaging, but, more often, the direction of the short jet of calcific stenosis cannot be identified. Even when jet direction is seen in a single tomographic plane, the orientation of the jet in the elevational plane remains unknown.

Pragmatically, the solution to the problem of aligning the ultrasound beam parallel to an aortic jet of unknown direction is to perform a careful search from several acoustic windows with optimal patient positioning and multiple transducer angulations. The highest-velocity signal obtained then is assumed to represent the most parallel intercept angle. At a minimum, the aortic jet should be interrogated from an apical approach with the patient in a steep left lateral decubitus position on an examination bed with an apical cutout, from a high right parasternal position with the patient in a right lateral decubitus position, and from the suprasternal notch with the patient supine and the neck extended. Even then, the possibility of underestimation of jet velocity due to a nonparallel intercept angle cannot be excluded. In some cases, the highest-velocity signal may be recorded from a subcostal or left parasternal window.

When the continuous-wave beam is aligned with the aortic jet, a smooth velocity curve is seen with a well-defined peak velocity and spectral darkening along the outer edge of the velocity curve. Audibly, the signal is high frequency and tonal. The spectral recording should be made with an appropriate velocity scale (at least 1 m/s higher than the observed maximum jet velocity), with wall filters set at a high level, and with gain adjustment to provide clear definition of the maximum velocity. Maximum velocity is measured at the edge of the dark velocity envelope. The velocity-time integral is measured by digitizing the velocity curve over systole.

Care is needed to correctly identify the origin of the high-velocity jet. Other high-velocity systolic jets (Table 11-4 and Fig. 11-11) may be mistaken for aortic stenosis if inadequate attention is paid to timing, shape, and associated diastolic flow curves. In some cases, 2D-"guided" continuous-wave Doppler may be helpful in correct identification of the jet, followed by recording with a nonimaging transducer for optimal signal quality.

OUTFLOW TRACT DIAMETER. Left ventricular outflow tract diameter is measured in midsystole, just proximal to and parallel with the plane of the stenotic aortic valve, from the inner edge of the septal endocardial echo to the leading edge of the base of the anterior mitral leaflet. A parasternal long-axis view provides the most accurate measurement because it depends on the axial (rather than lateral) resolution of the ultrasound

TABLE 11-4

Other High-Velocity Systolic Jets that May Be Mistaken for Aortic Stenosis

Subaortic obstruction (fixed or dynamic)
Mitral regurgitation
Tricuspid regurgitation
Ventricular septal defect
Pulmonic or branch pulmonary artery stenosis
Peripheral vascular stenosis (e.g., subclavian artery)

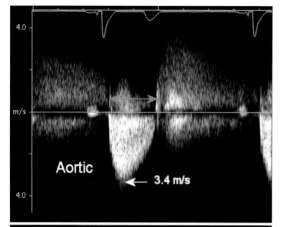

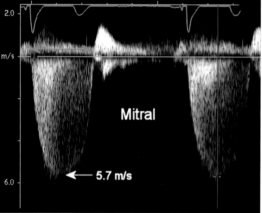

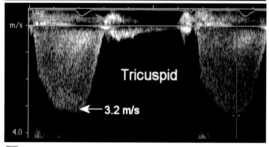

FIGURE 11-11. From an apical approach, three different high-velocity systolic jets directed away from the transducer were recorded in this patient with moderate aortic stenosis, mild mitral regurgitation, and severe pulmonary hypertension. These three flow signals can be differentiated based on timing, shape, and associated diastolic flow signals.

beam. Outflow tract CSA is assumed to be circular so that

$$CSA_{LVOT} = \pi(D/2)^2 \qquad (11\text{--}16)$$

Note that small errors in outflow tract diameter measurement may lead to large errors in calculated cross-sectional area. Furthermore, of the measurements made for evaluating aortic stenosis severity, outflow tract diameter shows the greatest intraob-

server and interobserver variability. Several measurements should be averaged to minimize this potential source of error.

OUTFLOW TRACT VELOCITY. The outflow tract systolic velocity signal is recorded from an apical approach using pulsed Doppler echo. Either an anteriorly angulated four-chamber view or an apical long-axis view can be used. A sample volume 3 to 5 mm in length is positioned just proximal to the region of acceleration into the stenotic jet. Correct positioning is ensured by starting with the sample volume *in* the jet and slowly repositioning it apically until a smooth velocity curve with a well-defined peak velocity and little spectral broadening is seen. The presence of an aortic valve closing (but not opening) click indicates that the sample volume is immediately adjacent to the valve. A transducer position is chosen initially that indicates a parallel alignment between the ultrasound beam and the long axis of the outflow tract on 2D imaging. Then, transducer position and angulation are adjusted, based on the audible Doppler signal and the velocity curve, to record the highest-velocity signal proximal to the flow acceleration region. In addition, the sample volume is moved laterally across the outflow tract in each apical view to document a flat flow velocity profile.

The rationale for this protocol for sample volume positioning is that the outflow tract diameter and velocity signals need to be recorded *at the same* anatomic site for accurate transaortic stroke volume calculations. Necessarily, these two recordings are made nonsimultaneously from different acoustic windows because of the need for a parallel orientation between the Doppler beam and the direction of blood flow for accurate velocity measurement versus a perpendicular orientation between the 2D echo beam and the outflow tract for accurate diameter measurement. Measuring both immediately adjacent to the stenotic valve provides a reference point that ensures that both measurements are made at the same spatial location.

The maximum outflow tract velocity is measured at the edge of the most intense spectral signal. The time-velocity integral is measured by tracing the modal velocity of the systolic flow curve. Wall filters are set low enough that the systolic ejection period is clearly defined.

Coexisting Valvular Disease

A high percentage (approximately 80%) of patients with predominant aortic stenosis also have aortic regurgitation, most often mild or moderate in severity. The degree of regurgitation can be evaluated as described in Chapter 12.

Although coexisting aortic regurgitation results in an increase in the transaortic pressure gradient (due to increased transaortic volume flow), valve area calculations are accurate because the stroke volume in the continuity equation still represents transaortic stroke volume.

Coexisting mitral regurgitation also is common due to mitral annular calcification in adults with calcific aortic stenosis. Again, mitral regurgitant severity can be evaluated as described in Chapter 12. Particular attention should be directed toward aortic valve area calculations when mitral regurgitation is present. Otherwise, severe aortic stenosis may be missed if the transaortic pressure gradient is low due to low transaortic volume flow.

Patients with rheumatic aortic stenosis may have significant mitral stenosis, mitral regurgitation, or mixed mitral disease. Evaluation of aortic stenosis severity is unaffected by these coexisting lesions other than the aforementioned potential for a low transaortic pressure gradient if the transaortic volume flow rate is depressed.

Response of the Left Ventricle to Valvular Aortic Stenosis

The left ventricular response to the chronic pressure overload of valvular aortic stenosis is concentric hypertrophy—an increase in left ventricular mass due to increased wall thickness without chamber dilation. Hypertrophy tends to normalize left ventricular wall stress, since

$$\text{Wall stress} \cong (R/Th) \times P \qquad (11\text{--}17)$$

where R is ventricular radius, Th is wall thickness, and P is left ventricular pressure. The relative wall thickness (the ratio of wall thickness to radius) is a useful and simple measure of the degree of hypertrophy. Left ventricular mass (which can be indexed for body size) can be calculated from tracings of endocardium and epicardium at end-diastole, as described in Chapter 6.

In aortic stenosis, left ventricular systolic function tends to be preserved until late in the disease course. When left ventricular systolic dysfunction does occur, it may be due to the increased afterload of outflow obstruction and thus is reversible after valve replacement. Ventricular systolic function can be evaluated qualitatively or quantitatively, as described in Chapter 6. Even a qualitative evaluation has significant prognostic implications in unoperated adults with aortic stenosis.

Interestingly, there appear to be gender differences in the response of the left ventricle to aortic stenosis. Women tend to have more hypertrophied, smaller ventricles with preserved systolic function, while men tend to show less increase in wall thickness, more left ventricular dilation, and a higher prevalence of systolic dysfunction.

Clinical Applications in Specific Patient Populations

Symptomatic Aortic Stenosis

Doppler echocardiography is the diagnostic test of choice for symptomatic adults with suspected aortic stenosis in whom valve replacement is being considered (Table 11–5). A complete echocardiographic examination includes evaluation of stenosis severity, assessment of left ventricular systolic function, and evaluation of coexisting valvular lesions, as described previously. While all the clinical and Doppler echo data should be considered in clinical decision making for each individual patient, a generalized diagnostic approach based on the Doppler data can be derived for this patient population. As for any generalization, exceptions do occur in clinical practice, so this diagnostic approach serves more as a useful frame of reference than as a rigid patient management scheme (Figs. 11–12 and 11–13).

For initial evaluation of aortic stenosis severity, aortic jet maximum velocity is the simplest and most useful quantitative measure. This is not surprising, because maximum velocity is predictably related to maximum pressure gradient (via the simplified Bernoulli equation), which, in turn, is linearly related to mean pressure gradient in native valvular aortic stenosis. Thus maximum velocities, maximum gradients, and mean gradient measurements are redundant, simply describing the same data in different ways.

When the aortic jet velocity is greater than 4 m/s, the presence of severe aortic valve disease is confirmed, and valve replacement is needed. Note that some subjects with a jet velocity greater than 4 m/s may have only moderate stenosis with coexisting moderate regurgitation. However, if symptoms consistent with aortic valve disease are

TABLE 11–5
Echocardiographic Approach to Valvular Aortic Stenosis

1. Valve anatomy, etiology of stenosis
2. Exclude other causes of left ventricular outflow obstruction
3. Stenosis severity
   a. Jet velocity
   b. Mean pressure gradient
   c. Continuity equation valve area
4. Degree of coexisting aortic regurgitation
5. Left ventricular hypertrophy and systolic function

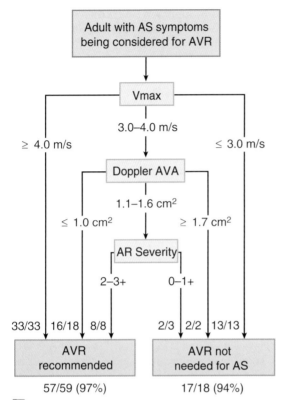

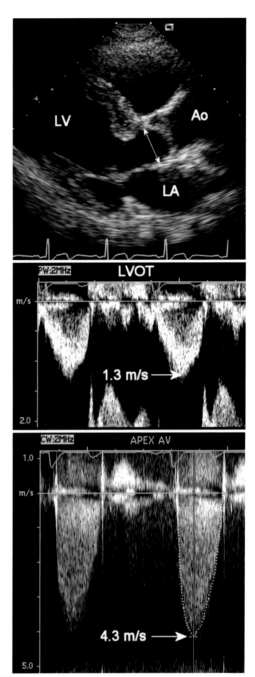

FIGURE 11–12. Diagnostic approach for evaluation of adults with aortic stenosis symptoms being considered for valve replacement. The number of subjects in each group (denominator) and the number in whom this echo approach was correct (numerator) are shown. Overall diagnostic accuracy of this approach is 96%. (From Otto CM, Pearlman AS: Arch Intern Med 148:2553–2560, 1988; copyrighted 1988, American Medical Association. All rights reserved.)

present, the high jet velocity confirms the clinical diagnosis, and valve replacement for mixed stenosis and regurgitation is needed. In these subjects, findings at cardiac catheterization are similar, with a high pressure gradient despite only a moderate reduction in valve area.

When the aortic jet velocity is less than 3 m/s, significant aortic valve disease is unlikely, and valve replacement is not needed. Caution is needed in this situation to ensure that the jet velocity measurement is accurate—a nonparallel intercept angle between the aortic jet and the Doppler beam can result in underestimation of jet velocity and the erroneous conclusion that severe stenosis is not present. If severe left ventricular systolic dysfunction is present, severe aortic stenosis may be present despite a low velocity (and low gradient). In these patients, calculation of valve area is needed.

In symptomatic adults with an aortic jet velocity between 3 and 4 m/s, further evaluation of

FIGURE 11–13. In this 26-year-old pregnant woman with a systolic murmur, the parasternal long-axis view shows a congenitally abnormal aortic valve with systolic doming and an outflow tract diameter of 2.1 cm. LV outflow velocity was recorded with pulsed Doppler from an apical approach and the aortic jet velocity was recorded with continous-wave Doppler from an apical approach. The jet velocity of 4.3 m/s corresponds to a maximum transaortic pressure gradient of 74 mm Hg and a mean gradient of 44 mm Hg. Aortic valve area, calculated with the continuity equation, is 1.1 cm^2 and the velocity ratio is 0.30.

stenosis severity is needed. These patients may have only moderate stenosis with normal transaortic volume flow, mild stenosis with coexisting aortic regurgitation, or severe stenosis with low transaortic volume flow. In aortic stenosis, low transaortic volume flow is not necessarily obvious on 2D imaging. For example, a hypertrophied left ventricle with normal systolic function but a small ventricular chamber will have a small stroke volume. Thus calculation of aortic valve area with the continuity equation is especially important in patients with only a moderate increase in jet velocity (3 to 4 m/s) and a corresponding modest mean pressure gradient (20 to 40 mm Hg). In addition, evaluation of the degree of coexisting aortic regurgitation is needed because valve replacement may be warranted in the symptomatic patient with only mild-to-moderate aortic stenosis and significant aortic regurgitation.

This diagnostic approach has been shown to be accurate and cost-effective in evaluating symptomatic adults with valvular aortic stenosis. Again, it must be emphasized that this approach is only as accurate as the Doppler echo data on which it is based. Careful attention to technical details is needed during the Doppler examination. In cases where the clinical situation is discrepant with the echo findings, other diagnostic tests such as cardiac catheterization may be helpful. Coronary angiography is needed in most patients if valve replacement is planned (for possible coronary artery bypass grafting) and often is needed if valve replacement is *not* planned to evaluate alternate etiologies for the patient's symptoms.

Asymptomatic Aortic Stenosis: Disease Progression and Prognosis

In observing individual patients over time, the reproducibility of a technique, as well as its accuracy, is important. Reproducibility of Doppler echo data includes

- recording variability (e.g., intercept angle, wall filters, signal strength, acoustic window),
- measurement variability (e.g., identification of the maximum velocity, outflow tract diameter), and
- physiologic variability (e.g., interim changes in heart rate, stroke volume, or pressure gradient).

Aortic jet maximum velocity measurement is reproducible with an intraobserver variability of 3.2% and an interobserver variability of 3.1%. Outflow tract velocity, recorded by two experienced sonographers, also is reproducible with intraobserver and interobserver variability of 3% and 3.9%. Measurement of outflow tract diameter shows the greatest variability, with intraobserver and interobserver mean coefficients of variation of 5.1% and 7.9%. These variabilities indicate that for values at the middle of the range, a change greater than measurement variability is greater than 0.2 m/s for maximum jet velocity, greater than 0.1 m/s for outflow tract velocity, greater than 0.2 cm for outflow tract diameter, and greater than 0.15 cm^2 for aortic valve area.

Doppler echo has been used to follow disease progression in asymptomatic adults with valvular aortic stenosis. Several observations from these studies are noteworthy. First, prognosis depends on the presence or absence of clinical symptoms and not on hemodynamic severity per se. There is significant overlap in all measures of hemodynamic severity between symptomatic and asymptomatic adults, and it is not unusual to see asymptomatic individuals with a jet velocity greater than 4 m/s. Second, the rate of hemodynamic progression is variable from patient to patient. However, on average, jet velocity increases by 0.3 m/s per year, mean pressure gradient increases by about 7 mm Hg per year, and valve area decreases by about 0.1 cm^2 per year. Third, while hemodynamic progression may present as an increase in aortic jet velocity (and transaortic pressure gradient), disease progression can occur with no change in jet velocity if there is a concurrent decrease in transaortic volume flow rate (Fig. 11–14).

In patients with asymptomatic aortic stenosis, clinical outcome is highly dependent on Doppler jet velocity. In those with an initial jet velocity less than 3 m/s, the rate of death or symptom onset requiring valve replacement is 8% per year, compared to 17% per year for those with a jet velocity between 3 and 4 m/s and 40% per year for those with a jet velocity greater than 4 m/s (Fig. 11–15). Although it could be argued that once the baseline examination has established the diagnosis, the patient can be followed clinically, because the timing of valve replacement is determined by symptom onset, adults with aortic stenosis often have significant comorbid disease so that knowledge of hemodynamic severity can be important in patient management. Thus in the clinically stable patient, repeat echocardiography every 2 to 3 years is indicated when the jet velocity is less than 3 m/s, with annual examinations appropriate in those with higher jet velocities.

Evaluation of Aortic Stenosis with Left Ventricular Systolic Dysfunction

In the patient with significant left ventricular systolic dysfunction and aortic valve stenosis,

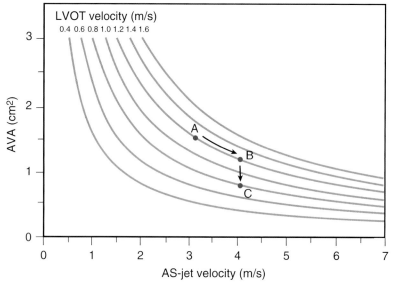

■ **FIGURE 11-14.** Graph of the relationship between aortic valve area (AVA) and aortic stenosis jet velocity for left ventricular outflow tract (LVOT) velocities ranging from 0.4 to 1.6 m/s. In the example shown, a patient initially has a jet velocity of 3 m/s and a valve area of 1.5 cm² *(A)*. As stenosis severity increases, jet velocity increases to 4.0 m/s and valve area decreases to 1.2 cm² *(B)*. However, with further disease progression *(C)*, jet velocity was unchanged at 4 m/s, but valve area decreased to 0.8 cm² in the setting of decreased transaortic volume flow (LVOT velocity 1.2 to 0.8 m/s).

evaluation of stenosis severity is problematic. Even with severe stenosis, pressure gradients may be low due to the low transaortic volume flow rate. Conversely, while valve area is less flow-dependent than pressure gradients, valve area can vary in parallel with flow rate and thus calculated valve area may appear to be reduced when ventricular dysfunction is present, even if stenosis is not severe. Several approaches to this difficult problem have been proposed. One approach is to assess the degree of change in

valve area with an increase in flow rate, for example, with dobutamine stress echocardiography (Fig. 11-16). The hypothesis is that an increase in valve area reflects flexible leaflets, whereas a fixed valve area indicates stiff leaflets that cannot open any further. However, this approach has several limitations including interpretation of the data if flow rate is unchanged and the lack of outcome studies. A more detailed discussion of this problem can be found in Suggested Readings 15 to 19.

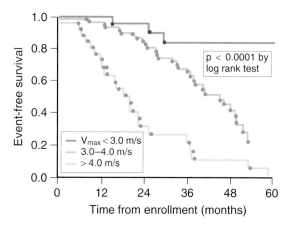

■ **FIGURE 11-15.** Cox regression analysis showing event-free survival in aortic stenosis groups defined by aortic jet velocity at entry (*P* < .0001 by log rank test). (From Otto CM, Burwash IG, Legget ME, et al: Circulation 95:2262–2270, 1997. Used with permission.)

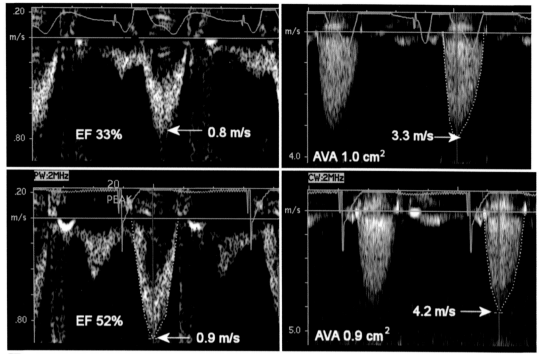

■ **FIGURE 11–16.** Dobutamine stress echocardiography was performed in this 56-year-old man with a dilated cardiomyopathy and a calcific aortic stenosis with resting data *(top)* and stress data *(bottom)* for LV outflow velocity *(left)* and aortic jet velocity *(right)*. At rest, his left ventricular ejection fraction was 33% with an aortic jet velocity of 3.3 m/s and a continuity equation valve area of 1.0 cm². With dobutamine at 20 µg/kg/min, ejection fraction increased to 52% with an increase in transvalvular volume flow rate as evidenced by the increase in outflow tract velocity. Aortic jet velocity increased to 4.2 m/s and continuity equation valve area showed no significant change at 0.9 cm². This response to dobutamine suggests fixed valve obstruction, as did the severe valve calcification seen on 2D imaging. He underwent aortic valve replacement and, at 1 year after surgery, has had a marked decrease in symptoms and an increase in ejection fraction to 41%.

MITRAL STENOSIS

Diagnostic Imaging of the Mitral Valve

Echocardiography in the patient with mitral stenosis includes evaluation of

- valve anatomy, mobility, and calcification;
- mean transmitral pressure gradient;
- 2D echo mitral valve area;
- Doppler pressure half-time valve area;
- pulmonary artery pressures; and
- coexisting mitral regurgitation.

Rheumatic Disease

Rheumatic disease predominantly affects the mitral valve and is the most common cause of mitral stenosis. Rheumatic valvular disease is characterized by commissural fusion, which results in bowing or doming of the valve leaflets in diastole (Fig. 11–17). The base and midsections of the leaflets move toward the ventricular apex, while the motion of the leaflet tips is restricted due

to fusion of the anterior and posterior leaflets along the medial and lateral commissures. Thickening at the leaflet tips occurs frequently, but the remainder of the leaflets can show variable degrees of thickening and/or calcification. If the base and midportions of the leaflets are relatively thin, leaflet mobility is normal other than the fused commissures. The rheumatic process also typically affects the subvalvular region with fusion, shortening, fibrosis, and calcification of the mitral chordae.

In rheumatic mitral stenosis, 2D echo allows detailed evaluation of mitral valve morphology, including assessment of leaflet thickness, leaflet mobility, the degree of calcification, and the extent of subvalvular involvement on transthoracic parasternal and apical views (Fig. 11–18). Occasionally, if transthoracic images are suboptimal, transesophageal imaging may be needed for evaluation of mitral valve anatomy, although definition of subvalvular disease may be limited due to shadows and reverberations from calcification of the mitral valve and annulus.

Mitral Stenosis

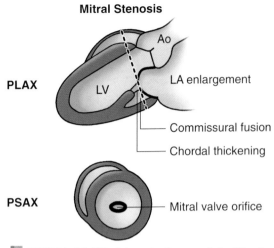

FIGURE 11-17. Schematic diagram of the 2D echo findings in mitral stenosis. In the parasternal long-axis view (PLAX), commissural fusion with diastolic doming of the mitral leaflets is seen, as well as chordal thickening and fusion. In a parasternal short-axis view (PSAX), at the mitral valve orifice, the area of opening can be planimetered. The plane of the short-axis view is indicated by a *dashed line* on the long-axis image.

Mitral Annular Calcification

Mitral annular calcification is a common finding on echocardiography in elderly subjects. Mild annular calcification appears as an isolated area of calcification on the left ventricular side of the posterior annulus, near the base of the posterior mitral leaflet. In more severe mitral annular calcification, increased echogenicity is seen in a hemielliptical pattern involving the entire posterior annulus. The area of fibrous continuity between the anterior mitral leaflet and the aortic root rarely is involved. The echocardiographic finding of mitral annular calcification, like aortic valve sclerosis, indicates a higher risk of adverse cardiovascular outcomes, even when valve function is relatively normal. Mitral annular calcification may result in mild-to-moderate mitral regurgitation due to increased rigidity of the mitral annulus. Occasionally, the calcification extends into the base of the mitral leaflets themselves, resulting in functional mitral stenosis due to narrowing of the diastolic flow area (Fig. 11–19). Calcific mitral stenosis can be distinguished from rheumatic disease by careful imaging techniques to demonstrate thin and mobile mitral leaflet tips without commissural fusion.

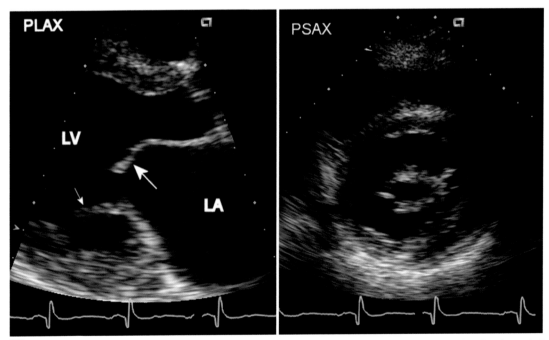

FIGURE 11-18. Parasternal long-axis view *(left)* of a patient with mild rheumatic mitral stenosis showing the typical doming of the anterior mitral leaflet due to commissural fusion. Left atrial enlargement is present. The short-axis view *(right)* allows accurate planimetry of the mitral orifice area if care is taken to identify the smallest opening by scanning slowly from apex toward the base.

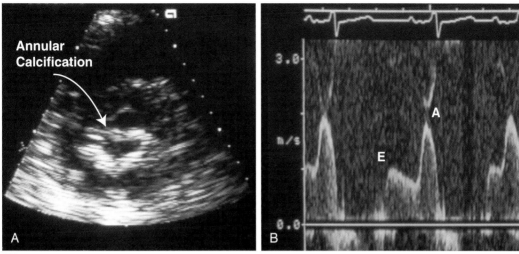

FIGURE 11-19. In an elderly patient with severe mitral annular calcification, involvement of the mitral leaflets by the calcific process in seen in the parasternal short-axis view *(left)*. The Doppler velocity curve across the valve shows a prolonged pressure half-time of 227 ms consistent with a functional mitral valve area of 1.0 cm². (From Otto CM: Mitral stenosis. In: Otto CM (ed): Valvular Heart Disease, 2nd ed. Philadelphia: WB Saunders, 2004, Fig. 10–2.)

Differential Diagnosis

In patients referred for echocardiography with suspected mitral stenosis, the initial differential diagnosis includes other causes of pulmonary congestion (Table 11–6). Standard echo Doppler evaluation will reveal whether left ventricular systolic dysfunction, aortic valve disease, or mitral regurgitation is present. The possibility of diastolic left ventricular dysfunction also should be considered. The rare case of an atrial myxoma or other atrial tumor obstructing left ventricular inflow, thus mimicking the clinical presentation of mitral stenosis, can easily be diagnosed by 2D imaging (see Chapter 15). Rarely, a patient with mild obstruction due to cor triatriatum may present as an adult.

Quantitation of Mitral Stenosis Severity

Pressure Gradients

The mean diastolic transmitral pressure gradient (Fig. 11–20) can be determined from the transmitral velocity curve using the simplified Bernoulli equation:

$$\Delta P_{\mathrm{mean}} = 4(v_1^2 + v_2^2 + v_3^2 + \cdots v_n^2)/n \quad (11\text{-}17)$$

With severe stenosis, the mean pressure gradient may be as high as 20 to 30 mm Hg, but it may be as low as 5 to 15 mm Hg. The variability in pressure gradients in severe mitral stenosis is due to the dependence of pressure gradients on volume flow rate as well as valve area. Severe mitral stenosis may be associated with a low stroke volume (due to the limitation of left ventricular diastolic filling), resulting in a relatively low mean gradient. If volume flow rate increases, for example, with exercise, an increase in transmitral gradient is seen. As for other types of valvular stenosis, calculation of valve area, considering both pressure gradient and volume flow rate, is helpful in quantitation of mitral stenosis severity.

Mitral Valve Area

TWO-DIMENSIONAL ECHO VALVE AREA. Compared with valvular aortic stenosis, the 3D anatomy of rheumatic mitral stenosis is simpler

TABLE 11-6
Echocardiographic Differential Diagnosis of Left Ventricular Inflow Obstruction
Mitral valve stenosis
Rheumatic mitral stenosis
Calcific mitral stenosis (rare)
Congenital mitral stenosis
Left atrial tumor (myxoma)
Left atrial thrombus
Left ventricular diastolic dysfunction
Congenital disease
Congenital mitral stenosis
Cor triatriatum

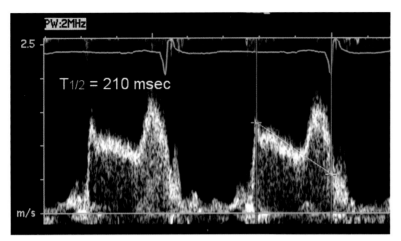

■ **FIGURE 11–20.** Transmitral flow curve in the same patient as in Figure 11–18. Using this velocity curve, pressure gradients can be calculated with the Bernoulli equation and valve area by the pressure half-time method. Note the well-defined maximal velocity and the clearly defined, linear deceleration slope. An *A* velocity is seen because sinus rhythm is present.

with a planar elliptical orifice that is relatively constant in position in mid-diastole (Fig. 11–21). Thus, 2D short-axis imaging of the diastolic orifice allows direct planimetry of valve area. This approach has been well validated compared with measurement of valve area at surgery and in comparison with catheterization-determined valve areas. Because the shape of the mitral valve inflow region is similar to a funnel, with the narrowest cross-sectional area at the leaflet tips, it is important to begin the 2D scan at the apex, slowly moving the image plane toward the mitral valve to identify the smallest orifice. With a low overall 2D gain setting, the inner edge of the black-white interface is traced. Given the accuracy of this tech-

nique, 2D echo mitral valve area (MVA) should be measured in patients with mitral stenosis whenever image quality is adequate.

PRESSURE HALF-TIME VALVE AREA. Calculation of mitral valve area by the pressure half-time method is based on the concept that the *rate* of pressure decline across the stenotic mitral orifice is determined by the cross-sectional area of the orifice: the smaller the orifice, the slower the rate of pressure decline (Figs. 11–22 and 11–23). The influence of left atrial and left ventricular compliance on the rate of pressure decline is assumed to be negligible—an assumption that is not always warranted, especially immediately after percutaneous commissurotomy.

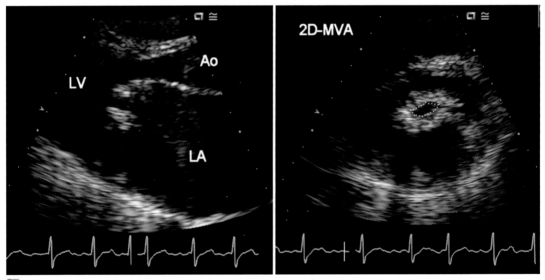

■ **FIGURE 11–21.** Long-axis *(left)* and short-axis *(right)* views of severe mitral stenosis with thickened and calcified leaflet tips. Note the diastolic doming and severe commissural fusion. Valve area by 2D planimetry is 0.6 cm². In addition, severe left atrial enlargement is present.

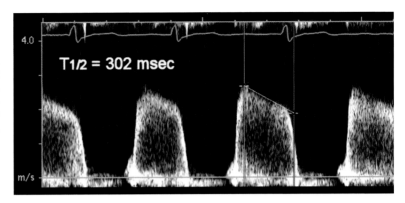

FIGURE 11–22. Pressure half-time measurement in the patient with severe mitral stenosis shown in Figure 11–21. The pressure half-time of 302 ms corresponds to a valve area of 0.7 cm². The patient is in atrial fibrillation so no *A* velocity is seen.

The pressure half-time is defined as the time interval (in milliseconds) between the maximum early diastolic transmitral pressure gradient and the time point where the pressure gradient is half the maximum value. Initially, the pressure half-time concept was evaluated using invasive measurements of left atrial and left ventricular pressure. Pressure half-time was found to be constant for a given individual, even with exercise-induced changes in volume flow rate, suggesting that this measurement is a constant measure of stenosis severity for a given valve area.

This concept then was adapted to transmitral Doppler flow velocity curves. Given the quadratic relationship between velocity and pressure gradients, the half-time is determined from a Doppler spectral velocity curve as the time interval from the maximum mitral velocity (V_{max}) to the point where the velocity has fallen to $V_{max}/\sqrt{2}$. Initial studies comparing Doppler half-time data with invasively determined Gorlin valve areas found a linear relationship, with a half-time of approximately 220 ms corresponding to a valve area of 1 cm². The empirical formula

$$MVA = 220/T_{1/2} \qquad (11–18)$$

was proposed and has been shown to correlate well with invasive valve areas in several clinical studies (Table 11–7).

CONTINUITY EQUATION MITRAL VALVE AREA. The continuity principle for calculation of valve area also can be applied to the mitral orifice:

$$MVA = \text{transmitral SV}/ \text{VTI}_{MS\text{-jet}} \qquad (11–19)$$

where SV is stroke volume (cm³), VTI is the velocity-time integral (cm) in the mitral stenosis jet, and MVA (cm²) is the mitral valve area. Stroke volume can be determined from the left ventricular outflow tract cross-sectional area and velocity-time integral (in the absence of aortic or mitral regurgitation) or from the pulmonary artery diameter and velocity-time integral. Note that stroke volume measured at either of these sites will represent transmitral volume flow accurately only if there is no significant mitral regurgitation.

In theory, transmitral volume flow rate can be calculated accurately in mitral stenosis even when mitral regurgitation is present using the proximal isovelocity surface area method. The color Doppler flow parameters are adjusted to demonstrate a well-defined hemispherical aliasing surface

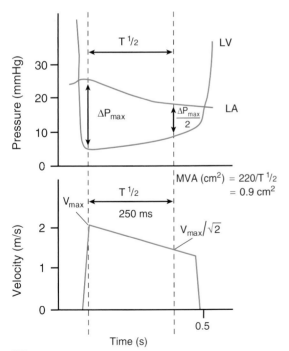

FIGURE 11–23. Schematic diagram of the relationship between left atrial and left ventricular pressures and the Doppler velocity curve in mitral stenosis. Maximum velocity and the diastolic slope are identified as shown, yielding a pressure half-time of 226 ms corresponding to a mitral valve area of 1 cm². There is no *A* velocity because atrial fibrillation is present.

TABLE 11-7

Selected Studies of Mitral Valve Area Determination

First Author/ Year	Comparison	N	Study Group	R	Range (cm²)	SEE (cm²)
Gorlin/1951	MVA by Gorlin formula vs. direct autopsy or surgery	11	Mitral stenosis	0.89	0.5–1.5	0.15
Libanoff/1968	$T_{1/2}$ at rest vs. Exercise	20	Mitral valve disease	0.98	20–340 ms	21 ms
Henry/1975	2D echo vs. direct measurement at surgery	20	MS pts undergoing surgery	0.92	0.5–3.5	–
Holen/1977	MVA by Doppler vs. Gorlin	10	Mitral stenosis	0.98	0.6–3.4	0.18
Hatle/1979	$T_{1/2}$ vs. Gorlin MVA	32	Mitral stenosis	−0.74	0.4–3.5	–
Smith/1986	2D echo vs. Gorlin	37	MS alone	0.83	0.4–2.3	0.26
		35	Prior commissurotomy	0.58		0.28
	$T_{1/2}$ MVA vs. Gorlin	(37)	MS alone	0.85		0.22
		(35)	Prior commissurotomy	0.90		0.14
Come/1988	$T_{1/2}$ MVA vs. Gorlin	37	Pre-MBC	0.51	0.6–1.3	–
			Post-MBC	0.47	1.2–3.8	–
	Gorlin vs. Gorlin		Repeat-cath	0.74	0.4–1.4	–
Thomas/1988	Predicted vs. actual $T_{1/2}$	18	Pre-MBC	0.93–0.96		
			Post-MBC	0.52–0.66		
Chen/1989	$T_{1/2}$ MVA vs. Gorlin	18	Pre-MBC	0.81	0.4–1.2	0.11
			Immediately post-MBC	0.84	1.3–2.6	0.20
			24–48 h post-MBC	0.72	1.3–2.6	0.49
Faletra/1996	2D echo vs. direct measurement	30	Mitral stenosis undergoing surgical mitral valve replacement	0.95	0.6–2.0	0.06
	$T_{1/2}$ vs. direct measurement	30		0.80		0.09
	Continuity equation vs. direct measurement	30		0.87		0.09
	Flow area vs. direct measurement	30		0.54		0.10

MBC, mitral balloon commissurotomy; Gorlin, Gorlin formula valve area; MS, mitral stenosis; MVA, mitral valve area; 2D, two-dimensional; $T_{1/2}$, pressure half-time.
Data from Gorlin et al: Am Heart J 41:1–29, 1951; Libanoff et al: Circulation 38:144–150, 1968; Henry et al: Circulation 51:827–831, 1975; Holen et al: Acta Med Scand 201:83–88, 1977; Hatle et al: Circulation 60:1096–1104, 1979; Smith et al: Circulation 73:100–107, 1986; Come et al: Am J Cardiol 61:817–825, 1988; Thomas et al: Circulation 78:980–993, 1988; Chen et al: J Am Coll Cardiol 13:1309–1313, 1989; Faletra F et al: J Am Coll Cardiol 28:1190–1197, 1996.

area on the left atrial side of the mitral orifice. The velocity at this location equals the Nyquist limit (the "aliasing" velocity). The cross-sectional area of the aliased boundary can be calculated as the surface area of a hemisphere with diameter measured from the color flow image. Multiplying cross-sectional area times the known velocity yields the volume flow rate, which then can be used in conjunction with the transmitral velocity time interval in the continuity equation. One difficulty with this approach is that the volume flow rate must be integrated over the diastolic filling period; a single color image yields only the volume flow rate at one time point in diastole. Because of this

problem, the proximal isovelocity method has not been widely applied in mitral stenosis.

Technical Considerations and Potential Pitfalls

As for any intracardiac blood flow, accurate pressure gradient calculations depend on accurate velocity measurements, which require a near-parallel intercept angle between the direction of blood flow and the Doppler beam (Table 11–8). The mitral stenosis jet nearly always can be recorded from an apical approach, but careful transducer positioning and angulation are needed to record an optimal signal. Color flow imaging may be helpful in defining the jet direction in a

TABLE 11-8

Pitfalls in Evaluation of Mitral Stenosis Severity

Pressure Gradient

Intercept angle between mitral stenosis jet and ultrasound beam
Beat-to-beat variability in atrial fibrillation
Dependence on transvalvular volume flow rate (e.g., exercise, coexisting mitral regurgitation)

2D Valve Area

Image orientation
Tomographic plane
2D gain settings
Intra- and interobserver variability in planimetry of orifice
Poor acoustic access
Deformed valve anatomy post-valvuloplasty

$T_{1/2}$ Valve Area

Definition of V_{max} and early diastolic slope
Nonlinear early diastolic velocity slope
Sinus rhythm with a wave superimposed on early diastolic slope
Influence of coexisting aortic regurgitation
Changing left ventricular and left atrial compliances immediately after commissurotomy

Continuity Equation Mitral Valve Area

Accurate measurement of transmitral stroke volume

given tomographic plane. Depending on the maximum jet velocity, the velocity curve can be recorded with conventional pulsed, high-pulse-repetition-frequency, or continuous-wave Doppler ultrasound. Pulsed Doppler recordings may show better definition of the maximum velocity and early diastolic slope than continuous-wave Doppler recordings because of a better signal-to-noise ratio.

Direct planimetry of mitral valve area on 2D short-axis images has proven to be a valid technique in most clinical situations. However, definition of valve area may be difficult if image quality is poor or if there is extensive distortion of the valve anatomy. Valve area can be underestimated if gain settings are too high and can be overestimated if the smallest area at the leaflet tips is not recorded. Low gain settings and careful scanning in a short-axis plane from the apex toward the base help avoid these potential problems.

Pressure half-time valve area calculations have significant limitations in certain clinical settings. When coexisting aortic regurgitation is present, left ventricular filling occurs both antegrade across the mitral valve and retrograde across the aortic

valve (Fig. 11–24). This may result in a more rapid rise in left ventricular diastolic pressure than if there were no aortic regurgitation, resulting in a shorter half-time measurement. Conversely, if severe aortic regurgitation impairs mitral leaflet opening, functional mitral stenosis may be superimposed on anatomic mitral stenosis, with lengthening of the half-time measurement. In clinical practice, if the 2D echo shows rheumatic mitral stenosis and only mild-to-moderate aortic regurgitation is present, the half-time method remains a useful approach for evaluation of stenosis severity. If aortic regurgitation is severe, or if the mitral valve anatomy is atypical, the potential influence of coexisting lesions should be considered.

A major assumption of the half-time method is that left atrial and left ventricular compliances do not significantly affect the rate of pressure gradient decline across the stenotic orifice. While this assumption appears to be warranted in clinically stable patients with mitral stenosis, it is *not* justified in the period immediately after catheter mitral valvuloplasty. After relief of mitral stenosis, the fall in left atrial pressure and the increase in left ventricular filling are accompanied by directionally opposite changes in left atrial and left ventricular compliance. During the 24 to 72 hours

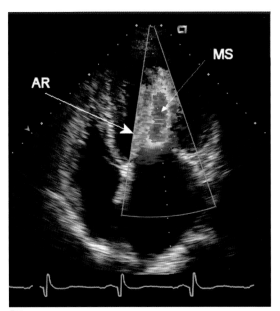

■ **FIGURE 11–24.** Color flow imaging in an apical four-chamber view shows the mitral stenosis (MS) jet and the aortic regurgitation (AR) jet in this patient with rheumatic disease. Although the aortic regurgitation usually does not affect left ventricular pressures enough to invalidate the pressure half-time method, care is needed to correctly identify the separate signals on pulsed and continuous-wave Doppler recordings.

after the procedure, equilibrium has not been reached, and the pressure half-time may not be an accurate reflection of orifice area. After this adjustment period, compliances stabilize, and the pressure half-time method again provides useful information.

Even under physiologically stable conditions, accurate pressure half-time measurements require careful recording of the mitral stenosis velocity curve. It is important that the intercept angle be parallel to flow and *constant* throughout diastole to avoid artifactual distortion in the shape of the curve. The maximum early diastolic velocity and the early diastolic deceleration slope should be well defined. In addition, pressure half-times are most easily and reproducibly measured if the deceleration slope is linear. If a linear slope cannot be obtained even after careful adjustment of transducer position and angulation, the half-time measurement should be made using the mid-diastolic slope of the curve.

In atrial fibrillation, several beats are averaged, since mean gradient will vary with the RR interval. While the half-time will be relatively constant despite variation in the length of diastole, only beats where the diastolic filling period is long enough to show the early diastolic slope clearly are appropriate for measurement. Although the pressure half-time method is accurate when sinus rhythm is present, the increase in velocity due to atrial contraction may obscure the early diastolic slope, particularly at high heart rates, so that half-time measurements may not be possible unless a slow heart rate allows clear definition of the middiastolic slope.

Continuity equation mitral valve area determinations are most accurate in patients without significant coexisting mitral regurgitation. In this subgroup, continuity equation mitral valve area calculations provide a useful alternative to the pressure half-time method, especially in situations of altered chamber compliances. The accuracy of the continuity equation method, as in aortic stenosis, depends on a parallel intercept angle between the mitral stenotic jet and the ultrasound beam and a careful stroke volume calculation from diameter and velocity recordings. Accurate pulmonary artery diameter measurement for stroke volume calculations can be difficult in adult patients due to poor acoustic access. Left ventricular outflow tract diameter nearly always can be depicted reliably. However, many patients with mitral stenosis have some degree of coexisting aortic or mitral regurgitation so that transaortic stroke volume does not equal transmitral stroke volume.

Consequences of Mitral Stenosis

Left Atrial Enlargement and Thrombus

Chronic pressure overload of mitral stenosis leads to gradual enlargement of the left atrium. Left atrial size can become extremely large in long-standing severe mitral stenosis. In conjunction with a low volume flow rate due to the stenotic valve, left atrial enlargement results in stasis of blood flow and thrombus formation. Thrombi are located preferentially in the left atrial appendage but also can occur in the body of the atrium as protruding or as laminated thrombus along the atrial wall or interatrial septum (Fig. 11–25). Left atrial thrombi are most common when atrial fibrillation is present but may occur even in sinus rhythm.

Transthoracic echo has a high specificity for detection of left atrial thrombus (i.e., if it is visualized, it most likely is a real finding), but the sensitivity is less than 50%. In part, this relates to the difficulty of imaging the left atrial appendage in adults. Sometimes the left atrial appendage can be visualized in a laterally angulated parasternal short-axis view at the aortic valve level or from an apical two-chamber view angulated slightly superiorly; however, often the atrial appendage cannot be visualized at all. When the atrial appendage is

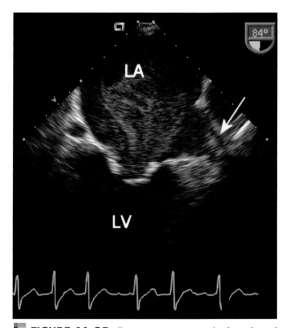

FIGURE 11–25. Spontaneous contrast in the enlarged left atrium and an echodensity suggestive of a thrombus in the atrial appendage of a patient with mitral stenosis, seen on transesophageal imaging.

seen, image quality usually is too poor to allow reliable exclusion of atrial thrombus due to poor ultrasound tissue penetration and beam width artifact at the depth of the left atrium from surface imaging.

Transesophageal echo has a high sensitivity (>99%) and specificity (>99%) for detection of left atrial thrombus. The left atrial appendage can be depicted well in multiple image planes using a multiplane probe. In addition, the higher transducer frequencies (5 to 7 MHz) and lower imaging depths result in high-resolution images. While thrombus in the appendage often protrudes into the chamber, laminated thrombus in the body of the atrium may be more difficult to recognize, especially along the interatrial septum.

Pulmonary Hypertension

In mitral stenosis, increased left atrial pressure results in pulmonary venous hypertension and consequent pulmonary artery hypertension. Initially, the increase in pulmonary artery pressure is "passive"–the pressure difference across the pulmonary bed (pulmonary artery minus left atrial pressure) is normal. In this situation, although pulmonary pressures are elevated, pulmonary vascular resistance is normal, and pulmonary pressures will fall toward normal after relief of mitral stenosis. With long-standing pulmonary venous hypertension, irreversible changes in the pulmonary vascular bed occur, leading to elevated pulmonary vascular resistance and persistent pulmonary hypertension after relief of mitral stenosis.

The presence of pulmonary hypertension can be suspected in mitral stenosis when there is midsystolic partial closure (or "notching") of the pulmonic valve M-mode, a short interval between the onset of flow and maximum velocity, or midsystolic abrupt deceleration in the right ventricular outflow velocity curve. With severe pulmonary hypertension, 2D echo may show right ventricular hypertrophy and enlargement, paradoxical septal motion, and tricuspid regurgitation secondary to annular dilation.

The degree of pulmonary hypertension can be quantitated from the velocity in the tricuspid regurgitant jet and the appearance of the inferior vena cava. The simplified Bernoulli equation is used to calculate the right ventricular to right atrial maximum systolic pressure difference from the continuous-wave Doppler tricuspid regurgitant jet recording. This difference is added to an estimate of right atrial pressure based on the size and respiratory variation of the inferior vena cava as it enters the right atrium as described in Chapter 6. Pulmonary hypertension out of proportion to the degree of mitral stenosis raises the possibility of a coexisting pulmonary disease process.

Mitral Regurgitation

Some degree of coexisting mitral regurgitation is common in patients with mitral stenosis. Mitral regurgitant severity can be evaluated using standard techniques (see Chapter 12) and is an important factor in deciding on appropriate therapy. For example, significant mitral regurgitation is a contraindication to surgical or percutaneous commissurotomy. Coexisting mitral regurgitation elevates the transmitral pressure gradient (due to increased transmitral volume flow rate), but both 2D echo and pressure half-time valve area measurements remain accurate.

Other Coexisting Valvular Disease

The rheumatic disease process also can affect the aortic valve (second in frequency to the mitral valve) and, less commonly, the tricuspid valve. Aortic valve involvement may result in stenosis and/or regurgitation that can be evaluated with appropriate 2D and Doppler echo techniques. Evaluation of aortic regurgitation by color flow imaging may be complicated in the presence of mitral stenosis due to merging of the two diastolic flow disturbances in the left ventricle. Imaging the aortic regurgitant jet in short axis just proximal to the aortic valve and using other Doppler methods for evaluation of regurgitant severity will avoid this potential problem.

Rheumatic tricuspid stenosis may be difficult to appreciate on 2D imaging. Doppler flow patterns are similar to mitral stenosis, and the same quantitative methods for evaluation of stenosis severity can be applied. Even in the absence of rheumatic involvement of the tricuspid valve, significant tricuspid regurgitation is common (due to pulmonary hypertension and annular dilation) in patients with mitral stenosis. Careful evaluation of tricuspid regurgitation severity is especially important preoperatively in case tricuspid annuloplasty is needed at the time of mitral valve surgery.

Left Ventricular Response

The left ventricle in mitral stenosis is small with normal wall thickness and normal systolic function, although diastolic function is impaired due to the restriction of flow across the mitral orifice. The presence of left ventricular dilation suggests that significant coexisting mitral or aortic regurgitation or primary myocardial dysfunction (cardiomyopathy or ischemic disease) is present.

Clinical Applications in Specific Patient Populations

Diagnosis, Hemodynamic Progression, and Timing of Intervention

Echo Doppler is the standard clinical method for evaluation of the presence and severity of valvular mitral stenosis (Table 11–9). Disease progression can be followed and the timing of intervention can be determined using Doppler echo and clinical data alone. Evaluation by cardiac catheterization rarely is needed.

Pre- and Postpercutaneous Commissurotomy

In the potential candidate for percutaneous balloon mitral commissurotomy, echo Doppler evaluation of mitral valve morphology is important in patient selection both in terms of predicted hemodynamic results and in terms of the risk of procedural complications. Mitral valve morphology may be described by a qualitative assessment, an additive scoring system (Tables 11–10 and 11–11), or quantitative measurements of leaflet mobility. Whatever approach is used, the important features to consider are leaflet mobility, leaflet thickness, leaflet and commissural calcification, and subvalvular involvement (Fig. 11–26). In general, the best hemodynamic results are seen

TABLE 11-9

Echocardiographic Approach to Mitral Stenosis

1. Valve morphology
2. Exclude other causes of clinical presentation
3. Mitral stenosis severity
   a. Mean transmitral pressure gradient
   b. 2D valve area
   c. $T_{1/2}$ valve area
4. Coexisting mitral regurgitation
5. Left atrial enlargement
6. Pulmonary artery pressure (from TR jet and IVC)
7. TEE for evaluation of left atrial clot if MBC is planned
8. Coexisting tricuspid regurgitation severity

MBC, mitral balloon commissurotomy; IVC, inferior vena cava; TR, tricuspid regurgitation; TEE, transesophageal echocardiography.

with thin, mobile leaflets that have commissural fusion but little calcification or subchordal thickening. However, some patients with a relatively unfavorable morphology do have relief of mitral stenosis with percutaneous commissurotomy. It is noteworthy that patients with the most heavily calcified and deformed valves (and the most

TABLE 11-10

Mitral Valve Morphology by Two-dimensional Echocardiography

Grade	Mobility	Subvalvular Thickening	Thickening	Calcification
1	Highly mobile valve with only leaflet tips restricted	Minimal thickening just below the mitral leaflets	Leaflets near normal in thickness (4–5 mm)	A single area of increased echo brightness
2	Leaflet mid and base portions have normal mobility	Thickening of chordal structures extending up to one third of the chordal length	Mid-leaflets normal, considerable thickening of margins (5–8 mm)	Scattered areas of brightness confined to leaflet margins
3	Valve continues to move forward in diastole, mainly from the base	Thickening extending to the distal third of the chords	Thickening extending through the entire leaflet (5–8 mm)	Brightness extending into the mid-portion of the leaflets
4	No or minimal forward movement of the leaflets in diastole	Extensive thickening and shortening of all chordal structures extending down to the papillary muscles	Considerable thickening of all leaflet tissue (>8–10 mm)	Extensive brightness throughout much of the leaflet tissue

The total echocardiographic score is derived from an analysis of mitral leaflet mobility, valvar and subvalvar thickening, and calcification are graded from 0 to 4 according to the above criteria. This gives a total score of 0 to 16.
From Wilkins GT, Weyman AE, Abascal VM, et al: Br Heart J 60:299–308, 1988.

TABLE 11-11
The French Three-Group Grading of Mitral Valve Anatomy

Echocardiographic Group	Mitral Valve Anatomy
Group 1	Pliable noncalcified anterior mitral leaflet and mild subvalvular disease (i.e., thin chordae ≥10 mm long)
Group 2	Pliable noncalcified anterior mitral leaflet and severe subvalvular disease (i.e., thickened chordae <10 mm long)
Group 3	Calcification of mitral valve of any extent, as assessed by fluoroscopy, whatever the state of the subvalvular apparatus

Reprinted from Iung B, Cormier B, Discimetiere P, et al: J Am Coll Cardiol 27:407–414, 1996. Copyright 1996, with permission from American College of Cardiology Foundation.

severe stenosis) are more likely to suffer procedure-related morbidity and mortality.

Another factor to consider in this patient population is the degree of coexisting mitral regurgitation, since percutaneous commissurotomy is contradicted if moderate or severe regurgitation is present. In addition, because any left atrial thrombi may be dislodged by the catheters during the procedure, transesophageal echocardiography is needed to evaluate for left atrial thrombus before the procedure.

After percutaneous commissurotomy, echo Doppler allows identification of complications, permits assessment of hemodynamic results, and provides a baseline for future disease progression (Figs. 11–27 and 11–28). Potential complications include (1) an increase in the severity of mitral regurgitation, and (2) the presence of an atrial septal defect (usually small) at the transseptal catheter puncture site (Fig. 11–29). Hemodynamic results can be evaluated with standard echo Doppler techniques, again with an awareness of the potential inaccuracies in the half-time method in the immediate postcommissurotomy period. Doppler evaluation of postprocedure pulmonary artery systolic pressure also can be helpful.

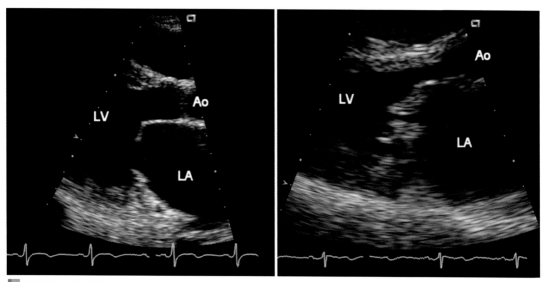

■ **FIGURE 11–26.** Parasternal long-axis views in two mitral stenosis patients, one with favorable *(left)* and one with unfavorable *(right)* mitral valve morphology for balloon valvuloplasty. The favorable mitral valve morphology is characterized by relatively thin, flexible valve leaflets as evidenced by the "doming" of the anterior leaflet and little calcification or subvalvular involvement. The same view in *(right)* a different patient shows leaflets that are extensively calcified and immobile, with less diastolic doming and with extensive subvalvular involvement.

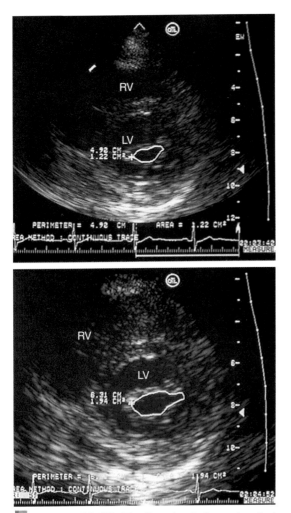

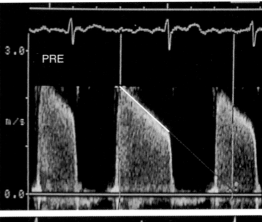

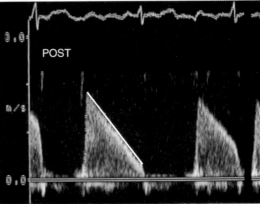

■ FIGURE 11-28. Doppler velocity curves across a stenotic mitral valve before *(top)* and after *(bottom)* percutaneous mitral valvuloplasty. Pressure half-time decreased from 297 to 130 ms, indicating an increase in valve area from 0.7 to 1.7 cm².

■ FIGURE 11-27. Two-dimensional short-axis mitral valve area before (1.2 cm²) and 2 years after (1.9 cm²) balloon mitral valvuloplasty.

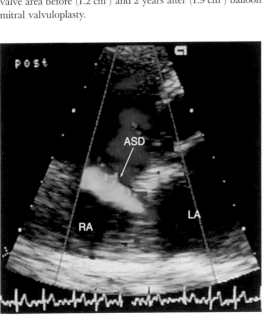

■ FIGURE 11-29. Parasternal short-axis echocardiographic image showing a small atrial septal defect with left to right flow, typically seen after balloon mitral valvuloplasty. LA, left atrium; RA, right atrium; Ao, aorta; LA, left atrium. (From Otto CM: Surgical and percutaneous intervention for mitral stenosis. In: Otto CM (ed): Valvular Heart Disease, 2nd ed. Philadelphia: WB Saunders, 2004, Fig. 11–10.)

Predictors of long-term outcome after balloon mitral comissurtomy include mitral valve area, severity of mitral regurgitation, and the mitral morphlogy score (Fig. 11–30).

Evaluation of the Pregnant Patient with Pulmonary Congestion

When echocardiography is requested in a pregnant patient with pulmonary congestion, the possibility of valvular mitral stenosis should be considered. Symptoms due to mitral stenosis often occur initially during pregnancy due to increased metabolic demands and volume flow rate, and the murmur may not be appreciated on auscultation. Careful imaging of the valve and recording of the transmitral flow velocity curve allows exclusion or confirmation of this possibility.

TRICUSPID STENOSIS

Tricuspid stenosis is uncommon in adult patients; in nearly all cases, it is due to rheumatic disease in association with rheumatic mitral involvement. Carcinoid heart disease affects both tricuspid and pulmonic valves and can lead either to stenosis or to regurgitation. Right atrial tumors, large vegetations, or a large atrial thrombus (which may have embolized from the venous bed) can obstruct right ventricular inflow and mimic tricuspid stenosis.

Two-dimensional echo images show thickening and shortening of the tricuspid valve leaflets (Figs. 11–31 and 11–32). Commissural fusion and dias-

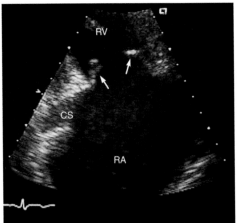

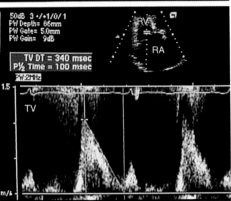

■ **FIGURE 11–31.** Two-dimensional right ventricular inflow view *(top)* and Doppler flow curve *(bottom)* views in a patient with rheumatic tricuspid valve disease. The leaflets are thickened, shortened, and immobile, resulting in a fixed orifice in systole and diastole. Right ventricular and right atrial enlargement secondary to volume overload are evident.

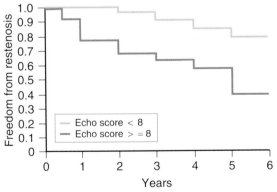

■ **FIGURE 11–30.** Freedom from restenosis in a series of 181 patients with initially successful mitral valvuloplasty and adequate echocardiographic data in those with an echo score less than 8 (n = 73) or 8 or greater. Restenosis was defined as a valve area less than 1.5 cm² and a 50% loss of the initial gain in valve area. (From Wang A, Krasuski RA, Warner JJ, et al: Serial echocardiographic evaluation of restenosis after successful percutaneous mitral commissurotomy. J Am Coll Cardiol 39(2):328–334, 2002.)

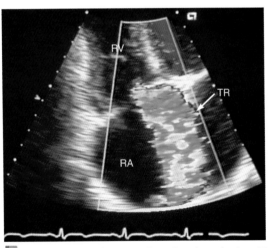

■ **FIGURE 11–32.** Color flow Doppler of tricuspid regurgitation in the same patient as in Figure 11–31 showing severe tricuspid regurgitation in an apical four-chamber view.

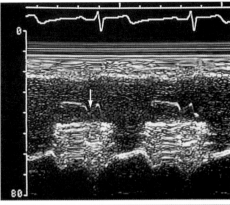

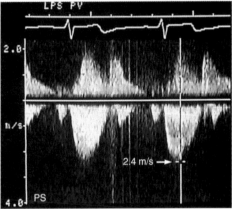

■ **FIGURE 11–33.** M-mode recording *(above)* of the pulmonic valve in a patient with mild pulmonic stenosis showing an increased *a* wave (note timing relative to the QRS complex and P wave). Continuous-wave Doppler from a left parasternal approach shows a pulmonary artery systolic velocity curve with a maximum velocity of 2.4 m/s corresponding to a maximum pressure gradient of 24 mm Hg *(below)*.

tolic bowing indicate rheumatic disease. Doppler recordings of the transvalvular flow velocity allow calculation of mean gradient and pressure half-time valve area as described for the mitral valve.

PULMONIC STENOSIS

Pulmonic stenosis in adults is most often due to congenital disease, either residual stenosis after reparative surgery in childhood or clinically insignificant obstruction. Pulmonic stenosis may occur in conjunction with other congenital lesions such as ventricular inversion (congenitally corrected transposition of the great arteries) or tetralogy of Fallot.

Two-dimensional echo imaging of the pulmonic valve shows thickened leaflets with systolic bowing. On Doppler interrogation, the antegrade velocity is increased with corresponding maximum and mean pressure gradients via the Bernoulli equation (Figs. 11–33 and 11–34). Pulmonic valve area is not usually calculated, but the continuity equation principle can be applied in this situation, using an appropriate intracardiac location for stroke volume determination. Post-stenotic pulmonary artery dilation may be present. Differentiation of valvular pulmonic stenosis from subvalvular or supravalvular obstruction can be difficult by 2D echo. Careful examinations with color flow and conventional pulsed Doppler can be very helpful in defining the site of the poststenotic flow disturbance (and thus the site of obstruction).

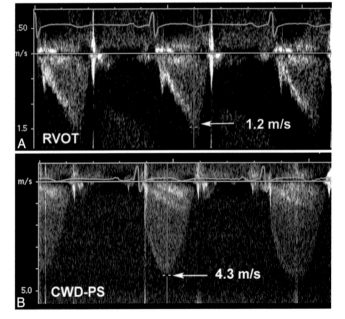

■ **FIGURE 11–34.** Doppler evaluation of a patient with severe pulmonic stenosis shows a right ventricular outflow tract velocity of 1.2 m/s using pulsed Doppler *(top)* and a pulmonary valve velocity of 4.3 m/s using continuous wave Doppler *(bottom)*. Because the proximal velocity is elevated, the equation $\Delta P = 4 \ (V_{max}^2 - V_{prox}^2)$ is used to calculate the peak transpulmonic gradient at 68 mm Hg. The best alignment between the Doppler beam and the pulmonic flow signal was from a subcostal window in this patient. (From Otto CM: Right sided valve disease. In: Otto CM (ed): Valvular Heart Disease, 2nd ed. Philadelphia: WB Saunders, 2004, Fig. 16–10.)

SUGGESTED READING

Basic Principles

1. Yoganathan AP, Cape EG, Sung H-W, et al: Review of hydrodynamic principles for the cardiologist: Applications to the study of blood flow and jets by imaging techniques. J Am Coll Cardiol 12:1344–1353, 1988.

   Review of basic principles of blood flow, including Bernoulli relationships, volume flow calculation, and the fluid dynamics of jets.

2. Thomas JD, Weyman AE: Fluid dynamics model of mitral valve flow: Description with in vitro validation. J Am Coll Cardiol 13:221–233, 1989.

   Fluid dynamic model of the mitral valve with emphasis on the implications for Doppler and invasive pressure gradient and valve area calculations.

3. Baumgartner H, Stefenelli T, Niederberger J, et al: "Overestimation" of catheter gradients by Doppler ultrasound in patients with aortic stenosis: A predictable manifestation of pressure recovery. J Am Coll Cardiol 33:1655–1661, 1999.

   Clinical differences between Doppler and catheter gradients in patients with aortic stenosis are most important when aortic diameter is small (<3 cm). Other factors that affect the degree of pressure recovery include orifice velocity, valve area, and jet eccentricity.

4. Bermejo J, Antoranz JC, Burwash IG, et al: In-vivo analysis of the instantaneous transvalvular pressure difference-flow relationship in aortic valve stenosis: Implications of unsteady fluid-dynamics for the clinical assessment of disease severity. J Heart Valve Dis 11:557–566, 2002.

   Detailed analysis of the pressure-flow relationships in aortic stenosis demonstrating that late-systolic reversal of the transaortic pressure gradient limits accurate measurement of the systolic ejection period from invasive data. Unsteady fluid dynamics support aortic valve area as a precise method to describe stenosis severity.

Aortic Stenosis

5. Hatle L, Angelsen BA, Tromsdal A: Non-invasive assessment of aortic stenosis by Doppler ultrasound. Br Heart J 43:284–292, 1980.

   Original description of noninvasive calculation of transaortic pressure gradients from continuous-wave Doppler using the Bernoulli equation in patients with aortic stenosis.

6. Currie PJ, Seward JB, Reeder GS, et al: Continuous-wave Doppler echocardiographic assessment of severity of calcific aortic stenosis: a simultaneous Doppler-catheter correlative study in 100 adult patients. Circulation 71:1162–1169, 1985.

   Validation of Doppler transaortic pressure gradients with simultaneous invasive and Doppler data. A classic.

7. Otto CM, Pearlman AS, Comess KA, et al: Determination of the stenotic aortic valve area in adults using Doppler echocardiography. J Am Coll Cardiol 7:509–517, 1986.

   One of the early descriptions of the continuity equation for evaluation of aortic stenosis severity.

8. Zoghbi WA, Farmer KL, Soto JG, et al: Accurate noninvasive quantification of stenotic aortic valve area by Doppler echocardiography. Circulation 73:452–459, 1986.

   One of the early descriptions of the continuity equation for evaluation of aortic stenosis severity.

9. Shavelle DM, Otto CM: Aortic stenosis: Echocardiographic evaluation of disease severity, disease progression and role of echocardiography in clinical decision making. In: Otto CM (ed): The Practice of Clinical Echocardiography, 2nd ed. Philadelphia: WB Saunders, 2002, pp. 469–500.

   Advanced discussion of the echocardiographic approach to evaluation of aortic stenosis severity with a review of the impact of echocardiographic findings on the clinical decision-making process; 178 references.

10. Otto CM: Aortic stenosis. In: Otto CM (ed): Valvular Heart Disease, 2nd ed. Philadelphia: WB Saunders, 2004.

    Clinical review of the pathophysiology, clinical presentation, natural history, therapy, and long-term outcome of adults with valvular aortic stenosis; 297 references.

11. Otto CM, Burwash IG, Legget ME, et al: A prospective study of asymptomatic valvular aortic stenosis: clinical, echocardiographic, and exercise predictors of outcome. Circulation 95:2262–2270, 1997.

    In a prospective echocardiographic study of 123 adults with initially asymptomatic aortic stenosis, the rate of hemodynamic progression was an increase in mean gradient of 7 ± 7 mm Hg/y, an increase in jet velocity of 0.32 ± 0.34 m/s/y, and a decrease in valve area of 0.12 ± 0.19 cm²/y. Kaplan-Meier survival without symptoms prompting valve replacement at 2 years was $84\% \pm 16\%$ for a jet velocity less than 3 m/s, $66\% \pm 13\%$ for a jet velocity of 3 to 4 m/s, and only $21\% \pm 18\%$ for a jet velocity greater than 4 m/s.

12. Rosenhek R, Klaar U, Schemper M, et al: Mild and moderate aortic stenosis. Natural history and risk stratification by echocardiography. Eur Heart J 25(3):199–205, 2004.

    In 176 adults with mild to moderate aortic stenosis (aortic jet velocity 2.5 to 3.9 m/s) followed for 48 ± 19 months, event-free survival was $60 \pm 5\%$ at 5 years. Predictors of outcome on multivariate analysis were the degree of valve calcification, coexisting coronary artery disease, and aortic jet velocity. With moderate to severe valve calcification, event free survival at 5 years was $42 \pm 7\%$ compared to $82 \pm 5\%$ in those with no calcification or mild calcification.

13. Burwash IG, Hay KM, Chan KL: Hemodynamic stability of valve area, valve resistance, and stroke work loss in aortic stenosis: a comparative analysis. J Am Soc Echocardiogr 15:814–822, 2002.

    Doppler measures of aortic stenosis severity were measured under varying flow conditions during dobutamine stress echocardiography in 30 adults. Although both valve area and valve resistance varied with volume flow rate, the changes with flow were more predictable for valve area. These data suggest valve area is the most appropriate clinical measure of stenosis severity.

14. Bermejo J, Odreman R, Feijoo J, et al: Clinical efficacy of Doppler-echocardiographic indices of aortic valve stenosis: A comparative test-based analysis of outcome. J Am Coll Cardiol 41:142–151, 2003.

    The steady component of stroke work loss can be estimated from systolic blood pressure (SBP) and the mean transaortic gradient (ΔP_{mean}) as:

    $$\% \ SWL = \Delta P_{mean}/(\Delta P_{mean} + SBP) \times 100\%$$

    For a normal valve, stroke work loss is close to 0%, with increasing values indicating more severe stenosis. Note that for a given transaortic pressure gradient, a higher blood pressure will correspond to a larger stroke work loss (i.e., more severe stenosis). Thus, stroke work loss takes into account 2 components of the systolic load faced by the ventricle—both the valve obstruction and the systemic vascular resistance. A stroke work loss greater than 25% is associated with symptom onset and adverse clinical outcomes

15. Gilon D, Cape EG, Handschumacher MD, et al: Effect of three-dimensional valve shape on the hemodynamics of aortic stenosis. Three-dimensional echocardiographic stereolithography and patient studies. J Am Coll Cardiol 40:1479, 2002.

    Pressure recovery is greatest for valves characterized by a long tapering dome (such as in congenital unicuspid valves) compared to a flat aortic valve geometry.

16. Burwash IG, Pearlman AS, Kraft CD, et al: Flow dependence of measures of aortic stenosis severity during exercise. J Am Coll Cardiol 24:1342–1350, 1994.

    In 110 exercise Doppler studies in adults with aortic stenosis, volume flow rate increased 24%, mean gradient increased 36%, valve area increased 14%, valve resistance increased 13%, and stroke work loss increased 17% on average. These findings demonstrate that all measures of stenosis severity are flow-dependent to some extent.

17. deFilippi CR, Willett DL, Brickner ME, et al: Usefulness of dobutamine echocardiography in distinguishing severe from non-severe valvular aortic stenosis in patients with depressed left ventricular function and low transvalvular gradients. Am J Cardiol 75:191–194, 1995.

    Dobutamine stress echocardiography in adults with aortic stenosis and left ventricular systolic dysfunction is proposed as a method for distinguishing between severe aortic stenosis with increased left ventricular afterload (valve area will not increase with increased transaortic flow) versus moderate aortic stenosis with primary myocardial dysfunction (valve area will increase with increased transaortic flow). Interpretation of results when there is no change in flow rate is problematic.

18. Monin JL, Monchi M, Gest V, et al: Aortic stenosis with severe left ventricular dysfunction and low transvalvular pressure gradients: Risk stratification by low-dose dobutamine echocardiography. J Am Coll Cardiol 37:2101–2107, 2001.

    In 45 patients with severe aortic stenosis (valve area ≥1.0 cm²) and a mean ejection fraction of 29%, those with contractile reserve (an increase in stroke volume by at least 20%) on dobutamine stress echocardiography had a survival of 88% with valve replacement, compared to 13% with medical therapy. In those without contractile reserve, survival was poor (approximately 30%) with either medical or surgical therapy.

19. Schwammenthal E, Vered Z, Moshkowitz Y, et al: Dobutamine echocardiography in patients with aortic stenosis and left ventricular dysfunction: predicting outcome as a function of management strategy. Chest 119:1766–1777, 2001.

    In 24 patients with severe aortic stenosis (valve area <0.9 cm²) and a mean ejection fraction of 28%, dobutamine stress echocardiography results were compared with clinical outcome. A concordant decision was defined as aortic valve replacement for a fixed valve area (increase by less than 0.3 cm² and remains <1.0 cm² at peak dose dobutamine) and medical therapy for those with an increase in valve area with dobutamine. Survival at 1.5 years was 81% with a concordant decision and 25% with a discordant decision.

Mitral Stenosis

20. Henry WL, Griffith JM, Michaelis LL, et al: Measurement of mitral orifice area in patients with mitral valve disease by real-time, two-dimensional echocardiography. Circulation 51:827–831, 1975.

    Validation of 2D echo planimetry of mitral valve area compared with measurements at operation. 2D echo valve area was within 0.3 cm² of surgical area in 12 of 14 (86%) patients.

21. Smith MD, Handshoe R, Handshoe S, et al: Comparative accuracy of two-dimensional echocardiography and Doppler pressure half-time methods in assessing severity of mitral stenosis in patients with and without prior commissurotomy. Circulation 73:100–107, 1986.

    In 74 patients with mitral stenosis, correlations were good for Doppler or 2D echo valve areas versus catheterization (r = 0.80 and 0.83), but Doppler correlated better (r = 0.90) than 2D echo (r = 0.58) in the 35 patients with prior valvuloplasty. Reproducibility was 0.14 cm² for 2D echo and 0.15 cm² for Doppler data.

22. Holen J, Aaslid R, Landmark K, Simonsen S: Determination of pressure gradient in mitral stenosis with a non-invasive ultrasound Doppler technique. Acta Med Scand 199:455–460, 1976.

    Original description of Doppler measurement of transmitral pressure gradients.

23. Libanoff AJ, Rodbard S: Evaluation of the severity of mitral stenosis and regurgitation. Circulation 33:218–226, 1966.

    Original description of pressure half-time with catheterization data.

24. Hatle L, Angelsen B, Tromsdal A: Noninvasive assessment of atrioventricular pressure half-time by Doppler ultrasound. Circulation 60:1096–1104, 1979.

    Application of pressure half-time concept to Doppler data.

25. Faletra F, Pezzano JA, Fusco R, et al: Measurement of mitral valve area in mitral stenosis: Four echocardiographic methods compared with direct measurement of anatomic orifices. J Am Coll Cardiol 28:1190–1197, 1996.

    Careful study demonstrating the accuracy of 2D planimetry, pressure half-time, and proximal flow convergence region methods for calculation of mitral valve area compared to direct measurement of the area of the excised mitral valves.

26. Binder TM, Rosenhek R, Porenta G, et al: Improved assessment of mitral valve stenosis by volumetric real-time three-dimensional echocardiography. J Am Coll Cardiol 36(4):1355–1361, 2000.

    Description of the use of real-time 3D echocardiography for improved visualization of the stenotic mitral valve orifice.

27. Gordon SP, Douglas PS, Come PC, Manning WJ: Two-dimensional and Doppler echocardiographic determinants of the natural history of mitral valve narrowing in patients with rheumatic mitral stenosis: Implications for follow-up. J Am Coll Cardiol 19:968–973, 1992.

    Doppler echocardiography in 140 patients with rheumatic mitral stenosis showed an average decrease in valve area of 0.09 ± 0.21 cm²/y. Predictors of more rapid progression were a higher initial gradient and echocardiographic score. In those with a morphology score greater than 8, valve area decreased by 0.3 ± 0.3 cm²/y compared to 0.0 ± 0.1 cm²/y in those with a score less than 8.

28. Sagie A, Freitas N, Padial LR, et al: Doppler echocardiographic assessment of long-term progression of mitral stenosis in 103 patients: Valve area and right heart disease. J Am Coll Cardiol 28:472–479, 1996.

    In 103 mitral stenosis patients, mitral valve area decreased by 0.09 cm²/y. Progression was most rapid in those with a larger initial valve area. These findings illustrate the utility of Doppler echocardiography in following disease progression in individual patients.

29. Vahanian A: Balloon valvuloplasty. Heart 85(2):223–228, 2001.

    Review of the approach, patient selection, and outcomes with balloon mitral valvuloplasty.

30. Reid CL: Echocardiography in the patient undergoing catheter balloon mitral commissurotomy. In: Otto CM (ed): The Practice of Clinical Echocardiography, 2nd ed. Philadelphia: WB Saunders, 2002, pp 435–451.

    Review of the use of echocardiography in patient selection, prediction of hemodynamic results, diagnosis of complications, and long-term outcome after mitral commissurotomy.

31. Iung B, Cormier B, Ducimetiere P, et al: Functional results 5 years after successful percutaneous mitral commissurotomy in a series of 528 patients and analysis of predictive factors. J Am Coll Cardiol 27:407–414, 1996.

    Stenotic mitral valves were classified by echocardiography as group I (flexible leaflets and mild subvalvular disease), group II (flexible leaflets and extensive subvalvular disease), and group III (calcified valves). Multivariate predictors of long-term functional results after percutaneous commissurotomy were echocardiographic group and cardiothoracic ratio before the procedure and valve area after the procedure.

32. Wang A, Krasuski RA, Warner JJ, et al: Serial echocardiographic evaluation of restenosis after successful percutaneous mitral commissurotomy. J Am Coll Cardiol 39(2):328–334, 2002.

    In a series of 310 patients undergoing percutaneous mitral valvuloplasty, the cumulative restenosis rate was 40% after 6 years. Overall, mitral valve area decreased by an average of 0.08 cm^2/yr by 2D planimetry and 0.06 cm^2/yr by the pressure half-time method. The only independent predictor of restenosis was a higher echocardiography mitral valve morphology score.

The Echo Exam *Aortic Stenosis*

Valve anatomy	Calcific
	Bicuspid (2 leaflets in systole)
	Rheumatic
Stenosis severity	Jet velocity (V_{max})
	Mean pressure gradient (ΔP_{mean})
	LVOT:AS velocity ratio
	Aortic valve area (AVA)
Co-existing AR	Qualitative evaluation of severity
LV response	LV hypertrophy
	LV dimensions or volumes
	LV ejection fraction
Other findings	Pulmonary pressures
	Mitral regurgitation

LV, left ventricle; AR, aortic regurgitation.

Example

An 82-year-old woman presents with dyspnea on exertion and is noted to have a 3/6 systolic murmur at the base, radiating to the carotids with a single S2 and a diminished carotid upstrokes. Echocardiography shows a calcified aortic valve with:

Aortic jet velocity (V_{max})	4.2 m/s
Velocity time integral (VTI_{AS})	68 cm
Mean gradient	45 mm Hg
LV outflow tract diameter ($LVOT_D$)	2.1 cm
LVOT velocity (V_{LVOT})	0.9 m/s
Velocity time integral (VTI_{LVOT})	14 cm

The *maximum jet velocity* of 4.2 m/s indicates severe stenosis which is confirmed by calculation of maximum and mean pressure gradients.

Maximum pressure gradient is calculated from maximum aortic jet velocity (V_{max}) as:

$$\Delta P_{max} = 4(V_{max})^2 = 4(4.2)^2 = 71 \text{ mm Hg}$$

Mean pressure gradient is calculated by tracing the outer edge of the CW Doppler velocity curve, with the echo instrument calculating and then averaging instantaneous pressure gradients over the systolic ejection period. The simplified method for estimation of mean gradient is

$$\Delta P = 2.4(V_{max})^2 = 2.4 \ (4.2)^2 = 42 \text{ mm Hg}$$

In order to correct for transvalvular volume flow rate, the velocity ratio and valve area are calculated:

Velocity ratio is $\quad V_{LVOT}/V_{max} = 0.9/4.2 = 0.21$ (dimensionless index)

Aortic valve area is

$$AVA = (CSA_{LVOT} \times VTI_{LVOT})/VTI_{AS\text{-}Jet}$$

Where cross-sectional area (CSA) of the LVOT is

$$CSA_{LVOT} = \pi(LVOT_D/2)^2 = 3.14(2.1/2)^2 = 3.46 \text{ cm}^2$$

Thus $\quad AVA = (3.46 \text{ cm}^2 \times 14 \text{ cm})/68 \text{ cm} = 0.71 \text{ cm}^2$

Simplified formula for valve area is

$$AVA = (CSA_{LVOT} \times V_{LVOT})/V_{max}$$

Thus

$$AVA = (3.46 \text{ cm}^2 \times 0.9 \text{ cm/s})/4.2 \text{ cm/s} = 0.74 \text{ cm}^2$$

This mean gradient (>40 mm Hg), velocity ratio (<0.25) and valve area (<1.0 cm^2) are all consistent with severe stenosis.

Quantitation of Aortic Stenosis Severity

Components	Modality	View	Recording	Measurements
LVOT diameter $LVOT_D$	2D	Parasternal long-axis	Adjust depth, optimize endocardial definition, zoom mode	Inner edge to inner edge of LVOT, parallel and adjacent to aortic valve, mid-systole
LVOT flow V_{LVOT} VTI_{LVOT}	Pulsed Doppler	Apical 4-chamber (anteriorly angulated)	Sample volume 2–3 mm, envelope of flow with defined peak, start with sample volume at valve and move apically	Trace modal velocity of spectral velocity curve
AS-Jet V_{max} $VTI_{AS\text{-}Jet}$	CW Doppler	Apical, SSN, other	Examination from multiple windows, careful positioning, and transducer angulation to obtain highest velocity signal	Measure maximum velocities at edge of intense velocity signal

The Echo Exam *Mitral Stenosis*

Valve anatomy	Valve thickness and mobility Calcification Commissural fusion Subvalvular involvement
Stenosis severity	2D valve area Mean pressure gradient Pressure half-time valve area
Left atrium	Size TEE for thrombus pre-valvuloplasty
Co-existing MR	Qualitative evaluation of severity
Pulmonary vasculature	Pulmonary systolic pressure Right ventricular size and function
Other findings	Aortic valve involvement Left ventricular size and systolic function

Example

A 26-year-old pregnant woman presents with dyspnea and is noted to have a diastolic murmur at the apex. Echocardiography shows rheumatic mitral stenosis with:

MVA_{2D} 0.8 cm^2
Mean ΔP 5 mm Hg
$T_{1/2}$ 260 ms

Mitral valve morphology score:

Leaflet thickness	2
Mobility	1
Calcification	1
Subvalvular	2
TOTAL	6

Tricuspid regurgitant jet velocity	3.1 m/s
Estimated RA pressure	10 mm Hg
Mitral regurgitation	Mild

Mean pressure gradient is calculated by tracing the outer edge of the CW Doppler velocity curve, with the echo instrument calculating and then averaging instantaneous pressure gradients over the systolic ejection period.

Doppler mitral valve area ($MVA_{Doppler}$) is calculated as

$$MVA_{Doppler} = 220/T_{1/2} = 220/260 = 0.85 \text{ cm}^2$$

The 2D mitral valve area and the pressure half-time valve area show reasonable agreement and both are consistent with severe mitral stenosis.

Pulmonary artery pressure (PAP) is

$$PAP = 4(V_{TR})^2 + RAP = 4(3.1)^2 + 10 \text{ mm Hg} = 48 \text{ mm Hg.}$$

Pulmonary pressure is moderately elevated consistent with a secondary response to severe mitral stenosis.

The mitral morphology score is low and only mild mitral regurgitation is present indicating a high likelihood of immediate and long-term success with balloon mitral valvuloplasty. A transesophageal echo is needed just before mitral valvuloplasty to evaluate for left atrial thrombus.

Quantitation of Mitral Stenosis Severity

Parameter	Modality	View	Recording	Measurements
2D valve area (MVA_{2D})	2D	Parasternal short-axis	Scan from apex to base to identify minimal valve area	Planimetry of inner edge of dark-light interface
Mean gradient (Mean ΔP)	HPRF Doppler	Apical 4-chamber or long-axis	Align Doppler beam parallel to MS jet. Adjust angle to obtain smooth envelope, clear peak and linear deceleration slope	Trace maximum velocity of spectral velocity curve
Pressure half-time ($T_{1/2}$)	HPRF Doppler	Apical 4-chamber or long-axis	Same as mean gradient. Adjust scale so velocity curve fills the screen. HPRF Doppler often has less noise than CW Doppler signal	Place line from maximum velocity along mid-diastolic linear slope

Classification of Aortic Stenosis Severity

	Mild	Severe
Jet velocity (m/s)	<3.0	>4.0
Mean gradient (mm Hg)	<20	>40
Velocity ratio	>0.50	<0.25
Valve area (cm^2)	>1.5	<1.0

Classification of Mitral Stenosis Severity

	Mild	Severe
Mean gradient (mm Hg)	<5	>15
Pulmonary pressure (mmHg)	<30	>60
Valve area (cm^2)	>1.5	<1.0

VALVULAR REGURGITATION

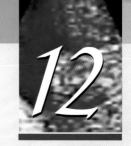

Echocardiographic evaluation of the patient with valvular regurgitation includes assessment of valve anatomy, the severity of regurgitation, chamber dilation due to the imposed volume overload, ventricular function, and the degree of pulmonary hypertension. In some clinical situations, the clinical significance of valvular regurgitation is related to the *presence* of abnormal regurgitation, regardless of severity. For example, detection of aortic regurgitation in a patient with chest pain and an enlarged aortic root heightens the suspicion of aortic dissection. Detection of regurgitation also may be important in terms of endocarditis risk and the need for prophylactic antibiotics in patients with a cardiac murmur. In other situations (e.g., endocarditis with acute

mitral regurgitation), the *severity* of regurgitation is an essential factor in clinical decision making regarding surgical intervention. In chronic regurgitation due to primary valve disease, regurgitant severity and the *response of the left ventricle to chronic volume overload* are the most important factors in deciding on the timing of valve surgery.

BASIC PRINCIPLES

Etiology of Valvular Regurgitation

Valvular regurgitation may be due to congenital or acquired abnormalities of the valve leaflets or to abnormalities of the associated supporting structures. For example, aortic root dilation can result in aortic regurgitation even with anatomically normal valve leaflets. Similarly, left ventricular dilation can result in mitral regurgitation even with normal valve leaflets and chordae. Echocardiographic examinations allow definition of the etiology of valvular regurgitation in most cases. Even when a single definite etiology is not evident, the differential diagnosis of the etiology of regurgitation often can be narrowed to the few most likely possibilities. The examination also may provide clues as to whether regurgitation is acute or chronic in duration.

If transthoracic images are not diagnostic for evaluation of aortic or mitral valve anatomy and the etiology of regurgitation, transesophageal imaging may be helpful. With aortic root disease, visualization of the ascending aorta often is suboptimal on transthoracic imaging, so transesophageal echocardiography typically is needed to fully define the extent and severity of disease

Fluid Dynamics of Valvular Regurgitation

The fluid dynamics of a regurgitant valve (Fig. 12–1) are, in many ways, similar to the fluid dynamics of a stenotic valve and are characterized by a

- regurgitant orifice area,
- high-velocity regurgitant jet,
- proximal flow convergence region,
- downstream flow disturbance, and
- increased antegrade flow volume.

Even though the anatomy of inadequate valve closure may be quite complex, the valve can be thought of as having a regurgitant orifice, which in simple physiologic terms is characterized by a high-velocity laminar jet (Table 12–1). The instantaneous velocity in this jet (v) is related to the instantaneous pressure difference (ΔP) across the valve, as stated in the simplified Bernoulli equation: $\Delta P = 4v^2$. Recording this high-velocity jet with continuous-wave Doppler allows assessment of the time course of the difference in pressure

Valvular Regurgitation

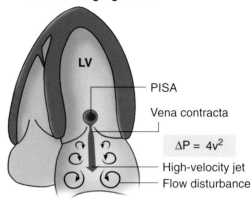

FIGURE 12–1. Schematic drawing of a regurgitant jet showing the proximal isovelocity surface area (PISA), the jet through the regurgitant orifice, and the flow disturbance in the receiving chamber.

between the two chambers on either side of the valve.

On the upstream side of the regurgitant valve, flow acceleration proximal to the regurgitant orifice is present, and a proximal isovelocity surface area (PISA) can be defined similar to that seen on the left atrial side of the stenotic mitral valve. The PISA, multiplied by the aliasing velocity, provides a method for quantitative evaluation of regurgitant stroke volume. The narrowest segment of the regurgitant jet, the vena contracta, occurs just distal to the regurgitant orifice, with vena contracta diameter reflecting regurgitant orifice area.

As the high-velocity jet enters the chamber receiving the regurgitant flow, the flow pattern becomes disturbed with nonlaminar flow, multiple blood flow velocities, and multiple blood flow directions. The *size* of the downstream regurgitant flow disturbance is affected by both physiologic and technical factors and thus is less useful for quantitation of regurgitant severity (Table 12–2). In addition, the *shape* and *direction* of the regurgitant jet are affected by the anatomy and

TABLE 12–1	
Relationship between Fluid Dynamics of Valvular Regurgitation and Diagnostic Approach	
Fluid Dynamic Characteristic	**Diagnostic Approach**
Conservation of mass through the regurgitant orifice	Continuity equation for regurgitant orifice area
High-velocity jet in regurgitant orifice	Pressure/velocity relationship of continuous-wave Doppler curve
Proximal flow convergence	Proximal isovelocity surface area
Downstream flow disturbance	Jet area in chamber receiving regurgitant flow
Increased volume flow across valve	Stroke volume across regurgitant minus competent valve

TABLE 12–2
Factors That Affect Regurgitant Jet Size and Shape

Physiologic

Regurgitant volume
Driving pressure
Size and shape of regurgitant orifice
Receiving chamber constraint
Wall impingement
Timing relative to the cardiac cycle
Influence of coexisting jets or flowstreams

Technical

Ultrasound system gain
Pulse repetition frequency
Transducer frequency
Frame rate
Image plane
Depth
Signal strength

Mitral Regurgitation

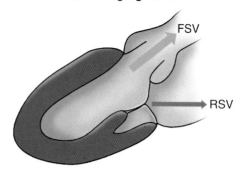

Total SV = Forward SV + Regurgitant SV

■ **FIGURE 12–2.** When mitral regurgitation is present, total stroke volume is the sum of the regurgitant (RSV) and forward stroke volumes (FSV).

orientation of the regurgitation orifice, the driving force across the valve, and the size and compliance of the receiving chamber. Jets are "pulled" toward adjacent walls (e.g., mitral regurgitation in the left atrium) if within a critical distance from the wall at the entry site and also are "pulled" toward other flowstreams (e.g., aortic regurgitation and mitral stenosis). Eccentric jets that adhere to the wall of the chamber will have a smaller color jet area on two-dimensional (2D) color flow imaging (and a smaller three-dimensional [3D] volume) because entrainment of additional fluid elements into the jet occurs on only one side, instead of on all sides, as with a central jet.

Volume Overload

In patients with regurgitant valves, the term *total stroke volume* refers to the total volume of blood pumped by the ventricle on a single beat. *Forward stroke volume* is the amount of blood delivered to the peripheral circulation, and *regurgitant volume* is the amount of backflow across the abnormal valve (Fig. 12–2).

Chronic valvular regurgitation results in progressive volume overload of the ventricle. Volume overload of the left ventricle results in chamber dilation with normal wall thickness so that total left ventricular mass is increased. An important clinical feature of chronic left ventricular volume overload is that an irreversible decrease in systolic function can occur in the absence of symptoms. In fact, an irreversible decrease in contractility can occur despite a normal ejection fraction due to the altered loading conditions of the ventricle when regurgitation is present.

Serial echocardiographic evaluation of left ventricular size and systolic function is a standard method of clinical evaluation, but two factors potentially limit the reliability of this approach. First, suboptimal image quality or recording techniques may result in erroneous measurements. Care is needed to ensure that the dimensions are measured perpendicular to the long and short axes of the left ventricle, and instrument settings must be adjusted for optimal endocardial definition. Accurate tracing of endocardial borders for calculation of ventricular volumes depends on clear endocardial definition, standard image planes without foreshortening of the long axis of the ventricle, and a trained and experienced individual tracing the borders at end-diastole and end-systole.

Second, the reproducibility of left ventricular measurements must be considered. Overall reproducibility includes variation in *recording* the data, variation in *measuring* the data, and *physiologic* variation (such as heart rate and loading conditions) that may affect the measurement. Reproducibility of 2D-guided M-mode measurements of the left ventricle suggests that an interval change of greater than 8 mm in end-systolic or end-diastolic dimensions represents a definite clinical change. Using 2D echocardiography, a change in ventricular volume or a change in ejection fraction greater than 10% on serial studies performed in the same laboratory indicates a significant change.

Detection of Valvular Regurgitation

Valvular regurgitation can be detected with either

■ color flow imaging, or
■ continuous-wave Doppler ultrasound.

While 2D imaging provides detailed information about valve anatomy and chamber dilation and function, it provides only indirect evidence for the presence or absence of valvular incompetence. The finding of an anatomically abnormal mitral valve in the presence of left atrial and left ventricular dilation suggests that mitral regurgitation may be present, but Doppler examination is necessary for direct confirmation or exclusion of the diagnosis. Although a few M-mode findings have been shown to be specific for diagnosing valvular regurgitation (e.g., high-frequency fluttering of the anterior mitral leaflet in aortic regurgitation), these findings are not sensitive enough to reliably exclude regurgitation when suspected on clinical grounds.

With color flow imaging, detection of regurgitation is based on identification of the flow disturbance downstream from the regurgitant orifice. When instrument settings and examination technique are optimal, color flow imaging is extremely sensitive (approximately 90%) and specific (nearly 100%) for detection of valvular regurgitation as compared with angiography. In fact, color flow imaging is so sensitive that regurgitation often is detected that is not audible by auscultation. These cases most often are true positives, as evidenced by angiographic confirmation. False-positive results can occur with color flow imaging when the origin or timing of the flow signal is mistaken. For example, normal pulmonary venous inflow into the left atrium may be mistaken for mitral regurgitation. False-negative results occur when signal strength is low due to poor acoustic access or attenuation due to the depth of interrogation. False-negative results also occur if color flow processing parameters are set incorrectly or if the examiner fails to evaluate the valve in more than one tomographic plane. Additional parameters important in detection of valvular regurgitation with color flow imaging include frame rate, Nyquist limit, color gain, and the color velocity/variance display.

Continuous-wave Doppler detection of valvular regurgitation is based on identification of the high-velocity jet through the regurgitant orifice. An advantage of continuous-wave Doppler is that beam width is broad at the level of the valves when studied from an apical approach. Identification of the regurgitant signal uses the velocity, shape, timing, and associated antegrade flow signal to correctly identify the origin of the signal (Fig. 12–3).

Valvular Regurgitation in Normal Individuals

A small degree of regurgitation, often termed *physiologic*, is present in a high percentage of otherwise

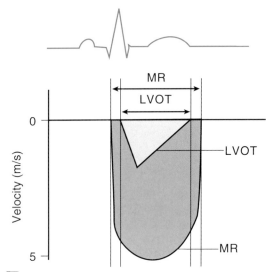

FIGURE 12–3. Relative timing of mitral regurgitation (MR) and left ventricular outflow tract (LVOT) flow signal. Mitral regurgitation extends from the onset of isovolumic contraction to the end of isovolumic relaxation. Left ventricular outflow is shorter, occurring only during ejection.

normal individuals (Fig. 12–4). Typically, physiologic regurgitation is

- spatially restricted to the area immediately adjacent to valve closure,
- short in duration, and
- represents only a small regurgitant volume.

When meticulously searched for, mitral regurgitation can be detected in 70% to 80%, tricuspid regurgitation in 80% to 90%, and pulmonic regurgitation in 70% to 80% of normal individuals. This small degree of regurgitation is normal and has no adverse clinical implications. Aortic regurgitation is found in only a small percentage (5%) of young individuals with an otherwise normal echocardiographic study, but the prevalence of detectable aortic regurgitation increases with age. The clinical significance of a small amount of aortic regurgitation is unknown.

APPROACHES TO EVALUATION OF THE SEVERITY OF REGURGITATION

The severity of valvular regurgitation typically is described using semiquantitative meaures as mild, moderate, or severe; for example, using color jet area (Table 12–3). Other semiquantitative measures include

- vena contracta width,
- pressure half-time (for aortic regurgitation), and
- distal flow reversals.

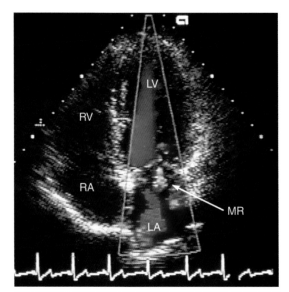

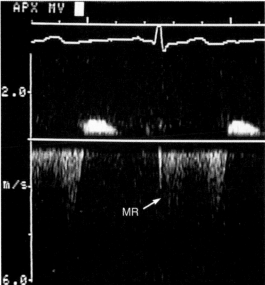

■ FIGURE 12–4. Example of "physiologic" mitral regurgitation recorded with color *(top)* and continuous-wave *(bottom)* Doppler in a normal individual. Note the low signal strength compared with antegrade flow and the incomplete systolic signal.

However, several quantitive measures of regurgitant severity have been well validated, including (Table 12–4)

- regurgitant volume,
- regurgitant fraction, and
- regurgitant orifice area.

Regurgitant volume (RV) is the retrograde volume flow rate across the valve, expressed either as an instantaneous flow rate in milliliters per second or (more correctly) averaged over the cardiac cycle in milliliters per beat. Regurgitant volume can be calcuated by three different approaches:

- PISA
- Volume flow rates across the regurgitant and a competent valve
- 2D total left ventricular stroke volume minus Doppler forward stroke volume

Regurgitant fraction (RF) is

$$RF = RV/SV_{total} \qquad (12\text{–}1)$$

Regurgitant orifice area (ROA) is calculated, using the continuity equation, from regurgitant volume and the velocity time integral of the regurgitant jet (VTI_{RJ}). Because the regurgitant volume (RV) proximal to and *in* the regurgitant orifice are equal,

$$RV = ROA \times VTI_{RJ} \qquad (12\text{–}2)$$

so that, solving for regurgitant orifice area,

$$ROA = RV/VTI_{RJ} \qquad (12\text{–}3)$$

with RV in cm^3, VTI_{RJ} in cm, and ROA in cm^2.

Color Doppler Imaging

Jet Area

Screening for significant regurgitation often is based on the size of the flow disturbance in the chamber receiving the regurgitant jet. The size of the flow disturbance is evaluated using color flow imaging in at least two views. For each tomographic image plane, it is noted whether an abnormal flow signal with appropriate timing (i.e., systole for mitral regurgitation, diastole for aortic regurgitation) is present or absent. The size of the jet, relative to the receiving chamber, provides a qualitative index of regurgitant severity on a 0 (mild) to 4+ (severe) scale. However, this index is most useful for identification of patients with mild regurgitation; there is substantial overlap in jet areas between patients with moderate and severe regurgitation (Figs. 12–5 and 12–6). Although the use of color flow imaging to define jet origin and direction is a useful qualitative descriptor in some cases, the length that a regurgitant jet extends into the receiving chamber is an unreliable indicator of disease severity and should no longer be used in patient management.

Because color flow imaging basically is pulsed Doppler ultrasound with somewhat different signal processing and display formats, it is important to remember that signal aliasing still occurs. However, flow imaging depends on the timing and spatial location of the Doppler signals and *not*

TABLE 12–3

Doppler Evaluation of Valvular Regurgitation

Method	Doppler Parameters	Limitations	Invasive Analog
Color flow imaging	Jet origin Jet direction Jet size	Variation with technical and physiologic factors	Angiography
Continuous-wave Doppler	Signal intensity Shape of velocity curve	Qualitative	Hemodynamics
Vena contracta width	Width of regurgitant jet at origin	Small values, careful measurement needed	None
Proximal isovelocity surface area (PISA)	Calculation of RV and ROA	Less accurate with eccentric jets Peak values only	None
Volume flow at two sites	Calculation of RV and ROA	Tedious	Invasive RV and RF
Distal flow reversals	Pulmonary vein (MR) or aorta (AR)	Qualitative, affected by LA pressure, AF (MR)	None

AR, aortic regurgitation; MR, mitral regurgitation; RV, regurgitant volume; ROA, regurgitant orifice area; RF, regurgitant fraction.

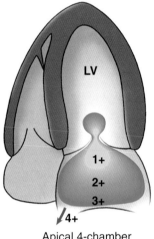

Apical 4-chamber

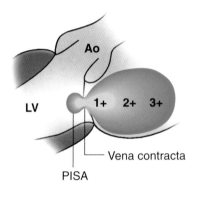

Parasternal long-axis

FIGURE 12–5. Color Doppler evaluation of mitral regurgitation. The parasternal and apical views provide information on jet geometry and direction. The vena contracta is imaged in a parasternal view, when possible, but may be well seen from apical views as well. The proximal flow convergence region typically is measured from an apical approach. Multiple views allow identification of eccentric jets. The colors indicate mild, moderate, and severe regurgitation. Severe (4+) mitral regurgitation is associated with systolic flow reversal in the pulmonary veins.

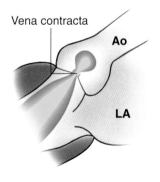

Long-axis

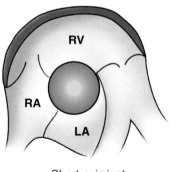

Short-axis just below aortic valve

FIGURE 12–6. Evaluation of aortic regurgitant severity using color flow mapping in parasternal long- and short-axis views. The vena contracta can be imaged in a long-axis or short-axis view. In the clinical setting, multiple views are used because jets often are eccentric in direction and asymmetric in shape.

TABLE 12–4

Selected Studies Validating Quantitative Evaluation of Regurgitant Severity Using Doppler Echocardiography

First Author/ Year	Method	Standard of Reference	N	R Value	SEE
Color Jet Area					
Spain/1989	Color jet area	Angio LV, TD-CO	15 MR pts	0.62 (RF)	–
Tribouilloy/ 1992	Regurgitant jet width at origin	Angio LV, TD-CO	31 MR pts	0.85 (RSV)	–
Enriquez-Sarano/1993	Color jet area	Doppler SV at two sites	80 MR pts	0.69 (RF)	4.4 cm^2
Vena Contracta					
Tribouilloy/ 2000	Vena contracta width	Doppler EROA and RV	79 AR pts	0.89 (EROA) 0.90 (RV)	0.08 cm^2 18 mL
Hall/1997	Vena contracta width	Doppler EROA and RV	80 MR pts	0.86 0.85 (RV)	0.15 cm^2 20 mL
PISA					
Recusani/ 1991	PISA (hemispherical)	Rotometer	In vitro, constant flow	0.94–0.99 (flow rate)	1–1.6 L/min
Utsunomiya/ 1991	PISA (hemispherical)	Actual flow rate stopwatch and cylinder	In vitro, pulsatile flow	0.99 (flow rate)	0.53 L/min
Vandervoort/ 1993	PISA	Actual flow rate	In vitro, steady flow	0.98–0.99 (flow rate)	–
Giesler/1993	PISA	LV angio, Fick CO	16 MR pts	0.88 (RSV)	17 mL
Chen/1993	PISA	Doppler SV at two sites	46 MR pts	0.94 (RSV)	18 mL
Continuous-Wave Doppler					
Teague/1986	AR half-time	Angio LV, Fick CO	32 AR pts	–0.88 (RF)	11%
Masuyama/ 1986	AR half-time	Angio LV, ID-CO	20 AR pts	–0.89 (RF)	–
Volume Flow at Two Sites					
Ascah/1985	Transmitral vs. transaortic SV	EM-flow	30 flow rates in canine model	0.83 (RF)	–
Kitabatake/ 1985	Transaortic vs. transpulmonic SV	Angio LV, TD-CO	20 AR pts	0.94 (RF)	–
Rokey/1986	Transmitral vs. transaortic SV	Angio LV, TD-CO	19 MR and 6 AR pts	0.91 (RF)	7%
Distal Flow Reversals					
Boughner/ 1975	Diastolic flow reversal in descending Ao	Angio LV, Fick CO	15 AR pts	0.91 (RF)	–
Touche/1985	Diastolic flow reversal in descending Ao	Angio LV, TD-CO	30 AR pts	0.92 (RF)	8.8%

Ao, aortic; AR, aortic regurgitation; CO, cardiac output; EM-flow, volume flow rate measured by electromagnetic flowmeter; ID, indicator dilation; LV, left ventricle; MR, mitral regurgitation; PISA, proximal isovelocity surface area method; RF, regurgitant fraction; RSV, regurgitant stroke volume; SV, stroke volume; TD, thermodilution.

Data from Bougher et al: Circulation 52:874–879, 1975; Touche et al: Circulation 72:819–824, 1985; Ascah et al: Circulation 72:377–383, 1985; Kitabatake et al: Circulation 72:523–529, 1985; Rokey et al: J Am Coll Cardiol 7:1273–1278, 1986; Teague et al: J Am Coll Cardiol 8:592–599, 1986; Masuyama et al: Circulation 73:460–466, 1986; Spain et al: J Am Coll Cardiol 13:585–590, 1989; Tribouilloy et al: Circulation 85:1248–1253, 1992; Enriquez-Sarano et al: J Am Coll Cardiol 21:1211–1219, 1993; Rescusani et al: Circulation 83:594–604, 1991; Utsunomiya et al: J Am Soc Echocardiol 4:338–348, 1991; Vandervoort et al: J Am Coll Cardiol 22:535–541, 1993; Giesler et al: AJC 71:217–224, 1993; Chen et al: J Am Coll Cardiol 21:374–383, 1993. Tribouilloy CM et al. Circuation 102:558–564, 2000; Hall SA et al. Circulation 95: 636–642, 1997.

absolute blood flow velocity. Thus, signal aliasing does not limit the utility of flow imaging and, in fact, may enhance the appreciation of abnormal flow patterns due to the presence of variance in the color flow signal. In addition, flow imaging can be performed from windows where the intercept angle between the ultrasound beam and the direction of regurgitant flow is nonparallel. Moreover, these windows often allow a shorter distance from the transducer to the flow region of interest, resulting in a better signal-to-noise ratio. For example, aortic regurgitation is best evaluated from the parasternal approach. Although the direction of an aortic regurgitant jet in the parasternal long-axis view is nearly perpendicular to the ultrasound beam, multiple flow directions within the jet allow detection of the diastolic flow disturbance. Of course, an accurate blood velocity determination cannot be made both because of the nonparallel intercept angle and because the velocity exceeds the Nyquist limit of the pulsed Doppler mode.

The appearance of a regurgitant jet with color flow imaging will vary depending on the ultrasound system, transducer frequency, and specific instrument settings. Correct visual interpretation depends on experience with a particular instrument and knowledge of the influence of instrument settings on the visual display. On most systems, a "variance" color scale results in a green regurgitant signal superimposed on the normal red-blue flow patterns. A "velocity" scale results in a mosaic of red, blue, and white pixels in the regurgitant jet. Because the goal of this application is to identify the location and timing of abnormal flow signals in a tomographic format, the exact color scale used is not particularly important as long as it displays the boundaries of the flow disturbance accurately.

With either a variance or a velocity color flow scale, it is obvious that an abnormal color pattern is not synonymous with abnormal flow given the physics of pulsed Doppler color flow imaging. An abnormal color pattern can be seen even with normal intracardiac flow patterns. For example, the normal antegrade flow velocity of laminar flow across the aortic valve exceeds the Nyquist limit, resulting in aliasing and an "abnormal" color pattern. Conversely, abnormal flow signals may not demonstrate variance or a mosaic pattern if the flow velocities are within the Nyquist limit for that interrogation depth. For example, the low velocities seen in pulmonic regurgitation result in a uniform color display even though the flow pattern is abnormal. Interpretation of the color images will be most consistent from study to study if instrument settings and flow maps are standardized for each laboratory.

Recommended instrument settings for color flow imaging are

- Nyquist limit at the maximum for the imaging depth (60 to 80 cm/s),
- color gain setting just below random speckle from nonmoving targets,
- maximum frame rate (e.g., narrow sector, decrease depth), and
- consistent color velocity/variance display scale.

Evaluation of the exact timing of a flow signal in relation both to valve closing and to the QRS complex can be helpful in correct identification of the signal. With color flow imaging, temporal resolution is sacrificed for spatial resolution because frame rates are far lower than the sampling rate of pulsed or continuous-wave Doppler. Simultaneous recording of an electrocardiographic lead is essential for frame-by-frame analysis of the color flow images to verify the timing of the disturbance. If the timing of a color flow velocity signal is unclear, use of 2D-guided color "M-mode" may be helpful by providing higher time resolution. With color M-mode Doppler, the signal is displayed at each depth along a single line of interrogation (y axis) versus time (x axis) at a higher sampling rate (Fig. 12–7). Thus, the color M-mode tracing allows evaluation of the timing of the flow disturbance in relation to valve opening and closing.

Vena Contracta

The vena contracta, the narrowest diameter of the flow stream, reflects the diameter of the regurgitant orifice with the advantages that it is independent of volume flow rate and driving pressure, and it is relatively unaffected by instrument settings. However, because vena contracta diameters have a narrow range of values, care is needed to obtain optimal images for measurement. In order to optimize both temporal and spatial resolution, the recommended approach to measurement of vena contracta is to use a view that is

- perpendicular to jet width,
- in zoom mode,
- narrow sector, and
- minimum depth.

Angulation out of the standard image planes may be needed to depict both the proximal acceleration region and downstream flow expansion for accurate identication of the vena contracta (Fig. 12–8).

Vena contracta diameter may vary with dynamic changes in regurgitant orifice area, for example, with late systolic mitral regurgitation due to mitral valve prolapse. However, vena contracta width remains accurate in the setting of acute regurgitation, when jet area may be misleading.

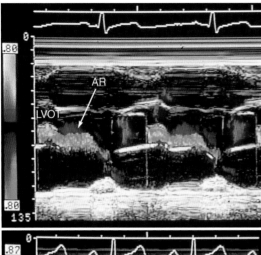

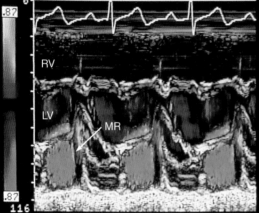

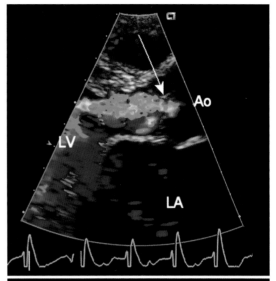

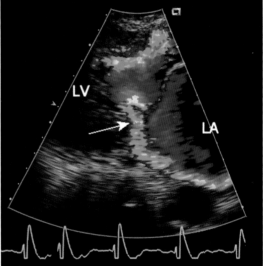

FIGURE 12–7. Color M-mode of aortic *(top)* and mitral *(bottom)* regurgitation shows the high time resolution of this approach.

Proximal Flow Convergence

Color flow imaging allows calcuation of the retrograde volume flow rate based on measurement of the flow convergence region proximal to the regurgitant orifice. Acceleration of flow occurs proximal to the valve plane with, conceptually, a series of isovelocity "surfaces" leading to the high-velocity jet in the regurgitant orifice. Immediately adjacent to the orifice, these surfaces are small with higher flow velocities; at increasing distances from the orifice, areas are larger and velocities are lower. Based on the principle of volume flow calculation by Doppler techniques, the volume flow rate (in this case, regurgitant flow) for a proximal isovelocity surface area (PISA), when averaged over the temporal flow period, is (Fig. 12–9)

Regurgitant volume
$$= \text{PISA} \times \text{aliasing velocity} \quad (12\text{–}4)$$

The velocity for a PISA can be determined from the color flow image as the aliasing velocity

FIGURE 12–8. Vena contracta measurement for aortic regurgitation *(top)* and mitral regurgitation *(bottom)* using a view perpendicular to the jet direction (parasternal) with a narrow sector and zoom mode. The long-axis view allows identification of the proximal flow convergence region and the downstream jet expansion, with the vena contracta identified as the narrowest segment joining them.

where a distinct red-blue interface is seen (Fig. 12–10). At this interface, the velocity is known, being equivalent to the Nyquist limit on the velocity color scale. The size of the PISA can be maximized to allow more accurate regurgitant flow rate calculations by decreasing the velocity range and/or by shifting the velocity baseline.

The shape of the isovelocity surface proximal to a regurgitant valve typically is hemispherical with a tendency toward a hemielliptical shape closer to the orifice. Assuming a hemispherical

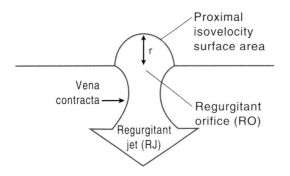

$$\text{Regurg. volume} = \text{PISA} \times \text{velocity}$$
$$\text{RO area} = \text{regurg. volume}/\text{VTI}_{RJ}$$

■ **FIGURE 12–9.** Proximal to a regurgitant orifice, flow accelerates resulting in concentric proximal isovelocity surface areas (PISAs). The radius (r) is used to calculate the PISA. The color Doppler aliasing velocity is used to calculate the regurgitant volume based on the aliasing velocity. In combination with the velocity-time integral (VTI) of the continuous-wave Doppler recording of the regurgitant jet (RJ), regurgitant orifice area (ROA) is calculated.

shape, the PISA is calculated from measurements of the distance from the aliasing velocity to the regurgitant orifice as

$$\text{PISA} = 2\pi r^2 \qquad (12\text{–}5)$$

Note that the PISA method for calculating regurgitant volume is analogous to calculation of stroke volume proximal to a stenotic valve. The differences between these approaches are (1) the differing shapes of the proximal velocity stream lines; (2) the use of color flow, rather than pulsed Doppler, to measure velocity at a given location; and (3) the need for temporal averaging when color data from single images are used.

The PISA method can be combined with the velocity-time integral of continuous-wave Doppler flow through the regurgitant orifice to calculate regurgitant orifice area using Eq. 12–3. Instead of averaging PISA over the duration of flow, most clinicians calculate the maximum instanteous regurgitant orifice area (ROA_{max} in cm^2) based on the maximum regurgitant volume (RV_{max}) flow rate (in milliliters per second) combined with maximum mitral regurgitant jet velocity (V_{MR} in centimeters per second):

$$\text{ROA}_{max} = \text{RV}_{max}/V_{MR} \qquad (12\text{–}6)$$

This approach assumes that RV_{max} and V_{MR} occur at the same time point in the cardiac cycle. The PISA should be recorded in a view parallel to the flow stream, typically an apical four-

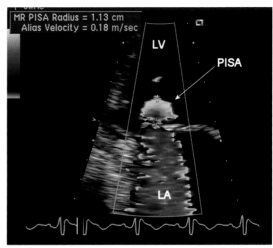

■ **FIGURE 12–10.** Proximal isovelocity surface area (PISA) in a patient with a dilated cardiomyopathy. The PISA has been optimized by decreasing the depth, narrowing the sector, and using the zoom mode. In addition the velocity color scale (no variance) has been adjusted to an aliasing velocity away from the transducer that maximizes the size of the PISA. The PISA radius of 1.1 cm (surface area = $2\pi r^2$ = 7.6 cm^2) at an aliasing velocity of 18 cm/s indicates an instantaneous regurgitant flow rate of 137 mL/s. The maximum mitral regurgitant jet velocity was 4.3 m/s, so that regurgitant orifice area is 0.32 cm^2, consistent with moderate mitral regurgitation.

chamber view for mitral regurgitation, using a narrow sector and zoom mode, with the aliasing velocity adjusted to optimize visualization of a hemispherical aliasing boundary. If the PISA is hemi-ellipitical or if the valve is nonplanar, an alternate approach should be used or appropriate corrections made in the calculations.

Continuous-Wave Doppler Approach

Several types of information regarding the severity of valvular regurgitation can be derived from the spectral display of the continuous-wave Doppler signal:

- Signal intensity relative to antegrade flow
- Antegrade flow velocity
- Time course (shape) of velocity curve

First, signal intensity is proportional to the number of blood cells contributing to the regurgitant signal. Because the ultrasound beam is relatively broad and signals from the entire length of the beam are recorded, much of the regurgitant jet can be encompassed in the beam with appropriate adjustment of beam direction. It is particularly helpful to compare the intensity of the regurgitant signal to antegrade flow across the same valve as a qualitative estimate of regurgitant

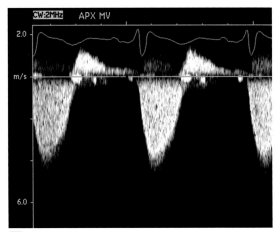

FIGURE 12–11. The continuous-wave Doppler mitral regurgitant signal, in the same patient as Figure 12–10, shows a dense signal, relative to antegrade mitral flow in diastole. The maximum velocity is only 4.3 m/s due to a low left ventricular systolic pressure and there is a rapid decline in velocity in late systole consistent with a left atrial *v* wave.

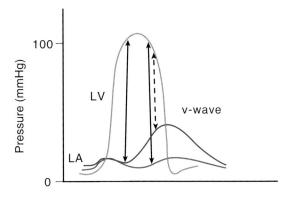

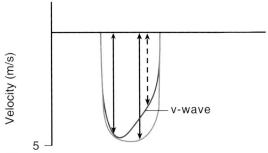

FIGURE 12–12. Left ventricular (LV) and left atrial (LA) pressures and the Doppler velocity curve in chronic (*solid lines*) and acute (*dashed lines*) mitral regurgitation are shown. Note that the shape of the velocity curve reflects the shape of the pressure difference between the left ventricle and the left atrium so that a late-systolic rise in left atrial pressure (*v* wave) is seen as a more rapid decrease in velocity in late systole on the Doppler curve.

severity (Fig. 12–11). A weak signal reflects mild regurgitation, whereas a signal nearly equal in intensity to antegrade flow reflects severe regurgitation. Moderate regurgitation has an intermediate signal strength relative to antegrade flow.

Second, the associated antegrade velocity across the regurgitant valve provides useful information. Regurgitation results in an increase in the antegrade volume flow rate across the valve, which is reflected in an increase in the antegrade velocity across the valve. The greater the severity of regurgitation, the higher is the antegrade velocity. Of course, the possibility of coexisting valvular stenosis also must be considered.

Third, the shape of the velocity curve depends on the time-varying pressure gradient across the regurgitant valve. Each instantaneous velocity is related to the instantaneous pressure gradient across the valve, as stated in the Bernoulli equation. Normal left ventricular systolic pressure is 100 to 140 mm Hg and normal left atrial pressure is 5 to 15 mm Hg, so the left ventricular to left atrial pressure difference in systole is 85 to 135 mm Hg. Thus, the mitral regurgitant velocity curve typically shows a maximum velocity of 5 to 6 m/s. When ventricular function is normal, there is rapid acceleration to peak velocity, with a maintained high velocity in systole and with rapid deceleration prior to diastolic opening of the mitral valve. An increase in end-systolic left atrial pressure (*v* wave) results in a late-systolic decline in the instantaneous pressure gradient and in the instantaneous velocity (Fig. 12–12).

Similarly, the shape of the aortic regurgitant velocity curve depends on the time course of the diastolic pressure difference across the aortic valve. When left ventricular end-diastolic pressure is low and aortic end-diastolic pressure is normal or mildly reduced, a large pressure difference (and high velocity) across the valve is present throughout diastole with a slow rate of pressure decline (Fig. 12–13). Acute or severe regurgitation results in more rapid equalization of left ventricular and aortic pressures with a more rapid velocity decline in diastole.

The utility of the continuous-wave Doppler curve depends, in large part, on technical factors in data recording as well as on correct data interpretation. The high-velocity regurgitant signal is optimized by use of

- sweep speed of spectral display at 100 mm/s,
- velocity range adjusted so that signal of interest fits but fills the screen,
- high-pass ("wall") filter set at the maximum level,

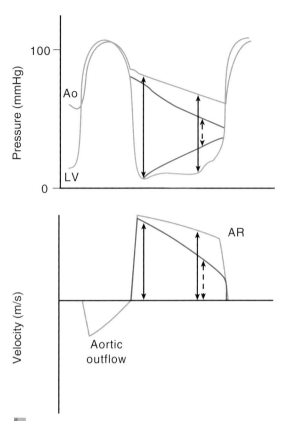

FIGURE 12–13. Left ventricular (LV) and central aortic (Ao) pressures and the corresponding Doppler velocity curve are shown for chronic (*green*) and acute (*blue*) aortic regurgitation. Again, the shape of the velocity curve is related to the instantaneous pressure differences across the valve, as stated in the Bernoulli equation. With acute aortic regurgitation, aortic pressure falls more rapidly and ventricular diastolic pressure rises more rapidly, resulting in a steeper deceleration slope on the Doppler curve.

- gain and dynamic range adusted to show dark outer edge of the velocity curve,
- examination from multiple acoustic windows, and
- careful transducer angulation.

Optimal patient positioning, examination from multiple windows, and transducer angulation are needed to ensure a near-parallel intercept angle between the direction of the ultrasound beam and the regurgitant jet, to avoid underestimation of velocities. Use of a dedicated, small, continuous-wave transducer often facilitates the examination and provides a better signal-to-noise ratio than 2D-guided continuous-wave Doppler. In addition, the 2D image may distract the examiner from searching for the highest-velocity signal. Color flow imaging is of limited value for locating the best continuous-wave signal because it provides only 2D information; jet direction in the eleva-

tional plane remains unknown. Temporal factors also affect data quality, and caution is needed in interpreting the shape of the velocity curve if jet direction (and thus Doppler-jet intercept angle) varies during the regurgitant flow period.

Distal Flow Reversals

When atrioventricular valve regurgitation is severe enough that a significant volume of blood is displaced by the regurgitant jet, flow reversal is seen in the veins entering the atrium. With severe tricuspid regurgitation, the normal pattern of systolic inflow into the right atrium from the superior and inferior vena cava is reversed. This can be demonstrated with a pulsed Doppler sample volume positioned in the central hepatic vein (Fig. 12–14). Severe mitral regurgitation results in reversal of the normal patterns of systolic inflow into the left atrium from the pulmonary veins. This may be difficult to demonstrate on a transthoracic study due to signal attenuation at the depth of the pulmonary vein but is easily recorded from a transesophageal approach (Fig. 12–15).

Regurgitation of a semilunar valve results in reversal of flow in the associated great vessel as blood flows from the great vessel, across the incompetent valve, and into the ventricle. The distance from the valve plane that this flow reversal extends in the great vessel is proportional to regurgitant volume. For example, with severe aortic regurgitation, holodiastolic flow reversal is seen in the proximal abdominal aorta. With moderate regurgitation, holodiastolic flow reversal only extends to the descending thoracic aorta.

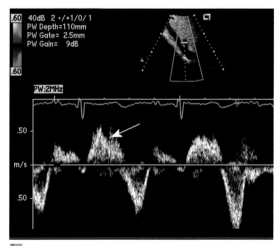

FIGURE 12–14. With the sample volume (SV) positioned in the central hepatic vein from a subcostal approach, systolic (*arrow*) flow reversal in the hepatic vein velocity curve is seen when severe tricuspid regurgitation is present. Forward flow into the right atrium in diastole also is seen.

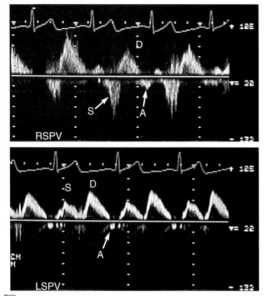

FIGURE 12–15. With severe mitral regurgitation, systolic flow reversal in the right superior pulmonary vein Doppler velocity curve *(top)* and blunting of systolic flow in the left superior pulmonary vein *(bottom)* are seen on transesophageal imaging in a patient with an eccentric, anteromedially directed regurgitant jet. D, diastolic flow; A, atrial reversal.

Volume Flow at Two Intracardiac Sites

Regurgitant stroke volume can be calculated using 2D diameter measurements in conjunction with pulsed Doppler flow velocities at two intracardiac sites. Total stroke volume is calculated from antegrade flow across the regurgitant valve as the cross-sectional area of flow times the velocity-time integral of transvalvular flow. Forward stroke volume is calculated as antegrade flow across a different (and nonregurgitant) valve (Fig. 12–16).

For example, with aortic regurgitation, transaortic stroke volume (SV) represents total left ventricular stroke volume and can be calculated as

$$SV_{total} = CSA_{LVOT} \times VTI_{LVOT} \qquad (12\text{-}7)$$

where CSA is cross-sectional area, VTI is the velocity-time integral, and LVOT is the left ventricular outflow tract. Forward stroke volume is represented by left ventricular inflow across the mitral annulus (MA), because the amount of blood filling the ventricle equals the amount of blood delivered to the body on each beat, and can be calculated as

$$SV_{forward} = CSA_{MA} \times VTI_{MA} \qquad (12\text{-}8)$$

With aortic regurgitation, alternate sites for measurement of forward stroke volume are the pul-

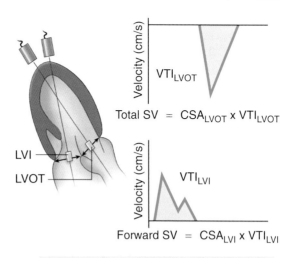

Total SV $= CSA_{LVOT} \times VTI_{LVOT}$

Forward SV $= CSA_{LVI} \times VTI_{LVI}$

Regurg. SV $=$ Total SV $-$ Forward SV

FIGURE 12–16. Calculation of aortic regurgitant stroke volume (SV) by measurement of transvalvular volume flow rate at two intracardiac sites is illustrated. Transaortic flow, representing total stroke volume, is calculated from the cross-sectional area (CSA) and velocity-time integral (VTI) of the left ventricular outflow tract (LVOT). Transmitral flow, representing forward stroke volume, is calculated from the cross-sectional area and velocity-time integral of left ventricular inflow (LVI) across the mitral annulus. Regurgitant stroke volume is the difference between total and forward stroke volume.

monary artery and right ventricular inflow region. Regurgitant volume is

$$RV = SV_{total} - SV_{forward} \qquad (12\text{-}9)$$

Regurgitant fraction and regurgitant orifice area then are calculated with Eqs. 12–1 and 12–3, respectively. Alternatively, total stroke volume can be derived from 2D or 3D imaging of the left ventricle with identification of endocardial borders at end-diastole and end-systole.

Calculation of regurgitant volume and regurgitant fraction from volume flow at two intracardiac sites has been shown to be accurate in animal models and in selected patient series. However, small errors in diameter measurement lead to large errors in cross-sectional area calculations due to the quadratic relationship between the two ($CSA = \pi r^2$). Other potential pitfalls in volume flow measurement are discussed in detail in Chapter 6. This method clearly can provide accurate quantitation of regurgitant severity when image quality is excellent; in other cases, it is helpful to compare the antegrade velocity-time integral (or peak velocity) for the regurgitant valve to the antegrade flow across a competent valve as an indicator of their relative stroke volumes.

Limitations and Alternate Approaches

Echocardiography is the clincial standard for evaluation of valvular regurgitation. The diagnostic value of the echocardiographic study is increased when the interpretation integrates data from several potential measures of regurgitant severity into a summary statement. Rather than being redundant, the different approaches to regurgitant severity serve as cross-checks on each other. Errors or limitations of one approach will be recognized when other approaches, with better data quality, show discrepant results. Because valvular regurgitant is dynamic and varies with loading conditions, it is essential to record blood pressure at the time of the echocardiographic examination.

When transthoracic echocardiographic data are suboptimal, transeophageal echocardiography is the next step. If further data are needed for clinical decision making, other approaches can be considered. Ventricular size and systolic function can be measured with radionuclide, angiographic, or magnetic resonance imaging approaches. A semiquantitative index of regurgitant severity is provided by contrast angiography (Fig. 12–17). Regurgitant volume and fraction can be calculated from invasive measures of total and forward stroke volume or by magnetic resonance imaging, but these approaches are rarely needed.

AORTIC REGURGITATION

The echocardiographic approach to the patient with aortic regurgitation includes not only evaluation of the presence of regurgitation but also determination of the etiology and severity of regurgitation along with the effect of the regurgi-

TABLE 12–5
Etiology of Aortic Regurgitation (Examples)

Leaflet Abnormalities

Congenital bicuspid valve
Calcific valve disease
Rheumatic valve disease
Myxomatous valve disease
Endocarditis
Nonbacterial thrombotic endocarditis

Aortic Root Abnormalities

Hypertensive aortic root dilation
Cystic medial necrosis
Marfan syndrome
Aortic dissection

tant lesion on ventricular size and function and any other associated abnormalities.

Diagnostic Imaging of the Valve Apparatus

Aortic regurgitation may be due either to abnormalities of the aortic root or to abnormalities of the leaflets themselves (Table 12–5). The disease processes that cause valvular aortic stenosis (*congenital bicuspid valve, calcific valve disease,* and *rheumatic disease*) also can result in aortic regurgitation due to alterations in leaflet flexibility or shape leading to inadequate diastolic coaptation of the leaflets. The 2D echocardiographic findings for these diagnoses are discussed in Chapter 11.

Other diseases that cause aortic regurgitation include *myxomatous valve disease,* which can affect the aortic valve as well as the mitral valve. The leaflets are thickened and redundant on 2D echocardiography with slight sagging of the leaflets into the left ventricular outflow tract in diastole. The normal hemi-cylindrical configuration of each leaflet in diastole is distorted so that the short-axis view intersects the center of the leaflet *en face,* resulting in the false appearance of an ill-defined echogenic "mass."

Endocarditis results in aortic regurgitation either by leaflet perforation due to the infectious process or to deformity of diastolic leaflet closure due to the presence of a valvular vegetation (Fig. 12–18). Less common abnormalities of the aortic valve leaflets leading to aortic regurgitation include congenital leaflet fenestrations, involvement by nonbacterial thrombotic endocarditis (Libman-Sachs vegetations in systemic lupus erythematosus), infiltrative diseases (e.g., amyloid), collagen-vascular disorders, mucopolysaccharidosis, or glycogen storage diseases.

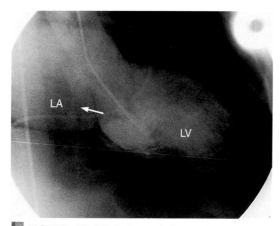

■ **FIGURE 12–17.** Left ventricular angiogram at end-systole showing severe mitral regurgitation with complete, dense opacification of the left atrium on the first beat.

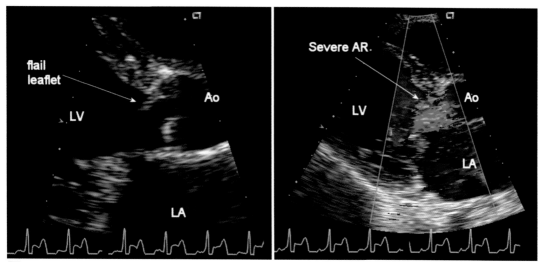

■ **FIGURE 12–18.** Flail aortic valve leaflet due to endocarditis *(left)* with a broad eccentric jet of aortic regurgitation on color flow imaging *(right)* in a parasternal long-axis view.

Abnormalities of the aortic root can result in aortic regurgitation, even when the leaflets themselves are normal, by alterations in the geometry of the structures supporting the leaflets. The aortic annulus is not a discrete planar ring of fibrous tissue but rather a complex crown-shaped structure where the leaflets attach to the aortic valve with the three "points" of the crown at the commissures and the three lowest points at the midsection of each leaflet. Dilation of this area at the base of the aortic root—often termed *annular dilation*—results in aortic regurgitation due to inadequate coaptation of the stretched leaflets. Note that adjacent leaflets normally overlap (apposition zone) so that mild degrees of annular dilation may not result in valvular incompetence. Annular dilation may be due to a variety of causes, including chronic *hypertension, cystic medial necrosis,* or *Marfan syndrome.* Marfan syndrome is characterized by effacement of the normal sinotubular junction with dilation of the annulus and sinuses of Valsalva (see Chapter 16). In cystic medial necrosis, the sinotubular junction usually is identifiable, although dilation may involve the base of the root as well as the ascending aorta. Many other diseases cause aortic root dilation, with consequent aortic regurgitation, including rheumatoid arthritis, ankylosing spondylitis, and mycotic aneurysm. Aortic regurgitation due to syphilitic aortitis is rare in the United States. When present, it typically is characterized by extensive calcification of the dilated aortic root. *Aortic dissection* can result in aortic regurgitation either by annular dilation resulting in inadequate coaptation or by the false channel of the dissection undermining

the aortic annulus and resulting in a flail leaflet (see Chapter 16).

The *differential diagnosis* for the echocardiographer in evaluation of a patient referred for suspected aortic regurgitation depends on the specific indications for the examination. If a diastolic murmur has been noted on auscultation, differential diagnoses include pulmonic regurgitation, mitral or tricuspid stenosis, and (rarely) a coronary arteriovenous fistula. In some cases, only the diastolic portion of a continuous murmur (e.g., a patent ductus arteriosus) may have been appreciated. If aortic regurgitation is suspected because of a concern for aortic dissection, the differential diagnosis should focus on examination of the ascending aorta.

Left Ventricular Response

When exposed to chronic volume overload from aortic regurgitation, progressive dilation and increased sphericity of the left ventricle occur. Initially, left ventricular systolic function remains normal. Note that ejection fraction remains normal (not hypernormal), since the total left ventricular stroke volume is ejected across the aortic valve into the high-impedance systemic vasculature (unlike the situation with chronic mitral regurgitation). With chronic gradually increasing aortic regurgitation, the left ventricle remains compliant in diastole so that end-diastolic pressure remains normal. Typically, left ventricular size slowly increases over a period of years without impairment of systolic function. However, left ventricular systolic dysfunction eventually occurs in the presence of hemodynamically significant chronic volume overload, and in some individuals, irreversible left ventricular systolic dysfunction supervenes even in the absence of clinical symptoms.

In contrast to chronic regurgitation, in acute aortic regurgitation, the short interval from onset of volume overload to clinical presentation means that significant left ventricular dilation has not yet occurred. The physiologic differences between acute and chronic aortic regurgitation are reflected both in the 2D echocardiographic findings and in the Doppler examination (Table 12–6).

Indirect Signs of Aortic Regurgitation

In addition to anatomic abnormalities of the aortic valve and the secondary left ventricular dilation that occurs in response to volume overload, several indirect signs may be seen in patients with aortic regurgitation:

- Increased E-point septal separation (EPSS)
- High-frequency fluttering of the anterior mitral leaflet
- "Reverse doming" of the anterior mitral leaflet
- Jet lesion on septum or mitral valve

If the regurgitant jet impinges on the anterior mitral valve leaflet, it causes impaired leaflet opening, resulting in an increased distance between the maximal anterior motion of the mitral valve in early diastole (the E point) and the most posterior motion of the interventricular septum (e.g., increased E-point septal separation). High-frequency fluttering of the anterior mitral valve leaflet resulting from impingement of the regurgitant jet also may be appreciated on M-mode (with its high sampling rate), although it is rarely appreciated on 2D imaging (due to the relatively low frame rate) (Fig. 12–19).

On 2D long- and short-axis imaging, the anterior mitral leaflet may appear curved in diastole

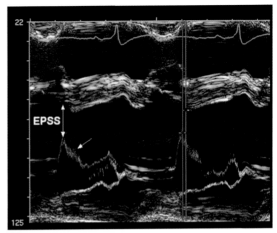

■ **FIGURE 12–19.** M-mode tracing showing increased E-point septal separation (EPSS) and high-frequency fluttering of the anterior mitral leaflet *(arrow)* due to impingement by an aortic regurgitant jet.

with the concavity toward the ventricular septum, with the region of abnormal curvature corresponding to the direction of the regurgitant jet. In short-axis views, a discrete area of reversed curvature corresponding to the spatial location of the regurgitant jet may be seen. This contrasts with the normal linear appearance of the anterior leaflet in diastole in long-axis views and the normal diastolic curvature toward the ventricular septum in the short-axis view. This observation has been termed *reverse doming*, because the curvature of the anterior leaflet is opposite to that seen in rheumatic mitral stenosis. With chronic regurgitation, the focal blood flow disturbance impinging on the septum or anterior mitral leaflet may result in a raised fibrotic lesion–identifiable by the pathologist postmortem as a jet lesion– which appears as an area of increased echogenicity on 2D imaging.

While none of these indirect signs of aortic regurgitation provides quantitative data, their presence may suggest a previously unsuspected diagnosis and prompt a directed Doppler examination. Recognition of the impact of aortic regurgitation on mitral leaflet motion and the appearance of jet lesions avoids misinterpretation of these findings.

Evaluation of Aortic Regurgitant Severity

Screening Examination

Screening for aortic regurgitation with color flow imaging and continuous wave Doppler ultrasound is part of a routine echocardiographic examination (Fig. 12–20). Parasternal views in both long and

TABLE 12–6

Chronic versus Acute Aortic Regurgitation

Parameter	Chronic	Acute
Etiology (examples)	Bicuspid valve	Endocarditis
	Hypertension	Aortic dissection
Left ventricular size	Dilated	Normal
Left ventricular end-diastolic pressure	Normal	Elevated
Pulse pressure	Wide	Narrow
Continuous-wave Doppler slope	Flat	Steep

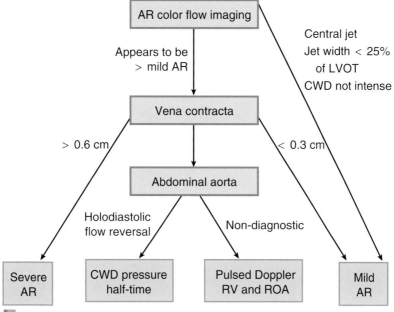

FIGURE 12–20. Approach to echocardiographic quantitation of aortic regurgitant severity.

short axis are helpful and may allow identification of the exact origin of the regurgitant jet as well as assessment of its width and cross-sectional area. Mild aortic regurgitation fills only a small area of the left ventricular outflow tract, whereas moderate-to-severe regurgitation fills a larger percentage of the outflow tract diamter or area (Figs. 12–21 and 12–22). Eccentric jets may traverse the outflow tract obliquely, which makes measure-ment of jet size more difficult. A central jet that fills less than 25% of the outflow tract is consistent with mild regurgitation.

Continuous-wave Doppler is used to record the antegrade aortic velocity signal from an apical approach with careful angulation to identify an aortic regurgitant signal, if present. A weak or absent diastolic signal confirms that significant regurgitation is not present.

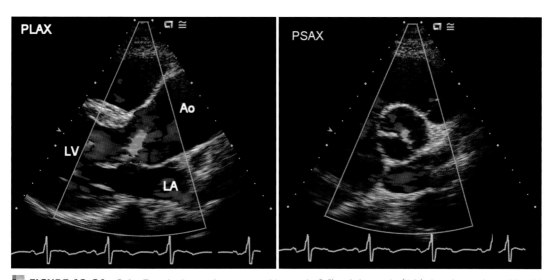

FIGURE 12–21. Color Doppler images in parasternal long-axis *(left)* and short-axis *(right)* views in a patient with mild aortic regurgitation. In long axis, a narrow eccentric jet is seen, which in short axis has a small cross-sectional area at the regurgitant orifice relative to the area of the outflow tract.

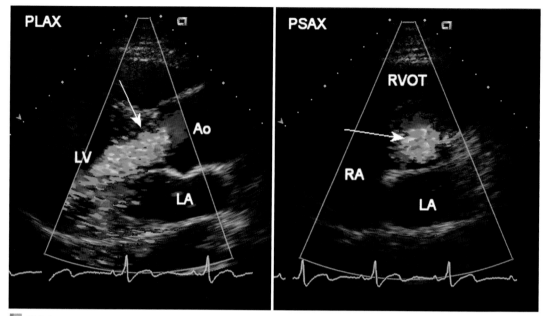

FIGURE 12–22. Color Doppler images in parasternal long- *(left)* and short-axis *(right)* views in a patient with severe aortic regurgitation. The flow disturbance fills the outflow tract in both views.

Vena Contracta

If the screening examination suggests more than mild aortic regurgitation, the next step is measurement of the vena contracta width, followed by further quantitation of regurgitant severity in some patients (Table 12–7). The vena contracta is visualized using color flow in a parastenal long-axis view in the zoom mode, with a narrow sector, to optimize temporal and spatial resolution. Careful angulation medially and laterally from the long-axis plane may be needed to clearly identify the narrowest segment of the regurgitant jet (see Fig. 12–8). A vena contracta width less than 0.3 cm is consistent with mild regurgitation and no further evalution is needed. A wider vena contracta width or poor data quality prompts further evaluation of regurgitant severity. With eccentric jets, diameter is measured perpendicular to the long axis of the jet, not the long axis of the outflow tract.

Aortic Flow Reversal

With severe aortic regurgitation, holodiastolic flow reversal is seen in the proximal abdominal aorta, recorded from the subcostal window (Fig. 12–23). This observation is analogous to the phys-

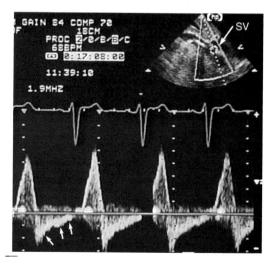

FIGURE 12–23. Two-dimensional image showing the pulsed Doppler sample volume (SV) position in the descending aorta from a subcostal approach *(top)*. The Doppler velocity curve *(bottom)* shows holodiastolic flow reversal *(arrows)* consistent with severe aortic regurgitation.

TABLE 12–7		
Quantitative Evaluation of Aortic Regurgitant Severity (ASE Guidelines)		
Parameter	**Mild**	**Severe**
Jet width/LVOT	<25%	≥65%
Vena contracta (cm)	<0.3	>0.6
Pressure half-time (ms)	>500	<200
Regurgitant volume (mL/beat)	<30	≥60
Regurgitant fraction (%)	<30	≥50
Regurgitant orifice area (cm²)	<0.10	≥0.30

ical examination finding of diastolic reversal in the femoral arteries (DeRosier's sign). Holodiastolic flow reversal in the abdominal aorta is sensitive (100%) and specific (97%) for diagnosing severe aortic regurgitation. False-positive results may be due to the presence of a patent ductus arteriosus, where the diastolic flow is from aorta to pulmonary artery rather than to the left ventricle. More proximal holodiastolic flow reversal, in the descending thoracic aorta, also is sensitive for detection of severe aortic regurgitation but is less specific, also being seen in some subjects with only moderate regurgitation (Fig. 12–24).

Continuous-Wave Doppler

The continuous-wave Doppler spectral recording of aortic regurgitation has its onset at aortic valve closure (during isovolumic relaxation) with a rapid increase in velocity to a maximum of 3 to 5 m/s, followed by a gradual decline in velocity during diastole. The velocity abruptly decelerates during isovolumic contraction, reaching baseline

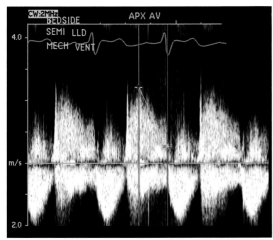

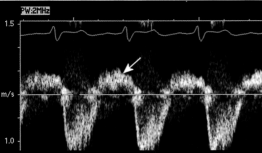

▪ **FIGURE 12–24.** Severe acute aortic regurgitation with a dense continuous-wave Doppler signal with a steep deceleration slope *(top)* and holodiastolic flow reversal in the descending thoracic aorta recorded from a suprasternal notch window *(bottom)* in the same patient as Figure 12–18.

at aortic valve opening. The intensity of the signal, relative to antegrade velocity, is an indicator of regurgitant severity. In moderate or severe regurgitation, the signal can easily be recorded throughout diastole, whereas mild regurgitation may not appear holodiastolic, with a recordable signal only at the beginning or end of diastole. This observation may be due to low signal strength or variation in jet direction during diastole resulting in significant intercept angle changes.

The shape of the continuous-wave Doppler time-velocity curve depends on the time-varying instantaneous pressure gradient across the valve in diastole, thus reflecting both severity and chronicity of regurgitation. Chronic severe aortic regurgitation results in an increased aortic pulse pressure with a low end-diastolic aortic pressure. The rapid rate of decline in aortic pressure is reflected in a more rapid decline in the Doppler velocity—that is, a steeper diastolic deceleration slope even if end-diastolic left ventricular pressure remains low (Fig. 12–25). Thus, diastolic deceleration slope provides a semiquantitative measure of aortic regurgitant severity. A flat slope (pressure half-time >500 ms) is consistent with mild regurgitation and a steep slope (pressure half-time <200 ms) indicates severe regurgitation.

However, in addition to aortic regurgitant severity, other factors that affect either left ventricular or aortic diastolic pressure also affect the course of the pressure difference (and velocity) across the regurgitant valve. With *acute* regurgitation, even if only moderate in severity, left ventricular compliance has not yet adapted, as occurs in response to chronic volume overload, so a significant increase in end-diastolic pressure is seen. In extreme cases, aortic and left ventricular end-diastolic pressure may equalize at end-diastole, resulting in a triangular-shaped continuous-wave velocity signal with a linear deceleration slope from maximum velocity to the baseline. Other factors that affect left ventricular diastolic pressure (e.g., systolic dysfunction, ischemia) or aortic diastolic pressure (e.g., sepsis, patent ductus arteriosus) also will affect the shape of the aortic regurgitant velocity curve.

The continuous-wave signal for aortic regurgitation usually is best recorded from an apical window to obtain a parallel intercept angle between the jet and the blood flow direction. Occasionally, an eccentric jet, directed either anteriorly or posteriorly, will be best recorded from a parasternal approach. If signal strength from the suprasternal notch is adequate, a signal similar to that recorded from the apex (but, of course, inverted) is seen.

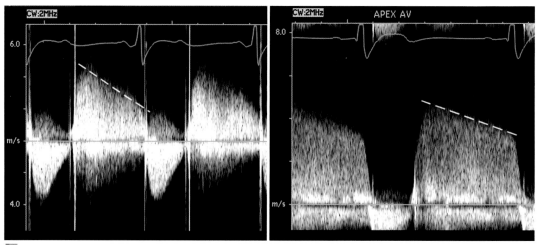

FIGURE 12-25. Continuous-wave Doppler recording in two patients, one with acute aortic regurgitation due to aortic dissection (*left*) and one with chronic regurgitation due to calcific aortic valve disease (*right*) showing the differences in the deceleration slope in these clinical situations.

Regurgitant Volume and Fraction

Aortic regurgitant volume and fraction can be calculated as the difference between transaortic and transmitral volume flow. In addition, in the specific case of aortic regurgitation, both forward and total stroke volume can be calculated at a single anatomic site: the proximal descending thoracic aorta. When aortic regurgitation is present, significant systolic expansion of the aorta occurs, so the antegrade flow velocity integral must be multiplied by the systolic cross-sectional area. The flow velocity integral of the reversed flow in diastole is multiplied by diastolic cross-sectional area. Either 2D short-axis imaging or an M-mode through the aortic arch can be used for measurement of systolic and diastolic cross-sectional areas. Note that this quantitative approach is the logical extension of the semiquantitative approach, which relies on the *presence* and spatial extent of holodiastolic flow reversal in the aorta in patients with aortic regurgitation.

Clinical Utility

Diagnostic Utility for Aortic Regurgitation

An echocardiogram may be requested to either confirm or exclude a clinical diagnosis of aortic regurgitation. Given the high sensitivity and specificity of this approach, the resulting diagnostic data are highly reliable. In addition, information on the etiology of valve disease, associated conditions, and the degree of left ventricular dilation is obtained.

If aortic regurgitation is detected in the course of an echocardiogram ordered for some other indication, it is incumbent on the echocardiographer to search carefully for the etiology of regurgitation. The finding of regurgitation may be the first clue that aortic root disease or a disease process affecting the aortic leaflets is present.

Timing of Surgical Intervention for Chronic Asymptomatic Aortic Regurgitation

Timing of surgical intervention in the asymptomatic patient is a problem because measures of left ventricular systolic function are dependent on loading conditions, which are altered by the presence of valvular regurgitation. End-systolic volume or dimension provides a relatively load-independent measure of ventricular performance. Several studies examining outcome after valve replacement for aortic regurgitation have shown that a left ventricular end-systolic dimension of less than 55 mm is predictive of preserved (or improved) left ventricular systolic function and an excellent prognosis after valve replacement (Fig. 12-26). While a prospective, randomized trial of surgical intervention in the asymptomatic patient has not been performed, a consensus has developed that surgical intervention is indicated for progressive left ventricular dilation or other evidence of decreased systolic function (see Suggested Reading 15). Annual echocardiography is recommended for evaluation of changes in left ventricle size and systolic function and to optimize the timing of valve replacement

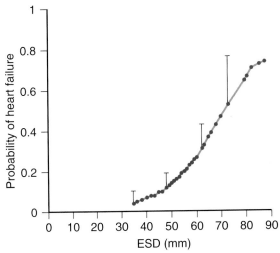

FIGURE 12–26. In a prospective study of 87 adults with aortic regurgitation, the probability of heart failure after aortic valve replacement (*y*-axis) plotted against preoperative end systolic diameter (ESD, *x*-axis). (From Tornos MP, Olona M, Permanyer-Miralda G, et al: Heart failure after aortic valve replacement for aortic regurgitation: Prospective 20-year study. Am Heart J 136(4 Pt 1):681–687, 1998.)

in the asymptomatic patient with significant regurgitation.

Monitoring the Effect of Medical Therapy

Several echocardiographic studies have shown that afterload reduction therapy for patients with chronic asymptomatic aortic regurgitation can prevent progressive left ventricular dilation and hypertrophy. In a randomized trial of nifedipine versus digoxin, afterload reduction decreased the rate of progression to symptoms or left ventricular systolic dysfunction. Thus, echocardiography now is a standard approach to evaluation of the effect of afterload reduction on ventricular dimensions, mass, and systolic function in patients with chronic aortic regurgitation.

In sequential studies, the accuracy of detecting a change in left ventricular dimension is greatest when similar examination techniques are used and when the studies are compared "side by side." With slow disease progression, similar directional changes on serial studies at several time points are more reliable than a single interval change.

Alternate Approaches

Alternate approaches to follow-up in patients with chronic aortic regurgitation include resting and exercise radionuclide ventriculography, magnetic resonance imaging, and cardiac catheterization.

MITRAL REGURGITATION

Diagnostic Imaging of the Mitral Valve Apparatus

Functionally, the mitral valve apparatus consists of several components:

- Left atrial wall
- Mitral annulus
- Anterior and posterior leaflets
- Chordae
- Papillary muscles
- Left ventricular myocardium underlying the papillary muscles

Dysfunction or altered anatomy of any one of these components can result in mitral regurgitation (Fig. 12–27). Mitral annular dilation may be due to either left atrial or left ventricular dilation and results in mitral regurgitation because of incomplete leaflet coaptation. The normal mitral apparatus is a saddle-shaped ellipse with its most apical points seen in the apical four-chamber view and its most basal points seen in the long-axis view. As noted for the aortic valve, the mitral leaflets have a normal area of overlap (or apposition) so that some degree of mitral annular dilation may be tolerated without significant regurgitation.

The mitral annulus area normally is smaller in systole than in diastole. Increased rigidity of the annulus, as seen with *mitral annular calcification*, impairs systolic contraction of the annulus leading to mitral regurgitation. Mitral annular calcification has a typical appearance on 2D imaging as an area of increased echogenicity on the left ventricular side of the annulus immediately adjacent to the attachment point of the posterior leaflet (Fig.

Mechanisms of Mitral Regurgitation

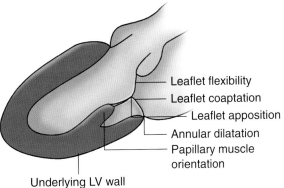

Leaflet flexibility
Leaflet coaptation
Leaflet apposition
Annular dilatation
Papillary muscle orientation
Underlying LV wall

FIGURE 12–27. Schematic diagram illustrating how abnormalities of any part of the complex mitral valve apparatus can result in mitral regurgitation.

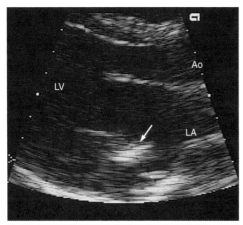

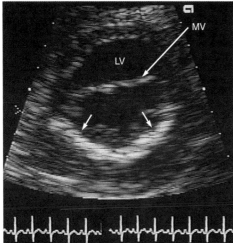

FIGURE 12-28. Two-dimensional parasternal long-axis *(top)* and short-axis *(bottom)* views of mitral annular calcification *(arrows)*. MV, mitral valve leaflet.

12-28). Acoustic shadowing, due to the presence of calcium, is seen. In short-axis views, the annular calcium may be focal or extensive, involving the entire U-shaped posterior annulus. The region of anterior mitral leaflet–aortic root continuity is involved only rarely. Mitral annular calcification is commonly seen in elderly subjects and in younger patients with renal failure or hypertension.

Diseases of the mitral valve leaflets include myxomatous disease, rheumatic disease, endocarditis, Marfan syndrome, and rare disorders such as infiltrative diseases (amyloid, sarcoid, mucopolysaccharidosis) and collagen-vascular disorders (systemic lupus erythematosus, rheumatoid arthritis). *Myxomatous* mitral valve disease is characterized by thickened, redundant leaflets and chordae with excessive motion and sagging of portions of the leaflets into the left atrium in systole (Fig. 12–29). The severity of disease is variable,

ranging from mitral valve prolapse, in which there is only minimal displacement of the leaflets into the left atrium in systole, to severe involvement of both leaflets by myxomatous disease with frankly prolapsed or flail leaflet segments. *Chordal disruption* or *elongation* leads to mitral regurgitation because of inadequate tensile support of the closed leaflets in systole. Chordal elongation results in severe bowing of the leaflet, or leaflet segment, into the left atrium, with the tip of the leaflet still directed toward the ventricular apex. With chordal rupture, there is a flail segment of the leaflet such that the leaflet is displaced into the left atrium in systole, with the tip of the leaflet pointing away from the ventricular apex (Fig. 12–30).

Rheumatic mitral regurgitation, like rheumatic mitral stenosis, is characterized by some degree of commissural fusion and thickening of the leaflet tips with leaflet motion is restricted by the disease process. *Endocarditis* results in mitral regurgitation

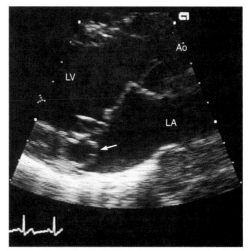

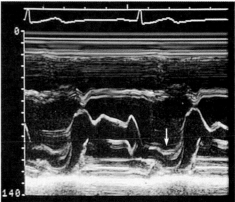

FIGURE 12-29. Parasternal long-axis *(top)* and M-mode recording *(bottom)* in a young woman with mitral valve prolapse. Posterior leaflet prolapse is seen both on 2D imaging and on M-mode *(arrows)*.

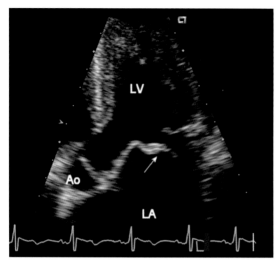

FIGURE 12–30. Apical four-chamber view demonstrating a partial flail anterior mitral leaflet (*arrow*) in a young man with myxomatous mitral valve disease. Note that the tip of the flail segment points away from the left ventricle apex.

by leaflet destruction, perforation, or deformity. *Marfan syndrome* is associated with a long redundant anterior leaflet that sags into the left atrium in systole. *Infiltrative diseases* result in irregular leaflet thickening and inadequate coaptation. Of note, *age-related degenerative changes* in the mitral leaflets often are seen (with or without associated mitral annular calcification) and appear as irregular areas of thickening and increased echogenicity of the mitral leaflets.

Ischemic mitral regurgitation may be due to regional left ventricular dysfunction with abnormal contraction of the papillary muscle or underlying ventricular wall. In patients with a myocardial infarction, myocadial scarring results in mitral regurgitation at rest. In patients with normal resting myocardial function but inducible ischemia with stress, mitral regurgitation may be intermittent. Ischemic mitral regurgitation is characterized by restricted leaflet motion, with tethering of valve closure resulting in the appearance of "tenting" of the mitral valve in systole (Fig. 12–31).

Papillary muscle rupture can occur as a complication of acute myocardial infarction. If the entire papillary muscle is disconnected from the underlying left ventricular wall, few patients survive due to acute severe mitral regurgitation. Echocardiographic evaluation in those who do survive shows a mass (the ruptured papillary muscle) attached to flail segments of anterior and posterior leaflets (since each papillary muscle attaches to both leaflets) (see Fig. 8–24). The ruptured papillary muscle head is seen in the left atrium in systole and in the left ventricle in diastole. Severe mitral regurgitation is present on Doppler examination.

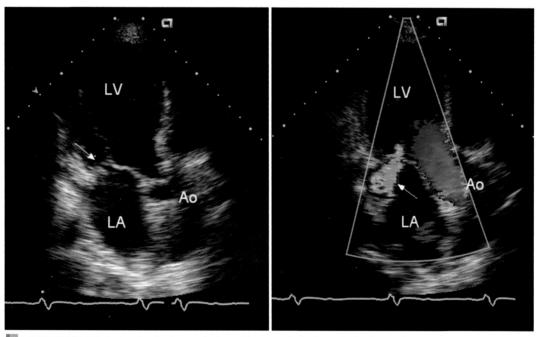

FIGURE 12–31. Ischemic mitral regurgitation with a posteriorly directed mitral regurgitant jet due to papillary muscle dysfunction seen in an apical long-axis view. Note the tethering of the posterior leaflet on the 2D image.

Partial rupture of a papillary muscle, defined as rupture of one of several "heads" or as partial disconnection of the base of the papillary muscle, is seen more often than complete rupture as patients are more likely to survive long enough to undergo diagnostic evaluation. In this situation, the echocardiogram shows a thin, attenuated, excessively mobile papillary muscle and, if one head has ruptured, a mass attached to the leaflet with prolapse into the left atrium in systole.

Mitral regurgitation due to left ventricular dilation and systolic dysfunction, in patients with normal valve leaflets and chordae, often is called *functional mitral regurgitation* (Fig. 12–32). The mechanism of functional mitral regurgitation remains controversial, with some studies suggesting abnormal orientation of the papillary muscles and others suggesting annular dilation.

Obviously, while mitral regurgitation due to conditions with unique anatomic features can be reliably diagnosed by echocardiographic imaging (rheumatic or myxomatous disease), there is considerable overlap in the anatomic features of other conditions (degenerative versus infiltrative leaflet abnormalities). In some cases, it is difficult to determine if mitral regurgitation is the cause or consequence of ventricular dilation and systolic dysfunction. When etiology is unclear, the echocardiographer can describe the valve anatomy and indicate possible reasons for the findings even though the specific tissue diagnosis remains unknown.

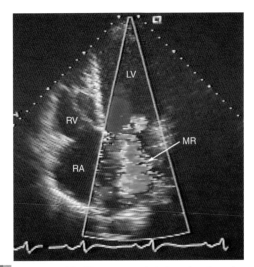

FIGURE 12–32. In an apical four-chamber view, a central mitral regurgitant jet due to dilated cardiomyopathy is seen. Because the leaflets and chordae are normal, this is often called *functional mitral regurgitation.*

Response of the Left Ventricle, Left Atrium, and Pulmonary Vasculature

Mitral regurgitation results in left ventricular volume overload due to the increase in total left ventricular stroke volume as blood is ejected both forward into the aorta and retrograde across the mitral valve. With acute mitral regurgitation, the left ventricle empties more completely (e.g., ejection fraction increases) such that forward cardiac output is maintained. With compensated chronic regurgitation, left ventricular diastolic volume increases and ejection fraction is normal such that end-systolic volume is within the normal range or only mildly increased. Although it might seem that afterload is decreased in patients with mitral regurgitation due to ejection into the low pressure left atrium, the effect of decreased ejection force is counterbalanced by increased ventricular chamber size without an increase in wall thickness. Thus with chronic mitral regurgitation, afterload is normal and ejection fraction typically is in the normal range.

With chronic regurgitation, progressive left ventricular dilation eventually occurs as the regurgitant volume (and thus total left ventricular stroke volume) increases. As with aortic regurgitation, an irreversible decline in left ventricular contractility can occur in the absence of symptoms. The left atrium gradually dilates to accommodate the regurgitant volume while maintaining a normal left atrial pressure. Left atrial compliance increases, that is, the left atrial pressure-volume relationship is shifted downward and to the right. With acute mitral regurgitation, the regurgitant volume is delivered into a small, noncompliant left atrium, resulting in a significant increase in left atrial pressure and a *v* wave in the left atrial pressure curve.

Pulmonary artery pressure increases passively in response to both the chronic mildly elevated left atrial pressure seen with chronic mitral regurgitation and the acute severe elevation seen with acute regurgitation. When left atrial pressure is chronically elevated, pulmonary vascular resistance may increase. Echocardiographic evaluation of the patient with mitral regurgitation includes noninvasive measurement of pulmonary artery pressure from the tricuspid regurgitant jet velocity and an estimate of right atrial pressure.

Evaluation of Mitral Regurgitant Severity

Screening Examination

The basic screening examination for mitral regurgitation includes color flow imaging and continuous-wave Doppler ultrasound (Fig. 12–33).

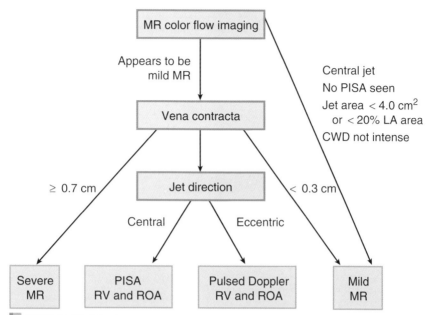

FIGURE 12–33. Approach to quantitation of mitral regurgitant severity. Evaluation of systolic flow reversal in the pulmonary veins provides useful additional information in patients with sinus rhythm. Transesophageal imaging often is needed for complete evaluation of mitral regurgitant severity in patients with moderate-to-severe disease.

JET AREA. Color Doppler imaging is performed in several tomographic planes in order to build a mental 3D reconstruction of the extent of the flow disturbance in the left atrium. The shape and direction of the jet also are evaluated; an eccentric jet suggests pathologic regurgitation and provides clues about the mechanism of regurgitation. Abnormalities of the posterior leaflet tend to result in an anteriorly directed jet (Fig. 12–34), while anterior leaflet or papillary

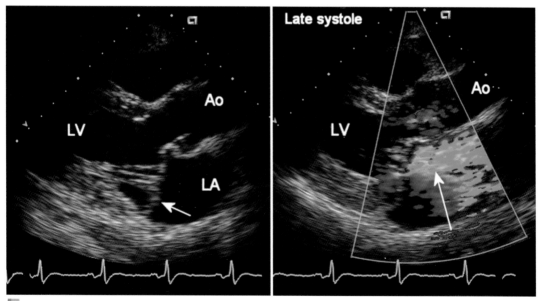

FIGURE 12–34. This young woman with posterior leaflet prolapse *(left)* has an anteriorly directed mitral regurgitant jet *(right)*. On frame-by-frame analysis and on continuous-wave Doppler, mitral regurgitation occurred only in the second half of systole.

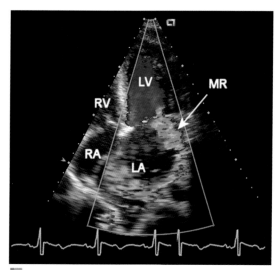

FIGURE 12–35. Eccentric posterior and laterally directed jet of mitral regurgitation (*arrow*) in the apical four-chamber view in the patient with a partial flail anterior leaflet, also shown in Figure 12–30.

muscle dysfunction tend to result in a posteriorly directed jet (Fig. 12–35). Dilation of the left ventricle or mitral annulus results in a central, symmetric regurgitant jet.

In addition to parasternal long- and short-axis views, apical four-chamber and long-axis views may be useful because they are nearly orthogonal to each other. However, signal attenuation at the depth of the left atrium may limit the utility of apical views if ultrasound penetration is suboptimal. A central jet with an area less than 4.0 cm² or less than 20% of the left atrial area in a nonoblique view, is consistent with mild mitral regurgitation.

CONTINUOUS-WAVE DOPPLER. The continuous-wave Doppler spectral recording of mitral regurgitation shows a rapid increase in velocity during isovolumic contraction (proportional to the rate of rise in left ventricular pressure or *dP/dt*) from baseline to a maximum velocity of 5 to 6 m/s. The velocity stays high throughout systole with a curve paralleling the rise and fall of left ventricular pressure given a normal left atrial pressure. During isovolumic relaxation, the velocity rapidly returns to baseline.

With acute mitral regurgitation (Table 12–8), an increase in left atrial pressure during late systole—a *v* wave—may be present due to a steep pressure-volume relationship of the nondilated left atrium. In this situation, the pressure gradient between the left ventricle and the left atrium is high initially but then begins to equalize in late systole as left atrial pressure rises. The corresponding Doppler velocity curve shows a high initial velocity with a more rapid fall in velocity in mid- to late systole. This pattern of Doppler velocities also is termed a *v wave* (see Fig. 12–11).

Signal intensity of the mitral regurgitant signal, in comparison with antegrade flow, is related to mitral regurgitation severity. In addition, significant regurgitation is associated with an increase in the antegrade velocity due to increased transmitral volume flow.

Vena Contracta

If color Doppler imaging shows an eccentric jet or a large jet area or if continous-wave Doppler suggests more than mild mitral regurgitation, the examination should include measurement of vena contracta diameter (Table 12–9). In patients with mitral regurgitation, vena contracta width is optimally visualized in a parasternal long-axis or short-axis view, although apical four-chamber and long-axis views may be used if parastenal images are inadequate. The apical two-chamber view is not reliable because the jet width may be broad in this image plane, even though regurgitation is not severe. Vena contracta width also can be

TABLE 12–8		
Chronic versus Acute Mitral Regurgitation		
Parameter	**Chronic**	**Acute**
Etiology (examples)	Myxomatous valve disease Annular dilation	Endocarditis Papillary muscle rupture Chordal rupture
Left ventricular size	Dilated	Normal
Left ventricular systolic function	Hyperdynamic early, may be normal or depressed with long-standing disease	Hyperdynamic
Left atrial size	Enlarged	Normal
Continuous-wave Doppler curve	High velocity throughout systole	Late systolic velocity decline (*v* wave)

TABLE 12–9		
Quantitative Evaluation of Mitral Regurgitant Severity (ASE Guidelines)		
Mitral Regurgitation	**Mild**	**Severe**
Jet area (cm^2)	<4 cm^2 or <20% LA area	>40% LA area
Vena contracta (cm)	<0.3	≥0.7
Regurgitant volume (mL)	<30	≥60
Regurgitant fraction (%)	<30	≥50
Regurgitant orifice area (cm^2)	<0.20	≥0.40

measured with transesophageal imaging. A vena contracta width greater than 0.3 cm indicates that further quantitation of regurgitant severity is needed.

Proximal Isovelocity Surface Area

With a central regurgitant jet, regurgitant volume and orifice area can be calculated by the PISA approach. The PISA is optimally imaged in an apical four-chamber view using a narrow sector, minimal depth, and zoom mode. The PISA also can be imaged from a transesophageal approach. The aliasing velocity is adjusted to provide a clearly identified hemispherical PISA, typically at a Nyquist limit of 20 to 40 cm/s. Instantaneous regurgitant volume flow rate is calculated as indicated in Eq. 12–4. The maximum velocity of the mitral regurgitant jet on continuous wave Doppler recording is then used in Eq. 12–6 to determine regurgitant orifice area.

Regurgitation Volume and Orifice Area

The PISA approach is less accurate with eccentric jets or when the isovelocity surface area is not hemispherical. In these situations, quantitation of mitral regurgitation by pulsed Doppler volume flow rates is more appropriate. Mitral regurgitant volume (RV_{mitral}) can be calculated from transmitral stroke volume (SV_{mitral}) (total left ventricular stroke volume) and transaortic stroke volume (forward stroke volume) measured in the left ventricular outflow tract (SV_{LVOT}) (Fig. 12–36):

$$RV_{mitral} = SV_{mitral} - SV_{LVOT}$$

Alternate sites for measurement of forward stroke volume are the tricuspid valve and the pulmonary artery. Regurgitant orifice area then can be calculated (Eq. 12–3) using this regurgitant volume and the velocity time integral of the continous-wave Doppler mitral regurgitant jet.

Pulmonary Vein Flow Reversal

As the mitral regurgitant jet enters the left atrium, it necessarily displaces blood that was already in the chamber. When severe regurgitation is present, systolic flow reversal in the pulmonary veins is seen. On transthoracic echocardiography, the flow pattern in the right inferior pulmonary vein can be recorded from the apical four-chamber view in most patients, although the signal-to-noise ratio may be suboptimal at this depth in some adult patients. On transesophageal echocardiography, the flow pattern in the pulmonary veins can be recorded at high resolution. Examination of all four pulmonary veins is especially helpful with an eccentric regurgitant jet, since the pattern of systolic flow reversal may not be uniform.

False-negative results occur when the left atrium is severely enlarged and compliant so that all the excess volume is contained in the left atrium without displacement into the pulmonary veins. False-positive results occur when an eccentric jet is directed into a pulmonary vein, causing flow reversal even when regurgitation is not severe. Pulmonary vein flow reversal in systole is more helpful when sinus rhythm is present. False-positive results also may be seen in patients in atrial fibrillation. Other physiologic factors also affect the atrial inflow patterns, including respiratory phase, cardiac rhythm, atrial and venous compliance, ventricular diastolic filling, and age. Thus, while the presence and severity of venous systolic flow reversal is a useful adjunct in evaluation of atrioventricular valve regurgitant severity, it certainly is not a pathognomonic finding.

Clinical Utility

Diagnosis and Severity of Mitral Regurgitation

Determination of the etiology of mitral regurgitation using 2D imaging often has important clinical implications. Evaluation of regurgitant severity also is of clinical importance, although a high degree of sophistication in echocardiographic interpretation is needed for this application (Fig. 12–37). In assessing the severity of regurgitation,

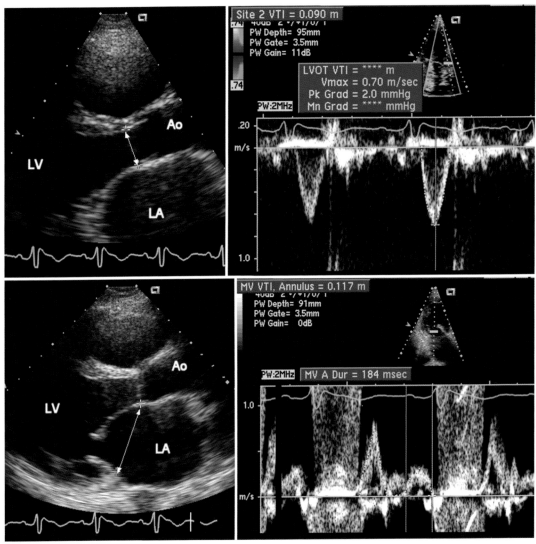

■ FIGURE 12–36. Quantitative evaluation of mitral regurgitant severity by calculation of transmitral and transaortic volume flow rates. Mitral annulus diameter and the velocity-time integral (VTI) of flow across the mitral annulus are used to calculate total stroke volume. Forward stroke volume is determined from the cross-sectional area and velocity-time integral of left ventricular outflow tract flow.

the echocardiographer should first describe the individual findings and then integrate these findings into a consistent overall interpretation. In addition, the degree of pulmonary hypertension, left atrial size, left ventricular size and systolic function, and any associated abnormalities are added to the Doppler findings before arriving at a final interpretation.

Examples of clinical situations in which decisions can be based on echocardiographic and Doppler data include acute mitral regurgitation after myocardial infarction, mitral valve endocarditis, and chronic mitral regurgitation due to myxomatous mitral valve disease. The decision

whether or not to perform valve surgery (repair or replacement) usually can be made based on clinical and echocardiographic data without invasive studies in these patient groups. Only in cases where there is a discrepancy between the clinical impression and the echocardiographic findings (or when coronary angiography is indicated) are further diagnostic tests warranted.

Diagnosis of Mitral Valve Prolapse

Mitral valve prolapse or myxomatous mitral valve disease is a pathologic condition characterized histologically by increased mucopolysaccharides, thickening, and disarray of the mitral valve leaflet.

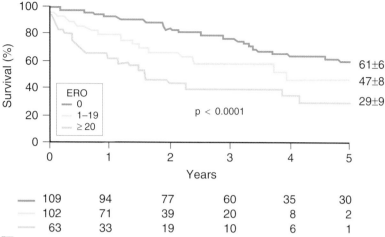

FIGURE 12–37. Actuarial survival in 165 patients with mitral regurgitation after acute myocardial infarction, compared to 109 acute myocardial infarction patients without mitral regurgitation. Patients with ischemic mitral regurgitation are stratified by effective regurgitant orifice area (ERO) as less than or greater than/equal to 0.2 cm². (From Grigioni F, Enriquez-Sarano M, Zehr KJ, et al: Ischemic mitral regurgitation: Long-term outcome and prognostic implications with quantitative Doppler assessment. Circulation 103(13):1759–1764, 2001.)

Grossly, the leaflets and chordae are thick and redundant but with reduced tensile strength so that they are prone to progressive elongation or rupture. Two-dimensional imaging demonstrates thick, redundant leaflets and chordae with systolic displacement of the leaflets into the left atrium in systole. Over time, a partial flail leaflet due to chordal rupture may develop. A subset of patients with this disease have a high incidence of significant mitral regurgitation and often go on to require mitral valve surgery. Patients with myxomatous mitral valve disease also may have aortic or tricuspid valve involvement.

In contrast, other patients with mitral valve prolapse have a more benign long-term outcome, suggesting that myxomatous mitral valve disease encompasses a spectrum of disease severity. These patients have echocardiographic findings closer to the range of normal variation in mitral valve anatomy and dynamics so that strict echocardiographic criteria must be used to avoid a false-positive diagnosis of mitral valve prolapse. For example, in an apical four-chamber view, the closure plane of the mitral leaflets may appear "flat" relative to the mitral annulus even in subjects with normal valve leaflets since the most apical points of the saddle-shaped annulus are seen in this view. In addition, normal leaflet closure may appear displaced to the atrial side of the annulus if image planes are oblique relative to the annular plane. Displacement of the leaflets into the left atrium in systole is most reliably

assessed in parasternal and apical long-axis views. In addition, it is helpful to describe valve anatomy (leaflet size, thickness, redundancy, chordal involvement) as well as the pattern of valve motion.

Follow-up of Chronic Asymptomatic Mitral Regurgitation

Sequential echocardiographic studies can be used to follow asymptomatic patients with mitral regurgitation. While mitral regurgitation severity and mitral valve anatomy are important data, the most important factor in patient evaluation is left ventricular size and systolic function. Current data suggest that evidence of progressive ventricular dilation, an end-systolic dimension greater than 45 mm, or any reduction in left ventricular systolic function should prompt consideration of surgical intervention regardless of the symptomatic status of the patient to prevent irreversible ventricular dysfunction postoperatively (Fig. 12–38).

Decision Making Concerning Mitral Valve Repair or Replacement

Once the decision has been made that surgical intervention is needed, the echocardiographic images are invaluable in considering whether mitral valve repair or reconstruction is possible. The study should be reviewed with the surgeon, focusing on the exact etiology of mitral regurgitation, the degree of annular dilation, the relative

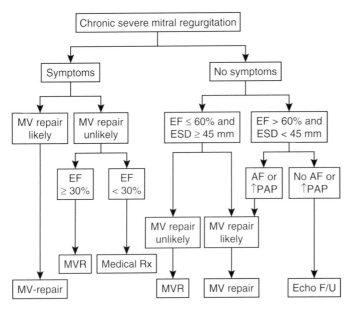

FIGURE 12–38. Clinical decision algorithm for timing of surgical intervention in patients with chronic severe mitral regurgitation. MV, mitral valve; MVR, mitral valve replacement; EF, ejection fraction; AF, atrial fibrillation; PAP, pulmonary artery pressure; ESD, end systolic dimension; Rx, therapy; F/U, follow-up. (From Otto CM (ed): Valvular Heart Disease, 2nd ed. Philadelphia: WB Saunders, 2004, Figure 15–13.)

involvement of anterior and posterior leaflets, the chordal and papillary muscle structural integrity, and overall ventricular size and systolic function. Typically, posterior leaflet prolapse and annular dilation are most amenable to repair, while more complex or extensive disease requires more complex procedures with a lower likelihood of successful repair. Often, transesophageal imaging is needed for preoperative evaluation when surgical intervention is contemplated.

Intraoperative Evaluation of Mitral Valve Repair

In the patient undergoing surgical mitral valve repair, transesophageal echocardiography is used to assess results after the procedure. Baseline transesophageal images are obtained in the operating room to reconfirm regurgitant severity under the loading conditions of general anesthesia and to serve as a baseline for comparison to the postrepair echocardiogram, with blood pressure recorded with the echocardiographic images at both time points. After valve repair, the patient is weaned from cardiopulmonary bypass, and valve anatomy and mitral regurgitant severity are reassessed. Preferably, regurgitant severity is evaluated under physiologic loading conditions with similar hemodynamics to those recorded during the baseline study (Fig. 12–39). If significant residual mitral regurgitation is present, a second bypass pump run may be done as part of the same procedure to allow a second attempt at repair or mitral valve replacement. Other complications of the valve repair also may be identified, including dynamic left ventricular outflow tract obstruction, functional mitral stenosis, and worsening of left ventricular systolic dysfunction.

TRICUSPID REGURGITATION

Diagnostic Imaging of the Tricuspid Valve Apparatus

Tricuspid regurgitation occurs with abnormalities of the supporting structures (annulus, right ventricle) or the leaflets themselves. Tricuspid regurgitation secondary to *annular dilation* often is due either to primary right ventricular dilation and systolic dysfunction or to *pulmonary hypertension*. Left-sided heart disease leading to pulmonary hypertension—especially mitral stenosis or regurgitation—often results in significant tricuspid regurgitation, presumably based on right ventricular dilation and systolic dysfunction.

Abnormalities of the tricuspid valve leaflets also are a cause of tricuspid regurgitation. *Rheumatic disease* involves the tricuspid valve in approximately 20% to 30% of cases, nearly always occurring in conjunction with mitral and aortic valve involvement. Rheumatic tricuspid disease typically is mild and may be difficult to appreciate on 2D echocardiography unless careful attention is directed toward imaging the valve leaflets and searching for evidence of commissural fusion. Rheumatic tricuspid regurgitation is more common than rheumatic tricuspid stenosis.

Carcinoid heart disease is a rare condition, but the echocardiographic findings are pathognomonic. Carcinoid heart disease (seen with metastatic carcinoid tumor to the liver) is charac-

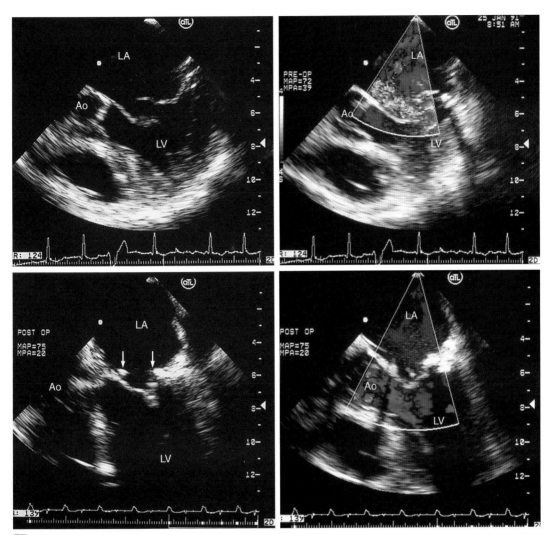

FIGURE 12–39. Two-dimensional *(left)* and color Doppler *(right)* intraoperative transesophageal images in a patient with myxomatous mitral valve disease before *(top)* and after *(bottom)* mitral valve repair. Before repair, severe mitral prolapse with a partial flail leaflet segment and moderate-to-severe mitral regurgitation are present. After repair, only minimal regurgitation is detected at similar loading conditions. A mitral annuloplasty ring *(arrows)* is seen.

terized by thickened, shortened, and immobile tricuspid valve leaflets with resultant tricuspid regurgitation or, less often, tricuspid valve stenosis (see Fig. 15–9). The pulmonic valve also may be involved. *Endocarditis* may involve the tricuspid valve, resulting in tricuspid regurgitation, and is most common in patients with a history of intravenous drug abuse.

Ebstein's anomaly of the tricuspid valve is a congenital abnormality in which one or more leaflets of the tricuspid valve are displaced from the tricuspid annulus toward the ventricular apex (see Fig. 17–9). Most often, the septal leaflet is involved, either in isolation or in association with apical displacement of posterior and anterior leaflets. The degree of apical displacement is extremely variable. While the normal tricuspid valve insertion plane is slightly more apical than the mitral valve attachment plane, Ebstein's anomaly should be considered when the separation between mitral and tricuspid valve planes is greater than 1 cm. The portion of the right ventricle excluded from the pumping chamber is said to be *atrialized*, since it effectively functions as part of the right atrium. The right atrium may appear severely enlarged due to "atrialization" of the base of the ventricle *plus* dilatation of the atrium due to tricuspid regurgitation. Right ventricular enlargement is seen as well if significant tricuspid regurgitation is present.

Right Ventricular and Right Atrial Dilation

Hemodynamically significant tricuspid regurgitation results in progressive right ventricular and right atrial enlargement due to volume overload. This dilation may complicate assessment of the etiology of regurgitation because the dilation itself may further increase regurgitant severity.

Right ventricular volume overload is associated with a pattern of abnormal septal motion characterized on M-mode recording by posterior motion of the septum in diastole (since right ventricular filling exceeds left ventricular filling) and anterior motion of the septum in systole, often referred to as *paradoxical septal motion*. On 2D short-axis imaging, the ventricular septum appears "flattened" in diastole as the increased transtricuspid stroke volume fills the right ventricle. In systole, the ventricular septum moves toward the center of gravity of the heart (normally toward the middle of the left ventricle), which is the midline of the right ventricle if severe right ventricular dilation is present.

The differential diagnosis of 2D findings of right ventricular dilation and paradoxical septal motion includes other causes of right ventricular volume overload such as an atrial septal defect, partial anomalous pulmonary venous return, pressure overload due to pulmonic valve disease, or pulmonary hypertension either due to left-sided heart disease or intrinsic lung disease.

Evaluation of Tricuspid Regurgitation Severity

Tricuspid regurgitation can be evaluated with color Doppler imaging to assess jet area. Mild regurgitation is characterized by a flow disturbance in systole localized to the area adjacent to the valve closure plane (jet area <5 cm^2). Moderate regurgitation fills between 5 and 10 cm^2 of the right

atrium, while severe regurgitation fills more than 10 cm^2 of an enlarged right atrium (Figs. 12–40 and 12–41). Useful views for evaluation of tricuspid regurgitation include parasternal short-axis view, the right ventricular inflow view, and the apical four-chamber view. Mild-to-moderate tricuspid regurgitation often is directed along the interatrial septum and must be distinguished from normal caval inflow or from atrial septal defect flow.

Measurement of the width of the vena contracta may be helpful; a jet width greater than 0.7 cm is sensitive (89%) and specific (93%) for severe tricuspid regurgitation. Calculation of regurgitant volume or orifice area by the PISA or pulsed Doppler methods is rarely performed for tricuspid regurgitation.

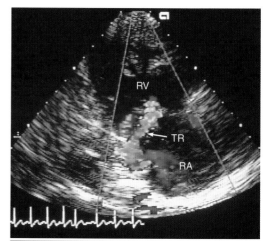

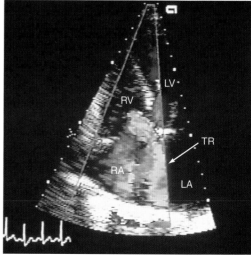

FIGURE 12–41. Color flow imaging in parasternal right ventricular inflow *(top)* and apical four-chamber *(bottom)* views in a patient with moderate tricuspid regurgitation (TR).

Flow Mapping for TR

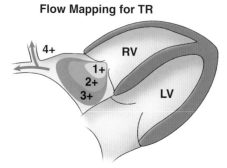

FIGURE 12–40. Schematic diagram of flow mapping for semiquantitative evaluation of tricuspid regurgitant severity. Severe (4+) tricuspid regurgitation is associated with systolic reversal in the hepatic veins.

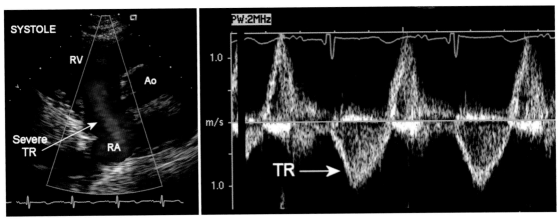

FIGURE 12–42. Severe tricuspid regurgitation with normal right ventricular and pulmonary systolic pressures is characterized by low velocity, laminar flow on color flow imaging *(left)* and on pulsed Doppler *(right)*.

Severe tricuspid regurgitation results in systolic flow reversal in the inferior and superior vena cava, analogous to the physical finding of a systolic pulsation in the neck veins. Inferior vena caval flow is best recorded in the central hepatic vein, which provides a flow channel parallel to the ultrasound beam from a subcostal approach and has no venous valves between the recording site and the right atrium (see Fig. 12–14).

The absolute value of the maximum velocity in the tricuspid regurgitant continuous-wave Doppler spectral recording reflects the maximum pressure difference across the tricuspid valve and *not* the severity of regurgitation. Severe regurgitation with a normal right ventricular systolic pressure (as seen with tricuspid valve endocarditis) has a low maximum velocity (Fig. 12–42). Mild tricuspid regurgitation in the presence of pulmonary hypertension (as seen with primary pulmonary hypertension) has a high maximum velocity. However, the *intensity* of the continuous-wave signals relative to the antegrade flow signal intensity does relate to regurgitant severity. In addition, the shape of the velocity-time curve indicates the time course of the instantaneous pressure differences across the valve. A right atrial *v* wave seen in acute regurgitation results in a more rapid decline in velocity in late systole similar to that seen in acute mitral regurgitation.

Clinical Utility

Evaluation of tricuspid regurgitation by Doppler echocardiography is the standard clinical approach to this problem. Even cardiac catheterization is of limited value because the catheter placed across the tricuspid valve to perform the right ventricular angiogram may itself induce regurgitation.

Evaluation of tricuspid regurgitant severity is particularly important in the patient undergoing mitral valve surgery. Many of these patients have significant coexisting tricuspid regurgitation, and many of the clinical symptoms will persist postoperatively if this condition is not recognized and treated (with tricuspid annuloplasty) at the time of surgery.

In patients undergoing tricuspid valve repair or surgery for endocarditis, intraoperative transesophageal echocardiography can be used to optimize the surgical approach and assess the functional consequences of the repair procedure.

PULMONIC REGURGITATION

Pulmonic regurgitation most often is an incidental benign finding, with a small amount of diastolic backflow across the pulmonic valve seen in most normal individuals (Fig. 12–43). Pathologic pulmonic regurgitation usually is a result of congenital pulmonic valve disease, either untreated mild disease or residual regurgitation after pulmonic valve surgery. Acquired pulmonic regurgitation is rare, being due to endocarditis, carcinoid syndrome, or myxomatous valve disease.

Evaluation of pulmonic valve anatomy may be limited in adult patients by poor acoustic access. With congenital disease, thickened, deformed leaflets are seen. In endocarditis, a valvular vegetation may be identified, although the pulmonic valve is involved least often. Carcinoid syndrome results in shortening and thickening of the pulmonic valve leaflet, similar to the involvement of the tricuspid valve, and may lead to stenosis and/or regurgitation. Myxomatous valve disease is rare, resulting in thickening, redundancy, and systemic sagging of the pulmonic valve leaflets.

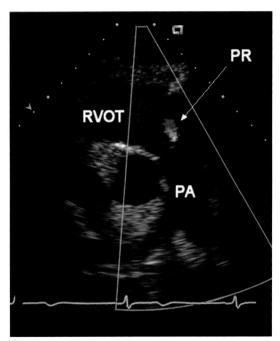

FIGURE 12–43. Color flow imaging in a right ventricular outflow view showing a small amount of pulmonic regurgitation.

Pulmonic regurgitation is diagnosed by documenting diastolic flow in the right ventricular outflow tract with conventional pulsed or color Doppler flow imaging. The width of the diastolic flow on color imaging provides a semiquantitative index of pulmonic regurgitant severity. The intensity and shape of the continuous-wave Doppler signal also provide an indication of regurgitant severity, analogous to the findings in aortic regurgitation. Holodiastolic flow reversal may be noted in the main pulmonary artery when significant regurgitation is present and must be distinguished from diastolic flow reversal due to a patent ductus arteriosus.

In adults, evaluation of pulmonic regurgitation is of most importance in patients with uncorrected or residual congenital heart disease (see Fig. 17–34). In these patients, the severity of pulmonic regurgitation may be a factor in deciding whether to perform further surgical procedures and in the specific design of the surgical procedure.

When pulmonic regurgitation is present, even if only mild in degree, the velocity in the pulmonic regurgitant curve reflects the pulmonary artery to right ventricular diastolic pressure difference. The instantaneous end-diastolic pulmonary artery to right ventricular gradient (calculated as $4v^2$) can be added to an estimate of right ventricular diastolic pressure (from inferior vena cava size and respiratory variation) to provide an estimate of diastolic pulmonary artery pressure. This approach to estimation of pulmonary artery pressure complements systolic pressure estimation from the tricuspid regurgitant jet and serves as an internal validity check when both can be recorded accurately.

SUGGESTED READING
Quantitation of Valvular Regurgitation

1. Zoghbi WA, Enriquez-Sarano M, Foster E, et al: Recommendations for evaluation of the severity of native valvular regurgitation with two-dimensional and Doppler echocardiography. J Am Soc Echocardiogr 16:777–802, 2003.

    Clear recommendations and detailed description of methods for quantitation of valvular regurgitation by echocardiography. Essential reading for all echocardiographers.

2. Robert BJ, Grayburn PA: Color flow imaging of the vena contracta in mitral regurgitation: Technical considerations. J Am Soc Echocardiogr 16:1002–1006, 2003.

    Summary of the hemodynamics of valve regurgitation and the approach to recording and measuring the vena contracta. The authors emphasize the use of axial beam resolution, a narrow sector, fast frame rate, and zoom mode to improve accuracy of this approach.

3. Heinle SK: Quantitation of valvular regurgitation: Beyond color flow mapping. In: Otto CM (ed): The Practice of Clinical Echocardiography, 2nd ed. Philadelphia: WB Saunders, 2002, pp 367–388.

    Detailed review of newer approaches to quantitation of valvular regurgitation including the proximal isovelocity surface area approach, vena contracta imaging, and conservation of momentum; 134 references.

4. Rokey R, Sterling LL, Zoghbi WA, et al: Determination of regurgitant fraction in isolated mitral or aortic regurgitation by pulsed Doppler two-dimensional echocardiography. J Am Coll Cardiol 7:1273–1278, 1986.

    Calculation of regurgitant volume and regurgitant fraction by Doppler at two intracardiac sites (mitral and aortic) was compared with invasive determinations in 25 patients (r = 0.91, SEE = 7%).

5. Recusani F, Bargiggia GS, Yoganathan AP, et al: A new method for quantification of regurgitant flow rate using color Doppler flow imaging of the flow convergence region proximal to a discrete orifice: An in vitro study. Circulation 83:594–604, 1991.

    The proximal isovelocity surface area method was used to calculate volume flow rate and then combined with continuous-wave Doppler data to calculate orifice areas in an in vitro study (r = 0.75–0.96).

6. Reimold SC, Ganz P, Bittl JA, et al: Effective aortic regurgitant orifice area: Description of a method based on conservation of mass. J Am Coll Cardiol 18:761–768, 1991.

    Description of a method for calculating regurgitant orifice area based on the continuity equation using a Doppler catheter system (for regurgitant volume flow measurement) and continuous-wave Doppler recordings of the regurgitant jet (for transvalvular mean velocity measurement) in an in vitro model and in 23 patients.

7. Takenaka K, Dabestani A, Gardin JM, et al: A simple Doppler echocardiographic method for estimating severity of aortic regurgitation. Am J Cardiol 57:1340–1343, 1986.

Holodiastolic flow reversal in the proximal abdominal aorta is a sensitive (100%) and specific (97%) method for separating subjects with 3–4+ from those with 0–2+ aortic regurgitation. The single false-positive result was a patient with a patent ductus arteriosus.

8. Grayburn PA, Handshoe R, Smith MD, et al: Quantitative assessment of the hemodynamic consequences of aortic regurgitation by means of continuous wave Doppler recordings. J Am Coll Cardiol 10:135–141, 1987.

Relationship between the shape of the aortic regurgitant jet on continuous-wave Doppler recordings and intracardiac dynamics is explored. All 10 patients with a diastolic decay slope >3.0 m/s² had 3+ to 4+ aortic regurgitation, although 9 of 21 (43%) of those with a slope <3.0 m/s² also had severe aortic regurgitation.

9. Heinle SK, Hall SA, Brickner E, et al: Comparison of vena contracta width by multiplane transesophageal echocardiography with quantitative Doppler assessment of mitral regurgitation. Am J Cardiol 81:175–179, 1998.

The vena contracta width could be identified on transesophageal color flow imaging in 97% of patients with native mitral valve regurgitation. A vena contracta width ≥0.5 cm indicates severe mitral regurgitation (regurgitant volume >60 mL and an effective regurgitant orifice area ≥0.4 cm²). Conversely, a vena contracta width ≤0.3 cm indicates mild regurgitation.

10. Seiler C, Aeschbacher BA, Meier B: Quantitation of mitral regurgitation using the systolic/diastolic pulmonary venous flow velocity ratio. J Am Coll Cardiol 31:1383–1390, 1998.

In patients in sinus rhythm with isolated mitral regurgitation (no aortic regurgitation, LV ejection fraction >45%), the ratio of the systolic to diastolic velocity time integral of flow in the pulmonary vein correlated moderately well with other quantitative measures of regurgitant severity. Although a systolic/diastolic pulmonary vein flow ratio less than 0 had a specificity of 96% for identification of severe mitral regurgitation, sensitivity was only 52%.

11. Gottdiener JS, Panza JA, St John SM, et al: Testing the test: the reliability of echocardiography in the sequential assessment of valvular regurgitation. Am Heart J 144:115–121, 2002.

Qualitative assessment of valvular regurgitation based on the ratio of color jet area to left atrial size, for mitral regurgitation, and color jet width to outflow tract diameter, for aortic regurgitation, shows an average test-retest variability of 25% to 30%.

12. Reimold SC, Maier SE, Fleischmann KE, et al: Dynamic nature of the aortic regurgitant orifice area during diastole in patients with chronic aortic regurgitation. Circulation 89:2085–2092, 1994.

Using 2D/Doppler echocardiography (continuity equation) and cine phase contrast magnetic resonance imaging, regurgitant orifice area was found to vary directly with regurgitant fraction (r = 0.86) in 17 patients with chronic aortic regurgitation. However, the regurgitant orifice area decreased during diastole in 88% of patients. This dynamic component decreased with increasing regurgitant fraction (r = −0.90).

13. Thomas JD, O'Shea JP, Rodriguez L, et al: Impact of orifice geometry on the shape of jets: An in vitro Doppler color flow study. J Am Coll Cardiol 17:901–908, 1991.

Jet momentum, defined as the product of the volume flow rate across the orifice, and velocity predict the appearance of jets in vitro. However, this approach assumes axial symmetry of the jet. In this paper, the authors use an in vitro model to show that jets from irregular orifices became nearly axisymmetrical within a few orifice diameters of jet origin.

14 Cape EG, Yoganathan AP, Weyman AE, Levine RA: Adjacent solid boundaries alter the size of regurgitant jets on Doppler color flow maps. J Am Coll Cardiol 17:1094–1102, 1991.

Influence of impinging walls on jet geometry and area is described. Jets deflected toward adjacent walls have smaller jet areas than jets that are centrally located in the receiving chamber.

Clinical Applications

15. Meier DJ, Landolfo CK, Starling MR: Role of echocardiography in the timing of surgical intervention for chronic mitral and aortic regurgitation. In: Otto CM (ed): The Practice of Clinical Echocardiography, 2nd ed. Philadelphia: WB Saunders, 2002, pp 389–416.

Detailed review of the literature on the natural history, postoperative outcome and optimal timing of surgical intervention for chronic valvular regurgitation. Algorithms are proposed for timing of surgical intervention based on a combination of clinical findings, ejection fraction, and end-systolic left ventricular dimension. Additional predictors of outcome also are discussed; 171 references.

16. Otto CM: Evaluation and management of chronic mitral regurgitation. N Engl J Med 345:740–746, 2001.

Concise review of the approach to diagnosis and treatment of chronic mitral regurgitation with areas of clinical uncertainty highlighted.

17. Szlachcic J, Massie BM, Greenberg B, et al: Intertest variability of echocardiographic and chest x-ray measurements: Implications for decision making in patients with aortic regurgitation. J Am Coll Cardiol 7:1310–1317, 1986.

Excellent discussion of the factors affecting intertest variability in sequential examinations of cardiac size. The 95% level prediction limits were ±8 mm for left ventricular dimensions and 12% for fractional shortening, so a difference greater than these limits indicates an interval change between studies.

18. Bonow RO, Lakatos E, Maron BJ, Epstein SE: Serial long-term assessment of the natural history of asymptomatic patients with chronic aortic regurgitation and normal left ventricular systolic function. Circulation 84:1625–1635, 1991.

Clinical study in 104 asymptomatic patients with aortic regurgitation demonstrating that the initial end-systolic dimensions, rate of change in end-systolic dimension, and resting ejection fraction are predictive of long-term outcome.

19. Borer JS, Hochreiter C, Herrold EM, et al: Prediction of indications for valve replacement among asymptomatic or minimally symptomatic patients with chronic aortic regurgitation and normal left ventricular performance. Circulation 97:525–534, 1998.

In 104 asymptomatic patients with aortic regurgitation followed for 7.4 ± 3.7 yr, 28 (72%) developed symptoms warranting valve replacement, 7 (18%) developed asymptomatic excessive left ventricular dilation, and 4 (10%) experienced sudden death. The overall rate of endpoints was 6.2% per year, with the strongest multivariate predictor of clinical outcome being change in left ventricular ejection fraction from rest to exercise, normalized for the exercise change in end-systolic wall stress.

20. Scognamiglio R, Rahimtoola SH, Fasoli G, et al: Nifedipine in asymptomatic patients with severe aortic regurgitation and normal left ventricular function. N Engl J Med 331:689–694, 1994.

    In a randomized trial of 143 asymptomatic patients with aortic regurgitation, after 6 years only 15% ± 3% of the patients receiving afterload reduction (nifedipine) had undergone valve replacement for symptoms or left ventricular dysfunction compared to 34% ± 6% of the patients treated with digoxin.

21. Reimold SC, Orav EJ, Come PC, et al: Progressive enlargement of the regurgitant orifice in patients with chronic aortic regurgitation. J Am Soc Echocardiogr 11:259–265, 1998.

    In a prospective study of 59 patients with audible aortic regurgitation murmurs, aortic regurgitant jet width increased by 0.04 ± 0.01 cm/year, and regurgitant orifice area increased by 0.01 ± 0.01 cm²/yr. Rate of progression was not related to the cause of aortic regurgitation, gender, or baseline regurgitant severity.

22. Burger AJ, Sherman HB, Charlamb MJ, et al: Low prevalence of valvular heart disease in 226 phentermine-fenfluramine protocol subjects prospectively followed for up to 30 months. J Am Coll Cardiol 34:1153–1158, 1999.

    In 226 obese subjects enrolled in a prospective study who had taken appetite suppressant drugs, the prevalence of significant aortic regurgitation was and mitral regurgitation was only 6.6% and 1.3%.

23. Weissman NJ, Panza JA, Tighe JF, et al. Natural history of valvular regurgitation 1 year after discontinuation of dexfenfluramine therapy. A randomized, double-blind, placebo-controlled trial. Ann Intern Med 134:267–273, 2001.

    After discontinuation of appetite suppression therapy, there is no evidence for progressive valve disease and there may be regression of aortic regurgitation in some patients.

24. Griffin BP, Stewart WJ: Echocardiography in patient selection, operative planning, and intraoperative evaluation of mitral valve repair. In: Otto CM (ed): The Practice of Clinical Echocardiography, 2nd ed. Philadelphia: WB Saunders, 2002, pp 417–434.

    Detailed review of the use of echocardiography in patients undergoing mitral valve repair procedures with numerous practical tips and excellent illustrations; 87 references.

25. Stewart WJ, Currie PJ, Salcedo EE, et al: Intraoperative Doppler color flow mapping for decision-making in valve repair for mitral regurgitation: Technique and results in 100 patients. Circulation 81:556–566, 1990.

    Intraoperative echo in 100 patients undergoing mitral valve repair showed a satisfactory repair in 92, persistent significant mitral regurgitation in 4, dynamic outflow obstruction in 3, and a persistent flail leaflet in 1 patient. Further mitral valve surgery was performed at the same operation in 6 of the 8 patients with unsatisfactory results; the other 2 required reoperation for persistent regurgitation.

26. Weisenbaugh T, Skudicky D, Sareli P: Prediction of outcome after valve replacement for rheumatic mitral regurgitation in the era of chordal preservation. Circulation 89:191–197, 1994.

    In 61 patients with rheumatic mitral regurgitation, preoperative end-systolic diameter was the only independent predictor of postoperative death. There was an increased probability of death or severe heart failure with a preoperative end-systolic diameter greater than 50 mm, with a .98% accuracy of this breakpoint for predicting outcome.

27. He S, Fontaine AA, Schwammenthal E, et al: Integrated mechanism for functional mitral regurgitation–leaflet restriction versus coapting force: In vitro studies. Circulation 96:1826–1834, 1997.

    Use of 3D echocardiography to study the complex interrelationships of the mitral valve apparatus.

28. Grigioni F, Enriquez-Sarano M, Zehr KJ, et al: Ischemic mitral regurgitation: long-term outcome and prognostic implications with quantitative Doppler assessment. Circulation 103:1759–17641, 2001.

    Quantitative Doppler measures of mitral regurgitant severity, including regurgitant volume and regurgitant orifice area, are predictors of clinical outcome after myocardial infarction.

29. Breithardt OA, Sinha AM, Schwammenthal E, et al: Acute effects of cardiac resynchronization therapy on functional mitral regurgitation in advanced systolic heart failure. J Am Coll Cardiol 41:765–770, 2003.

    Quantitative Doppler measures of mitral regurgitant severity, including regurgitant fraction and regurgitant orifice area, were used to demonstrate an improvement in functional mitral regurgitation after biventricular pacing in patients with dilated cardiomyopathy.

Alternate Approaches to Evaluation of Valvular Regurgitation

30. Otto CM: Cardiac catheterization and angiography and other diagnostic approaches. In: Otto CM (ed): Valvular Heart Disease, 2nd ed. Philadelphia: WB Saunders, 2004, pp 93–135.

    Chapters reviewing the role of computed tomography, radionuclide studies, magnetic resonance imaging, and cardiac catheterization in the evaluation of patients with valvular heart disease. A useful reference for making recommendations about additional diagnostic testing when echocardiography is inconclusive.

31. Baim DS, Grossman W: Cardiac Catheterization, Angiography, and Intervention, 6th ed. Baltimore: Lippincott Williams and Wilkins, 2000.

    Textbook of cardiac catheterization techniques emphasizing clinical applications. Chapters on hemodynamic principles and profiles in valvular heart disease are especially helpful.

The Echo Exam *Aortic Regurgitation*

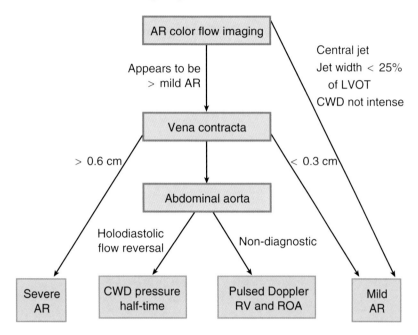

Quantitative Evaluation of Aortic Regurgitant Severity (ASE Guidelines)

Parameter	Mild	Severe
Jet width/LVOT	<25%	≥65%
Vena contracta (cm)	<0.3	>0.6
Pressure half-time (ms)	>500	<200
Regurgitant volume (mL/beat)	<30	≥60
Regurgitant fraction (%)	<30	≥50
Regurgitant orifice area (cm²)	<0.10	≥0.30

Quantitation of Aortic Regurgitation Severity

Parameter	Modality	View	Recording	Measurements
Vena contracta width	Color flow imaging	Parasternal long-axis	Angulate, decrease depth, narrow sector, zoom	Narrowest segment of regurgitant jet between proximal flow convergence and distal jet expansion
Descending aortic diastolic flow reversal	Pulsed Doppler	Subcostal and SSN	Sample volume 2–3 mm, decrease wall filters, adjust scale	Holodiastolic reversal of flow
CW Doppler signal (intensity, slope, VTI)	CW Doppler	Apical	Careful positioning, and transducer angulation to obtain clear signal	Compare signal intensity of retrograde to antegrade flow, measure half time from slope of signal edge
Volume flow at two sites (RV, RF,) ROA	2D and pulsed Doppler	Parasternal (2D) and apical	LVOT diameter and VTI Mitral annulus diameter and VTI	Calculations in example

Etiology	Valve abnormality
	Aortic root disease
Severity of regurgitation	Vena contracta width
	Descending aorta holosystolic flow reversal
	CW Doppler deceleration slope
	Calculation of RV, RF, and ROA
Coexisting aortic stenosis	Aortic jet velocity
Left ventricular response	LV dimensions or volumes
	LV ejection fraction
	dP/dt
Other findings	Aortic coarctation (with bicuspid valve)

Example

A 37-year-old man presents with an asymptomatic diastolic murmur. Echocardiography shows a bicuspid aortic valve with more than mild aortic regurgitation with:

Vena contracta width	5 mm
Descending aorta	Holodiastolic flow reversal in descending thoracic, but not proximal abdominal, aorta
CW Doppler	AR signal less dense than antegrade flow
	Pressure half-time = 400 ms
	$VTI_{AR} = 204$ cm
LVOT diameter ($LVOT_D$)	2.8 cm
VTI_{LVOT}	24 cm
Mitral annulus diameter	3.1 cm
VTI_{MA}	12 cm

The vena contracta width indicates more than mild aortic regurgitation, but this could be moderate or severe.

Holodiastolic flow reversal in the proximal abdominal aorta would be consistent with severe AR. Flow reversal in the descending thoracic aorta indicates at least moderate AR but is less specific for severe AR.

CW Doppler signal density indicates at least moderate AR and a pressure half-time >200 but <500 ms is also consistent with moderate or severe aortic regurgitation.

Next, regurgitant volume (RV), regurgitant fraction (RF) and regurgitant orifice area (ROA) are calculated.

Using the LVOT and mitral annulus diameters (MA_D), the circular cross-sectional areas of flow are calculated:

$$CSA_{LVOT} = \pi(LVOT_D/2)^2 = 3.14(2.8/2)^2 = 6.2\,cm^2$$

$$CSA_{MA} = \pi(MA_D/2)^2 = 3.14(3.1/2)^2 = 7.5\,cm^2$$

Stroke volume across each valve ($cm^3 = ml$), then is

$$SV_{LVOT} = (CSA_{LVOT} \times VTI_{LVOT}) = 6.2\,cm^2 \times 24\,cm$$
$$= 149\,cm^3$$

$$SV_{MA} = (CSA_{MA} \times VTI_{MA}) = 7.5\,cm^2 \times 12\,cm = 91\,cm^3$$

Regurgitant volume (*RV*) is calculated from transaortic flow (TSV, total stroke volume) and transmitral flow (FSV, forward stroke volume), as

$$RV = TSV - FSV = 149\,mL - 91\,mL = 58\,mL$$

Regurgitant fraction (RF) is

$$RV = RSV/TSV \times 100\% = 58\,mL/149\,mL \times 100\% = 39\%$$

Regurgitant orifice area (*ROA*) is

$$ROA = RSV/VTI_{AR} = 58\,cm^2/204\,cm \times 100\% = 0.28\,cm^2$$

The RV, RF, and ROA all are consistent with moderate (but nearly severe) aortic regurgitation.

The Echo Exam *Mitral Regurgitation*

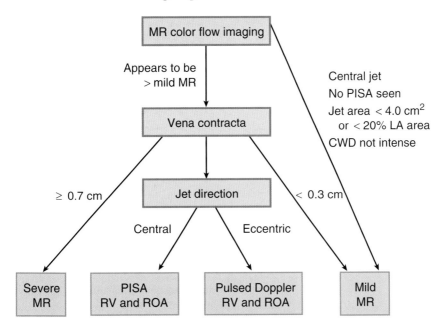

Quantitative Evaluation of Mitral Regurgitant Severity (ASE Guidelines)

Mitral Regurgitation	Mild	Severe
Jet area (cm²)	<4 cm² or <20% LA area	>40% LA area
Vena contracta (cm)	<0.3	≥0.7
Regurgitant volume (mL)	<30	≥60
Regurgitant fraction (%)	<30	≥50
Regurgitant orifice area (cm²)	<0.20	≥0.40

Quantitation of Mitral Regurgitation Severity

Parameter	Modality	View(s)	Recording	Measurements
Vena contracta width	Color flow imaging	Parasternal long-axis	Angulate, decrease depth, narrow sector, zoom	Narrowest segment of regurgitant jet between proximal flow convergence and distal jet expansion
Color flow imaging	Color flow imaging	Parasternal and apical	Narrow sector, decrease depth	Central vs. eccentric, anterior vs. posterior
CW Doppler signal	CW Doppler	Apical	Careful positioning, and transducer angulation to obtain clear signal	Compare signal intensity of retrograde to antegrade flow
Proximal isovelocity surface area	Color flow imaging	A4C or A-long axis	Decrease depth, narrow sector, zoom, adjust aliasing velocity	Adjust aliasing velocity so PISA is hemi-spherical, measure from aliasing boundary to orifice
Volume flow at two sites	2D and pulsed Doppler	Parasternal (2D) and apical	LVOT diameter and VTI Mitral annulus diameter and VTI	See calculations for aortic regurgitation example, with substitution of transmitral flow for TSV and transaortic flow for FSV
Pulmonary vein systolic flow reversal	Pulsed Doppler	A4C on TTE but TEE often needed	Pulmonary vein flow in all four veins	Qualitative; caution in patients in atrial fibrillation

Etiology	Primary valve disease
	Secondary (functional)
Severity of regurgitation	Vena contracta width
	Jet direction (central, eccentric)
	CW Doppler signal
	Calculation of RV, RF, and ROA
	Central jet: PISA method
	Eccentric jet: Volume flow at two sites
	Pulmonary vein flow reversal
Left ventricular response	LV dimensions or volumes
	LV ejection fraction
	dP/dt
Pulmonary vasculature	Pulmonary systolic pressure
	Right ventricular size and systolic function
Other findings	Left atrial size

Example

A 52-year-old man with a dilated cardiomyopathy presents with worsening heart failure symptoms. Echocardiography shows a dilated left ventricle with an ejection fraction of 32% and a central jet of mitral regurgitation with:

Vena contracta width	8 mm
CW Doppler	MR signal as dense as antegrade flow with no evidence for a v wave
	dP/dt =840 mm Hg/s
	Maximum MR velocity = 4.6 m/s
	VTI_{MR} =150 cm
PISA radius	1.2 cm
Aliasing velocity	30 cm/s

Right superior pulmonary vein   Systolic flow reversal

The vena contracta width indicates severe mitral regurgitation.

CW Doppler signal density indicates moderate to severe MR and the absence of a v-wave suggests a chronic disease process. The dP/dt is <1000 mm Hg/s consistent with decreased left ventricular contractility.

Color flow indicates a central jet so the proximal isovelocity surface area (PISA) method can be used to quantitate regurgitant severity.

The *proximal isovelocity surface area (PISA)* is calculated from the radius measurement as

$$PISA = 2\pi r^2 = 2\pi(1.0\,cm)^2 = 6.3\,cm^2$$

The maximum *instantaneous regurgitant volume (RV_{inst})* is calculated from PISA and the aliasing velocity ($V_{aliasing}$) as

$$RV_{inst} = PISA \times V_{aliasing} = 6.3\,cm^2 \times 30\,cm/s = 189\,cm^3/s$$

Maximum regurgitant orifice area (instantaneous) then is calculated from the RV and MR jet velocity (where 4.6 m/s = 460 cm/s)

$$ROA_{max} = RV_{max}/V_{MR} = (189\,cm^3/s)/460\,cm/s = 0.41\,cm^2$$

This ROA is consistent with severe mitral regurgitation.

Regurgitant volume over the systolic flow period can be estimated as

$$RV = ROA \times VTI_{MR} = 0.41\,cm^2 \times 150\,cm = 62\,cm^3 \text{ or ml}$$

This regurgitant volume also is consistent with severe mitral regurgitation.

If the jet is eccentric, quantitation should be performed using transaortic (forward) stroke volume and trans-mitral (total) stroke volume calculations, as illustrated for aortic regurgitation

PROSTHETIC VALVES

Echocardiographic evaluation of prosthetic valves is similar, in many respects, to evaluation of native valvular disease. However, there are some important differences. First, there are several types of prosthetic valves with differing fluid dynamics for each basic design and differing flow velocities for each valve size. Second, the mechanisms of valve dysfunction are somewhat different from those for native valve disease. Third, the technical aspects of imaging artificial devices–specifically, the problem of acoustic shadowing–significantly affect the diagnostic approach when prosthetic valve dysfunction is suspected (Table 13–1).

Echocardiographers increasingly are asked to evaluate prosthetic valve function, given the increasing number of prosthetic valves implanted annually and the greater longevity of patients with prosthetic valves. Both an understanding of the basic approach to echocardiographic evaluation (as outlined in this chapter) and detailed knowledge of the specific flow dynamic for the size and type of prosthesis in an individual patient (see Suggested Reading) are needed for appropriate patient management.

BASIC PRINCIPLES

Types of Prosthetic Valves and Fluid Dynamics

The three basic types of prosthetic valves (Figs. 13–1 and 13–2; Table 13–2) are

- tissue valves, or bioprostheses,
- homograft valves, and
- mechanical valves.

Bioprosthetic Valves

Tissue valves are composed of three biologic leaflets with an anatomic structure similar to the native aortic valve. With traditional stented prosthetic valves, the leaflets (typically porcine), or pericardium (usually bovine or equine) shaped to mimic normal leaflets, are mounted on a cloth-covered rigid support that functions as the crown-shaped aortic annulus with a raised "stent" at each of the three commissures. Variations in the support structure and leaflet types abound in commercially available valves; newer valves may include anticalcification treatments. Current generation stented tissue valves include the Edwards Perimount and the Medtronic Mosaic valve. Older examples of stented heterografts include Carpentier-Edwards porcine valves, Hancock porcine valves, and Ionescu-Shiley bovine pericardial valves.

Tissue valves also have been developed that use a flexible cuff of fabric or tissue, instead of rigid stents, to support the valve leaflets with the goal of optimizing valve hemodynamics. Examples include the St. Jude Toronto SPV valve and the Carpentier-Edwards freestyle valve. Stented tissue valves are simpler to implant, requiring only suturing at the planar sewing ring. In contrast, implantation of stentless valves is more complex

355

TABLE 13-1

Comparison of Different Valve Types

Normal	Native Valve	Bioprosthesis	Mechanical Valve
Fluid dynamics	Central orifice, laminar flow, blunt flow profile	Central orifice, laminar flow, blunt flow profile	Complex fluid dynamics depending on valve type
Antegrade velocity	Normal	Increased	Increased
Normal regurgitation	Mild, central	Mild, central	Mild, oblique jets
Mechanisms of dysfunction	Multiple	Tissue degeneration, endocarditis, pannus ingrowth, sewing ring dehiscence	Mechanical failure, endocarditis, pannus ingrowth, thrombus, sewing ring dehiscence
Technical aspects of imaging	Calcification may cause acoustic shadows in some cases	Acoustic shadow from sewing ring	Extensive reverberations and acoustic shadowing

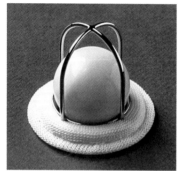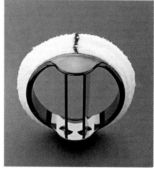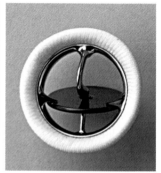

■ **FIGURE 13-1.** Photographs of three different mechanical valves: a ball-cage type valve (Starr-Edward mitral, *left*), a bileaflet valve (St. Jude Medical–heart valve, *center*), and a tilting-disk valve (Medtronic Hall valve, *right*). (Courtesy of Baxter Healthcare Corporation, Santa Ana, CA; St. Jude Medical, St. Paul, MN; and Medtronic, Inc., Minneapolis, MN.)

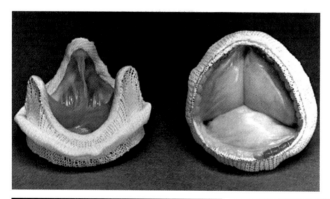

■ **FIGURE 13-2.** Examples of three tissue valve prostheses. A conventional stented Carpentier Edwards porcine valve (*top*), a stentless St Jude Toronto tissue valve (*bottom right*) (St. Jude Medical, St Paul, MN), and the Edwards Perimount pericardial valve (*bottom left*) (Edwards Lifesciences). (From Otto CM: Prosthetic valves. In: Otto CM (ed): Valvular Heart Disease, 2nd ed. Philadelphia: WB Saunders, 2004, Figure 15–13.)

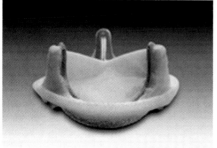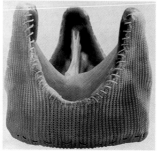

TABLE 13-2	
Examples of Valve Types and Names	
Homografts	Cryopreserved by tissue bank
Heterografts	
Stented	Carpentier-Edwards
	Edwards Perimount
	Medtronic Mosaic
Stentless	St. Jude Toronto stentless porcine valve (SPV)
	Edwards Freestyle
Mechanical	
Ball-cage	Starr-Edwards
Floating-disk	Beall (no longer used)
Tilting-disk	Omniscience
	Bjork-Shiley
Bileaflet	St. Jude

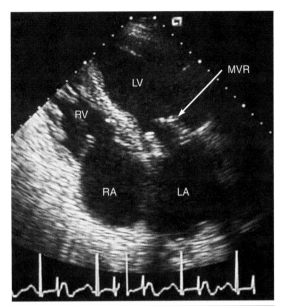

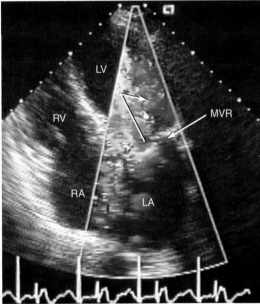

with the surgical technique affecting the three-dimensional (3D) anatomy of the valve.

All these tissue valves are similar in that the trileaflet valve opens to a circular orifice (in systole in the aortic position or in diastole in the mitral position). The normal flow pattern is similar to that of a native valve, specifically, laminar flow with a relatively blunt flow profile. Regardless of valve type, the orientation of a mitral prosthesis valve results in the inflow stream being directed anteriorly and medially toward the ventricular septum in most patients instead of toward the ventricular apex, as is seen for normal native valves. This results in a reversed vortex of blood flow in mid-diastole, as seen in an apical four-chamber view (Fig. 13–3).

Conventional tissue valves also differ from native valves in the presence of the support structure, which both limits acoustic access and results in a "normal" valve area that is smaller than the native valve (with corresponding higher "normal" antegrade flow velocities) due to limitation of the flow area by the supporting structure. These limitations are largely avoided with the newer stentless valves, which appear similar to a normal native valve and have hemodynamics more closely approximating normal valve function. As is seen with native valves, a small degree of valve regurgitation is found in a high percentage of normally functioning bioprosthetic valves.

Homograft Valves

Homograft valves are cryopreserved human aortic valves harvested at autopsy. Typically, the valve, ascending aorta, and anterior mitral leaflet are preserved as a block, to be trimmed appropriately at the time of implantation. Aortic homo-

■ FIGURE 13–3. Apical four-chamber view (*top*) in a patient with a porcine mitral valve replacement (MVR) showing color flow (*bottom*) toward the apex along the ventricular septum with flow toward the base along the lateral wall–the opposite of the normal pattern shown in Figure 2–32.

grafts are used in the aortic or pulmonic position but are rarely used for atrioventricular valve replacement (because a supporting prosthetic structure would be needed). While the fluid dynamics of a homograft are similar to those of a native valve, flow velocities are slightly higher and valve areas slightly smaller than for a normal native valve due to the space occupied by the homograft annulus in the patient's outflow tract.

Mechanical Valves

A variety of mechanical valves currently are available. In addition, several other types of valves, which were implanted in the past, are still in situ in some patients. The basic types of mechanical valves are

■ a ball-cage valve in which a spherical occluder is contained by a metal "cage" when the valve is open and fills the orifice in the closed position (like on a snorkel);

■ a tilting-disk valve where a single circular disk opens at an angle to the annulus plane, being constrained in its motion by a smaller "cage," a central strut, or a slanted slot in the valve ring; and

■ a bileaflet valve where two semicircular disks hinge open to form two large lateral orifices and a smaller central orifice (Fig. 13–4).

ANTEGRADE FLOW PROFILES. As might be expected, the spatial flow profiles across each of these valve types vary substantially, and none is analogous to flow across the normal native valve. With a ball-cage valve in the open position, blood flows across the sewing ring and around the ball occluder on all sides. When the valve closes, a small amount of regurgitation is seen circumferentially around the ball as it seats in the sewing ring.

The fluid dynamics of a tilting-disk valve are characterized by two orifices in the open position, one larger than the other (major versus minor), with an asymmetric flow profile as blood accelerates along the tilted surface of the open disk. Subtle variations in this flow pattern depend on the shape of the disk (convex versus concave surface) as well as the sewing ring design.

Bileaflet mechanical valves have complex fluid dynamics that affect the Doppler echocardiographic evaluation of these valves. With the leaflets open, there are two large lateral valve orifices with a small narrow central "slitlike" orifice. The flow velocity profile shows three peaks corresponding to these three orifices, with higher velocities in the center of each orifice. Of note, the local acceleration forces within the narrow central orifice result in localized high-pressure gradients in this region of the valve. These local gradients often are substantially higher than the overall pressure gradient across the valve.

NORMAL MECHANICAL VALVE REGURGITATION. With a tilting-disk valve, when the disk closes to occlude the valve annulus, regurgitation occurs at the closure line with the major regurgitant jet directed away from the sewing ring at the edge of the major orifice (Fig. 13–5). Note that the orientation of the prosthetic valve in the annulus can be variable, depending on surgical preference,

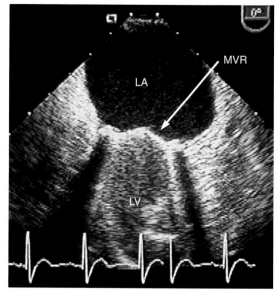

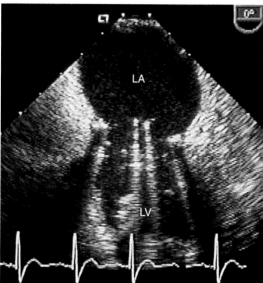

FIGURE 13–4. Bileaflet mitral valve prosthesis seen in systole (*above*) and diastole (*below*) from a transesophageal approach. In systole, the two leaflets close with a slightly obtuse closure angle. In diastole, the sewing ring and two parallel open leaflets are seen. Reverberations from the leaflets and shadowing from the sewing ring are prominent in both systole and diastole.

so that the open disk position and the orientation of the regurgitant jet vary correspondingly. Additional smaller regurgitant jets circumferentially around the annulus normally are present. With a single-disk valve and a central strut (e.g., Medtronic-Hall), a small central jet of regurgitation also occurs around the central hole of the disk, as might be expected. When a bileaflet valve closes, two crisscross jets of regurgitation are seen

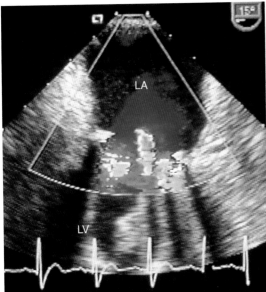

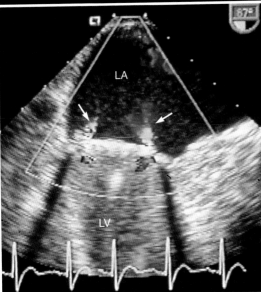

■ **FIGURE 13–5.** Color flow image of a bileaflet mitral valve prosthesis in diastole (*above*), showing acceleration of flow across the valve with two large lateral orifices and a small central orifice. In systole (*below*), two normal jets of regurgitation are seen.

in the plane parallel to the leaflet opening plane. In the perpendicular plane, two smaller diverging regurgitant jets are seen. The total volume of regurgitation is small with normal prosthetic valve function.

Valved Conduits

Valved conduits are used in congenital heart surgery and in ascending aortic repairs when both a new passageway for blood flow and a valve are needed. The conduit may be biologic (i.e., a homo-

graft) or artificial (i.e., Gore-Tex or Dacron) material. A conduit may incorporate either a tissue or a mechanical valve with fluid dynamics similar to those for a valve implanted in the native annulus.

Mechanisms of Prosthetic Valve Dysfunction

The types of disease processes that affect prosthetic valves are distinctly different from those seen with native valvular heart disease and can be classified into three groups:

■ Structural failure
■ Thromboembolic complications
■ Endocarditis

Primary Structural Failure

Failure of a bioprosthetic valve to open or close properly (mechanical failure) usually is the result of slowly progressive tissue degeneration with fibrocalcific changes of the leaflets resulting in increased resistance to opening (stenosis) or failure to coapt during valve closure (regurgitation). Typically, failure of tissue valves occurs 10 or more years after valve implantation. Acute bioprosthetic valve stenosis is rare. Acute bioprosthetic regurgitation can occur with a leaflet tear, usually adjacent to a region of calcification.

Failure of a mechanical valve can occur due to faulty design or wear and tear of the prosthetic material resulting in disk escape or incomplete valve closure. However, these complications were seen only with older generation valves (which may still be persent in a few patients). Current generation mechanical valves are reliable and very durable. More often, mechanical valve stenosis or regurgitation is due to thrombus formation or pannus ingrowth around the valve, impairing disk excursion or closure.

With both bioprosthetic and mechanical valves, paravalvular regurgitation can occur around the sewing ring due to loss of suture material postoperatively, most often related to fibrocalcific disease in the valve annulus. The new onset of paravalvular regurgitation late after surgery raises the possibility of an infectious process (endocarditis) resulting in valve dehiscence.

Thromboembolic Complications

Prosthetic valves, particularly mechanical valves, are prone to thrombus formation which may result in systemic embolic events or valve dysfunction. Echocardiographic evaluation for prosthetic valve thrombus is limited, except with very large masses, due to shadowing and reverberations. In addition, clinical events may be associated with clots smaller than the limits of clinical ultrasound resolution. Thus, echocardiography cannot exclude the possibility of thrombus on a prosthetic valve; in patients with embolic events, the prosthetic valve itself is a cardiac "source of embolus."

Endocarditis

Infection of a valve prosthesis is a serious clinical problem, so suspected endocarditis is a frequent indication for echocardiography in patients with prosthetic valves. Endocarditis on a bioprosthesis may result in vegetations similar to those seen on a native valve. However, with a mechanical valve, the infection often is paravalvular, and no discrete vegetation may be present.

Technical Aspects of Echo Evaluation

The most technically limiting aspect of echo-cardiographic evaluation of prosthetic valves is the problem of acoustic shadowing. The sewing rings of both bioprosthetic and mechanical valves and the occluders of mechanical valves are strong echo reflectors, resulting in acoustic shadows and reverberations (Fig. 13–6). These reverberations and shadows obscure the motion of the valve structures themselves and block detection of imaging and Doppler abnormalities in the acoustic shadow region. During the examination, considerable effort is directed toward utilizing windows and views that avoid these imaging artifacts. Transesophageal echocardiography is particularly useful in evaluation of prosthetic mitral valves because it provides acoustic access from the left atrial side of the valve.

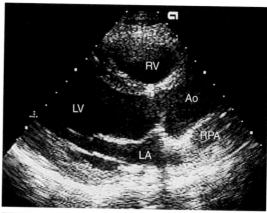

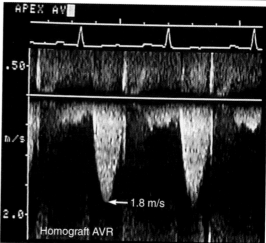

FIGURE 13–7. Aortic valve homograft in a parasternal long-axis view showing an appearance similar to a native valve other than thickening and increased echogenicity of the aortic root. Continuous-wave Doppler shows a mildly increased antegrade velocity across the homograft compared with a native valve. RPA, right pulmonary artery.

ECHOCARDIOGRAPHIC APPROACH

Imaging

Bioprosthetic Valves

Aortic homografts appear similar to native aortic valves except for some increased thickness in the left ventricular outflow tract and the ascending aorta at the proximal and distal suture sites (Fig. 13–7). Typically, the homograft is implanted using the mini-root technique with the homograft replacing a segment of the native aorta. This approach necessitates reimplantation of the coronary arteries. In the past, the aortic homograft sometimes was positioned inside the patient's native aorta with appropriate trimming to maintain patency of the coronary ostia. In patients with endocarditis, the attached anterior mitral leaflet of the homograft may be used to patch a ventricular septal defect or abscess cavity. The echocardio-

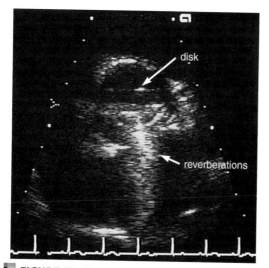

FIGURE 13–6. Parasternal short-axis view of a bileaflet mechanical aortic valve in systole. The anterior disk is seen as a clear line. The posterior disk and posterior sewing ring are obscured by reverberations from the valve.

graphic appearance of a homograft is very similar to that of a native aortic valve, except for the associated surgical changes. Standard parasternal long- and short-axis image planes provide optimal visualization of valve leaflet anatomy and motion.

Stented tissue prosthetic valves have a trileaflet structure similar to a native aortic valve. An M-mode through the leaflets shows the typical "boxlike" opening in systole (for the aortic position) or diastole (for the mitral position) as is seen with a normal native aortic valve. However, with conventional valve designs, the echogenic sewing ring and struts may limit visualization of the leaflets with the specific ultrasound appearance of the supporting structures depending on the specific model. Because there is marked variability in surgeons' valve preferences, it is helpful to obtain photographs of the valves most commonly encountered at your institution (Fig. 13–8). *Stentless bioprosthetic valves* have an echocardiographic appearance very similar to a native aortic valve, other than increased echogenicity in the aortic root in the early postoperative period (Fig. 13–9). This valve is best identified by reviewing the chart or asking the patient about any cardiac surgical procedures before beginning the study.

Improved images of prosthetic tissue valves can be obtained from a transesophageal approach, particularly for valves in the mitral position, since the ultrasound beam has a perpendicular orientation to the leaflets with no intervening structures from this approach. With aortic valve prostheses, transesophageal imaging is less rewarding because the posterior part of the sewing ring shadows the valve leaflets. When images of the leaflets themselves are suboptimal, Doppler data can provide valuable information.

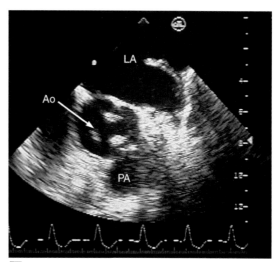

FIGURE 13–8. Transesophageal view of a porcine aortic valve replacement in a short-axis view showing the three normal stents that support the valve leaflets.

Conventional bioprosthetic valves have an average longevity of approximately 10 years, with slowly progressive tissue failure being the primary reason for reoperation. Typically, the leaflets develop fibrocalcific changes that result in leaflet deformity (leading to regurgitation) and/or increased stiffness (leading to stenosis). Echocardiographically, increased echogenicity and irregularity of the leaflets may be noted, although images of the leaflets often are suboptimal due to shadowing and reverberation.

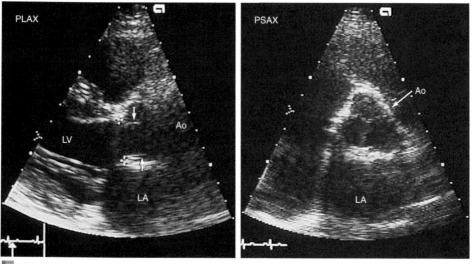

FIGURE 13–9. Parasternal long-axis (*left*) and short-axis (*right*) views of a stentless tissue valve in the aortic position. The valve appearance is similar to a native trileaflet aortic valve other than slightly increased echogenicity in the aortic root.

Mechanical Valves

Ultrasound imaging of mechanical valves from a transthoracic approach is frustrating because of severe reverberations and acoustic shadowing. While imaging may provide clues as to the type of valve prostheses (e.g., "low-profile" bileaflet or tilting-disk valve versus "high-profile" ball-cage valve), obviously it is simpler to ascertain the exact valve type and size from the patient's medical record or valve identification card. Assessing motion of the valve occluder often is difficult. For example, the leading edge of a tilting-disk valve results in a strong reverberation across the image obscuring motion of the disk itself. In addition, an oblique image plane often is obtained relative to the prosthetic valve, since orientation of the prosthesis within the annulus is not standard. With a tomographic plane perpendicular to the open bileaflet valve, the two leaflets can be identified clearly, an image plane that is best identified on multiplane transesophageal imaging.

Technical limitations make identification of prosthetic valve endocarditis or thrombosis problematic because the abnormalities may be obscured by reverberations or hidden by acoustic shadowing. Transesophageal imaging can be helpful in identifying thrombus or infected vegetations on the atrial side of a mitral prosthesis, because the left atrium is "masked" by the prosthetic valve from both parasternal and apical windows. In a patient with a mechanical aortic valve, the subaortic region can be evaluated well from a transthoracic approach from parasternal and apical windows. In this situation, transesophageal images are less helpful due to shadowing of the outflow tract by the posterior aspect of the prosthesis.

Valved Conduits

Ultrasound imaging of a bioprosthetic or mechanical valve in a conduit (e.g., right ventricular to pulmonary artery) may be difficult due to ultrasound attenuation by the conduit prosthetic material. Of note, stenosis in a valved conduit can occur as a result of stenosis of the valve prosthesis or fibrotic ingrowth along the length of the conduit. In addition, residual or progressive stenosis at the proximal or distal anastomosis site can occur. Imaging the narrowing in the conduit often is difficult, but a careful Doppler examination may allow detection of the abnormal flow velocities. Continuous-wave Doppler is used to assess the maximum flow velocity, while pulsed Doppler or color flow imaging is used to localize the level of obstruction along the length of the conduit.

Doppler Evaluation

Normal Doppler Findings

PROSTHETIC VALVE "CLICKS." The motion of the occluder of a mechanical valve (or the tissue leaflets of a biologic valve) creates a brief intense Doppler signal that appears as a dark narrow band of short duration on the spectral display (Fig. 13–10). Audibly, this signal is similar to the valve "click" appreciated on auscultation. However, unlike auscultation, usually both opening and closing valve clicks are seen on spectral Doppler analysis. The Doppler signals associated with valve opening and closing are similar to those seen with native valves but are of greater intensity. The motion of the occluder also may result in color flow artifacts, with color signals covering large areas of the image that are inconsistent from beat to beat.

ANTEGRADE VELOCITIES/PRESSURE GRADIENTS. Compared with a normal native valve, all prosthetic valves are inherently stenotic to some extent. Specifically, the expected antegrade velocities and pressure gradients across a normally functioning prosthetic valve are higher than the corresponding values for a native valve. Similarly, the effective orifice area of a prosthetic valve is smaller than the orifice area of a normal native valve.

The expected velocities, pressure gradients, and valve areas depend on the specific type, size, and position of the prosthetic valve. While manufacturers have data on in vitro flow characteristics for each valve, in vivo echocardiographic data are sparse owing to the large number of valve

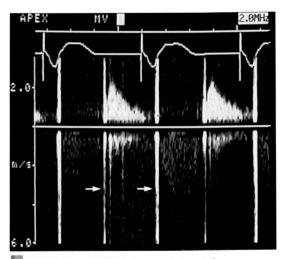

I FIGURE 13–10. Left ventricular inflow across a mechanical mitral valve replacement showing an increased antegrade velocity (compared with a native valve) and prominent valve clicks (*arrows*).

types and sizes. Even in a large study, only a few patients have the same valve type, position, and size. In the available Doppler studies of normal prosthetic valves, data often are presented in various ways. Some studies report the mean ±1 SD for each variable; others include the range as well. While compilation of the normal values from all these studies is not possible from the published data, estimates of the expected normal velocities, pressure gradients, and valve areas for several commonly seen prosthetic valves are shown in Tables 13–3 and 13–4.

In general, larger valve sizes have lower velocities and gradients, and larger effective orifice areas. Mitral prosthesis have lower velocities and gradients than aortic prostheses. Note that many

of the smaller prosthetic aortic valves have hemodynamics that are consistent with clinical stenosis even with normal valve function. The lower velocities and pressure gradients with mitral valve prostheses are due, in part, to larger valve sizes but also to passive flow at a lower pressure gradient from the atrium into the ventricle in diastole compared with active ejection and a higher left ventricular to aortic pressure gradient in systole for aortic prostheses.

As indicated by the ranges and standard deviations in the tables, there is a wide range of reported "normal" values for a given prosthetic valve type and size. Anatomic features and the details of implantation in each patient may account for some of this variability. However, the

TABLE 13–3

Normal Doppler Data for Prosthetic Aortic Valves

Valve Type	Size (mm)	V_{max} (m/s)	Mean Gradient (mm Hg)	Velocity Ratio	AVA (cm^2)
Mechanical Valves					
Bileaflet (St. Jude)	19	3.0 (2.0–4.5)	20 (10–30)	0.37	1.0
	21	2.7 (2.5–3.5)	14 (10–30)	0.40	1.3
	23	2.5 (2.0–3.5)	12 (10–30)	0.37	1.3
	25	2.4 (2.0–3.5)	12 (5–30)	0.42	1.8
	27	2.2 (2.0–3.1)	11 (5–20)	0.46	2.4
	29	2.0 (2.0–2.5)	10 (5–15)	0.49	2.7
	31	2.1 (1.5–2.5)	10 (5–15)	0.49	3.1
Tilting-disk (Bjork-Shiley, Medtronic Hall)	19	21 ± 7			
	21	2.8 ± 0.9	16		
	23	2.6 ± 0.4	14 ± 5		
	25	2.1 ± 0.3	13 ± 3		
	27	1.9 ± 0.2	10 ± 3		
	29	1.9 ± 0.2	7 ± 6		
Ball-cage (Starr-Edwards)		3.1 ± 0.5	24 ± 4		
Tissue Valves					
Stented porcine tissue (Hancock or Carpentier-Edwards)	19	2.8 ± 0.7	16 ± 2		1.5 ± 0.1
	21	2.6 ± 0.4	15 ± 6		1.8 ± 0.2
	23	2.6 ± 0.4	13 ± 6		2.1 ± 0.2
	25	2.5 ± 0.4	11 ± 2		
	27	2.4 ± 0.4	10 ± 1		
	29	2.4 ± 0.4	12		
Pericardial valve (CE Perimount)		1.5 ± 0.9	4.4 ± 1.8		2.5 ± 0.6
Mosaic valve (Medtronic) 23 mm		2.3 ± 1.2	12 ± 3		
Nonstented tissue valves					
SPV-Toronto (St. Jude)		2.2 ± 0.4	3 (2–20)		1.8–2.3
Ao-homograft		1.8 ± 0.4	7 ± 3		2.2 (1.7–3.1)

Note: Values shown are mean ± 1 SD or mean (range).
Velocity ratio, LV outflow velocity/aortic jet velocity.
Data from Reisner et al: J Am Soc Echo 1:201, 1988; Zabalgoitia et al: Curr Prob Cardiol 5:271, 1992; Sagar et al: J Am Coll Cardiol 7:68, 1986; Baumgartner et al: Circulation 82:1467, 1990; Chafizadeh et al: Circulation 83:213, 1991; Jaffe et al: Am J Cardiol 63:1466, 1989; Firstenberg et al: Ann Thorac Surg 71:S285, 2001; Nardi et al: J Heart Valve Dis 10:100, 2001.

TABLE 13–4				
Normal Doppler Data for Prosthetic Mitral Valves				
Valve Type	V_{max} (m/s)	Mean Gradient (mm Hg)	$T_{1/2}$ (m/s)	MVA (cm²)
Mechanical				
Bileaflet (St. Jude)	1.6 ± 0.3	4 ± 1	77 ± 17	2.9 ± 0.6
Tilting-disk (Bjork-Shiley)	1.6 ± 0.3	3 ± 2	90 ± 22	2.4 ± 0.6
Ball-cage (Starr-Edwards)	1.9 ± 0.5	5 ± 2	110 ± 27	2.0 ± 0.5
Porcine Tissue				
Ionescu-Shiley	1.5 ± 0.3	3 ± 1	93 ± 25	2.4 ± 0.8
Carpentier-Edwards	1.8 ± 0.2	6 ± 2	90 ± 25	2.5 ± 0.7
Hancock	1.5 ± 0.3	4 ± 2	129 ± 31	1.7 ± 0.4
CE Pericardial		4 ± 2		2.6 ± 0.6

Values shown are mean ± 1 SD.
Data from Reisner, Meltzer: J Am Soc Echocardiogr 1:201, 1988; Zabalgoitia: Curr Prob Cardiol 5:271, 1992.

impact of transvalvular volume flow rate on transvalvular velocities and pressure gradients should not be underestimated. Even with a normally functioning prosthesis, a high cardiac output (e.g., postoperative, pregnancy, or sepsis) results in a high velocity and pressure gradient. This variability in "normal" velocities can be compensated for by calculating effective orifice area to "correct" for volume flow rate.

A useful clinical approach is to obtain a baseline Doppler echo study in each patient after valve replacement (but not in the immediate postoperative period). The values obtained then serve as the "normal" reference for that patient. This facilitates detection of changes in prosthetic valve function over time, with each patient serving as his or her own control. In some patients with a stentless valve in the aortic position, high velocities are seen early postoperatively with a progressive decline in velocity to the normal range at 1- to 2-year follow-up, presumably related to geometric remodeling of the annulus and outflow tract region.

NORMAL REGURGITATION. Normal prosthetic valve function implies a small degree of valvular regurgitation in virtually all mechanical valves and in a high percentage (30% to 50%) of bioprosthetic valves. The patterns of regurgitation detected corresponds to the fluid dynamics of each valve type. Color flow imaging shows the spatial distribution of normal prosthetic regurgitation with patterns specific to each valve type.

On a transthoracic study, it may be difficult to separate normal from pathologic prosthetic regurgitation, especially for the mitral position. On color flow imaging, normal prosthetic regurgitation tends to be a uniform color with little variance, whereas pathologic regurgitation shows aliasing and variance with a "confetti-like" appearance to the flow pattern. On continuous-wave Doppler examination, normal prosthetic regurgitation has a low signal strength, may persist through only part of the cardiac cycle, and is spatially localized. Note that pathologic regurgitation may appear "mild" by both continuous-wave and color Doppler criteria due to acoustic shadowing of the flow signal. In some cases, consideration of other echocardiographic and clinical factors may allow differentiation of pathologic from physiologic prosthetic regurgitation. However, if pathologic regurgitation is suspected, transesophageal imaging is needed in many aortic valve and all mitral valve cases.

On transesophageal imaging, the normal patterns of prosthetic regurgitation for each valve type can be identified, keeping in mind that normal regurgitation tends to be relatively uniform in color, even though the jet area may appear relatively large. Physiologic regurgitation originates within the sewing ring with typical patterns for each valve type. Pathologic regurgitation is typically characterized by

■ an eccentric or large jet,
■ marked variance on the color flow display,
■ a jet that often originates around the valve sewing ring, and
■ visualization of a proximal flow acceleration region on the left ventricular side of the mitral valve.

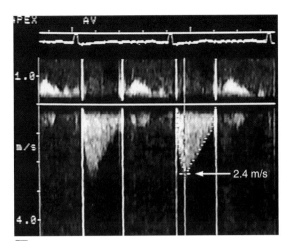

FIGURE 13–11. Antegrade velocity across a normal aortic valve replacement. The antegrade velocity is increased compared with a native valve, the shape of the flow curve is triangular, and prominent prosthetic valve clicks are present.

Prosthetic Valve Stenosis

PRESSURE GRADIENTS. The principles applied to evaluation of native valve stenosis also have been used for suspected stenosis of prosthetic valves. From a continuous-wave Doppler recording of the antegrade velocity across the valve, obtained at a parallel intercept angle, maximum instantaneous and mean pressure gradients can be calculated using the Bernoulli equation $(4v^2)$. Although the maximum velocity across a pros-

thetic valve is higher than that for a native valve, the shape of the velocity curve is triangular (in contrast to the rounded contour seen in aortic stenosis). Thus, the calculated mean gradient typically is less for a prosthetic valve than for a native valve with the same maximum antegrade velocity (Fig. 13–11).

Maximum and mean pressure gradients across bioprosthetic valves calculated by Doppler echo compare well with directly measured pressure gradients (Table 13–5). The situation is more complex for mechanical valves because of the differing fluid dynamics of each type of prosthesis. In theory, the pressure gradient across a given degree of stenosis will be identical whether the stenosis consists of a single orifice or multiple orifices, with the Bernoulli relationship being valid for each orifice. Thus, a maximum pressure gradient of 36 mm Hg will correspond to a single or multiple 3-m/s jets across the valve. However, while this theory holds true when local acceleration and viscous forces can be ignored, local higher-pressure gradients do occur with some valve types. This phenomenon has been studied most thoroughly for the bileaflet valve.

With the valve leaflets open, the bileaflet valve has a narrow, slitlike central orifice flanked by two larger semicircular orifices (Fig. 13–12). The walls of this narrow central orifice are formed by the parallel valve disks, which are nearly perpendicular to the sewing ring of the valve. Within this narrow central flow stream, acceleration forces

---

TABLE 13–5

Validation of Doppler Echo Prosthetic Mean Valve Gradients Compared with Invasive Data (Selected Series)

First Author/ Year	Valve Type/Position	*n*	*r*	SEE (mm Hg)	Mean Difference
Sagar/1986	Hancock & B.S./mitral	19	0.93	2.5	
Sagar/1986	Hancock & B.S./aortic	11	0.94	7.4	
Wilkins/1986	Starr-Edwards, B.S./ porcine/mitral	11	0.96	–	
Burstow/1989	Mixed/aortic	20	0.94	3	
	Mixed/mitral	20	0.97	1.2	
Baumgartner/1990	St. Jude	In vitro	0.98	1.9	10 ± 3 mm Hg
	Hancock	In vitro	0.98	1.4	2 ± 1 mm Hg
Stewart/1991	Bioprosthetic/aortic	In vitro	0.78–0.98		Overestimation by Doppler
Baumgartner/1992	St. Jude	In vitro	0.98	2.0	13 ± 8 mm Hg
	Medtronic-Hull	In vitro	0.99	0.5	0.8 ± 0.6
	Starr-Edwards	In vitro	0.97	2.0	8 ± 4 mm Hg
	Hancock	In vitro	0.99	1.5	1.9 ± 1.6

B.S., Bjork-Shiley tilting-disk mechanical valve.
References as in Suggested Reading and Sager KB, et al: J Am Coll Cardiol 7:681–687, 1986.

Bi-leaflet Mechanical Valve

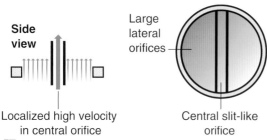

Side view

Large lateral orifices

Localized high velocity in central orifice

Central slit-like orifice

■ **FIGURE 13–12.** Schematic drawing of a bileaflet mechanical valve in the open position in side (*left*) and frontal (*right*) views. Two large lateral orifices flank a central slitlike orifice that is associated with localized high-velocity flow (and a localized pressure gradient).

result in a localized high-pressure gradient (and corresponding high velocity) with rapid pressure recovery distal to the valve. Therefore, the pressure difference measured between the upstream side of the valve and this central orifice is greater than the pressure difference between the upstream and downstream sides of the valve. Because continuous-wave Doppler ultrasound records the highest velocity along the length of the ultrasound beam, it is this higher localized velocity that is recorded. While this high localized gradient is measured correctly, the gradient of interest is the upstream-to-downstream valve gradient. This explains the observation that even though the correlation between Doppler and invasive pressure gradient measurements is high, the slope of the regression line indicates that the Doppler approach consistently "overestimates" the overall transvalvular gradient. This overestimation is large enough that an erroneous diagnosis of severe stenosis might be made if the phenomenon of pressure recovery is not recognized.

Interestingly, the overestimation of pressure gradients across bileaflet valves becomes less significant in the presence of prosthetic valve stenosis. The proposed mechanism for this observation is a gradual reduction in the size of the central orifice as leaflet opening is reduced. Clinically, this poses a dilemma in that a high velocity across a bileaflet valve might represent overestimation of the pressure gradient with normal valve function or a correct estimate of a high gradient with a stenotic valve. Again, a baseline study in the postoperative period provides a standard of comparison when subsequent valve dysfunction is suspected.

Valve Areas. Even when accurately measured, the physiologic limitation of transvalvular velocities across prosthetic valves is that velocities vary with volume flow rate for a given orifice area.

A normally functioning valve prosthesis in an individual patient may have

■ a high transvalvular velocity if cardiac output is elevated (e.g., with exercise, anemia, fever), or

■ a low transvalvular velocity if cardiac output is depressed (e.g., left ventricular dysfunction).

For these reasons, a flow-independent measure of prosthetic valve function is more useful clinically.

Aortic. Bioprosthetic aortic valves have fluid dynamics similar to those of a native aortic valve, and it is logical to assume that continuity equation valve area calculations are valid in this situation (Fig. 13–13). In fact, direct comparisons of Doppler echo (AVA_{prost}) and invasive valve areas in patients with suspected stenosis of bioprosthetic aortic valves have shown a reasonable correlation. As for a native aortic valve, the components of the continuity equation are the left ventricular outflow tract velocity-time integral (VTI_{LVOT}), the left ventricular outflow tract cross-sectional area (CSA_{LVOT}), and the aortic jet velocity-time integral (VTI_{Ao}). The continuity equation, then, is

$$AVA_{prost} = (CSA_{LVOT} \times VTI_{LVOT})/VTI_{Ao}$$

Left ventricular outflow tract velocity is recorded from an apical approach using pulsed Doppler echo with the sample volume positioned proximal to the prosthetic valve, avoiding the small region of flow acceleration immediately adjacent to the valve. Aortic jet velocity is recorded with continuous-wave Doppler from whichever window gives the highest-velocity signal, as for native valve stenosis. Left ventricular outflow tract diameter is measured in a parasternal long-axis view in mid-systole from the septal endocardium to the anterior mitral leaflet parallel to and immediately adjacent to the aortic valve (Fig. 13–14). Direct measurement of outflow tract diameter is preferable to use of the implanted prosthetic valve size, since valve size relates to the external diameter of the sewing ring, not the effective diameter of the subvalvular flow region. As usual, a circular cross-sectional left ventricular outflow tract area is calculated as $\pi(D/2)^2$ from this diameter measurement.

The use of the continuity equation for mechanical aortic valves is more problematic. Presumably, if the transvalvular velocity-time integral is an accurate reflection of transvalvular volume flow rate, then calculated valve areas should be accurate. Remember that the continuity equation assumes a flat flow velocity profile *in* the stenotic orifice (or vena contracta), as well as proximal to the valve. Clearly, this assumption is not true for bileaflet valves. The local high velocities in the

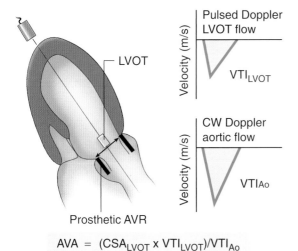

$$AVA = (CSA_{LVOT} \times VTI_{LVOT})/VTI_{Ao}$$

▌ FIGURE 13–13. The continuity equation can be used for calculation of aortic valve area (AVA) for an aortic valve replacement (AVR). Left ventricular outflow tract (LVOT) flow is recorded from an apical approach using pulsed Doppler with the sample volume positioned just proximal to the prosthetic valve. LVOT diameter is measured from a parasternal long-axis view for calculation of a circular cross-sectional area (CSA) of flow. Continuous-wave (CW) Doppler is used to record the flow signal across the prosthetic valve from whichever window yields the highest-velocity jet.

central orifice will result in a significant error in measurement of volume flow rate across the valve orifice, with a consequent underestimation of valve area. However, for tilting-disk and ball-cage valves, limited data suggest that the continuity equation may be reasonably accurate, despite complex fluid dynamics, because the continuous-wave velocity signal provides an approximation of the spatial mean flow velocity across the valve (Table 13–6).

Another approach to evaluation of suspected prosthetic aortic valve stenosis is to measure the "step-up" in velocity across the valve. The ratio of the outflow tract velocity to aortic jet velocity reflects the degree of stenosis—if no obstruction is present, these velocities will be nearly equal with a ratio close to 1; as the degree of narrowing increases, the aortic jet velocity will increase with no change in outflow tract velocity resulting progressively in a ratio of <1. Since all prosthetic valves are inherently stenotic to some degree, the "normal" velocity ratio across an aortic prosthesis ranges from 0.35 to 0.50, compared with 0.75 to 0.90 for a normal native aortic valve.

The velocity ratio has several advantages because

■ it takes volume flow rate into account,
■ it does not require an outflow tract diameter measurement,
■ it is easily measured and reproducible, and

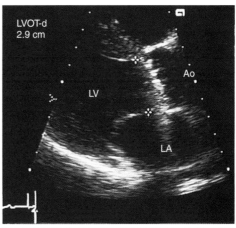

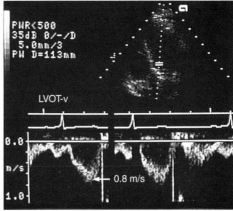

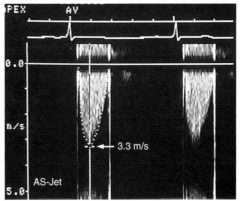

▌ FIGURE 13–14. Continuity equation prosthetic valve area is calculated from a parasternal long-axis midsystolic diameter (2.9 cm) measurement (*above*), the pulsed Doppler left ventricular outflow tract velocity (0.8 m/s) recorded from an apical approach (*center*), and the continuous-wave Doppler signal of flow across the valve (3.3 m/s) recorded from whichever window gives the highest velocity (*below*). Even though the antegrade velocity is increased compared with a native valve, the calculated valve area is 1.6 cm².

■ a baseline "normal" value can be established for comparison on follow-up studies.

Some investigators advocate measuring the velocity ratio with increases in flow rate (e.g., with

TABLE 13–6

Validation of Doppler Echo Prosthetic Valve Areas (Selected Series)

First Author/ Year	Valve Type/ Position	n	Comparison	r	SEE	Mean Difference
Sagar/1986	Hancock and B.S./ mitral	12	$T_{1/2}$ vs. Gorlin	0.98	0.1 cm^2	
Wilkins/1986	Porcine/mitral	8	$T_{1/2}$ vs. Gorlin	0.65	–	–
Rothbart/1990	Bioprosthetic/aortic	22	Cont eq vs. Gorlin at cath	0.93	–	–
Chafizadeh/ 1991	St. Jude/aortic	67	Cont eq vs. actual orifice area	0.83		Doppler effective orifice area less than actual orifice area
Baumgartner/ 1992	St. Jude	In vitro	Cont eq vs. Gorlin	0.99	0.08	0.4–0.6 cm^2
	Medtronic-Hall	In vitro		0.97	0.10	0–0.25 cm^2
	Hancock aortic	In vitro		0.93	0.10	0–0.25 cm^2

B.S., Bjork-Shiley tilting-disk mechanical valve; Cont eq, continuity equation valve area with Doppler and 2D echo data; Gorlin, Gorlin formula valve area using invasive data; $T_{1/2}$, Doppler pressure half-time method.
References as in Suggested Reading and Sager KB, et al: J Am Coll Cardiol 7:681–687, 1986.

exercise) to increase its specificity in excluding prosthetic valve stenosis.

Pragmatically, even if Doppler velocities and continuity equation valve areas overestimate the degree of prosthetic valve stenosis, in an individual patient a *change* in velocity or valve area is valuable in patient management decisions.

MITRAL. Prosthetic mitral valve areas can be estimated using the pressure half-time approach as for native mitral valve stenosis. The expected normal half-time for a prosthetic valve is longer than for a native valve, with the specific value depending on valve type and size. For bioprosthetic mitral valves, valve area can be estimated from the same formula as for native valves:

$$MVA = 220/T_{1/2}$$

where the pressure half-time ($T_{1/2}$) is measured in milliseconds, as described in Chapter 11.

Somewhat surprisingly, the empirical constant 220 also appears to provide a reasonable approximation of mitral valve area for mechanical prostheses. With a bileaflet valve, the higher localized velocities in the central slitlike orifice affect the accuracy of pressure gradient calculations. However, the pressure half-time measurement is less affected because it depends on the *time course* of the velocity decline relative to the maximum velocity rather than on the velocities themselves.

Continuity equation valve area also can be calculated for a mitral prosthesis (in the absence of mitral regurgitation) using the antegrade stroke volume across the aortic or pulmonic valve in the equation.

The antegrade velocity curve across a mitral bioprosthesis may be recorded from an apical approach using pulsed, high pulse-repetition frequency, or continuous-wave Doppler ultrasound. Care in positioning the transducer is needed because inflow may be directed obliquely into the ventricular chamber. Some echocardiographers find it helpful to use the color flow image to aid in alignment of the Doppler beam parallel to the inflow stream. In many patients after mitral valve replacement, the inflow stream is directed anteriorly and medially toward the ventricular septum. In these patients, a low parasternal window may provide an optimal intercept angle for recording antegrade velocity. As for native mitral valve stenosis, Doppler acquisition parameters are adjusted to show a smooth velocity deceleration slope and a band of velocity signals along the edge of the curve.

Prosthetic Valve Regurgitation

DETECTION OF REGURGITATION. The echocardiographic approaches described for evaluation of native valve regurgitation in Chapter 12 also apply to evaluation of prosthetic valve regurgitation. The major differences between evaluation of native or prosthetic valves are

■ the prosthetic valve has a higher antegrade velocity,
■ the degree of normal prosthetic regurgitation is greater than the trivial amounts of native

valve regurgitation seen in normal individuals, and

■ acoustic shadowing, reverberations, and beam width artifact make evaluation of a prosthetic valve more difficult.

These differences decrease the sensitivity of transthoracic echocardiography for detection of prosthetic regurgitation so that transesophageal imaging is needed more frequently.

Transthoracic color Doppler flow imaging for detection of prosthetic valve regurgitation can be helpful, particularly if a view can be obtained where the ultrasound beam has access to the chamber receiving the regurgitant flow without first traversing the valve prosthetic. For the aortic valve, both parasternal and apical views are helpful because the ultrasound signal reaches the left ventricular outflow tract region without intercepting the valve prosthesis, avoiding the problem of acoustic shadowing (Fig. 13–15). For the mitral valve, the parasternal approach may be helpful if a view can be obtained where the left atrial side of the valve is not shadowed by the valve prosthesis. Apical views often are limited due to acoustic shadowing, but occasionally, a paraprosthetic jet can be identified from this approach. In addition to acoustic shadowing, color artifacts are prominent in patients with prosthetic valves, which may obscure detection of abnormal flow signals.

Continuous-wave Doppler also is helpful for detection of prosthetic regurgitation with the advantage of a wide beam size at the depth of a prosthetic valve and a high signal-to-noise ratio, enhancing the likelihood that a weaker signal or eccentric jet (i.e., paraprosthetic regurgitation) will be identified. The timing of the presumed regurgitant signal is extremely important for correct identification of the origin of the Doppler signal. Many laboratories find it helpful to examine the prosthetic valve with continuous-wave Doppler starting with the ultrasound beam aligned in the flow direction of the valve and then slowly scanning in progressively larger circles to identify any potential paraprosthetic jets (Fig. 13–16).

Due to the problems of acoustic shadowing and reverberations, even the most carefully performed transthoracic examinations have a low sensitivity for detection and quantitation of prosthetic regurgitation. Especially for the mitral position, the transesophageal approach provides both improved image quality and the opportunity to interrogate the valve from the left atrial side–that is, the acoustic shadow now will obscure the left ventricle rather than the left atrium. Thus, when prosthetic mitral valve regurgitation is suspected, a transesophageal study should be considered (Fig. 13–17). A transthoracic study showing prosthetic regurgitation can be clinically useful (high positive predictive value) but rarely allows for accurate quantitation of mitral regurgitant severity. A transthoracic study that does not show prosthetic regurgitation does not exclude this possibility (low negative predictive value).

SEVERITY AND ETIOLOGY OF PROSTHETIC REGURGITATION. When prosthetic regurgitation is detected, the first step in evaluation and inter-

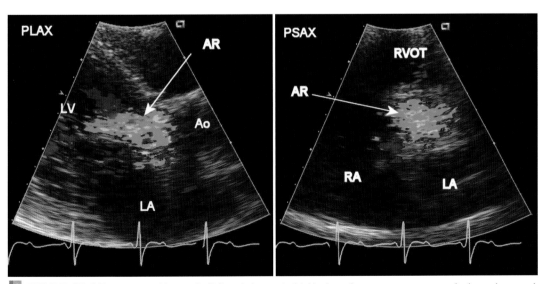

FIGURE 13–15. Parasternal long-axis (*left*) and short-axis (*right*) views demonstrate severe prosthetic aortic regurgitation. Transthoracic imaging is diagnostic because the prosthesis does not shadow the outflow tract from this window.

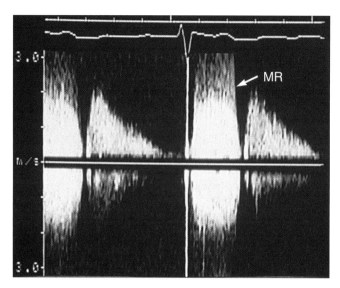

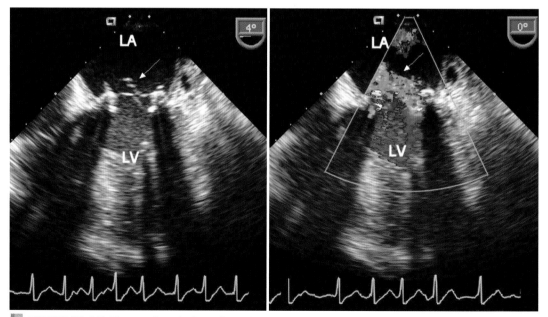

FIGURE 13–16. Continuous-wave Doppler recording of prosthetic mitral regurgitation obtained from an apical window. The regurgitant signal starts immediately after the mitral closure click and continues up to the onset of antegrade flow across the prosthesis in diastole. The jet is eccentric and not parallel with the ultrasound beam, so flow signals appear as both sides of the baseline.

pretation is whether "normal" or pathologic prosthetic regurgitation is present. While the normal backflow across the valve represents a small volume of blood, the color jets on transesophageal imaging can be fairly large in area. Distinguishing features are the characteristic pattern for each valve type, a uniform color pattern rather than the mosaic flow disturbance seen with pathologic regurgitation, and the absence of other features (increased antegrade velocity, chamber sizes and function, pulmonary hypertension) to suggest significant regurgitation.

Pathologic regurgitation of bioprosthetic valves most often is due to degenerative changes of the leaflets. This can be slowly progressive, with gradually increasing severity of a central regurgitant stream, or can occur abruptly, with cusp rupture adjacent to a fibrocalcific nodule. Mechanical valves can have prosthetic regurgitation due to incomplete closure resulting from pannus ingrowth around the sewing ring or from thrombus formation (Fig. 13–18).

Paraprosthetic regurgitation is most common with mechanical valves but also can occur with

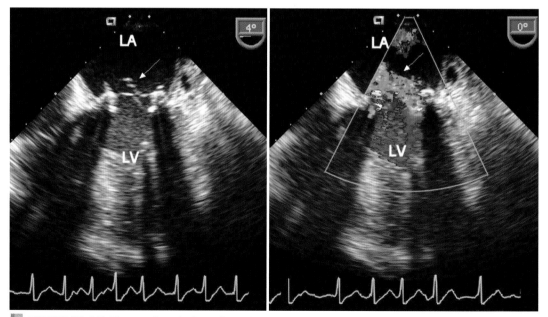

FIGURE 13–17. Transesophageal echocardiography showing a stented tissue mitral valve prosthesis with a flail leaflet (*arrow*), due to endocarditis, on 2D imaging (*left*). Color flow shows an eccentric jet of regurgitation through the valve with a wide vena contracta consistent with severe prosthetic regurgitation (*right*).

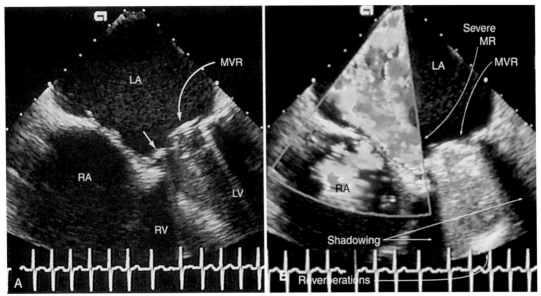

■ **FIGURE 13–18.** Transesophageal view of a patient with suspected prosthetic mitral regurgitation. The 2D images (*left*) showed an area of abnormal motion on real time imaging at the medial aspect of the sewing ring (*small arrow*) and color flow imaging (*right*) documented severe paraprosthetic mitral regurgitation with a large color flow jet filling the entire enlarged left atrium and with systolic flow reversal in the pulmonary veins. MVR, mitral valve replacement. (From Otto CM: Prosthetic valves. In: Otto CM (ed): Valvular Heart Disease, 2nd ed. Philadelphia: WB Saunders, 2004, p 461.)

bioprosthetic valves. Distinguishing prosthetic from paraprosthetic regurgitation is difficult on transthoracic imaging; in most cases, transesophageal echocardiography is needed. The etiology of paraprosthetic regurgitation may be a scarred and/or calcified annulus resulting in disruption of the sutures securing the valve or a paravalvular abscess with tissue destruction (Fig. 13–19). The regurgitant jet originates external to the sewing ring, with an eccentric jet extending into the receiving chamber. A single or multiple paraprosthetic jets may be present. Color flow imaging may show proximal flow acceleration (on the left ventricular side of the mitral valve) into the regurgitant orifice, facilitating identification of the paraprosthetic origin of the signal. Immediately after implantation, a small degree of paraprosthetic regurgitation may be normal on intraoperative transesophageal echocardiography and usually does not have long-term adverse clinical consequences.

Evaluation of the severity of prosthetic regurgitation is more challenging than for a native valve, and transesophageal imaging usually is needed. However, the following approaches remain useful:

■ The shape, origin, and orientation of the regurgitant jet

■ Vena contracta diameter (if visualized)
■ The intensity and shape of the continuous-wave Doppler signal (Fig. 13–20)
■ Evidence for distal flow reversals (e.g., descending aorta diastolic flow in aortic regurgitation) (Fig. 13–21)
■ The antegrade velocity across the prosthetic valve

Calculation of regurgitant volume and orifice area is more difficult because calculation of antegrade flow rates across a prosthetic valve is a problem and jets are usually eccentric, limiting the proximal isovelocity surface area (PISA) approach. However, clinical decision making usually is based on the presence of pathologic prosthetic regurgitation and its clinical consequences (hemolysis, heart failure, etc.), rather than on exact measures of severity.

Other Echocardiographic Findings

In addition to direct imaging or Doppler interrogation of the prosthetic valve, several other findings on the echocardiographic examination are integrated in the overall interpretation of prosthetic valve function:

■ Left ventricular size, hypertrophy, and systolic function

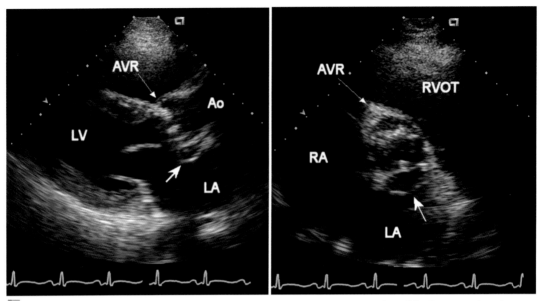

■ **FIGURE 13-19.** On transthoracic imaging in a patient with prosthetic valve endocarditis, the cause of aortic regurgitation is evident with an echolucent space (*arrows*) seen posterior to the tissue aortic valve prosthesis in both long-axis (*left*) and short-axis views (*right*). AVR, aortic valve replacement.

■ The antegrade velocity across the prosthetic valve
■ Pulmonary artery pressures

For example, persistent left ventricular hypertrophy after aortic valve replacement for aortic stenosis raises the possibility of prosthetic valve stenosis. In other cases, left ventricular dilation may suggest aortic or mitral prosthetic regurgitation with resultant volume overload. A hyperdynamic (but previously normal) left ventricle may indicate prosthetic mitral regurgitation. While it

may be difficult in some patients to separate persistent postoperative abnormalities from new pathologic findings, a change between examinations is of concern.

An increase in antegrade velocity may be due to increased volume flow because of prosthetic regurgitation rather than prosthetic stenosis. In this case, while the calculated gradient will be higher, the valve area will be unchanged. Alternatively, an increased flow velocity across the prosthetic valve may be due to a high cardiac output state (such as fever, anemia, or anxiety). In

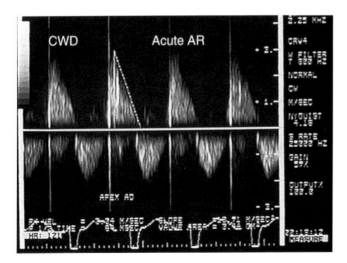

■ **FIGURE 13-20.** Continuous-wave Doppler (CWD) in a patient with prosthetic aortic regurgitation shows an aortic regurgitant signal of equal intensity to antegrade flow with a steep deceleration slope consistent with acute, severe aortic regurgitation (AR).

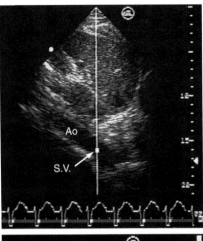

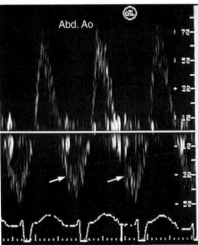

█ FIGURE 13–21. With a pulsed Doppler sample volume (SV) in the proximal abdominal aorta (*top*) in the same patient as in Figure 13–20, prominent holodiastolic (*arrow*) flow reversal (*bottom*) is seen, again consistent with severe aortic regurgitation.

this situation, antegrade velocities across the other cardiac valves will be increased proportionately.

Although pulmonary hypertension can persist after successful mitral valve surgery, *recurrent* pulmonary hypertension (after an initial postoperative decline) may relate to prosthetic valve dysfunction.

An incidental finding in some patients with a prosthetic valve is the phenomenon of *spontaneous contrast*. This phenomenon is similar to the spontaneous left atrial contrast seen in patients with an enlarged left atrium and low-velocity flow, which has been reported to be associated with a high propensity for thrombus formation. With a prosthetic valve, the appearance of echogenic particles downstream from the valve can occur even in the absence of a low flow state. The presumed mech-

anism of spontaneous contrast with a prosthetic valve is microcavitation due to impact of the occluder against the sewing ring and this phenomenon is more common with mechanical valves.

LIMITATIONS AND ALTERNATE APPROACHES

As repeatedly emphasized in this chapter, the major limitation of transthoracic echocardiography for evaluation of prosthetic valves is technical, specifically reverberations, artifacts, and acoustic shadowing. The last of these problems can be circumvented to some extent with the transesophageal approach by casting the shadow in the opposite direction. Reverberations and other ultrasound artifacts remain a problem with both approaches.

Other limitations are overestimation of transvalvular pressure gradients with bileaflet mechanical valves, limited validation of valve area calculations for mechanical valves, and the problem of differentiating "normal" from pathologic prosthetic valve regurgitation.

Importantly, the same factors that can lead to errors in evaluation of native valves also are significant limitations in evaluation of prosthetic valves. Most notably, these factors include ultrasound tissue penetration, Doppler intercept-angle assumptions, accurate diameter measurement, correct image orientation, and correct identification of the origin of Doppler signals.

When the echocardiographic examination is negative or yields results discordant with other clinical findings, other diagnostic procedures may be indicated. Cardiac catheterization can be performed with direct measurement of intracardiac pressures to confirm the pressure gradient across the valve and measure pulmonary artery pressures. In combination with cardiac output measurement, Gorlin formula valve area and pulmonary vascular resistance can be calculated. For some mechanical valves, catheterization may be complicated by a risk of inducing valve dysfunction if a catheter is passed retrograde across the valve. In these cases, evaluation of a mechanical aortic valve requires transseptal catheterization with measurement of left ventricular pressures by advancing the catheter across the mitral valve into the left ventricle. With a mitral valve prosthesis, transseptal catheterization is more reliable than the pulmonary wedge pressure in evaluating the left atrial to left ventricular pressure gradient.

Angiographic evaluation (left ventricle for mitral regurgitation, aortic root for aortic regurgitation) is helpful in evaluating prosthetic regurgitation on a semiquantitative (0 to 4+) scale or for calculating regurgitant volumes and fractions in conjunction with other quantitative cardiac output data.

Fluoroscopy of the valve is important for some valve types. For bileaflet and single-disk mechanical valves, the angle of opening can be measured from a view oriented perpendicular to the plane of the open leaflet(s). In a small number of now discontinued valve models, the occluder undergoes degeneration, resulting in a decrease in size that can be detected by fluoroscopic measurements. None of the valves prone to this type of wear (and subsequent leaflet escape) are currently implanted, and there are few patients with these prostheses still in place.

Neither magnetic resonance imaging nor computed tomographic imaging has proved particularly helpful in evaluation of prosthetic valves. Newer approaches to imaging regurgitant jets with these techniques may yield useful data in the future.

CLINICAL UTILITY

Prosthetic Valve Stenosis

Echocardiography is the initial diagnostic approach to evaluation of suspected prosthetic valve stenosis. The antegrade velocity and mean gradient across the prosthetic valve, particularly in comparison with previous data in that patient, may be diagnostic. Valve area can be calculated by the continuity equation for valves in the aortic (Fig. 13–22) or pulmonic position and by the pressure half-time method for valves in the mitral or tricuspid (Fig. 13–23) position. Despite the overestimation of the average transvalvular gradient that occurs with Doppler evaluation of bileaflet mechanical valves, this approach still is helpful in assessing changes over time in an individual patient.

The differential diagnosis of an increased antegrade velocity across the valve includes a high cardiac output state or coexisting valvular regurgitation, as well as prosthetic valve stenosis. A significant prosthetic or paraprosthetic regurgitant jet can increase the antegrade volume flow rate across the valve substantially, resulting in a high velocity and a high transvalvular gradient. Valve area, however, remains relatively normal.

With careful examination techniques, the antegrade velocity across the prosthetic valve can be recorded in nearly all patients. When signal strength is suboptimal, invasive evaluation may be required. This is most likely for evaluation of a prosthetic valve in a conduit (typically right ven-

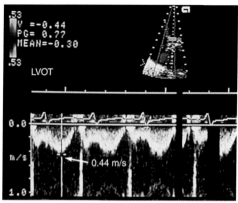

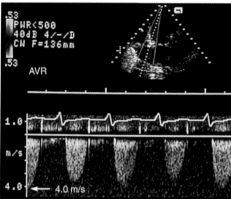

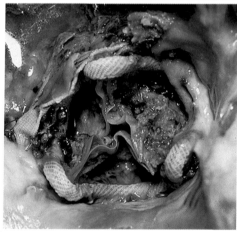

■ **FIGURE 13–22.** A 46-year-old man with chronic renal failure and a porcine valve replacement 8 years ago presented with presyncope. Echocardiography showed severely reduced left ventricular systolic function, a left ventricular outflow tract velocity of only 0.4 m/s (*top*), and an aortic jet of 4 m/s (*middle*). Continuity equation valve area was 0.5 cm². At autopsy, the porcine valve leaflets were severely calcified and stiff (*bottom*).

tricle or right atrium to pulmonary artery). In this situation, the valve is difficult to image due to shadowing by the vascular graft, and it is difficult to obtain a window where the Doppler beam is parallel to flow across the prosthetic valve.

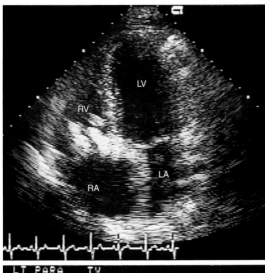

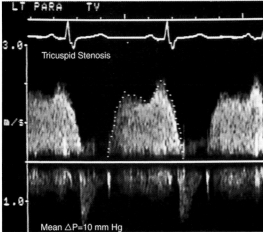

FIGURE 13–23. A 36-year-old man with a previous tricuspid valve replacement for endocarditis presented with right-sided heart failure. The apical four-chamber view showed a severely calcified porcine tricuspid valve replacement (*top*) with an increased antegrade velocity and prolonged pressure half-time (*bottom*).

Prosthetic Valve Regurgitation

Transthoracic echocardiography is accurate for the diagnosis of aortic prosthetic valve regurgitation and for the differentiation of normal from pathologic regurgitation (Fig. 13–24). However, because of acoustic shadowing, the sensitivity for detection of mitral prosthetic regurgitation is lower, and it is more difficult to distinguish normal from pathologic regurgitation. Transesophageal echocardiography imaging is needed when this diagnosis is suspected on clinical grounds. Transesophageal echocardiography has a high accuracy for detection of prosthetic regurgitation and reliably distinguishes transprosthetic from paraprosthetic regurgitation.

Prosthetic Valve Endocarditis

Detection of valvular vegetations on prosthetic valves is difficult with transthoracic echocardiography due to reverberations and acoustic shadowing (Figs. 13–25 and 13–26). Features that might increase the suspicion of prosthetic valve endocarditis on a transthoracic echocardiographic examination include Doppler evidence of valve dysfunction (either regurgitation due to incomplete closure or stenosis due to an infected pannus on the inflow surface of the valve), evidence of valve instability (i.e., "rocking"), an unexplained increase in pulmonary artery pressures, or an interval change in chamber dimensions. Prosthetic valve endocarditis often involves the sewing ring

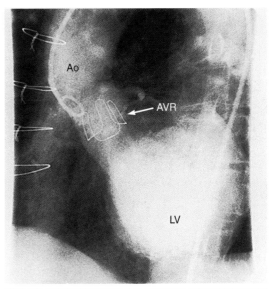

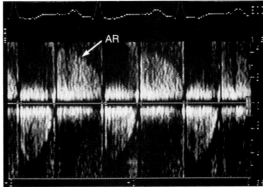

FIGURE 13–24. A 60-year-old man with a previous porcine aortic valve replacement presented with congestive heart failure. Angiography (*top*) showed severe prosthetic aortic regurgitation (the left ventricle is densely opacified with an aortic root contrast injection). Echocardiography was technically limited due to poor ultrasound tissue penetration, but the continuous-wave Doppler signal (*bottom*) is diagnostic for significant aortic regurgitation.

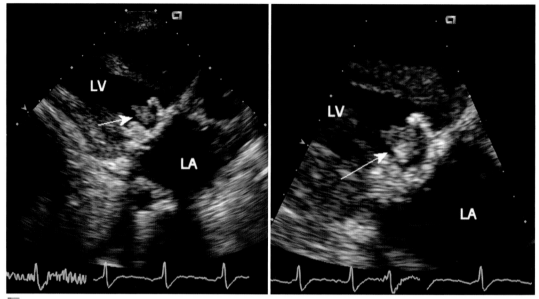

I FIGURE 13-25. Although transthoracic images often are nondiagnostic for prosthetic valve endocarditis, the large valvular vegetation on the stented tissue mitral prosthesis in this patient is obvious (*arrow*) in a low parasternal long-axis view. In the image on the right, the depth has been decreased to improve image resolution showing the vegetation within the struts of the prosthetic valve.

and annulus, resulting in formation of a paravalvular abscess ("ring" abscess) rather than the typical vegetation seen with native valve infection. Identification of an abscess may be limited on transthoracic echocardiography.

Thus, given the technical and pathologic peculiarities of evaluation of suspected prosthetic valve endocarditis, transesophageal imaging is needed in the majority of these patients. Transesophageal echocardiography has a high sensitivity for detec-

tion of prosthetic valve endocarditis and/or abscess formation. As for native valve endocarditis (see Chapter 14), cardiac abscesses may be echodense or relatively echo-free. Persistent infection also may result in an aneurysm instead of an abscess cavity (Fig. 13-27).

Prosthetic Valve Thrombosis

In patients with embolic events presumed secondary to prosthetic valve thrombosis, even

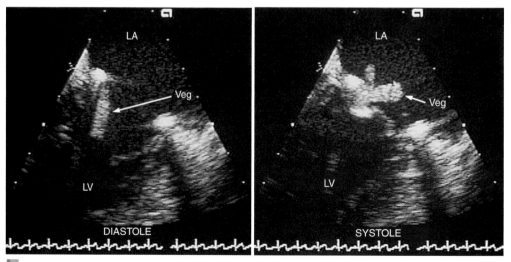

I FIGURE 13-26. Prosthetic valve endocarditis of a mitral porcine valve seen on transesophageal imaging with a large vegetation prolapsing into the left ventricle in diastole (*left*) and into the left atrium in systole (*right*).

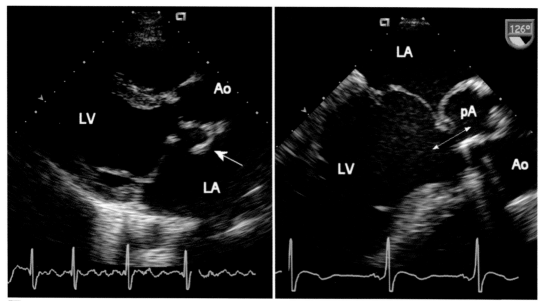

FIGURE 13–27. Aneurysm of the mitral aortic intravalvular fibrosa in a 28-year-old man with a mechanical aortic valve replacement. The transthoracic long-axis image (*left*) shows the pseudoaneurysm between the posterior aspect of the aortic prosthesis and the base of the anterior mitral leaflet (*arrow*). The corresponding transesophageal image (*right*) shows the narrow neck of the pseudoaneurysm (*double arrow*). Doppler color flow imaging showed flow into the pseudoaneurysm from the left ventricle in systole (with flow back into the left ventricle), and associated collapse of the pseudoaneurysm in diastole.

transesophageal echocardiographic results may be negative if the thrombi are small or if new thrombus has not formed since the embolic event. When thrombi are documented on transesophageal echocardiography, this finding may be important in patient management in some cases. However, an embolic event in a patient with a prosthetic valve (especially mechanical) presumably is related to the presence of a prosthetic valve even if transesophageal echocardiography is negative. Thus, the potential clinical implications of the study results should be considered *before* the examination. If the treatment and subsequent management would be the same whether or not a thrombus is documented, then transesophageal echocardiography may be unnecessary. If documentation of thrombus or exclusion of other possible abnormalities would affect patient management, then transesophageal echocardiography examination is appropriate. Of course, infected pannus due to prosthetic valve endocarditis cannot be differentiated from thrombus on ultrasound imaging. Careful clinical and bacteriologic correlation is needed whenever an abnormal valve-associated mass is observed (Fig. 13–28).

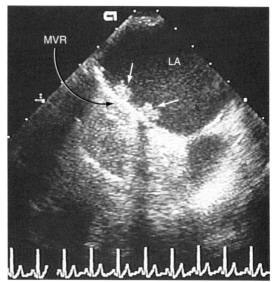

FIGURE 13–28. Transesophageal echocardiographic image showing pannus or thrombus formation (*arrows*) on the left atrial side of a St. Jude mechanical valve replacement. (From Otto CM: Prosthetic valves. In: Otto CM (ed):Valvular Heart Disease, 2nd ed. Philadelphia: WB Saunders, 2004, p 460.)

"Routine" Follow-up of Prosthetic Valve Function

While it is difficult to justify routine periodic echocardiographic examinations of prosthetic valve function in clinically stable patients, the importance of a baseline examination in each patient with a prosthetic valve should not be overlooked. There is wide variability in normal antegrade velocities and in the degree of "normal" regurgitation across prosthetic valves even for a given size, type, and position. Establishing baseline Doppler findings in each patient soon after implantation serves as a reference point in case prosthetic valve dysfunction is suspected in the future. Approximately 6 to 8 weeks after surgery is a reasonable time to obtain this baseline study because the patient has recovered from surgery, is returning to cardiology follow-up, and has stable hemodynamic status with a normal cardiac output. This timing of the examination also allows an initial evaluation of regression of left ventricular hypertrophy or dilation, recovery of left ventricular systolic function, changes in pulmonary artery pressures, and other long-term effects of the valve surgery.

SUGGESTED READING

General Reviews

1. Zabalgoitia M: Echocardiographic recognition and quantitation of prosthetic valve dysfunction. In: Otto CM (ed): The Practice of Clinical Echocardiography. Philadelphia: WB Saunders, 2002, pp 525–550.

   Advanced level review and discussion of echocardiographic evaluation of prosthetic valve dysfunction. Numerous tables summarize normal values for prosthetic valves and findings reported with abnormal valve function. Excellent photographs and echocardiographic images of each valve type. Complications reviewed include mechanical failure, thrombosis, endocarditis, patient-prosthesis mismatch, prosthetic stenosis, and regurgitation.

2. Vongpatanasin W, Hillis LD, Lange RA: Prosthetic heart valves. N Engl J Med 335:407–416, 1996.

   Concise review of the clinical aspects of prosthetic valve function and dysfunction. Excellent description and chart of the normal and abnormal auscultatory findings for each valve type.

3. Zoghbi WA: Echocardiographic recognition of unusual complications after surgery on the great vessels and cardiac valves. In: Otto CM (ed): The Practice of Clinical Echocardiography. Philadelphia: WB Saunders, 2002, pp 551–570.

   Discussion and examples of prosthetic valve complications including aortic pseudoaneurysms, left ventricular pseudoaneurysm, aneurysm of the mitral-aortic intravalvular fibrosa, and intracardiac fistula after valve surgery.

4. Otto CM: Prosthetic valves. In: Otto CM (ed): Valvular Heart Disease. Philadelphia: WB Saunders, 2004.

   Clinical review of prosthetic heart valves with sections on hemodynamics and long-term outcome for each valve type, medical management of patients with prosthetic valves, and evaluation and treatment of prosthetic valve dysfunction. Over 300 references.

Normal Doppler Flow Patterns

5. Yoganathan AP, Travis BR: Fluid dynamics of prosthetic valves. In: Otto CM (ed): The Practice of Clinical Echocardiography. Philadelphia: WB Saunders, 2002, pp 501–524.

   Review of the basic principles of fluid dynamics and the application of fluid dynamics to evaluation of prosthetic heart valves. Extensive tables summarize in vitro data for each valve type and size. Illustrations show the flow patterns for each valve type. Mathematical descriptions of fluid dynamics are included.

6. Reisner SA, Meltzer RS: Normal values of prosthetic valve Doppler echocardiographic parameters: A review. J Am Soc Echocardiogr 1:201–210, 1988.

   Summary of normal Doppler velocities across prosthetic valves, including data from 18 studies with a total of 1105 patients; 32 references.

7. Palka P, Harrocks S, Lange A , Burstow DJ, O'Brien MF: Primary aortic valve replacement with cryopreserved aortic allograft: an echocardiographic follow-up study of 570 patients. Circulation 105:61–66, 2002.

   Echocardiography was performed a mean of 6.8 years after aortic homograft valve replacement. Significant aortic regurgitation was present in 15% and aortic stenosis was present in 3%. The root replacement technique of homograft insertion was associated with the best long term hemodynamics.

8. Savoye C, Auffray JL, Hubert E, et al: Echocardiographic follow-up after Ross procedure in 100 patients. Am J Cardiol 85:854–857, 2000.

   Perioperative mortality for the Ross procedure in 105 patients (mean age 29 years) was 4.7%. Echocardiography at a mean interval of 2.8 years after pulmonic autograft replacement of the aortic valve showed low peak gradients (5.5 ± 3.5 mm Hg). There were no cases of more than mild aortic regurgitation but in 10% of patients, aortic sinus dimension increased by ≥20%.

Validation of Doppler Echo Pressure Gradients

9. Baumgartner H, Khan S, DeRobertis M, et al: Discrepancies between Doppler and catheter gradients in aortic prosthetic valves in vitro. A manifestation of localized gradients and pressure recovery. Circulation 82:1467–1475, 1990.

   In vitro study emphasizing the importance of pressure recovery downstream from the valve as a cause of discrepancies between Doppler and invasive pressure gradient measurements, with an overestimation of 13% ± 11% for mean gradients across the Hancock bioprosthetic valve. High localized gradients in the narrow central orifice at the valve plane of the St. Jude (bileaflet) valve were measured accurately by Doppler echo. However, this localized gradient was greater than the gradient measured 30 mm downstream from the valve.

10. Wilkins GT, Gillam LD, Kritzer GL, et al: Validation of continuous-wave Doppler echocardiographic measure-

ments of mitral and tricuspid prosthetic valve gradients: A simultaneous Doppler-catheter study. Circulation 74:786–795, 1986.

Simultaneous Doppler and catheter pressure gradients were measured across prosthetic mitral valves in 12 patients, showing an excellent correlation for both porcine and mechanical valves.

11. Burstow DJ, Nishimura RA, Bailey KR, et al: Continuous wave Doppler echocardiographic measurement of prosthetic valve gradients. A simultaneous Doppler-catheter correlative study. Circulation 80:504–514, 1989.

Simultaneous Doppler and catheter pressure gradients were measured in 36 patients. Correlations for maximum and mean pressure gradients were excellent for both aortic and mitral prostheses and for bioprosthetic and mechanical valves.

12. Stewart SFC, Nast EP, Arabia FA, et al: Errors in pressure gradient measurement by continuous-wave Doppler ultrasound: Type, size and age effects in bioprosthetic aortic valves. J Am Coll Cardiol 18:769–779, 1991.

Consistent overestimation of pressure gradients across prosthetic valves as measured by Doppler echocardiography was observed in detailed in vitro studies of four types of bioprosthetic valves. Pressure recovery downstream did not account for this overestimation. Instead, this error may be related to neglect of proximal velocities in the Bernoulli equation. For example, a mean proximal velocity of 0.66 ± 0.02 m/s at a mean flow rate of 5.6 L/min would result in an error of 1.74 ± 0.10 mm Hg for mean gradient and 3.48 ± 0.21 mm Hg for maximum gradient. These differences are even larger at higher flow rates.

13. Baumgartner H, Khan S, DeRobertis M, et al: Effect of prosthetic aortic valve design on the Doppler-catheter gradient correlation: An in vitro study of normal St. Jude, Medtronic-Hall, Starr-Edwards and Hancock valves. J Am Coll Cardiol 19:324–332, 1992.

This in vitro study shows that smaller valve sizes have higher antegrade velocities and pressure gradients than larger valve sizes. The 19-mm St. Jude and Hancock valves can have velocities as high as 4.7 m/s with a gradient of 89 mm Hg even with normal prosthetic valve function. Doppler gradients consistently overestimated catheter gradients for St. Jude and Starr-Edwards valves (differences as great as 44 mm Hg were seen). Agreement was closer for Hancock and Medtronic-Hall valves.

Prosthetic Valve Area

14. Chafizadeh ER, Zoghbi WA: Doppler echocardiographic assessment of the St. Jude medical prosthetic valve in the aortic position using the continuity equation. Circulation 83:213–223, 1991.

In 67 patients with recent implantation (and clinically normal valve function) of St. Jude aortic valve prostheses, continuity equation valve areas (0.73 to 4.23 cm^2) correlated well with the reported actual orifice area ($r = 0.83$). The Doppler velocity index—the ratio of left ventricular outflow tract to aortic jet velocity—provides a useful simple index of valve function and is less dependent on valve size.

15. Baumgartner H, Khan SS, DeRobertis M, et al: Doppler assessment of prosthetic valve orifice area: An in vitro study. Circulation 85:2275–2283, 1992.

Continuity equation valve areas correlated well with invasively derived Gorlin formula valve areas for St. Jude, Medtronic-Hall, and Hancock aortic valves in a pulsatile flow model. However, valve area of St. Jude valves was significantly underestimated due to the localized high velocities in the narrow central orifice. Valve areas decrease with low flow in Hancock valves consistent with incomplete opening of the leaflets at low flow rates.

16. Rothbart RM, Castriz JL, Harding LV, et al: Determination of aortic valve area by two-dimensional and Doppler echocardiography in patients with normal and stenotic bioprosthetic valves. J Am Coll Cardiol 15:817–824, 1990.

In 22 patients undergoing catheterization for suspected dysfunction of bioprosthetic aortic valves, Doppler continuity equation valve areas agreed well with invasively determined Gorlin valve areas.

17. Dumesnil JG, Honos GN, Lemieux M, Beauchemin J: Validation and applications of indexed aortic prosthetic valve areas calculated by Doppler echocardiography. J Am Coll Cardiol 16:637–643, 1990.

In 31 patients with a Medtronics Intact Bioprosthesis in the aortic position, both standard and simplified continuity equation valve areas correlated well with in vivo and known in vitro prosthetic valve areas ($r = 0.86$, SEE $= 0.16$ cm^2).

18. Baumgartner H, Schima H, Kuhn P: Effect of prosthetic valve malfunction on the Doppler-catheter gradient relation for bileaflet aortic valve prostheses. Circulation 87:1320–1327, 1993.

Malfunction of bileaflet mechanical valves was simulated in a pulsatile flow model by restricting opening of one leaflet. While Doppler and catheter gradients correlated well for each degree of prosthetic valve stenosis, the slope of the regression line progressively approached 1 with increasing stenosis. Thus, while Doppler overestimates bileaflet prosthetic valve gradients with normal valve function, the Doppler gradients are accurate when stenosis is present. The mechanism of this observation most likely is a reduction in the central orifice size. Clinically, these findings suggest that the development of stenosis of a bileaflet mechanical valve may not be reflected in increases in velocity across the prosthesis.

19. Chambers JB, Cochrane T, Black MM, Jackson G: The Gorlin formula validated against directly observed orifice area in porcine mitral bioprostheses. J Am Coll Cardiol 13:348–353, 1989.

In an in vitro pulsatile flow system, measured orifice area and the modified Gorlin relation (Q/V_{max}) correlated well ($r = 0.88$). Maximum valve orifice area, measured by a high-speed video camera, decreased at low flow rates for all four Carpentier-Edwards prostheses.

Natural History of Doppler Echo Findings

20. Bach DS, Goldman B, Verrier E et al. Eight-year hemodynamic follow-up after aortic valve replacement with the Toronto SPV stentless aortic valve. Semin Thorac Cardiovasc Surg 13:173–179, 2001.

In 470 patients with stentless aortic valve replacements, a progressive decrease in left ventricular mass and increase in left ventricular outflow tract diameter and valve area were seen over 8 years of follow-up. The prevalence of more than mild aortic regurgitation was only 2.5% at 6 years and 4.5% at 8 years.

21. Banbury MK, Cosgrove DM III, Thomas JD, et al: Hemodynamic stability during 17 years of the Carpentier-Edwards aortic pericardial bioprosthesis. Ann Thorac Surg 73:1460–1465, 2002.

Echocardiography in 85 patients showed that valve area and mean gradient remained stable over 17 years of follow up but there was a progressive increase in aortic regurgitation from none to 1–2+. However, at 17 years, less than 10% had developed 3 or 4+ aortic regurgitation.

22. Dellgren G, David TE, Raanani E, et al: Late hemodynamic and clinical outcomes of aortic valve replacement with the Carpentier-Edwards Perimount pericardial bioprosthesis. J Thorac Cardiovasc Surg 124:146–154, 2002.

    Echocardiography was performed in about ½ of a group of 254 patients at a mean of 5.6 years after valve replacement. The peak prosthetic valve gradient was 23.2 ± 9.6 with a mean gradient of 12.3 ± 4.8 mm Hg. Trivial to mild aortic regurgitation was present in 94%, with moderate-severe aortic regurgitation in 4% of survivors.

Exercise Studies with Prosthetic Valves

23. van den Brink RB, Verhuel HA, Visser CA, et al: Value of exercise Doppler echocardiography in patients with prosthetic or bioprosthetic cardiac valves. Am J Cardiol 69:367–372, 1992.

    In 61 asymptomatic patients with an aortic (n = 24) or mitral (n = 39) prosthetic valve, postexercise Doppler data could be obtained within 60 seconds in 92%. In the mitral group, heart rate increased from 80 ± 12 to 116 ± 14 bpm, mean gradient from 6 to 14 mm Hg, and pulmonary artery systolic pressure from 34 to 57 mm Hg. In the aortic group, heart rate increased from 74 ± 0 to 105 ± 18 bpm and mean gradient from 24 (range 12 to 50) to 39 (range 18 to 100) mm Hg.

24. Pibarot P, Dumesnil JG, Briand M, et al: Hemodynamic performance during maximum exercise in adult patients with the Ross operation and comparison with normal controls and patients with aortic bioprostheses. Am J Cardiol 86:982–988, 2000.

    Doppler echocardiography was used to evaluate rest and exercise hemodynamics in 20 adults after pulmonic autograft aortic valve replacement compared to 12 normal subjects. Aortic valve hemodynamics were similar in both groups but the pulmonic homograft had a smaller valve area index (1.10 ± 0.46 cm²/m² in the Ross group versus 1.95 ± 0.41 cm²/m² in the control group). The peak exercise gradient across the pulmonic homograft was 21 ± 14 mm Hg in the Ross group.

25. Silberman S, Shaheen J, Merin O, et al: Exercise hemodynamics of aortic prostheses: Comparison between stentless bioprostheses and mechanical valves. Ann Thorac Surg 72:1217–1221, 2001.

    In patients with a stentless aortic valve prosthesis there was little change in transvalvular gradient on dobutamine stress echocardiography, despite an increase in transvalvular flow rate. In contrast, there was a doubling of the transvalvular gradient with dobutamine in patients with a mechanical aortic valve.

Prosthetic Valve Regurgitation

26. Baumgartner H, Khan S, DeRobertis M, et al: Color Doppler regurgitant characteristics of normal mechanical mitral valve prostheses in vitro. Circulation 85:323–332, 1992.

    Patterns of normal regurgitation for bileaflet and tilting-disk mechanical mitral valves in a pulsatile flow model are described. Bileaflet valves showed two converging jets from the pivot points, a small central jet, and a variable number of peripheral jets. Normal bileaflet regurgitant jets showed little signal aliasing. Tilting-disk (with a central strut and hole) valves showed a large central jet and one or two small peripheral jets. The large central jet showed aliasing extending distally into the atrium.

27. Flachskampf FA, O'Shea JP, Griffin BP, et al: Patterns of normal transvalvular regurgitation in mechanical valve prostheses. J Am Coll Cardiol 18:1493–1498, 1991.

    In an in vitro system, bileaflet valves showed peripheral convergent jets in a plane parallel to the two disk axes and several diverging jets in the orthogonal place. Tilting-disk (with central strut and hole) valves showed a prominent central jet with minor jets along the periphery of the disk.

Transesophageal Echocardiography

28. Khandheria BK, Seward JB, Oh JK, et al: Value and limitations of transesophageal echocardiography in assessment of mitral valve prostheses. Circulation 83:1956–1968, 1991.

    In reviewing the clinical experience at the Mayo Clinic, 50 patients with a prosthetic mitral valve had a transesophageal study followed by confirmatory cardiac catheterization, surgery, or both. For mechanical valves, 10 of 25 (40%) were considered abnormal on transthoracic echocardiography, while 16 of 25 (64%) had abnormalities detected on transesophageal echocardiography. Findings were concordant at surgery in 20 of 23 (87%). For bioprosthetic valves, 9 of 25 (36%) had an abnormal prosthesis on transthoracic echocardiography, while 20 of 25 (80%) had an abnormal transesophageal echocardiography examination. Transesophageal echocardiographic findings were confirmed at surgery in all cases.

29. Karalis DG, Chandrasekaran K, Ross JJ Jr, et al: Single-plane transesophageal echocardiography for assessing function of mechanical or bioprosthetic valves in the aortic valve position. Am J Cardiol 69:1310–1315, 1992.

    In 89 patients, with 69 mechanical and 20 bioprosthetic aortic valves, transesophageal echocardiography was superior to transthoracic echocardiography for evaluation of prosthetic aortic regurgitation only when transthoracic echocardiographic image quality was poor. Transesophageal echocardiography was superior for detection of perivalvular abscess, subaortic perforation, valve dehiscence, and abnormal bioprosthetic valve cusps, as well as in differentiating valvular from paravalvular regurgitation.

30. Daniel WG, Mugge A, Grote J, et al: Comparison of transthoracic and transesophageal echocardiography for detection of abnormalities of prosthetic and bio-prosthetic valves in the mitral and aortic positions. Am J Cardiol 71:210–215, 1993.

    In 126 patients with 148 prosthetic valves (35 mechanical, 113 bioprosthetic), transesophageal echocardiography had a higher sensitivity (35 of 41, 85%) than transthoracic echocardiography (13 of 41, 32%) for detection of prosthetic valve endocarditis and thrombi. Transesophageal echocardiography also had a higher sensitivity for anatomic bioprosthetic valve abnormalities (87% versus 65%).

31. Barbetseas J, Crawford ES, Sail HJ, et al: Doppler echocardiographic evaluation of pseudoaneurysms complicating composite grafts of the ascending aorta. Circulation 85:212–222, 1992.

    Description of the echo Doppler findings in eight patients with pseudoaneurysms of ascending aortic grafts. An echo-free space adjacent (often posterior) to the aortic graft with flow from the graft lumen into the pseudoaneurysm is seen. Identification is facilitated by transesophageal echocardiography imaging when image quality is suboptimal on a transthoracic echocardiographic approach.

32. Garcia MJ, Vandervoort P, Stewart WJ, et al: Mechanisms of hemolysis with mitral prosthetic regurgitation. Study using transesophageal echocardiography and fluid dynamic simulation. J Am Coll Cardiol 27:399–406, 1996.

In 27 patients with prosthetic regurgitation, echocardiographic factors associated with hemolysis (present in 16 patients) were examined. Hemolysis was associated with a paravalvular origin of the regurgitant jet (8/16 with hemolysis versus 2/11 without hemolysis). In addition, patterns of flow fragmentation, collision, or rapid acceleration were associated with hemolysis.

The Echo Exam *Prosthetic Valves*

Transthoracic Examination

Imaging: Valve leaflet thickness and motion
LV size, wall thickness, and systolic function

Doppler: Antegrade prosthetic valve velocity
Evaluate for stenosis
Search carefully for regurgitation
Pulmonary artery pressures

Transthoracic Doppler Evaluation of Prosthetic Valves

Components	Modality	View	Recording	Measurements
Antegrade flow velocity	Pulsed or CW Doppler	Apical	Antegrade transmitral or transaortic velocity	Peak velocity (compare to normal values for valve type and size)
Measures of valve stenosis	Pulsed and CW Doppler	Apical	Careful positioning to obtain highest velocity signal	Mean gradient Aortic valves: ratio of LVOT to aortic velocity Mitral valve: pressure half-time
Valve regurgitation	Color imaging and CW Doppler	Parasternal apical, SSN	Jet origin, direction, and size on color	Vena contracta width
			CW Doppler of each valve	Intensity of CW Doppler signal
			Pulmonary vein flow	Pulmonary vein systolic flow reversal (MR)
			Descending aorta flow	Descending aorta flow reversal (AR)
Pulmonary pressures	CW Doppler	RV inflow and apical	TR-jet velocity IVC size and variation	Calculate PAP as $4v^2$ of TR jet plus estimated right atrial pressure

Transesophageal Examination

Imaging: Valve leaflet thickness and motion
Examine atrial side of mitral prostheses
LV size, wall thickness, and systolic function

Doppler: Antegrade prosthetic valve velocity
Evaluate for stenosis
Search carefully for regurgitation
Pulmonary artery pressures

Transesophageal Evaluation of Prosthetic Valves

Components	Modality	View	Recording	Limitations
Valve imaging	2D echo	High esophageal	Mitral valve in high esophageal four-chamber view Aortic valve in high esophageal long- and short-axis views	Aortic valve prosthesis may shadow anteior segments of the aortic valve With both aortic and mitral prostheses, the aortic shadow may obscure the mitral prosthesis
Antegrade flow velocity	Pulsed or CW Doppler	High esophageal or transgastric apical	Antegrade transmitral or transaortic velocity	Alignment of Doppler beam with transaortic valve flow may be problematic, compare with TTE data
Measures of valve stenosis	Pulsed and CW Doppler	High esophageal or transgastric apical	Careful positioning to obtain highest velocity signal	Mean gradient Aortic valves: ratio of LVOT to aortic velocity (alignment may be suboptimal) Mitral valve: pressure half-time
Valve regurgitation	Color imaging and CW Doppler	High esophageal with rotational scan	Document origin of jet and proximal flow acceleration, and jet size and direction	Measure vena contracta, record pulmonary venous flow pattern, search carefully for eccentric jets
Pulmonary pressures	CW Doppler	RV inflow and apical	TR-jet velocity IVC size and variation	Calculate PAP as $4v^2$ of TR jet plus estimated right atrial pressure. May be difficult to align Doppler beam parallel to TR jet, correlate with TTE data

Echocardiographic Signs of Prosthetic Valve Dysfunction

Increased antegrade velocity across the valve
Decreased valve area (continuity equation or $T_{1/2}$)
Increased regurgitation on color flow
Increased intensity of continuous-wave Doppler regurgitant signal
Progressive chamber dilation
Persistent left ventricular hypertrophy
Recurrent pulmonary hypertension

Example

A 62-year-old man with a mechanical mitral valve replacement 2 years ago for myxomatous mitral valve disease presents with increasing heart failure symptoms and a systolic murmur. He is in chronic atrial fibrillation.

Transthoracic echocardiography shows:

LA anterior-posterior dimension	5.7 cm
LV dimensions (systole/diastole)	6.2/3.8 cm
Ejection fraction	56%
Transmitral E-velocity	1.8 m/s
Mitral pressure half-time	100 ms
TR jet velocity	3.2 m/s
IVC size and variation	Normal

Color flow imaging shows ghosting and reverberations in the left atrial region but no definite regurgitant jet can be identified. Continuous-wave Doppler shows a mitral regurgitant signal that is incomplete in duration and not as dense as antegrade flow.

This transthoracic study is difficult to interpret without a previous study for comparison. The left atrial and left ventricular dilation and the borderline ejection fraction may be residual from before the valve surgery or could represent progressive changes after valve replacement. Pulmonary artery pressure (PAP) is moderately elevated at

$$PAP = 4(V_{TR})^2 + RAP = 4(3.2)^2 + 10 = 41 + 10$$
$$= 51 \text{ mm Hg}$$

Again, pulmonary hypertension may be residual or recurrent after valve surgery but the presence of pulmonary hypertension suggests the possibility of significant prosthetic mitral regurgitation. Although a clear regurgitant jet is not demonstrated due to shadowing and reverberations from the valve prosthesis, the high antegrade flow velocity with a short pressure half-time and detection of regurgitation with continuous wave Doppler indicate that further evaluation is needed.

Transesophageal echocardiography demonstrates a paravalvular mitral regurgitant jet with a proximal acceleration region seen at the lateral aspect of the annulus, a vena contracta width of 7 mm, and an eccentric jet directed along the posterior-lateral left atrial wall. The left pulmonary veins show definite systolic flow reversal, the right pulmonary veins show blunting of the normal systolic flow pattern. These findings are consistent with severe paraprosthetic regurgitation.

On transesophageal imaging the left ventricle was not well visualized due to shadowing and reverberations from the mitral prosthesis. Although transgastric short-axis views were obtained, ejection fraction could not be calculated. The maximum TR jet obtained on transesophageal echocardiography was 2.9 m/s. Because a higher jet was obtained on transthoracic imaging, the TEE jet most likely underestimates pulmonary pressures.

In summary, this patient has severe paraprosthetic mitral regurgitation with left atrial and left ventricular dilation, moderate pulmonary hypertension, and a borderline ejection fraction. As is typical with prosthetic valves, the combination of transthoracic and transesophageal echocardiography was needed for diagnosis.

ENDOCARDITIS

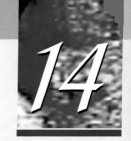

Echocardiography is an essential component of the evaluation of a patient with infective endocarditis. In combination with clinical and bacteriologic data, the echocardiographic finding of a valvular vegetation allows an accurate diagnosis of endocarditis. In addition, echocardiographic assessment of the degree of valve dysfunction and detection of complications, such as a paravalvular abscess or fistula, are needed for optimal patient care.

While transthoracic echocardiography is adequate in some cases, transesophageal imaging is more sensitive and specific, both for the detection of valvular vegetations and for detection of complications. Furthermore, demonstration of normal valve anatomy and function on transesophageal imaging reliably excludes endocarditis in patients in whom this diagnosis is suspected.

BASIC PRINCIPLES

The diagnosis of endocarditis is most secure when there is pathologic confirmation of a valvular vegetation with active infection, local tissue destruction, and/or paravalvular abscess formation. In the clinical setting, endocarditis is diagnosed based on a combination of echocardiographic, laboratory, and physical examination findings as detailed in Table 14–1. The major criteria for the diagnosis of endocarditis are persistent bacteremia with typical organisms and echocardiographic evidence of endocardial involvement. Minor criteria include less specific bacteriologic and echocardiographic findings, factors predisposing to endocarditis (such as preexisting valve disease

or intravenous drug use), vascular events (such as pulmonary or systemic emboli), immunologic phenomenon (such as glomerulonephritis), and signs of systemic infection (such as fever).

The goals of echocardiography in a patient with an infective endocarditis are

- to identify the presence, location, size, and number of valvular vegetations;
- to assess functional abnormalities of the affected valve(s), especially valvular regurgitation;
- to identify the underlying anatomy of the affected valve(s) and any coincident valvular disease;
- to assess the impact of valvular disease on chamber dimensions and function, most importantly left ventricular size and systolic function;
- to identify other complications of endocarditis (e.g., paravalvular abscess, pericardial effusion); and
- to provide prognostic data on the anticipated clinical course, risk of systemic embolization, and potential need for surgical intervention.

In a patient with a lower likelihood of endocarditis on clinical grounds, an echocardiogram often is requested to "rule out" endocarditis. In this setting, the goals of the echocardiographic examination are

- identification of any valvular vegetations, and
- assessment of valve anatomy and function with respect to anatomic or physiologic factors that increase the likelihood of endocarditis (e.g., bicuspid aortic valve, myxomatous mitral valve).

TABLE 14-1

Modified Duke Criteria for Infective Endocarditis

Pathologic Criteria

Microorganisms: demonstrated by culture of histology in a vegetation, *or* in a vegetation that has embolized, *or* in an intracardiac abscess

Pathologic lesions: vegetation or intracardiac abscess present, confirmed by histology showing active endocarditis

Clinical Criteria

Major Criteria

Positive blood culture for infective endocarditis
    Typical microorganism for infective endocarditis from two separate blood cultures
        Viridans streptococci,[†] *Staphylococcus aureus, Streptococcus bovis,* HACEK group, *or*
        Enterococci, in the absence of a primary focus, *or*
    Persistently positive blood culture, defined as recovery of a microorganism consistent with infective endocarditis
        from:
        Blood cultures drawn more than 12 hours apart, *or*
        All of three or a majority of four or more separate blood cultures, with first and last drawn at least 1 hour apart
        Positive blood culture for *Coxiella burnetii* or anti-phase I IgG antibody titer >1:800
Evidence of endocardial involvement
    Positive echocardiogram for infective endocarditis
        Oscillating intracardiac mass, on valve or supporting structures, *or* in the path of regurgitant jets, *or* on implanted
            material, in the absence of an alternative anatomic explanation, *or*
        Abscess, *or*
        New partial dehiscence of prosthetic valve, *or*
    New valvular regurgitation (increase or change in preexisting murmur not sufficient)

Minor Criteria

Predisposition: predisposing heart condition *or* intravenous drug use
Fever: ≥38.0°C (100.4°F)
Vascular phenomena: major arterial emboli, septic pulmonary infarcts, mycotic aneurysm, intracranial hemorrhage, conjunctival hemorrhages, Janeway lesions
Immunologic phenomena: glomerulonephritis, Osler's nodes, Roth spots, rheumatoid factor
Microbiologic evidence: positive blood culture but not meeting major criterion as noted previously[‡] or serologic evidence of active infection with organism consistent with infective endocarditis

Definite endocarditis: 2 major criteria *or* 1 major and 3 minor criteria *or* 5 minor criteria
Possible endocarditis: 1 major plus 1 minor, or 3 minor criteria

---

HACEK, *Haemophilus* spp., *Actinobacillus actinomycetemcomitans, Cardiobacterium hominis, Eikenella* spp., and *Kingella kingae.*
[†]Including nutritional variant strains.
[‡]Excluding single positive cultures for coagulase-negative staphylococci and organisms that do not cause endocarditis.
From Durack DT, Lukes AS, Bright DK: New criteria for diagnosis of infective endocarditis: Utilization of specific echocardiographic findings. Duke Endocarditis Service. Am J Med 96:200–209, 1994. With a modification by Li JS, Sexton DJ, Mick N, et al: Proposed modification to the Duke criteria for the diagnosis of infective endocarditis. Clin Infect Dis 30:633–638, 2000.

If an abnormality is identified, complete evaluation is directed toward the goals listed for clinical endocarditis.

ECHOCARDIOGRAPHIC APPROACH

Valvular Vegetations

Transthoracic Echocardiography

On two-dimensional (2D) echocardiography, the features that typify a valvular vegetation are

- ■ an abnormal echogenic, irregular mass;
- ■ attachment on the upstream side of the valve leaflet; and

- ■ a pattern of motion that is dependent on, but more chaotic than, normal valve motion.

For example, an aortic valve vegetation prolapses into the left ventricular outflow tract in diastole and extends into the aortic root in systole (Fig. 14–1). The mass is attached to the left ventricular side of the valve leaflet but shows motion in excess of normal valve excursion with rapid oscillations in diastole (best appreciated on M-mode recordings). A mitral valve vegetation is attached on the atrial side of the valve, prolapses into the left atrium in systole, and moves into the left ventricle, beyond the normal

Aortic Valve Vegetation

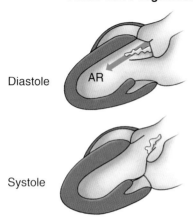

FIGURE 14–1. Schematic diagram of an aortic valve vegetation attached to the ventricular side of the leaflet with prolapse into the left ventricular outflow tract in diastole. AR, aortic regurgitation.

range of mitral valve opening, in diastole (Fig. 14–2).

Valvular vegetations vary in size from so small as to be undetectable with current imaging techniques to greater than 3 cm in length. Vegetations may be attached at any area of the leaflet, although lesions at the coaptation line are most common. More than one valve can be involved, either by direct extension of infection or as a separate process, emphasizing the caveat that each valve requires careful examination even if a vegetation has been identified on another valve. In most cases, endocarditis occurs on a previously abnormal valve.

Mitral Valve Vegetation

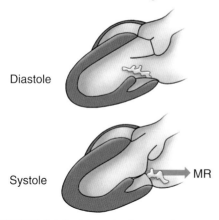

FIGURE 14–2. Schematic diagram of a mitral valve vegetation attached to the atrial side of the leaflet with prolapse into the left atrium in systole. MR, mitral regurgitation.

Multiple acoustic windows and 2D views are needed for detection of a valvular vegetation. Because the vegetation is a discrete structure, it may be seen only in certain tomographic planes. Slow scanning between the standard image planes—for example, between the parasternal long-axis view and the right ventricular inflow view—increases the likelihood of identifying a valvular vegetation. Orthogonal views further ensure that all segments of the valve leaflets are examined. In a patient with suspected endocarditis, a complete examination is needed with scanning from parasternal, apical, subcostal, and suprasternal notch views for careful evaluation of each valve. The reported sensitivity of transthoracic echocardiography for detection of valvular vegetations ranges from less than 50% to as high as 90% (Table 14–2). To some extent, the reported sensitivity of transthoracic echocardiography increased between the advent of 2D instruments in the late 1970s and the improved image quality with advances in instrumentation in the 1980s.

AORTIC VALVE. Aortic valve vegetations most often are detected in parasternal long- and short-axis views. Careful angulation from medial to lateral in the long-axis plane and from inferior to superior in the short-axis plane is needed because vegetations often are eccentrically located. Image quality is optimized by use of a minimum depth setting and adjustment of gain and processing parameters. An echogenic mass attached to the ventricular side of the leaflet with independent motion and prolapse into the outflow tract in diastole is diagnostic for a valvular vegetation (Fig. 14–3). Rapid oscillating motion may be best appreciated on an M-mode recording.

Less typically, a vegetation may be attached to the aortic side of the leaflet or may show little independent motion. A definitive diagnosis may be difficult if the underlying valve anatomy is abnormal. For example, a vegetation on a calcified aortic valve may be difficult to see. In these cases, the findings of independent motion and prolapse into the left ventricle in diastole are particularly helpful signs. Comparison with previous echocardiograms may allow recognition of recent changes, increasing the likelihood of valve infection, or may show no significant difference, decreasing the likelihood of an acute process.

Findings that may be mistaken for an aortic valve vegetation include beam-width artifact related to either a calcified nodule, a prosthetic valve, the normal leaflet apposition zone, or the normal leaflet thickening at the central coaptation

TABLE 14–2

Accuracy of Echocardiographic Diagnosis of Valvular Vegetations (Selected Studies)

First Author/ Year	Study Entry Criteria/ Standard of Reference	No. of Valves	Percent Prosthetic	Transthoracic Echo		Transesophageal Echo	
				Sensitivity	Specificity	Sensitivity	Specificity
Mugge/1989	Definite endocarditis *plus* surgery/ autopsy	91	4%	53/91 (58%)	–	82/91 (90%)	–
Jaffe/1990	Definite endocarditis *plus* surgery/ autopsy	38	6%	38/44 (86%)	–	–	–
Burger/1991	Suspected endocarditis and clinical outcome	101	–	35/39 (90%)	61/62 (98%)	–	–
Shively/1991	Suspected endocarditis and clinical outcome	6	8%	7/16 (44%)	49/50 (98%)	15/16 (94%)	50/50 (100%)
Pedersen/1991	Suspected endocarditis and clinical outcome	24	2%	5/10 (50%)	13/14 (93%)	10/10 (100%)	14/14 (100%)
Daniel/1993	Prosthetic valve with surgically confirmed endocarditis	33	0%	12/33 (36%)	–	27/33 (82%)	–
Sochowski/1993	Suspected endocarditis with initially negative TTE study	65	2%	–	–	Negative predictive value	= 56/65 (86%)
Shapiro/1994	Suspected endocarditis	68	–	23/34 (68%)	31/34 (91%)	33/34 (97%)	31/34 (91%)

Data from Mugge et al: J Am Coll Cardiol 14:631–638, 1989; Jaffe et al: J Am Coll Cardiol 15:1227–1233, 1990; Burger et al: Angiology 42:552–560, 1991; Shiveley et al: J Am Coll Cardiol 18:391–397, 1991; Pedersen et al: Chest 100:351–356, 1991; Daniel et al: Am J Cardiol 71:210–215, 1993; Sochowski, Chan: J Am Coll Cardiol 21:216–221, 1993; Shapiro et al: Chest 105:377, 1994.

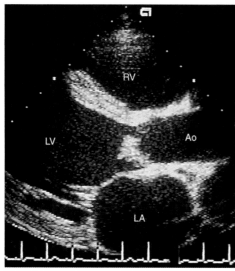

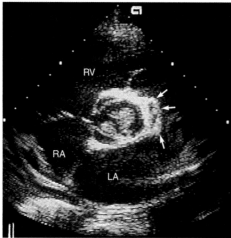

FIGURE 14–3. In a 29-year-old intravenous drug user with *S. aureus* endocarditis, aortic valve vegetations are seen in transthoracic parasternal long-axis *(top)* and short-axis *(bottom)* views. Irregularly shaped echogenic masses are attached to the ventricular side of the aortic valve leaflets with prolapse into the outflow tract in diastole (seen in the long-axis view) and extension into the aortic root in systole (seen in the short-axis view). Severe aortic regurgitation was present. The short-axis view also shows a paravalvular abscess *(three arrows)*.

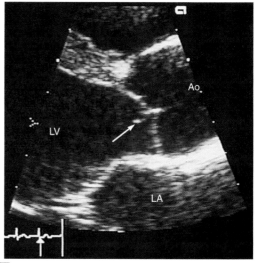

FIGURE 14–4. Lambl's excrescence or beam-width artifact at the aortic closure line that might be mistaken for a valvular vegetation.

region (the nodule of Arantius). Occasionally, a linear echo representing a normal variant called a *Lambl's excrescence* is seen. These small fibroelastic protrusions from the ventricular side of the leaflet closure zone occur with increasing frequency with age and are present in a high percentage of patients. As image quality improves, these normal structures are seen more frequently (Fig. 14–4).

Apical views of the aortic valve, both from an anteriorly angulated four-chamber view and from an apical long-axis view, may show an aortic valve vegetation. The finding of an abnormality in both parasternal and apical views decreases the likelihood of an ultrasound artifact, since the relationship of the ultrasound beam and aortic valve is entirely different from these two windows.

Two- or three-dimensional imaging of a definite or suspected aortic valve vegetation is accompanied by evaluation of the functional abnormalities due to valve destruction, as discussed in the following sections.

MITRAL VALVE. Mitral valve vegetations typically are located on the atrial side of the leaflets. Diagnostic features include rapid independent motion, prolapse into the left atrium in systole, and functional evidence of valve dysfunction. Parasternal long- and short-axis views with careful scanning across the valve apparatus in both image planes allows assessment of the presence, size, and location of any vegetation (Fig. 14–5). Apical four-chamber, two-chamber, and long-axis views again are helpful both in visualizing valve and vegetation anatomy and in distinguishing a true valve mass from an ultrasound artifact.

As for the aortic valve, beam-width artifacts can be mistaken for a vegetation. A particular artifact to be aware of is the appearance of a "mass" on the atrial side of the anterior mitral leaflet in the apical four-chamber view due to beam-width

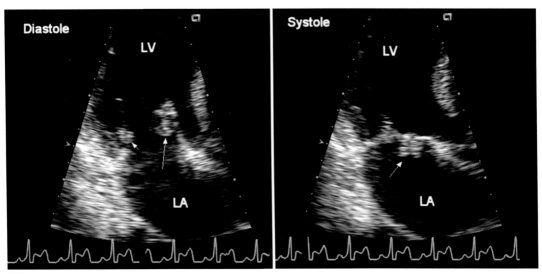

FIGURE 14–5. A typical-appearing mitral valve vegetation (VEG) seen in an apical long-axis view in diastole attached to the atrial side of the anterior mitral valve leaflet *(left)*. In systole *(right)*, the mass prolapses into the left atrium with motion in realtime independent of valve leaflet motion.

artifact from a calcified or prosthetic aortic valve. Other types of mitral valve pathology may be difficult to distinguish from a valvular vegetation, including a severely myxomatous leaflet, a partial flail leaflet, or a ruptured papillary muscle (Fig. 14–6). Again, comparison with previous studies may help differentiate an acute process from chronic underlying valve disease. With mitral valve endocarditis, mitral regurgitation typically, but not invariably, is present.

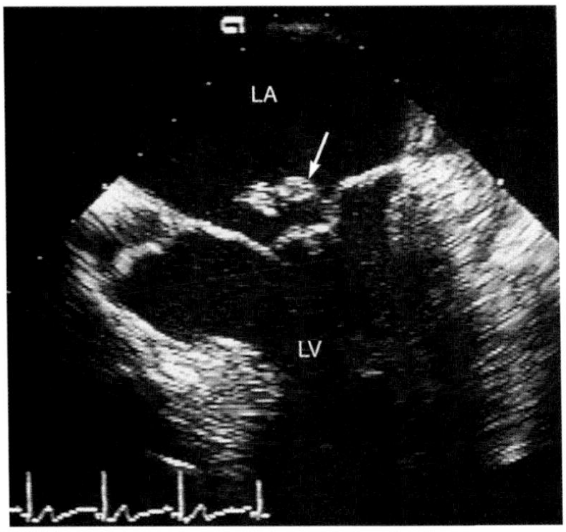

TRICUSPID VALVE. Tricuspid valve endocarditis occurs most often in intravenous drug abusers, is associated with large vegetations due to *Staphylococcus aureus* infection, and tends to have a better prognosis than left-sided valvular involvement.

The right ventricular inflow view often is diagnostic, showing a large, mobile mass of echoes attached to the atrial side of the leaflet with prolapse into the right atrium in systole (Fig. 14–7). Given the range of excursion and mobility of these vegetations, it is not surprising that septic pulmonary emboli are a frequent complication of tricuspid valve endocarditis.

The apical and subcostal four-chamber views allow further evaluation of the presence and extent of tricuspid valve infection. Assessment of tricuspid regurgitant severity and consequent right atrial and right ventricular dilation also can be performed from these windows.

Transesophageal Imaging

From the transesophageal approach, the aortic valve is examined in multiple image planes including a standard long-axis (typically at approximately 120° rotation) and short-axis (about 45° rotation) views. As with transthoracic imaging, careful scanning from medial to lateral in the long-axis view and from superior to inferior in the short-axis view is needed to fully evaluate valve

FIGURE 14–6. Abnormal valve (myxomatous) with a flail leaflet *(arrow)* but no vegetation on transesophageal imaging. Angulation showed this "mass" to be a flail leaflet. The patient had no clinical evidence of endocarditis.

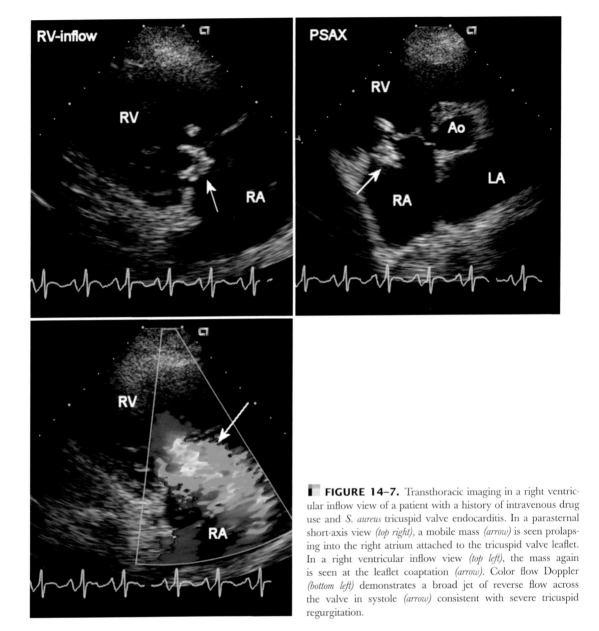

FIGURE 14–7. Transthoracic imaging in a right ventricular inflow view of a patient with a history of intravenous drug use and *S. aureus* tricuspid valve endocarditis. In a parasternal short-axis view *(top right)*, a mobile mass *(arrow)* is seen prolapsing into the right atrium attached to the tricuspid valve leaflet. In a right ventricular inflow view *(top left)*, the mass again is seen at the leaflet coaptation *(arrow)*. Color flow Doppler *(bottom left)* demonstrates a broad jet of reverse flow across the valve in systole *(arrow)* consistent with severe tricuspid regurgitation.

anatomy and to achieve a high sensitivity for detection of valvular vegetations (Figs. 14–8 and 14–9). When the image plane is oblique, an aortic leaflet may be seen *en face*, mimicking an aortic valve mass. Evaluation in more than one image plane and assessment of the pattern of motion (rapid oscillating independent motion versus motion *with* the valve) avoids this potential error. Because image quality tends to be superior from the transesophageal approach, small normal variants of valve anatomy may be appreciated and should not be interpreted as abnormalities. Image

quality may be enhanced by use of a higher-frequency transducer and magnification of the area of interest. Sometimes the aortic valve can be evaluated from a transgastric apical view; however, image quality may be no better than from a transthoracic approach due to the distance from the transducer to the aortic valve.

The mitral valve is well seen from a high esophageal position. Since the mitral valve plane is perpendicular to the ultrasound beam from this approach, excellent images can be obtained in multiple views by slowly rotating the multi-

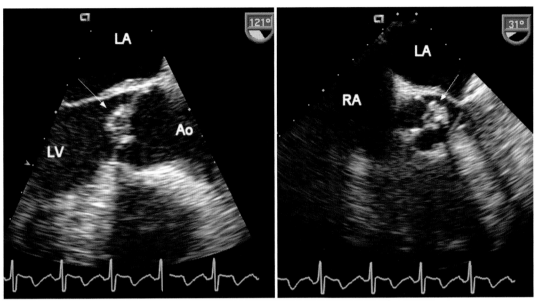

■ **FIGURE 14–8.** Transesophageal images of the aortic valve in a long-axis *(left)* and short-axis view *(right)* showing valvular vegetations *(arrow).*

plane transducer from 0 to 180°. Particular attention should be paid to standard four-chamber (at 0°), two-chamber (at 60°), and long-axis (at 120°) views. The degree of mitral regurgitation can be assessed with color flow imaging in these same views. Given the distance of the mitral valve from the chest wall in both parasternal and apical transthoracic views, transesophageal imaging often provides dramatically better images and important clinical data (Figs. 14–10 and 14–11).

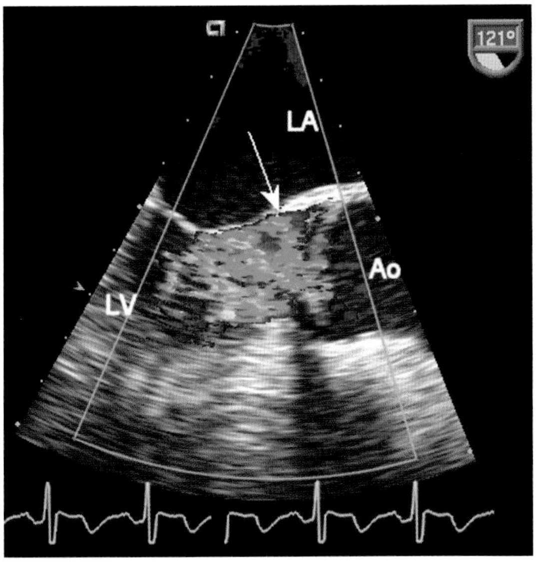

The tricuspid valve is seen in the transesophageal four-chamber view and from a transgastric approach. Because the tricuspid valve lies closer to the chest wall than the mitral valve, transthoracic imaging often is diagnostic. Transesophageal imaging is most valuable in these patients for detection of left-sided valve involvement (Fig. 14–12).

Diagnostic Accuracy of Echocardiography for Detection of Vegetations

While numerous studies have evaluated the sensitivity of echocardiography for diagnosis of valvular vegetation by comparing the echo findings with subsequent surgical or autopsy findings, there are fewer data on the specificity of echocardiography for valvular vegetations. This stems from two study design problems. First, most studies only include subjects with a definite diagnosis of endocarditis. Thus, there are no subjects without the disease in the study group. Second, when surgical or autopsy inspection of the valve is the standard of reference, only patients who are sick enough to need surgery or who have died are included in the study group. Direct inspection of valves that appeared normal on echocardiography rarely is available.

■ **FIGURE 14–9.** Color flow Doppler in the same patient as in Figure 14–8 in a tranesophageal long-axis view shows acute severe aortic regurgitation (AR) due to the valve destruction in this patient.

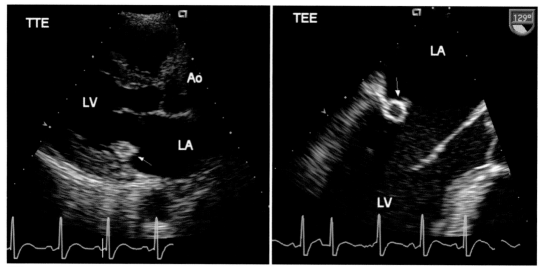

■ **FIGURE 14–10.** Transthoracic *(left)* and transesophageal *(right)* imaging in a patient with fungal endocarditis. The unusual appearing valvular vegetation *(arrow)* is seen on transthoracic imaging but is better defined on transesophageal imaging with a dense spherical mass with some small attached areas of independent motion *(arrows)*.

A few studies (for example, studies 3 through 5 in Table 14–2) have circumvented these study design problems by including all patients with *suspected* endocarditis (some have the disease and some do not) and using clinical outcome rather than direct valve inspection as the standard of reference. All these studies demonstrate a high specificity of transthoracic (93% to 98%) and transesophageal (100%) echocardiography in excluding the diagnosis of endocarditis. Another study (study 7 in Table 14–2) found that the negative predictive value of a negative transesophageal study also is high (86%).

The specificity of echocardiography depends on distinguishing a valvular vegetation from other intracardiac masses and from ultrasound artifacts.

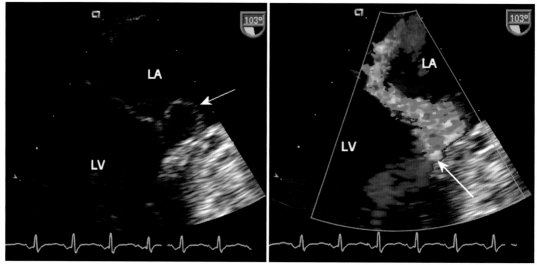

■ **FIGURE 14–11.** Transesophageal echocardiography in a 28-year-old man with systemic embolic events and blood culture results positive for *S. aureus*. There is an apparent prolapse of the lateral segment of the mitral leaflet in a two-chamber view *(left)*. Color flow Doppler *(right)* shows an eccentric jet of severe mitral regurgitation through this region with proxmial flow accleration and a wide vena contracta. These findings, in conjunction with the clinical symptoms and postive blood cultures, are consistent with a ruptured mitral valve psuedoaneurym due to infective endocarditis.

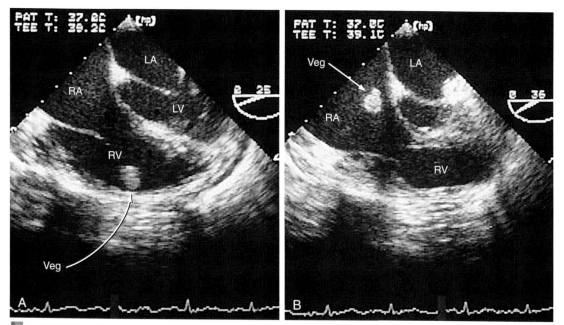

■ **FIGURE 14–12.** Transesophageal echocardiographic images showing a vegetation attached to the tricuspid valve in a patient with a history of intravenous drug use. The vegetation (VEG) is attached to the tricuspid valve leaflet but prolapses into the right ventricle in diastole *(left)* and back into the right atrium in systole *(right)*. (From Otto CM: Valvular Heart Disease, 2nd ed. Philadelphia: WB Saunders 2004, Figure 18–16.)

Echocardiographic findings that may be mistaken for a vegetation include

- papillary fibroelastoma,
- myxomatous mitral valve disease,
- nonbacterial thrombotic endocarditis,
- systemic lupus erythematosus,
- thrombus (especially with prosthetic valves),
- beam width artifact, and
- Lambl's excrescence or nodule of Arantius.

In a patient with abnormal valve leaflets (e.g., myxomatous, calcified), it may be difficult to distinguish the abnormal tissue from a valvular vegetation, particularly a partial flail leaflet or ruptured chord. A study performed before onset of the illness can provide a useful comparison. Mistaking ultrasound artifacts for a vegetation can be avoided by identification of the characteristic findings in more than one view. Note that not all valvular vegetations are "typical." Some may be on the downstream side of the valve or may show little independent motion. These atypical findings further decrease the sensitivity and specificity of echocardiography for valvular vegetations.

Endocarditis most often occurs on a previously abnormal valve or a prosthetic valve. Evaluation of the underlying valve disease is an important aspect of the ultrasound examination.

Functional Valvular Abnormalities Due to Endocarditis

Valve leaflet destruction by the infectious process and the distortion of leaflet closure by the vegetation mass result in valvular regurgitation. Regurgitation can occur at the closure line or through a perforation in the leaflet itself. The degree of regurgitation varies from none to mild, moderate, or severe.

Assessment of valvular regurgitation in endocarditis is performed using the pulsed, color flow, and continuous-wave Doppler approaches described in Chapter 12 with careful attention to the features that distinguish acute from chronic regurgitation. Because endocarditis often affects a previously abnormal valve, acute regurgitation may be superimposed on chronic regurgitation, resulting in mixed findings on echocardiography.

Valvular stenosis due to endocarditis is rare. Occasionally, a large vegetation will partially obstruct the orifice of the open valve, resulting in some degree of functional stenosis.

Note that not all patients with endocarditis have a new murmur (approximately 10% do not) and a few have no regurgitation detectable on Doppler examination. This is most likely to occur if the vegetation is located at the base of the leaflet, resulting in little distortion of leaflet closure. Echocardiographic recognition of the diagnosis in this subgroup is all the more important in that endocarditis often is not suspected clinically with the echocardiogram having been ordered for other reasons.

Other Echocardiographic Findings

In addition to direct assessment of valvular disease, the examination includes evaluation of cardiac chamber size and function. Acute aortic regurgitation results in only mild left ventricular dilation, but a subacute or acute course superimposed on mild-to-moderate chronic disease may result in significant ventricular dilation. Severe valve destruction may result in a flail aortic leaflet (see Figs. 14–8 and 14–9). Mitral regurgitation results in left atrial and left ventricular enlargement. Left ventricular systolic dysfunction may be seen either due to longstanding valvular disease or to the acute infectious process.

Pulmonary pressures may be elevated due to mitral regurgitation directly resulting in an elevated left atrial pressure or to aortic regurgitation with a high end-diastolic left ventricular pressure.

A small pericardial effusion often is seen with endocarditis. A larger effusion raises the concern of purulent pericarditis due to direct extension from a paravalvular abscess.

Diagnosis of Paravalvular Abscess and Intracardiac Fistula

Unlike abscesses elsewhere in the body, a cardiac abscess may be either echolucent or echodense on ultrasound examination. Typically, abscesses occur in the valve annulus adjacent to the infected leaflet tissue and are more common with aortic than with mitral valve endocarditis. For diagnosis of aortic annular abscess, findings include increased echogenicity or an echolucent area in the base of the septum or increased thickness of the posterior aortic root (Figs. 14–13 and 14–14). Involvement of the aortic annulus may extend into the contiguous anterior mitral valve leaflet with evidence of increased thickness of the leaflet tissue, a valvular vegetation, and/or leaflet perforation (Figs. 14–15 and 14–16). A sinus of Valsalva aneurysm can occur due to infection of the aortic wall and may be detected by echocardiography, before rupture occurs, as a dilated and distorted sinus. In effect, this represents an abscess that is in direct communication with the bloodstream.

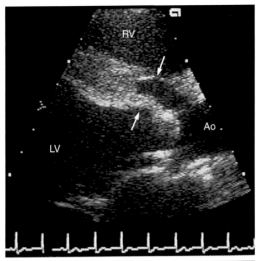

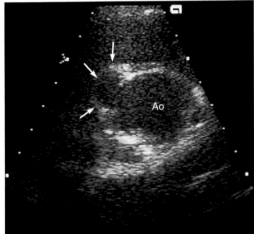

FIGURE 14–13. Transthoracic parasternal long-axis *(top)* and short-axis *(bottom)* views in a 34-year-old man with a bicuspid aortic valve and suspected endocarditis. Definite evidence for valvular vegetations and a paravalvular abscess *(arrows)* is seen. Doppler allowed assessment of the severity of aortic regurgitation.

Rupture of an aortic annular abscess can occur in several fashions. The region of the noncoronary cusp can rupture into the right ventricular outflow tract either in the sinus of Valsalva (an aortic to right ventricular connection) or from the left ventricular outflow tract through the septum into the right ventricle (a ventricular septal defect) (Figs. 14–17 and 14–18). An aortic to right ventricular fistula shows both systolic and diastolic left-to-right flow on Doppler interrogation, while a ventricular septal defect shows predominantly systolic flow. Rupture also can occur from the left ventricle into the mitral-aortic intervalvular

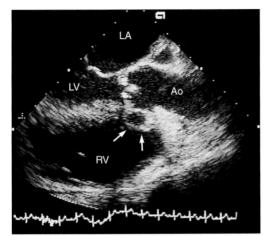

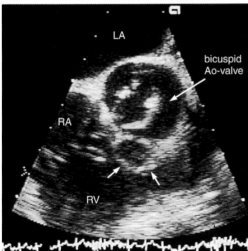

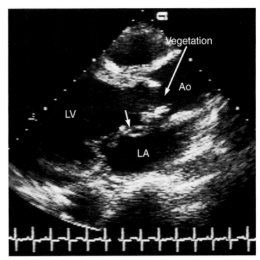

■ **FIGURE 14–15.** Aortic valve endocarditis with vegetations and extension into the base of the anterior mitral valve leaflet resulting in mitral leaflet perforation.

■ **FIGURE 14–14.** Transesophageal long-axis *(top)* and short-axis *(bottom)* views of the aortic valve in the same patient as in Figure 13–13. While the bicuspid valve, valvular vegetations, and paravalvular abscess *(arrows)* are more clearly seen, no additional diagnostic information was obtained compared with the transthoracic study. At surgery, a paravalvular abscess due to α-hemolytic *Streptococcus* was found.

the left or right atrium, or infection may extend directly into the interatrial septum.

A mitral annular abscess appears as increased thickening and echogenicity in the posterior aspect of the mitral annulus. Infection may extend into the basal segments of the ventricular myocardium or into the pericardial space. Again, identification may be difficult on echocardio-

fibrosa with flow into and out of the abscess cavity from the left ventricular outflow tract (Fig. 14–19).

The right coronary sinus region can rupture into the right ventricle or right atrium and can lead to involvement of the adjacent septal leaflet of the tricuspid valve. Again, rupture can occur either from the aorta or from the left ventricular outflow tract into the right side of the heart. Note that a small segment of ventricular septum (the atrioventricular septum) actually separates the left ventricle from the right *atrium* so that a ventriculoatrial communication can occur. The left coronary sinus of the aortic valve can rupture into

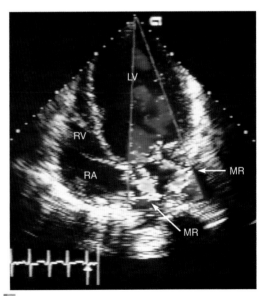

■ **FIGURE 14–16.** In the same patient as in Figure 14–15, the apical four-chamber color flow image showed two jets of mitral regurgitation—one through the leaflet perforation and one through the valve coaptation zone.

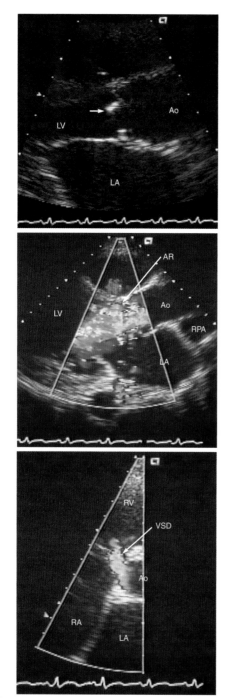

FIGURE 14-17. In a 50-year-old man with *S. aureus* endocarditis, echocardiography after 6 weeks of antibiotic therapy showed persistent aortic valvular vegetations *(top)* and severe aortic regurgitation *(middle)*. In addition, a ventricular septal defect was present just inferior to the aortic annulus, best seen in the parasternal short-axis view *(bottom)* with color flow from the left ventricular outflow tract to right ventricle immediately adjacent to the tricuspid valve.

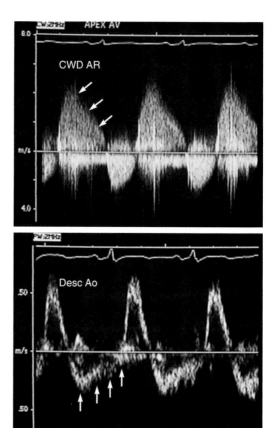

FIGURE 14-18. In the same patient as in Figure 14-17, evidence for acute severe aortic regurgitation is present including a dense continuous-wave Doppler signal *(top)* with a steep deceleration slope *(arrows)* and holodiastolic flow reversal in the proximal abdominal aorta *(bottom)*.

graphic imaging, and the diagnosis should be pursued with transesophageal echocardiography when suspected on clinical grounds. An unusual complication of mitral valve endocarditis is a persistent contour abnormality, in effect a pseudoaneurysm of the valve leaflet, which persists even after the infection is treated (Fig. 14-20).

Tricuspid valve endocarditis may be associated with a ring abscess, again manifested as increased thickening and echogenicity in the annulus region.

Diagnosis of paravalvular abscess by transthoracic echocardiography has a markedly lower sensitivity and specificity (Table 14-3), compared with transesophageal imaging, due to poor ultrasound tissue penetration resulting in suboptimal image quality. A high index of suspicion is needed by the echocardiographer, and subtle abnormalities that may suggest a valve abscess should not be ignored. However, even with careful imaging from several acoustic windows in multiple

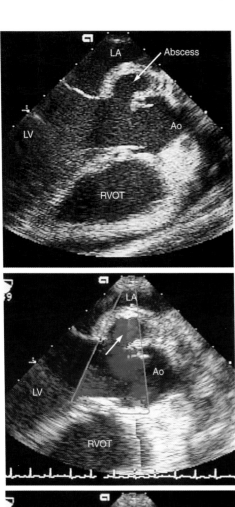

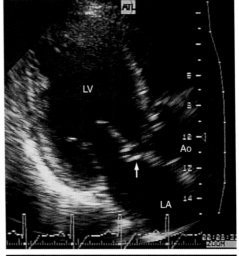

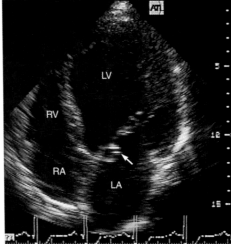

■ FIGURE 14-20. Chronic mitral valve pseudoaneurysm in a 69-year-old man with a remote history of bacterial endocarditis. In the apical long-axis *(top)* and four-chamber *(bottom)* views, a circular echolucent structure is seen at the base of the anterior mitral leaflet *(arrow)*.

■ FIGURE 14-19. In this 26-year-old woman with a history of intravenous drug use and *S. aureus* endocarditis, transesophageal echocardiography shows an abscess of the mitral-aortic intervalvular fibrosa *(top)*. This cavity communicated with the left ventricular outflow tract with flow into the abscess in systole *(middle)* with diastolic regurgitation *(bottom)* into the left ventricle.

tomographic planes, a definite diagnosis may not be possible. Transesophageal imaging is especially important in patients with prosthetic valve endocarditis as paravalvular abscesses are common and shadowing and reverberations from the valve prosthesis compromise the examination (see Chapter 13).

The superior image quality of transesophageal echocardiography is associated with a higher sensitivity (87%) and specificity (96%) for diagnosis of paravalvular abscess. In addition to 2D findings of abnormal areas of increased echogenicity or abnormal echolucent areas adjacent to the valve, color flow imaging and conventional pulsed Doppler may allow demonstration of flow into

TABLE 14-3

Accuracy of Echocardiographic Diagnosis of Paravalvular Abscess (Selected Series)

First Author/ Year	Study Entry Criteria	No. of Valves	Percent Prosthetic	Transthoracic Echo		Transesophageal Echo	
				Sensitivity	Specificy	Sensitivity	Specificity
Daniel/1991	Endocarditis with surgery or autopsy	137	25%	13/46 (28%)	90/91 (99%)	40/46 (87%)	87/91 (96%)
Jaffe/1990	Endocarditis with surgery or autopsy	7		5/7 (71%)			
Karalis/1992	Endocarditis with surgery or autopsy	55	46%	13/24 (54%)		24/24 (100%)	

Data from Daniel et al: N Engl J Med 324:795–800, 1991; Jaffe et al: J Am Coll Cardiol 15:1227–1233, 1990; Karalis et al: Circulation 86:353–362, 1992.

and out of these abnormal areas consistent with an abscess that partially communicates with the bloodstream.

LIMITATIONS/TECHNICAL CONSIDERATIONS

Active versus Healed Vegetations

Sequential echocardiographic studies in a patient undergoing treatment for endocarditis may show a gradual reduction in size, decrease in mobility, and increase in echogenicity of the valvular vegetation. However, vegetations may either abruptly "disappear" from the heart due to embolization or may remain unchanged in size or appearance long after the acute episode. Thus, a patient with active endocarditis may have no visible vegetation if recent embolization has occurred. Conversely, a patient with prior endocarditis may have a persistent vegetation without active infection. Echocardiography, by itself, can neither exclude nor establish a diagnosis of endocarditis. Correlation of the echocardiographic findings with the patient's clinical presentation (fevers, systemic emboli, new murmur, peripheral manifestation of endocarditis) plus the results of microbiologic cultures is needed for diagnosis as detailed in Table 14–1. Obviously, echocardiography provides no information regarding the causative organism. While certain etiologic agents (fungal endocarditis, *Haemophilus influenzae*) are associated with larger vegetations, this observation is not diagnostically useful in an individual patient.

Nonbacterial Thrombotic Endocarditis

The echocardiographic appearance of nonbacterial thrombotic endocarditis, as has been described

in patients with malignancy and in patients with systemic lupus erythematosus, is similar to that of infectious endocarditis. Although the vegetations of nonbacterial thrombotic endocarditis tend to be smaller, to be located near the leaflet base, and to show variable echo density and less independent motion, again, clinical and bacteriologic correlation is needed for a correct diagnosis (Fig. 14–21).

Diagnosis of Vegetations with Underlying Valve Disease

Endocarditis most often occurs on a previously abnormal valve, because the local flow distur-

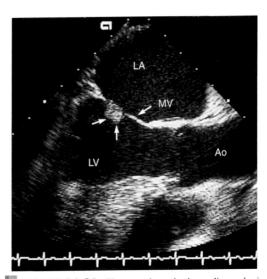

FIGURE 14–21. Transesophageal echocardiography in a 49-year-old woman with the antiphospholipid antibody syndrome and multiple embolic events shows a typical mass on the mitral valve *(arrows)* consistent with nonbacterial thrombotic endocarditis. She was afebrile and had negative blood culture results.

bance increases the likelihood of bacterial deposition. When the underlying disease is anatomically straightforward, such as a bicuspid aortic valve, this poses little problem in diagnosing superimposed valvular vegetations. Often, however, the presence of an abnormal valve makes exclusion or confirmation of a valvular vegetation more difficult. For example, with calcific aortic stenosis, the irregular areas of increased echogenicity on the valve leaflets could represent a vegetation or chronic fibrocalcific changes. Findings of independent rapid motion and prolapse into the outflow tract in diastole increase the likelihood of a vegetation, but the absence of these findings does not allow a definite conclusion as to the absence of a vegetation.

Another example is myxomatous mitral valve disease where an independently mobile mass of echoes attached to the leaflet and prolapsing into the left atrium in systole could represent either a valvular vegetation or a flail leaflet segment and attached chordae. When underlying valve disease is present, the improved images obtained by the transesophageal approach may increase the certainty of diagnosis. In any case, careful integration with other clinical findings usually leads to a correct diagnosis.

Endocarditis of Prosthetic Valves

Evaluation of prosthetic valves for suspected endocarditis is problematic for two reasons. First, infection often involves the area around the sewing ring of the prosthetic valve rather than resulting in a discrete valvular vegetation. Second, reverberations and shadowing by the prosthesis limit the ability of echocardiography to detect abnormalities. This is a particular problem with transthoracic imaging of mitral prostheses, where the left atrial side of the valve is "masked" by the prosthesis so that neither the paravalvular infection in the mitral annulus nor the resulting valvular incompetence can be detected (see Chapter 13). Acoustic shadowing is less of a problem with aortic valve prostheses because aortic regurgitation can be evaluated from both apical and parasternal windows without "masking" by the valve prosthesis. However, since the anterior part of the valve prosthesis shadows the more posterior portions, images of the valve leaflets may be suboptimal.

With suspected prosthetic valve endocarditis, the transthoracic examination may provide clues that suggest the diagnosis even when definitive findings are not present. For example, if color flow imaging is nondiagnostic due to shadowing and color flow artifacts, a careful continuous-wave Doppler examination may show a regurgitant

signal. Care is needed in assessment of the *severity* of regurgitation in this situation, and it may be prudent to state only that regurgitation is present but quantitation is not possible. Other clues to prosthetic valve dysfunction include an increased antegrade flow velocity across the prosthesis (reflecting increased antegrade volume flow due to prosthetic regurgitation) and an elevated tricuspid regurgitant jet velocity due to pulmonary hypertension.

Whenever prosthetic valve endocarditis is suspected, transesophageal imaging should be strongly considered (Figs. 14–22 to 14–24). If the transthoracic images are diagnostic, or if

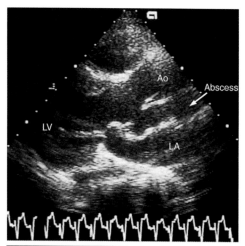

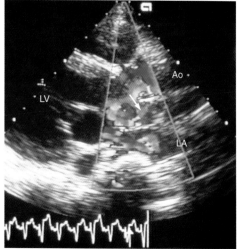

■ **FIGURE 14–22.** In a 24-year-old woman with an aortic homograft valve replacement for a previous episode of endocarditis, reinfection with *S. aureus* has resulted in a paravalvular abscess (or pseudoaneurysm) posterior to the homograft. The transthoracic parasternal long-axis view shows the abscess cavity *(top)* and color flow imaging shows flow from the aortic root into the abscess cavity *(bottom)*.

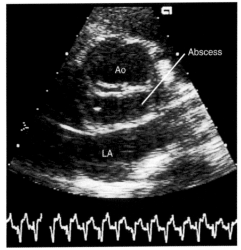

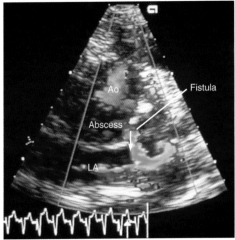

FIGURE 14–23. Short-axis views in the same patient as in Figure 13–24 show the proximity of the abscess cavity to the left atrium *(top)* and color flow Doppler shows a fistula from the abscess cavity into the left atrium *(bottom)*.

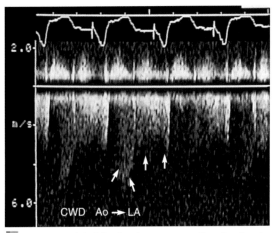

FIGURE 14–24. Continuous-wave Doppler in the same patient as in Figures 13–24 and 13–25 shows continuous high-velocity flow in systole and diastole *(arrows)* consistent with a fistula from a high-pressure (aorta) to low-pressure (left atrium) chamber.

In an individual patient, a *change* in the appearance or flow characteristics of a prosthetic valve is more diagnostic than an observation at one point in time. Review of previous studies (if available) performed when the patient clinically was well can improve the diagnostic yield of echocardiography.

CLINICAL UTILITY

Suspected Endocarditis

Although transesophageal echocardiography is more sensitive and specific than transthoracic echocardiography for detection of valvular vegetations, transthoracic echocardiography remains the initial procedure of choice in low risk patients due to the lower cost and risk of this approach (Fig. 14–25).

Transesophageal imaging clearly has a greater sensitivity for detection of vegetations and should be performed early in the disease course in high-risk patients with suspected endocarditis. High-risk patients include those with prosthetic valves, congenital heart disease, previous endocarditis, new heart failure, new atrioventricular block, and community acquired Staph bacteremia. Typically, transthoracic imaging also is needed in these patients. The transthoracic approach allows parallel alignment for continuous-wave Doppler evaluation of high-velocity flows, standard measurement of chamber dimensions, quantitation of left ventricular systolic function, and measurement of pulmonary artery pressures.

the results of transesophageal imaging will not change patient management, it may not be needed. Otherwise, this technique is warranted given its higher sensitivity and specificity for detection of prosthetic valve endocarditis, paravalvular abscess, and prosthetic mitral regurgitation.

Endocarditis rarely can result in prosthetic valve stenosis due to impingement of the infected mass on leaflet opening or to an infected pannus on the upstream side of the valve. Again, visualization of the infected mass may not be possible on transthoracic imaging. Prosthetic valve stenosis is recognized by findings of an increased transvalvular pressure gradient and a decreased valve area (by pressure half-time or by continuity equation).

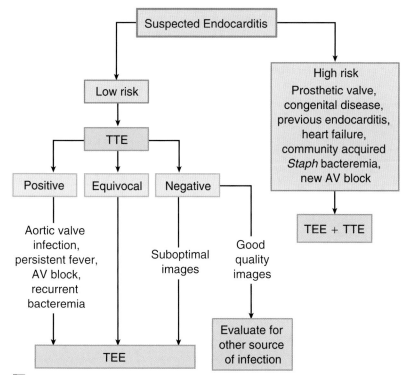

FIGURE 14–25. Flow chart for the suggested role of echocardiography in diagnosis of endocarditis. (From Otto CM: Valvular Heart Disease, 2nd ed. Philadelphia: WB Saunders, 2004, Figure 18–10.)

In lower risk patients, transesophageal echocardiography should be reserved for those with suboptimal images or equivocal findings on transthoracicic imaging. In patients with a definite vegetation on transthoracic imaging, transesophageal imaging is needed when the aortic valve is involved, due to the high risk or paravalvular abscess and in patients with persistent fever, recurrent bacteremia or new atrioventricular block—all signs of paravalvular abscess formation.

Cardiac Evaluation of the Patient with Endocarditis

In a patient with known endocarditis, an echocardiogram is an invaluable adjunct to clinical decision making concerning potential surgical intervention and prediction of short- and long-term prognosis. Echocardiography often allows clear definition of which (and how many) valves are affected.

Diagnosis of acute severe valvular regurgitation or a paravalvular abscess is a clear indication for surgical treatment. Associated left ventricular dysfunction, involvement of more than one valve, and secondary pulmonary hypertension as evaluated by echocardiography are important determinants of the surgical approach and timing of intervention.

The occurrence of a systemic embolic event generally is accepted as an indication for valve replacement; however, the importance of vegetation size and appearance by echocardiography remains controversial. If patients with embolization before echocardiography are excluded, several studies have shown a trend toward a higher incidence of systemic embolization with a vegetation diameter greater than 1 cm (Table 14–4). However, other studies contest this conclusion. Infection with *H. influenzae* and mitral valve involvement also have been shown to predict a higher rate of systemic emboli. Recent studies have suggested that sequential transesophageal echocardiographic evaluation of patients with endocarditis can predict whether antimicrobial therapy is effective by demonstrating progressive decreases in vegetation size. However, the cost-effectiveness (and patient acceptance) of this approach is unclear.

In the current era, with aggressive and prompt surgical intervention, severe regurgitation and heart failure do *not* predict mortality, since these patients undergo early valve replacement. With

TABLE 14-4

Size of Vegetation by Two-Dimensional Echocardiography versus Risk of Embolism

Study	n	Total No. of Emboli	No Veg or ≤10 mm	Veg >10 mm	P Value
Lutas, et al.	76	17	16% (8/50)	45% (9/26)	0.06[‡]
Buda, et al.*	42	14	26% (8/31)	55% (6/11)	0.08[‡]
Wann, et al.[†]	21	7	21% (3/14)	57% (4/7)	0.16[§]
Wong, et al.	31	6	20% (3/15)	19% (3/16)	0.64[§]
Jaffe, et al.	50	10	11% (2/18)	26% (8/32)	0.19[§]
Di Salvo, et al.	178	66	23% (26/111)	60% (40/67)	0.001[‡]
Total	398	120	21% (50/239)	44% (70/159)	<0.001[§]

*Excludes patients with right-sided endocarditis.
[†]Vegetation size graded qualitatively on 1+ to 3+ scale; 3+ was considered >10 mm.
[‡]Chi-square analysis.
[§]Fisher's exact test.
From Otto CM: Infective endocarditis. In: Otto CM (ed): Valvular Heart Disease, 2nd ed. Philadelphia: WB Saunders, 2004. Data from Lutas et al: Am Heart J 112:107, 1986; Buda et al: Am Heart J 112:1291, 1986; Wann et al: Circulation 60:728, 1979; Wong et al: Arch Intern Med 143:1874, 1983; Jaffe et al: J Am Coll Cardiol 12:1227, 1990; DiSalvo G et al: J Am Coll Cardiol 37:1069, 2001.

antibiotic therapy and appropriate surgical intervention, risk factors for in-hospital death are prosthetic valve infection, systemic embolism, and infection with *S. aureus*. Long-term outcome in survivors is related to the residual degree of valve damage, the effects of chronic valvular regurgitation on ventricular function and pulmonary artery pressures, and the risk of recurrent episodes of endocarditis.

SUGGESTED READING

General

1. Schiller NB: Clinical decision making in patients with endocarditis: The role of echocardiography. In: Otto CM (ed): The Practice of Clinical Echocardiography, 2nd ed. Philadelphia: WB Saunders, 2002, pp 469–500.

   Review of the current role of echocardiography in management of the patient with suspected or known endocarditis. In addition to a review of the literature, this chapter provides useful tips on the echocardiographic approach with clear illustrations.

2. Saunders GP, Yeon SB, Grunes J, et al: Impact of a specific echocardiographic report comment regarding endocarditis prophylaxis on compliance with American Heart Association recommendations. Circulation 106:300–303, 2002.

   The additional of a specific recommendation on the echocardiography report indicating whether endocarditis prophylaxis is indicated significantly improved compliance with established guidelines. Laboratories should consider making this a standard part of every echocardiography report.

3. Mylonakis E, Calderwood SB: Infective endocarditis in adults. N Engl J Med 345:1318–1330, 2001.

   Detailed review of clinical aspects of endocarditis including epidemiology, predisposing factors, microbiology, clinical symptoms *and signs, diagnosis, complications, and treatment. A very useful overview of the subject with 99 references.*

Clinical Diagnosis

4. Durack DT, Lukes AS, Bright DK: New criteria for diagnosis of infective endocarditis: Utilization of specific echocardiographic findings. Duke Endocarditis Service. Am J Med 96:200–209, 1994.

   Proposed criteria for the clinical diagnosis of endocarditis as detailed in Table 14–1 incorporate echocardiographic findings as key factor in the diagnosis. Includes validation of sensitivity and specificity of this approach compared to older diagnostic approaches. The Duke criteria are used at many medical centers.

5. Li JS, Sexton DJ, Mick N, et al: Proposed modifications to the Duke criteria for the diagnosis of infective endocarditis. Clin Infect Dis 30:633–638, 2000.

   Modification of the Duke criteria to eliminate nonspecific echocardiographic findings, add evidence for Q-fever as a major criteria, and change the major criteria for S. aureus *bacteremia to include any cause of bacteremia. Possible endocarditis is defined as one major plus one minor, or three minor criteria. Table 14–1 includes these modifications.*

6. Dodds GA, Sexton DJ, Durack DT, et al: Negative predictive value of the Duke criteria for infective endocarditis. Am J Cardiol 77:403–407, 1996.

   In 405 episodes of suspected endocarditis, 52 were classified as "rejected" endocarditis based on the Duke criteria. With clinical outcome used as the standard of reference, none of these patients subsequently developed endocarditis, although one had possible endocarditis at autopsy, indicating a negative predictive value of the Duke criteria of at least 92%.

Echocardiographic Diagnosis

7. Yvorchuk KJ, Chan KL: Application of transthoracic and transesophageal echocardiography in the diagnosis and

management of infective endocarditis. J Am Soc Echocardiogr 14:294–308, 1994.

Review article on the utility of echocardiography in patients with known or suspected endocarditis. An excellent synthesis of the literature with tables summarizing data, clear examples, and a proposed diagnostic approach; 61 references.

8. Daniel WG, Mugge A, Grote J, et al: Comparison of transthoracic and transesophageal echocardiography for detection of abnormalities of prosthetic and bioprosthetic valves in the mitral and aortic positions. Am J Cardiol 71:210–215, 1993.

Detection of prosthetic valve endocarditis was enhanced by transesophageal echocardiography. Of 148 prosthetic valves, 124 were abnormal at surgery or autopsy (33 endocarditis, 8 thrombi, and 83 degeneration). Endocarditis was correctly identified in 12 of 36 (36%) by transthoracic echocardiography and 27 of 33 (82%) by transesophageal echocardiography.

9. Lowry RW, Zoghbi WA, Baker WB, et al: Clinical impact of transesophageal echocardiography in the diagnosis and management of infective endocarditis. Am J Cardiol 73:1089–1091, 1994.

In 93 consecutive patients undergoing transesophageal echocardiography for suspected endocarditis, the negative predictive value of transesophageal echocardiography was 100% for native valves and 90% for prosthetic valves. Transesophageal echocardiography resulted in a change in the subsequent diagnostic or therapeutic plan in greater than 90% of patients.

10. Lindner JR, Case RA, Dent JM, et al: Diagnostic value of echocardiography in suspected endocarditis: an evaluation based on the pretest probability of disease. Circulation 93:730–736, 1996.

This study suggests that echocardiography is not necessary in patients with a low pretest likelihood of the diagnosis. In those with an intermediate or high pretest likelihood (positive blood cultures plus new murmur or predisposing heart disease), transthoracic echocardiography should be performed first. Transesophageal echocardiography is needed primarily when the transthoracic study is technically inadequate, indicates an intermediate probability of endocarditis, or when a prosthetic valve is present.

11. Heidenreich PA, Masoudi FA, Maini B, et al: Echocardiography in patients with suspected endocarditis: A cost-effectiveness analysis. Am J Med 107:198–208, 1999.

The effect of transthoracic (TTE) and transesophageal echocardiography (TEE) on quality adjusted life years (QALYs) was evaluated using a decision tree and Markov model. With a pretest likelihood between 4% and 60%, as commonly seen in clinical practice, TEE results in lower costs and improved outcomes compared to TTE. TTE alone was useful only in patients with a very low pretest likelihood of endocarditis.

12. Roe MT, Abramson MA, Li J, et al: Clinical information determines the impact of transesophageal echocardiography on the diagnosis of infective endocarditis by the duke criteria. Am Heart J 139:945–951, 2000.

In 114 cases of suspected endocarditis, the incremental value of TEE was examined. Compared to TTE results, superior image quality on TEE resulted in a change from probable to definite endocarditis in 11% of 80 cases of suspected native valve infection and 34% of 34 episodes of suspected prosthetic valve endocarditis. These findings emphasize the importance of TEE for accurate diagnosis of endocarditis, especially in patients with prosthetic valves.

Diagnosis of Paravalvular Abscess

13. Daniel WG, Mugge A, Martin RP, et al: Improvement in the diagnosis of abscesses associated with endocarditis by transesophageal echocardiography. N Engl J Med 324:795–800, 1991.

In 118 consecutive patients with endocarditis, 44 (37%) had surgical or autopsy evidence of abscess formation. Abscesses were more common with infection with Staphylococcus (52% of cases) and with aortic valve involvement. The hospital mortality rate in patients with an abscess was 23% versus 14% in the remainder of the study group. Transesophageal echocardiography was much more sensitive than transthoracic echocardiography for diagnosis of paravalvular abscess.

14. Karalis DG, Bansal RC, Huack AJ, et al: Transesophageal echocardiographic recognition of subaortic complications in aortic valve endocarditis: Clinical and surgical implications. Circulation 86:353–362, 1992.

Detailed description (with illustrations) of the patterns of paravalvular and subaortic abscess formation in patients with aortic valve endocarditis. The authors note that eccentric jets of mitral regurgitation in patients with aortic valve endocarditis raise the possibility of involvement (perforation) of the anterior mitral leaflet by the infectious process.

Risk of Embolic Events

15. Mügge A, Daniel WG, Frank G, Lichtlen PR: Echocardiography in infective endocarditis: Reassessment of prognostic implications of vegetation size determined by the transthoracic and the transesophageal approach. J Am Coll Cardiol 14:631–638, 1989.

In 105 patients with endocarditis, a vegetation size greater than 10 mm on transthoracic or transesophageal echocardiography was predictive of embolic events (22 of 47 with vegetation ≤10 mm, P < .01). Mitral valve endocarditis also was associated with a higher likelihood of embolism. Heart failure and survival were not related to vegetation size.

16. Steckelberg JM, Murphy JG, Ballard D, et al: Emboli in infective endocarditis: The prognostic value of echocardiography. Ann Intern Med 114:635–640, 1991.

In 207 patients with endocarditis, the likelihood of first embolic events was 6.2 per 1000 patient days (95% confidence interval, 4.2 to 9.2). The risk of embolic events was related to infection with Streptococcus viridans infections but not to vegetation size. The likelihood of embolization decreased over time, falling to 1.2 per 1000 patient days after 2 weeks of therapy.

17. Sanfilippo AJ, Picard MH, Newell JB, et al: Echocardiographic assessment of patients with infectious endocarditis: Prediction of risk for complications. J Am Coll Cardiol 18:1191–1199, 1991.

In 204 patients with endocarditis, multivariate predictors of complications (persistent fever, congestive heart failure, systemic emboli, surgery, and mortality) were vegetation size, extent, and mobility. The authors propose an echo score for vegetation appearance to predict the likelihood of complications.

18. Di Salvo G, Habib G, Pergola V, et al: Echocardiography predicts embolic events in infective endocarditis. J Am Coll Cardiol 37:1069–1076, 2001.

In 178 patients with endocarditis, embolic events occurred in 37% when a careful search for both clinical and silent embolic events was performed. On multivariate analysis, the only predictors of embolic events were vegetation length and mobility. In the 30 patients with large (>15 mm) mobile vegetations, embolic events occurred in 83%.

19. Vilacosta I, Graupner C, San Roman JA, et al: Risk of embolization after institution of antibiotic therapy for infective endocarditis. J Am Coll Cardiol 39:1489–1495, 2002.

In 217 episodes of left sided endocarditis, 13% had embolic events after initiation of antibiotic therapy (within 2 weeks in 65%). Risk factors for embolism were an increasing vegetation size despite antibiotic therapy, mitral valve involvement, infection with Staphylococcus and embolization before the onset of antibiotic therapy.

Long-term Outcome

20. Jaffe WM, Morgan DE, Pearlman AS, Otto CM: Infective endocarditis, 1983–1988: Echocardiographic findings and factors influencing morbidity and mortality. J Am Coll Cardiol 15:1227–1233, 1990.

In 70 patients with endocarditis, predictors of in-hospital mortality were prosthetic valve endocarditis, occurrence of a systemic embolic event, and infection with S. aureus. Abnormal (≥2+) valvular regurgitation was noted on transthoracic Doppler examination in 88% of patients.

21. Werner GS, Schulz R, Fuchs JB, et al: Infective endocarditis in the elderly in the era of transesophageal echocardiography: Clinical features and prognosis compared with younger patients. Am J Med 100:90–97, 1996.

Compared to younger patients, elderly patients (age >70 years) with endocarditis more often have predisposing valve conditions, including calcified and prosthetic valves, which decrease the sensitivity of transthoracic imaging for detection of valvular vegetations. The sensitivity of transthoracic echocardiography was only 45% in those older than age 70 compared to 75% in those younger than age 50 years in this study.

22. Erbel R, Liu F, Ge J, et al: Identification of high-risk subgroups in infective endocarditis and the role of echocardiography. Eur Heart J 16:588–602, 1995.

High-risk subgroups with endocarditis can be identified based on clinical and echocardiographic features. Factors associated with a poor clinical outcome include increased age, delayed diagnosis, infection with S. aureus, aortic valve involvement, large vegetations, embolic events, prosthetic valves, and failed antibiotic therapy.

23. Rohmann S, Erbel R, Darius H, et al: Prediction of rapid versus prolonged healing of infective endocarditis by monitoring vegetation size. J Am Soc Echocardiogr 4:465–474, 1991.

Increasing vegetation size during antibiotic therapy was associated with a higher rate of valve replacement, embolic events, paravalvular abscess formation, and mortality in 83 patients with echocardiographic evidence of endocarditis

24. Fowler VG, Li J, Corey R, et al: Role of echocardiography in evaluation of patients with Staphylococcus aureus

bacteremia: Experience in 103 patients. J Am Coll Cardiol 30:1072–1078, 1997.

In a consecutive series of patients with S. aureus bacteremia, definite endocarditis (Duke criteria) was present in only 25%. Transthoracic echocardiography had a low sensitivity (32%) but was 100% specific for detection of vegetations. Transesophageal echocardiography had a sensitivity of 100% and a specificity of 99% (one false-positive result). Death due to sepsis was significantly (P = .03) more likely in those with endocarditis (15%) compared to those with bacteremia alone (3%), even though evidence for eradication of the infection was similar in both groups.

25. Cabell CH, Pond KK, Peterson GE, et al: The risk of stroke and death in patients with aortic and mitral valve endocarditis. Am Heart J 142:75–80, 2001.

In 148 cases of definite endocarditis affecting the aortic (43%) or mitral (57%) valve, stroke occurred in 23% and 1-year mortality was 37%. Multivariate predictors of stroke were mitral valve involvement and vegetation length. Predictors of death were age and vegetation size.

Right-sided Endocarditis

26. Hecht SR, Berger M: Right-sided endocarditis in intravenous drug users: Prognostic features in 102 episodes. Ann Intern Med 117:560–566, 1992.

Clinical study of 132 patients with right-sided endocarditis emphasizes the high prevalence of S. aureus infection (82%), tricuspid valve involvement (96%), large vegetation size (>10 mm in 80%), and low mortality (7%) in right-sided (versus left-sided) endocarditis.

Nonbacterial Thrombotic Endocarditis

27. Roldan CA, Shively BK, Crawford MH: An echocardiographic study of valvular heart disease associated with systemic lupus erythematosus. N Engl J Med 335:1424–1430, 1996.

Valvular abnormalities were seen on echocardiography in two thirds of 69 patients with lupus. Valve thickening was most common, but vegetations were seen in 43% and significant valvular regurgitation was seen in 25%. Echocardiographic findings often changed on follow-up examination with some patients having resolution of valvular abnormalities and others having increased valve dysfunction.

28. Edoute Y, Haim N, Rinkevich D, et al: Cardiac valvular vegetations in cancer patients: A prospective echocardiographic study of 200 patients. Am J Med 102:252–258, 1997.

In 200 ambulatory patients with solid tumors, echocardiography showed valvular vegetations (most often on the aortic or mitral valve) in 19% of patients. Cardiac abnormalities were most common in patients with carcinoma of the pancreas and lung and with lymphoma. Systemic thromboembolism occurred in 11% of the total study group.

29. Roldan CA, Shively BK: Echocardiographic findings in systemic disease characterized by immune-mediated injury. In: Otto CM (ed): The Practice of Clinical Echocardiography, 2nd ed. Philadelphia: WB Saunders, 2002, pp 761–778.

Excellent summary of echocardiographic findings that might be mistaken for endocarditis including findings in patients with systemic lupus erythematosus, rheumatoid arthritis, ankylosing spondylitis, scleroderma, and other connective tissue disorders. Detailed tables and illustrations, 143 references.

Clinical Guidelines

30. Bayer AS, Bolger AF, Taubert KA, et al: Diagnosis and management of infective endocarditis and its complications. From the Ad Hoc Writing Group of the Committee on Rheumatic Fever, Endocarditis, and Kawasaki Disease; American Heart Association. Circulation 98:2936–2948, 1998.

American Heart Association scientific statement supporting use of the Duke criteria for diagnosis of infective endocarditis. The role of echocardiography is discussed in detail including a flow chart of the use of transthoracic versus transesophageal echocardiography when endocarditis is suspected. Medical and surgical therapy also are reviewed; 141 references.

The Echo Exam *Endocarditis*

Duke Criteria (Short Version)

Definite endocarditis = 2 major or
$\qquad\qquad\qquad$ 1 major + 3 minor or
$\qquad\qquad\qquad$ 5 minor criteria
Major criteria = Bactermia with a typical organism
$\qquad\qquad\quad$ Echo evidence of endocarditis
Minor criteria = Predisposing condition
$\qquad\qquad\quad$ Fever
$\qquad\qquad\quad$ Vascular phenomenon
$\qquad\qquad\quad$ Immunologic phenomenon
$\qquad\qquad\quad$ Other microbiologic evidence

Echocardiographic Approach

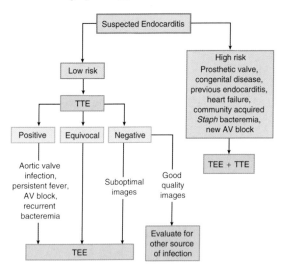

Detection of Valvular Vegetations

Start with standard views
Scan carefully between image planes
Use high-frequency transducer
Optimize image quality
Look for indirect signs (valve regurgitation, echolucent
$\quad$ space, etc.)
TEE whenever risk is high or TTE is nondiagnostic

Difficult Issues in Echo Evalation for Endocarditis

Active versus healed vegetation
Nonbacterial thrombotic endocarditis (NBTE)
Abnormal underlying valve anatomy
Prosthetic valve
Detection of abscess
Need for clinical and microbiologic correlation

Example

A 28-year-old man with a bicuspid aortic valve presents with a 2-week history of fever and fatigue. Physical examination shows a blood pressure of 120/40 mm Hg and a harsh diastolic murmur at the left sternal border. Blood cultures (3 sets) are positive for *Streptococcus viridans*. With a predisposing factor, fevers, and positive blood culture results with a typical organism, the pretest likelihood of endocarditis is very high (>90%)

Transthoracic echocardiography shows a bicuspid aortic valve with a mass on the ventricular side of the leaflets with independent motion. LV size and systolic function are normal. Color flow Doppler shows aortic regurgitation with an eccentric jet and a vena contracta width of 7 mm, CW Doppler shows a dense signal with a pressure half time of 120 msec, and there is holodiastolic flow reversal in the proximal abdominal aorta.

The TTE findings are diagnostic for endocarditis so that this patient now has two major Duke critiera and a diagnosis of *definite endocarditis*. With his bicuspid valve, there may have been some degree of underlying regurgitation. However, the normal ventricular size and the short half time of the CW aortic regurgitant jet are consistent with superimposed *acute* aortic regurgitation. Aortic regurgitation is *severe* as evidenced by a wide vena contracta and holodiastolic flow reversal in the aorta.

The following day, a prolonged PR interval (first degree AV block) is noted on the ECG and transesphageal echocardiography is performed. The TEE shows an echolucent area in the aortic annulus region consistent with abscess and the patient is referred for prompt surgical intervention.

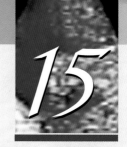

CARDIAC MASSES AND POTENTIAL CARDIAC "SOURCE OF EMBOLUS"

15

A cardiac mass is defined as an abnormal structure within or immediately adjacent to the heart. There are three basic types of cardiac masses:

- Tumor
- Thrombus
- Vegetation

Abnormal mass lesions must be distinguished from the unusual appearance of a normal cardiac structure, which may be mistakenly considered as an apparent "mass." Echocardiography allows dynamic evaluation of intracardiac masses with the advantage, compared with other tomographic techniques, that both the anatomic extent and the physiologic consequences of the mass can be evaluated. In addition, associated abnormalities (e.g., valvular regurgitation associated with a vegetation) and conditions that predispose to development of a mass (e.g., apical aneurysm leading to left ventricular thrombus or rheumatic mitral stenosis resulting in left atrial thrombus) can be assessed. Disadvantages of echocardiography include suboptimal image quality in some patients, a relatively narrow field of view compared with computed tomography (CT) or magnetic resonance imaging (MRI), and the possibility of mistaking an ultrasound artifact for an anatomic mass.

BASIC PRINCIPLES

The first step in assessing a possible cardiac mass is to ensure that the echocardiographic findings represent an actual mass rather than an ultrasound artifact. As discussed in detail in Chapter 1, artifacts can be caused by electrical interference, characteristics of the ultrasound transducer/system, or various physical factors influencing image formation from the reflected ultrasound signals. These include beam-width artifact, near-field "ring-down," and multipath artifact. Appropriate transducer selection, scanning technique, and evaluation from multiple examining windows will help to distinguish artifacts from actual anatomic structures.

Besides ultrasound artifacts, several normal structures and normal variants may be mistaken for a cardiac mass (see the Echo Exam section at the end of this chapter). In the ventricles, normal trabeculae, aberrant trabeculae or chordae (ventricular "webs" or false tendons) (Fig. 15–1), muscle bundles (such as the moderator band), or the papillary muscles may be mistaken for abnormal structures.

Valvular anatomy includes a wide range of normal variation, and the appearance of a normal (but often unrecognized) structure such as a nodule of Arantius on the aortic valve may be considered incorrectly to represent a cardiac mass.

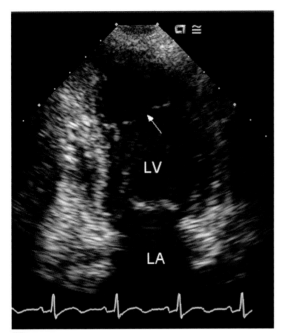

■ FIGURE 15-1. Left ventricular aberrant trabeculation or "web" seen in an apical four-chamber view in a 35-year-old woman with a normal echocardiogram.

The belly of a valve leaflet, if cut tangentially, may appear as a "mass" when it actually is a portion of the leaflet itself seen en face. In the atrium, normal ridges adjacent to the venous entry sites (Figs. 15–2 and 15–3), normal trabeculations (Fig.

15–4), postoperative changes (see Fig 9–29 post-transplant), and distortion of the free wall contour by structures adjacent to the atrium (Fig. 15–5) all may be diagnosed erroneously as a cardiac mass.

Definitive diagnosis of an intracardiac mass by echocardiography is based on:

■ Excellent image quality, which may require use of a high-frequency (5- or 7.5-MHz) short-focus transducer to evaluate the left ventricular apex from the transthoracic approach and the use of transesophageal imaging to evaluate posterior cardiac structures (e.g., left atrium, mitral valve).

■ Identification of the mass throughout the cardiac cycle, in the same anatomic region of the heart, from more than one acoustic window. This decreases the likelihood of an ultrasound artifact.

■ Knowledge of the normal structures, normal variants, and postoperative changes that may simulate a cardiac mass.

■ Integration of other echocardiographic findings (e.g., rheumatic mitral stenosis and left atrial enlargement in a patient with suspected left atrial thrombus) and clinical data in the final echocardiographic interpretation.

ECHOCARDIOGRAPHIC APPROACH

Once it is clear that a cardiac mass is present, the next step is to determine whether that mass most likely is a tumor, a vegetation, or a throm-

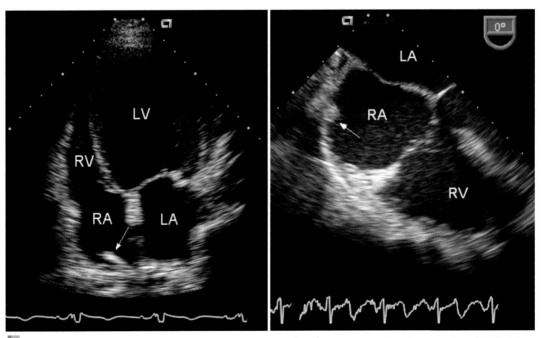

■ FIGURE 15-2. Normal appearance of the crista terminalis *(arrow)* in the right atrium in a transthoracic apical four-chamber view *(left)* and a transesophageal view *(right)*.

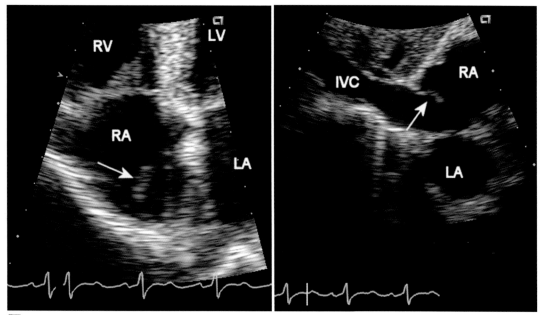

▌ FIGURE 15-3. Prominent valve at the entrance of the inferior vena cava into the right atrium seen in an apical four-chamber view *(left)* might be mistaken for a cardiac mass. A subcostal view *(right)* shows the inferior vena cava and valve more clearly.

bus. A definitive diagnosis generally cannot be made from the echocardiographic images alone, because the microscopic and bacteriologic characteristics of the structure cannot be determined. However, a reasonably secure diagnosis often can be made by integrating the clinical data, echo-

cardiographic appearance, and associated echo Doppler findings.

Infectious Cardiac Masses

Infectious cardiac masses include valvular vegetations, which are seen in patients with endocardi-

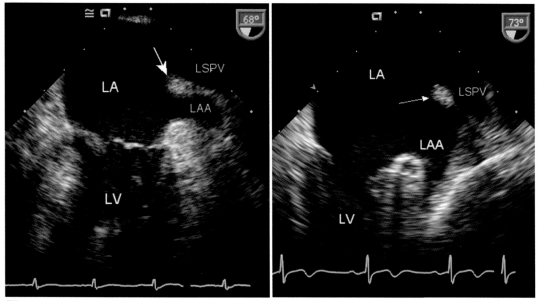

▌ FIGURE 15-4. The normal ridge between the left atrial appendage (LAA) and left superior pulmonary vein (LSPV) may be mistaken for an abnormal mass. Transesophageal views of this ridge in two different patients are shown. Sometimes this ridge is evident on transthoraic parasternal short-axis or apical two-chamber views.

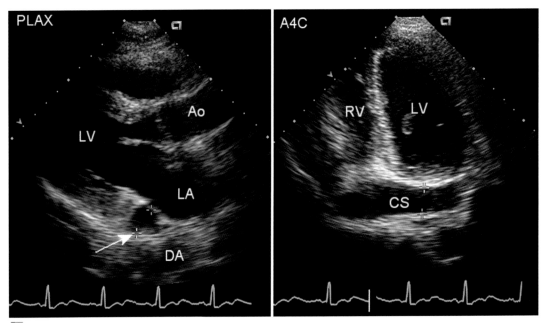

■ **FIGURE 15–5.** Persistent left superior vena cava resulting in a dilated coronary sinus (CS) posterior to the left atrium seen in a parasternal long-axis view *(left)*. If there is ultrasound "dropout" from the wall of the coronary sinus, the abnormal contour of the left atrium may be mistaken for a mass. In the posteriorly angulated apical four-chamber view, the dilated coronary sinus is seen *(right)*, which can be demonstrated to be connected to the right atrium by angulation back to a four-chamber view.

tis (bacterial or fungal). Noninfectious vegetations also occur in patients with nonbacterial thrombotic endocarditis (NBTE, or *marantic* endocarditis). Vegetations typically are irregularly shaped, attached to the upstream side of the valve leaflet (e.g., left atrial side of the mitral valve, left ventricular side of the aortic valve), and exhibit chaotic motion that differs from that of the leaflets themselves (see Figs. 14–1 and 14–2). Valvular regurgitation is a frequent but not invariable accompaniment of endocarditis. Valvular stenosis *due to* the vegetation is rare. Paravalvular abscess, which also presents as a cardiac mass, may be difficult to recognize on transthoracic imaging but can be diagnosed with a high sensitivity and specificity on transesophageal echocardiography. Infectious cardiac masses are discussed in detail in Chapter 14.

Cardiac Tumors

Nonprimary

Nonprimary cardiac tumors are approximately 20 times more common than primary cardiac tumors. Tumors can involve the heart by direct invasion from adjacent malignancies (lung, breast), by lymphatic spread, or by metastatic spread of distant disease (lymphoma, melanoma). In autopsy series of patients with a malignancy, cardiac involvement is present in approxi-

mately 10% of cases, although clinical recognition of cardiac involvement occurs less frequently. Melanoma has the highest rate of pericardial metastases, but since there are relatively few patients with melanoma, a cardiac tumor is more likely to represent a more prevalent malignancy, as shown in Table 15–1. Almost three-fourths of cardiac metastases are due to lung, breast, or hematologic malignancies. Lymphomas associated with acquired immunodeficiency syndrome have frequent and extensive cardiac involvement.

TABLE 15–1

Origin of Metastatic Cardiac Tumors in Adults (in Order of Frequency)

Lung
Lymphoma
Breast
Leukemia
Stomach
Melanoma
Liver
Colon

Data from Abraham KP, Reddy V, Gattuso P: Neoplasms metastatic to the heart: Review of 3314 consecutive autopsies. Am J Cardiovasc Pathol 3:195–198, 1990.

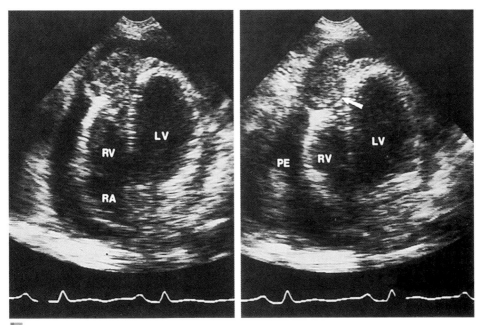

▪ **FIGURE 15–6.** Metastatic tumor to the heart with an irregular epicardial mass invading the myocardium at the right ventricular apex and an associated pericardial effusion.

Nonprimary cardiac tumors can affect the heart by

▪ invasion of the pericardium, epicardium, myocardium, or endocardium;
▪ production of biologically active substances; or
▪ toxic effects of treatment on the heart (e.g., radiation or chemotherapy).

Cardiac malignancies most often involve the pericardium and epicardium (approximately 75% of metastatic cardiac disease), presenting as a pericardial effusion, with or without tamponade physiology (Figs. 15–6 and 15–7). Because echocardiographic diagnosis of the *cause* of a pericardial effusion rarely is possible, the diagnosis of a pericardial effusion (and particularly tamponade) in a patient with a known malignancy should alert the clinician to the possibility of cardiac involvement. Confirmation of the diagnosis requires examination of pericardial fluid and, if necessary, pericardial biopsy. The differential diagnosis of a pericardial effusion in a patient with a known malignancy includes radiation pericarditis and idiopathic pericarditis (which is common in patients with cancer), as well as metastatic disease. Repeat echocardiographic evaluation of patients with a malignant pericardial effusion often is needed after the initial diagnosis for assessment of therapeutic interventions and follow-up for recurrent effusion.

Myocardial involvement by metastatic disease is less common than pericardial involvement, but

does occur, particularly with lymphoma or melanoma. Intramyocardial masses can project into or compress cardiac chambers, resulting in hemodynamic compromise. Endocardial involvement is rarely seen.

A specific type of cardiac involvement by tumor that should be recognized by the echocardiographer is extension of *renal cell carcinoma* up the

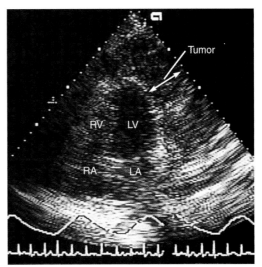

▪ **FIGURE 15–7.** Metastatic lymphoma has filled the pericardial space resulting in compression of the heart and tamponade physiology in the absence of free pericardial fluid.

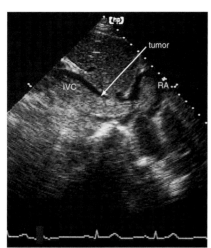

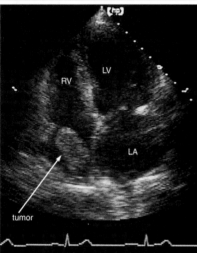

FIGURE 15–8. Renal cell carcinoma extending up the inferior vena cava (IVC) is seen on a subcostal view *(above)* and in an apical four-chamber view *(below)* protruding into the right atrium and across the tricuspid valve into the right ventricle. This tumor was resected *en bloc* at the time of surgery.

inferior vena cava (Fig. 15–8). A "fingerlike" projection of tumor may protrude into the right atrium from the inferior vena cava, and the tumor can be followed retrograde (from a subcostal approach) back to the kidney. Collaboration with the abdominal ultrasound laboratory is needed for full delineation of the tumor extent. Identification is important, because curative en bloc resection may be possible. *Uterine tumors* occasionally present in this fashion as well.

Tumors also can affect the cardiac structures indirectly, as is seen in *carcinoid heart disease* (Fig. 15–9). Metastatic carcinoid tissue in the liver produces biologically active substances, including serotonin, which cause abnormalities of the right-sided cardiac valves and endocardium. Typical

changes include thickening, retraction, and increased rigidity of the tricuspid and pulmonic valve leaflets, resulting in valvular regurgitation or, less often, valvular stenosis. Left-sided valvular involvement is rarely seen, possibly due to a lower concentration of the active molecules after passage through the lungs. While metastatic carcinoid disease is rare, the echocardiographic findings are pathognomonic and may lead to the diagnosis in a patient in whom it was not considered previously. Although only one-third of patients with carcinoid tumors have cardiac involvement, half the deaths in carcinoid patients are due to heart failure resulting from severe tricuspid regurgitation.

Primary

As for tumors elsewhere in the body, the distinction between benign and malignant primary cardiac tumors is based on pathologic examination of tissue and its tendency to invade adjacent tissue or metastasize to distant sites (Table 15–2). Although 75% of primary cardiac tumors are benign, a pathologically benign cardiac tumor can have "malignant" hemodynamic consequences if it obstructs the normal pattern of blood flow. Thus, the echocardiographic examination includes definition of both the anatomic extent of a cardiac tumor and its physiologic consequences.

BENIGN PRIMARY CARDIAC TUMORS. *Myxomas* account for 27% of primary cardiac tumors. Cardiac myxomas most often are single, arising from the fossa ovalis of the interatrial septum and protruding into the left atrium (in approximately 75% of cases) (Fig. 15–10). Other sites of origin include the right atrium (18%), the left ventricle (4%), and the right ventricle (4%). More than one site can occur in an individual patient (5% of cases).

The clinical presentation of a cardiac myxoma can include constitutional symptoms (fever, malaise), clinically evident embolic events, and symptoms of mitral valve obstruction. A myxoma also may be an unexpected finding on a study requested for other clinical indications.

A left atrial myxoma may nearly fill the left atrial chamber (Figs. 15–11 and 15–12), with prolapse of the tumor mass across the mitral annulus into the left ventricle in diastole (accounting for the tumor "plop" on auscultation). The mass often has an irregular shape characterized by protruding "fronds" of tissue or a "grape cluster" appearance. The echogenicity of the mass may be nonhomogeneous, and sometimes areas of calcification are noted.

The degree to which the tumor causes functional obstruction to left ventricular diastolic

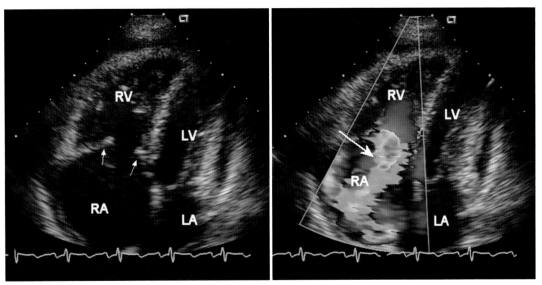

FIGURE 15–9. Carcinoid heart disease with thickening and shortening of the tricuspid leaflets *(arrows)* seen in an apical four-chamber view *(left)*. Mild stenosis and severe regurgitation of the tricuspid valve were present as seen on color flow imaging *(right)*.

filling can be evaluated qualitatively by color flow imaging and quantitatively by the pressure half-time method. Careful echocardiographic evaluation from multiple views, often including transesophageal, is needed in planning the surgical approach. Important goals of the echo examination are

■ to identify the site of tumor attachment,
■ to ensure that the tumor does not involve the valve leaflets themselves, and
■ to exclude the possibility of multiple masses.

Postoperatively, complete excision should be documented by echocardiography. Sequential

TABLE 15–2		
Primary Cardiac Tumors in Adults		
Benign		
Myxoma		27%
Lipoma		10%
Papillary fibroelastoma		10%
Hemangioma		3%
Mesothelioma of the AV node		1%
Malignant		
Angiosarcoma		9%
Rhabdomyosarcoma		5%
Mesothelioma		4%
Fibrosarcoma		3%
Malignant lymphoma		2%
Extraskeletal osteosarcoma		1%
Cysts		
Pericardial		18%
Bronchogenic		2%

AV, atrioventricular.
Data from McAllister HA, Fenoglio JJ: Tumors of the cardiovascular system. In: Atlas of Tumor Pathology, fasicle 15, second series. Bethesda, MD: Armed Forces Institute of Pathology, 1978.

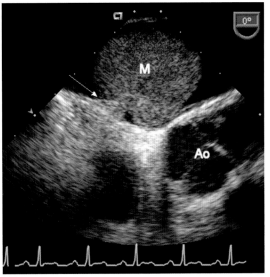

FIGURE 15–10. Left atrial myxoma arising from a thin stalk *(arrow)* attached to the fossa ovalis of the interatrial septum seen in a transesophageal view.

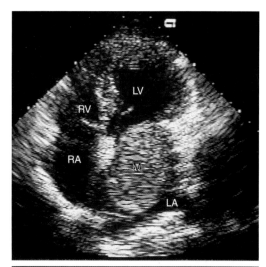

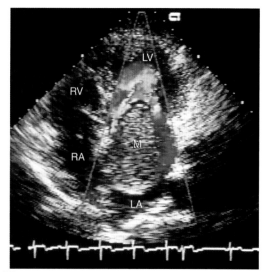

■ **FIGURE 15–12.** Color flow imaging also shows the partial obstruction to left ventricular diastolic filling due to the atrial myxoma (M) in the same patient as in Figure 15–11.

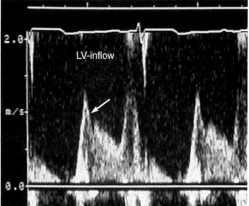

■ **FIGURE 15–11.** Large left atrial myxoma (M) in an 84-year-old woman with prolapse across the mitral annulus in diastole *(above)* in an apical four-chamber view. Doppler left ventricular filling *(below)* shows normal filling at valve opening *(arrow)* followed by obstruction as the myxoma obstructs the mitral orifice.

long-term follow-up is indicated because recurrent myxomas have been reported, particularly with a familial form of this disease, with multiple myxomas, or with a less than full-thickness excision.

The echocardiographic approach to myxomas arising in other locations is similar to that described for left atrial myxomas, except that the imaging and Doppler examination are tailored toward evaluating the specific region of tumor involvement in that patient. Again, it should be emphasized that the diagnosis of a myxoma, based on the clinical features, anatomic location, and echocardiographic appearance of the tumor, is only presumptive until confirmed histologically. A "typical" myxoma may turn out to be a meta-

static malignancy or a primary cardiac malignancy on pathologic examination. Hence the echocardiographic examination should be as complete as possible to exclude tissue invasion by the tumor, multiple sites of involvement, or atypical features.

A *papillary fibroelastoma* is a benign cardiac tumor that arises on valvular tissue, thus mimicking the appearance of a valvular vegetation. A papillary fibroelastoma appears as a small mass attached to the mitral or (less often) aortic valve with motion independent from the normal valve structures (Fig. 15–13). Unlike a vegetation, fibroelastomas are more often found on the downstream side of the valve (left ventricular side of mitral valve, aortic side of aortic valve). The histologic appearance is very similar to the smaller Lambl's excrescences, which can be seen on normal valves in the elderly. Usually a papillary fibroelastoma is of no clinical significance, but may cause consternation on the part of the physicians caring for the patient and lead to further diagnostic tests with their associated costs and complications. Occasional cases of superimposed thrombus formation resulting in systemic embolic events have been described.

Other benign cardiac tumors seen in adults include hemangiomas, and mesotheliomas of the atrioventricular node.

Lipomatous hypertrophy of the interatrial septum presents as a cardiac mass that may be mistaken for a tumor. Lipomatous hypertrophy typically involves the superior and inferior fatty portions

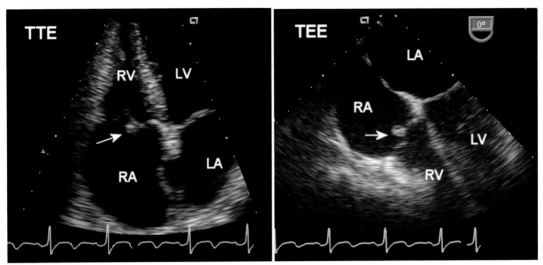

FIGURE 15-13. Small mass, suggestive of a papillary fibroelastoma *(arrow)*, attached to the septal leaflet of the tricuspid valve (with independent motion) as seen on transthoracic *(left)* and transesophageal imaging *(right)* in a 56-year-old woman referred for exercise echocardiography for atypical chest pain.

of the atrial septum, sparing the fossa ovalis region (Fig. 15–14). However, symmetric ellipsoid-shaped enlargements of the interatrial septum also have been described. If the etiology of atrial septal hypertrophy is unclear on echocardiography, CT scanning may establish the diagnosis of lipomatous hypertrophy by showing the characteristic radiographic density of adipose tissue.

MALIGNANT PRIMARY CARDIAC TUMORS. Malignant primary cardiac tumors are rare. In adults, angiosarcomas, rhabdomyosarcomas (Fig. 15–15), mesotheliomas, and fibrosarcomas are seen (see Table 15–1). The clinical presentation is variable, ranging from an "incidental" finding on echocardiography or nonspecific systemic symptoms (fever, malaise, fatigue) to signs and symptoms of cardiac tamponade. Because metastatic disease is far more likely than a primary cardiac origin, thorough evaluation must include a search for potential primary sites. Ultimately, the diagnosis depends on examination of tissue from the cardiac mass.

The echocardiographic examination focuses on

- the anatomic location and extent of the tumor involvement,
- the physiologic consequences of the tumor (e.g., valve regurgitation, chamber obliteration, obstruction), and
- associated findings (pericardial effusion, evidence of tamponade physiology).

FIGURE 15-14. Lipomatous hypertrophy *(arrows)* of the interatrial septum seen on transesophageal imaging with typical sparing of the thin fossa ovalis.

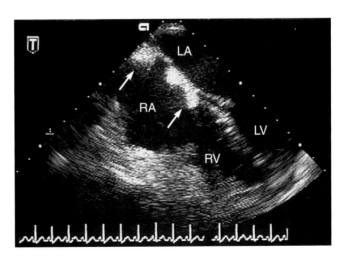

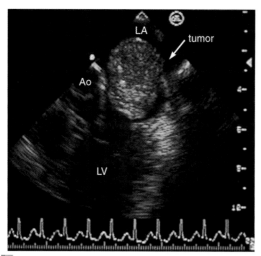

■ **FIGURE 15-15.** Large, recurrent left atrial rhabdomyosarcoma attached to the ridge between the left atrial appendage and left superior pulmonary vein. Note that this malignant tumor appears similar on echocardiography to a benign myxoma.

Along with other imaging techniques, the echocardiographic examination may help guide therapy by determining whether the tumor is resectable or whether palliative cardiac procedures are likely to be beneficial. Specific attention also is directed toward possible involvement of the valves, coronary arteries, or conducting system.

Technical Considerations/Alternate Approaches

Although echocardiography has definite advantages for evaluating cardiac tumors, it has significant disadvantages as well. These include (1) poor acoustic access, resulting in suboptimal image quality, which limits the confidence with which tumor location and extent can be defined or

results in a missed diagnosis (transesophageal imaging may obviate this limitation in some patients); (2) the need for a careful and meticulous examination to detect and fully evaluate the cardiac tumor (as for other applications, echocardiography is operator dependent, and a significant learning curve for obtaining optimal data can be observed); and (3) the limited "field of view" inherent in echocardiography (i.e., structures adjacent to the heart in the mediastinum and lung are difficult to evaluate). Other tomographic imaging techniques, specifically CT and MRI, have the advantage of a wide field of view so that the relationship between cardiac and extracardiac tumor involvement can be evaluated. Often judicious use of both echocardiographic techniques (to assess cardiac involvement in detail and to evaluate the physiologic consequences of the tumor mass) and CT or MRI (to assess potential extracardiac involvement) may be needed in an individual patient for optimal clinical decision making. Both CT and MRI may provide data on the tissue characteristics of the abnormal mass, which currently cannot be obtained with echocardiography (Fig. 15–16).

Left Ventricular Thrombus

Predisposing Conditions

Thrombus formation in the left ventricle tends to occur in regions of blood stasis or low-velocity blood flow. The most familiar example of blood flow stasis in the left ventricle is a ventricular aneurysm, in which low-velocity swirling blood flow patterns are seen. Stasis also may occur with less severe segmental wall motion abnormalities (e.g., apical akinesis) and with diffuse left ventricular dysfunction (e.g., dilated cardiomyopathy). Left ventricular thrombus formation is extremely rare in the absence of an akinetic or dyskinetic

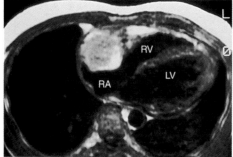
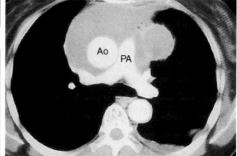

■ **FIGURE 15–16.** *Left,* MRI scan in a patient with angiosarcoma shows a large nonhomogeneous right atrial mass. *Right,* CT scan at the level of the pulmonary artery and ascending aorta in a different patient (who also had an angiosarcoma) shows extensive intrapericardial tumor involvement. These cases illustrate the advantage of the wide field of view of MRI and CT techniques compared with the narrow field of view of echocardiography.

apex or diffuse left ventricular dysfunction. Thrombus formation also often accompanies a left ventricular pseudoaneurysm. In this case, the thrombus lines an area of left ventricular rupture that has been contained by the pericardium (see Fig. 8–29).

Even when a definite left ventricular thrombus is not seen on an echocardiographic examination, the likelihood of thrombus formation remains high in patients with left ventricular aneurysm, apical akinesis, or diffuse left ventricular systolic dysfunction with an ejection fraction less than 20%. Doppler analysis of apical flow patterns has been suggested to help identify which of these patients are at highest risk of thrombus formation. Evidence of apical flow stasis or of continuous swirling of flow around the apex is thought to identify patients at particular risk for apical thrombus.

Identification of Left Ventricular Thrombi

The sensitivity of echocardiography for detecting left ventricular thrombi is extremely operator-dependent (Table 15–3). A careful and thorough examination requires not only standard views but also angulated apical views and the use of higher-frequency short-focus transducers to improve near-field resolution. It is advantageous to use a 5- or 7.5-MHz transducer from the standard apical four-chamber window and also to move the transducer slightly laterally while angulating it medially to obtain an apical short-axis view. Scanning across the apex in several views usually allows distinction of apical thrombi from prominent apical trabeculations or false tendons, which are bright linear structures that attach to mural trabeculae. Thrombus is often (though not always) somewhat more echogenic than the underlying myocardium, and has a contour distinct from the endocardial border.

The diagnosis of left ventricular thrombus is most secure when an echogenic mass is seen with a convex surface that is not a "ring-down" artifact, is clearly distinct from the endocardium, and is located in a region of abnormal wall motion (Fig. 15–17). The diagnosis of laminated thrombus is more of a problem unless a clear demarcation between the thrombus and the underlying myocardium is seen, but it can be suspected when the apex appears "rounded" and akinetic with apparent excessively thick apical myocardium.

Clinical Implications

In some cases, apical images are suboptimal despite careful examination technique. In this situation, definite exclusion of apical thrombus may not be possible. Even so, clinical management (e.g., chronic anticoagulation) may depend more

---

TABLE 15–3

Sensitivity and Specificity of Diagnostic Tests for Intracardiac Thrombus Formation

Test	Sensitivity	Specificity
LA thrombus		
Echo-TTE*	59–63%	95–99%
Echo-TEE[†]	100%	100%
Radionuclide angiography	67%	54%
CT[‡]	100%	91%
Angiography[‡]	70%	88%
LV thrombus		
Echo-TTE[§]	92–95%	86–88%
Radionuclide angiography[11]	77%	88%
MRI[¶]	93%	85%
Indium-111 platelet scintigraphy[#]	71%	100%

*Shrestha et al: Am J Cardiol 48:954–960, 1981; Chiang et al: J Ultrasound Med 6:525–529, 1987; Bansal et al: Am J Cardiol 64:243–246, 1989.
[†]Aschenberg et al: JACC 7, 163–166, 1986; Olson et al: J Am Soc Echo 5:52–56, 1992.
[‡]Tomoda et al: Am Heart J 100: 306, 1980.
[§]Visser et al: Chest 83:228–232, 1983; Stratton et al: Circulation 66:156–165, 1982.
[11]Stratton et al: Am J Cardiol 48:565–572, 1981.
[¶]Sechtem et al: Am J Cardiol 64:1195–1199, 1989.
[#]Stratton et al: Am J Cardiol 47:874–881, 1981; Seabold et al: J Am Coll Cardiol 9:1057–1066, 1987.
LA, Left atrium; LV, left ventricle; MRI, magnetic resonance imaging; TEE, transesophageal echocardiography; TTE, transthoracic echocardiography.

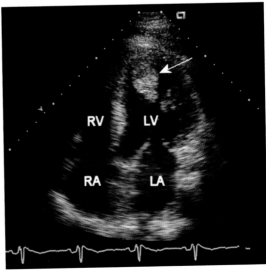

▪ **FIGURE 15–17.** Protruding thrombus *(arrows)* in an akinetic apex in a patient with a dilated cardiomyopathy seen in an apical four-chamber view.

on assessment of overall left ventricular function or the presence of an apical aneurysm than on the presence or absence of an echocardiographically documented thrombus.

The presence of a left ventricular thrombus on echocardiographic examination is a strong predictor of subsequent embolic events, particularly when the thrombus protrudes into the ventricular cavity or shows independent mobility. Sessile, nonprotruding thrombi may have lower embolic potential.

Alternate Approaches

Transthoracic echocardiography is the clinical procedure of choice for identification of left ventricular thrombi. Transesophageal imaging rarely is helpful and may be less sensitive, because the apex may not be depicted in standard image planes and the left ventricular apex is at a considerable distance from the transducer, thereby limiting resolution of structural detail. Left ventricular contrast angiography and radionuclide ventriculography both have a low sensitivity and specificity for diagnosing left ventricular thrombus. In the research setting, indium 114–labeled platelets with gamma-camera imaging have shown a high specificity, but this approach is not available for routine clinical use.

Left Atrial Thrombus

Predisposing Factors

Left atrial thrombi tend to form when there is stasis of blood flow in the left atrium. In general, low-velocity flow in the left atrium is associated with

- atrial enlargement,
- mitral valve disease, and
- atrial fibrillation.

The highest incidence of left atrial thrombus is in patients with rheumatic mitral stenosis and atrial fibrillation. However, in the presence of mitral stenosis or poor left ventricular function, even patients in sinus rhythm and those with only modest left atrial enlargement can have left atrial thrombi. Left atrial thrombi are less common in patients with mitral regurgitation, presumably because the high-velocity regurgitant jet mechanically disrupts the area of blood stasis within the left atrium.

Identification of Left Atrial Thrombi

Visualization of left atrial thrombi using transthoracic echocardiography is limited by two factors:

1. The left atrium is in the far field of the image from both parasternal and apical windows,

thus limiting resolution of left atrial structures and possible thrombi.
2. A large percentage of left atrial thrombi are found in the left atrial appendage, which is difficult to image from the transthoracic approach.

In some patients, the left atrial appendage can be imaged from a parasternal approach, starting in the short-axis view at the aortic valve level and angulating the transducer inferiorly and laterally to demonstrate the triangular appendage just inferior to the pulmonary artery. From the apical two-chamber view, the left atrial appendage may be visualized by slight superior angulation of the transducer. If a discrete echogenic mass is seen in the left atrium of a patient with mitral stenosis and atrial fibrillation, the specificity of this finding for left atrial thrombus is very high (Fig. 15–18). Of course, the differential diagnosis includes tumor, but this possibility is much less likely in this setting. Nonetheless, the sensitivity of transthoracic echocardiography for detection of left atrial thrombus remains modest at best. If *no* left atrial thrombus is seen in a patient in whom the diagnosis is suspected, a transthoracic echo study certainly does *not* exclude this possibility.

Transesophageal imaging has a much greater sensitivity and a high negative predictive value for the diagnosis of left atrial thrombi. Hence, transesophageal evaluation should be considered when the presence or absence of left atrial thrombus is important for patient management. From the transesophageal approach, the left atrium lies close to the transducer, and usually it can be demonstrated clearly with a 5- or 7.5-MHz transducer in at least two orthogonal views. Optimally, the left atrial appendage is evaluated by centering the appendage in the image plane at the 0° transducer position, using a small field of view and a high-frequency transducer. Then the image plane is slowly rotated through 180°, keeping the atrial appendage centered in the image, to evaluate for possible thrombus. In addition, the body of the left atrium and atrial septal region are evaluated using rotational scanning from 0° to 180° from a high esophageal position (Fig. 15–19).

Stasis of blood flow may be seen on transesophageal imaging as "spontaneous" echo contrast, that is, echogenic reflections from the low-velocity blood flow appearing as white swirls on the echocardiographic image (Fig. 15–20). While the appearance of "spontaneous" contrast depends on technical factors such as transducer frequency and instrument gain, as well as the pattern of blood flow, it clearly is associated with an increased risk of left atrial thrombus formation.

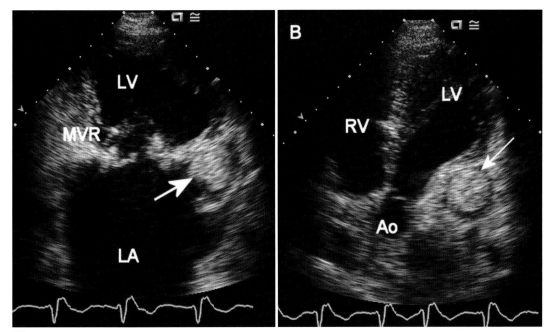

■ FIGURE 15–18. Transthoracic apical two-chamber view *(left)* showing a definite thrombus *(arrow)* in the left atrial appendage. The thrombus can also be seen in the atrial appendage in an anterioly angulated apical four-chamber view *(right)*. MVR, mitral valve replacement.

An increased risk of embolic complications that appears to be independent of associated atrial thrombus also has been reported. Doppler recordings of the pattern of blood flow in the left atrial appendage also may be helpful in identifying patients at highest risk of thrombus formation (Fig. 15–21). With a pulsed Doppler sample volume positioned approximately 1 cm from the entry of the appendage into the body of the left atrium, a normal contraction velocity is about

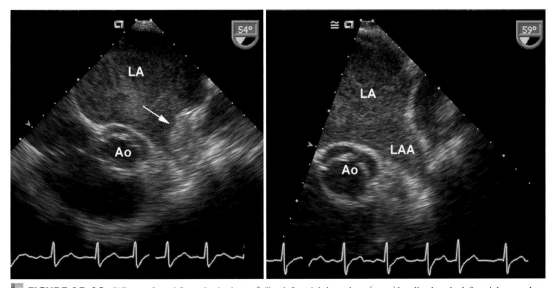

■ FIGURE 15–19. When referred for valvuloplasty *(left)*, a left atrial thrombus *(arrow)* localized to the left atrial appendage was seen on transesophageal echocardiography in a patient with mitral stenosis and atrial fibrillation. After 3 months of anticoagulation *(right)*, spontaneous contrast in the left atrium persists but there now is no thrombus. (From Otto CM: Valvular Heart Disease, 2nd ed. Philadelphia: WB Saunders, 2004, Fig. 10–4.)

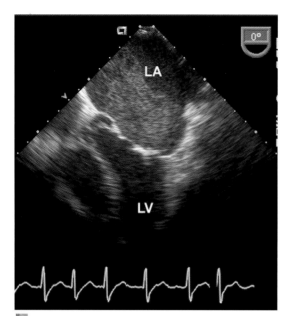

■ FIGURE 15–20. Spontaneous contrast in the left atrium seen on transesophageal echocardiography in a patient with severe rheumatic mitral stenosis and atrial fibrillation. This patient also had laminated thrombus in the body of the left atrium despite long-term anticoagulation. (From Otto CM: Valvular Heart Disease, 2nd ed. Philadelphia: WB Saunders, 2004, Fig. 10–3.)

0.4 m/s; values less than this are asssociated with an increased risk of thrombus formation.

Prognosis/Clinical Implications

The importance of a left atrial thrombus depends on the clinical setting. In a patient with new atrial fibrillation and an embolic stroke, the most likely cause of the stroke is a left atrial thrombus whether or not one is actually imaged, and thus the demonstration of a left atrial thrombus would be unlikely to change clinical management. In contrast, in a patient with rheumatic mitral stenosis, the presence of a left atrial thrombus is a contraindication to mitral balloon commissurotomy.

Alternate Approaches

While few direct comparisons of echocardiography versus CT or MRI have been performed, these imaging modalities have been reported to have a high sensitivity for detection of left atrial thrombus.

Right Heart Thrombi

Formation of thrombi in the right side of the heart is rare, although it has been reported in cases of severe right ventricular dilation and systolic dysfunction. A more likely source of thrombi seen within the right side of the heart is venous thrombi that have embolized and become entrapped in the tricuspid valve apparatus or right ventricular trabeculations during passage from the peripheral veins toward the pulmonary artery (Fig. 15–22). Thrombi also can form on indwelling catheters or pacer wires. While thrombi in the right side of the heart can sometimes be demonstrated by meticulous transthoracic imaging (Fig. 15–23), transesophageal echo is better able to resolve the presence, extent, and attachment of right-sided heart thrombi.

When mobile echogenic targets are seen within the right heart chambers, it is important to distinguish thrombi from Eustachian valve remnants, microbubbles, or reverberation artifacts. Eustachian valve remnants, which are persistent

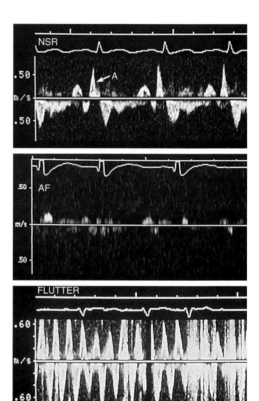

■ FIGURE 15–21. Left atrial appendage blood flow pattern recorded on transesophageal echocardiography in sinus rhythm *(top)*, atrial fibrillation *(middle)*, and atrial flutter *(bottom)*. Notice that both the P wave in sinus rhythm and the flutter waves are associated with a flow velocity out of the atrial appendage greater than 40 cm/s. In contrast, only very low flow velocities are seen in atrial fibrillation leading to stasis of blood in the atrial appendage. AF, atrial fibrillation; NSR, normal sinus rhythm.

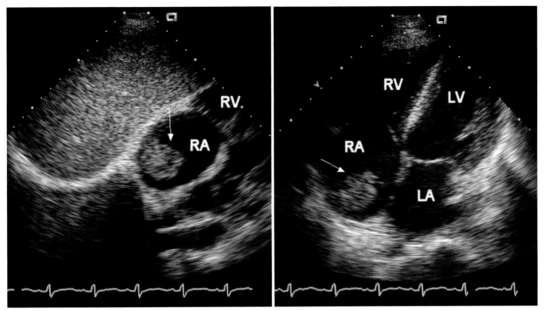

■ **FIGURE 15–22.** Right atrial thrombus *(arrows)* seen on a subcostal *(left)* and apical four-chamber view *(right)*. This may represents a thrombus-in-transit from a peripheral venous thrombosis.

portions of the embryologic valves of the sinus venosus, are typically mobile, thin linear structures attached at the junction of the inferior or superior cavae and the right atrial cavity. They may be extensive and can cross the atrium, attaching to the fossa ovalis, sometimes referred to as a Chiari network. They do not extend antegrade to cross the tricuspid valve in diastole, however. Microbubbles, which are encapsulated gas bubbles that can be seen in patients with indwelling venous access, appear as discrete echogenic targets that are usually located in different parts of the heart during successive cycles.

CARDIAC SOURCE OF EMBOLUS

Basic Principles

In a patient with a suspected cardiac origin of a systemic embolic event, echocardiographic evaluation is directed toward one or all of the following:

- Identification of an abnormal intracardiac mass (e.g., left ventricular thrombus, left atrial tumor, valvular vegetation),
- Identification of an abnormality that may predispose the patient to development of intracardiac thrombi (e.g., left ventricular aneurysm, mitral stenosis, atrial flow stasis),
- Identification of a cardiac abnormality that may serve as a potential conduit for systemic embolism (patent foramen ovale, atrial septal defect), or

- Evaluation for aortic atheroma, with or without protruding thombus.

Note that echocardiographic evaluation *after* an index embolic event may fail to demonstrate a

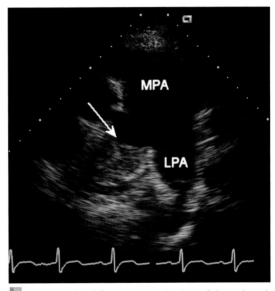

■ **FIGURE 15–23.** Transthoracic view of the main pulmonary artery (MPA) with bifurcation into the right and left pulmonary artery (LPA) demonstrates an echodensity nearly filling the right pulmonary artery *(arrow)* in this 63-year-old woman with recurrent pulmonary emboli referred for surgical thrombectomy.

cardiac thrombus even if it was the etiology of the clinical event, because now the thrombus has embolized and is no longer in the heart. Recurrent intracardiac thrombus formation may not yet have occurred.

Identifiable Cardiac Sources of Emboli

In patients with an abnormal intracardiac mass on echocardiography in the aftermath of a recent systemic embolic event, the likelihood is very high that a portion of the mass embolized, thereby causing the clinical event. Cardiac masses known to be associated with clinical systemic embolic events include

■ valvular vegetations,
■ left ventricular and atrial thrombi, and
■ cardiac tumors (especially left atrial myxomas).

Other potential pathways for systemic embolization (patent foramen ovale) and possible cardiac sources (atrial septal aneurysm, aortic atherosclerosis) are discussed in the following section.

In patients with suspected systemic embolic events, a definite cardiac source is documented by transthoracic echocardiography in approximately 10% to 15% of sequential cases. To some extent, the low prevalence of a definite source may relate to imaging *after* the event (when the mass is no longer in the heart). On the other hand, in many patients the source of embolus may have been noncardiac (e.g., atheromas with or without superimposed thrombus in the carotid arteries or ascending aorta), or the intracardiac thrombi may have embolized soon after formation. In this latter group, it is especially important to search for conditions that predispose to intracardiac thrombus formation, even though an intracardiac thrombus is not identified at the time of the examination.

Predisposing Conditions

Apical aneurysms have a high incidence of associated thrombus formation. Other segmental wall motion abnormalities and diffuse left ventricular systolic dysfunction also predispose to left ventricular thrombus formation. A left ventricular *pseudoaneurysm* is almost invariably accompanied by thrombus lining the pseudoaneurysm cavity.

Rheumatic mitral stenosis is associated with left atrial thrombus formation. *Atrial fibrillation,* even when it occurs without coexisting mitral valve disease, is strongly associated with systemic embolic events, presumably due to left atrial thrombi. In a patient with a systemic embolic event and either paroxysmal or sustained atrial fibrillation, left atrial thrombus formation is so likely that even if transesophageal echocardiography fails to demonstrate a left atrial clot, it still is appropriate to treat the patient with systemic anticoagulants to prevent recurrent atrial thrombus formation.

Intracardiac thrombi may occur in patients with *congenital heart disease*, particularly those with atrial dilation or ventricular dysfunction. Patients with a large atrial septal defect are at risk for "paradoxical" systemic embolization of peripheral venous thrombi. Thrombi can pass from the right to the left atrium even when the shunt is predominantly left to right, owing to streaming of flow or transient shifts in the right-to-left atrial pressure gradient. While patients with Eisenmenger's complex and a large ventricular septal defect are at risk of systemic embolization from peripheral venous thrombus formation, such paradoxical embolization is unlikely when the ventricular septal defect is small and there is a large pressure difference between the left and right ventricles.

Prosthetic valves are another potential source of embolic events; the incidence of clinical events is higher with mechanical compared with tissue valves. Demonstration of small thrombi on prosthetic valves is difficult even with transesophageal imaging, due to shadowing and reverberations from the prosthetic leaflets and sewing ring. Hence, the diagnosis often is presumptive when there is evidence of suboptimal anticoagulation at the time of the event or when other causes for the clinical event have been excluded even if the level of anticoagulation appears to have been adequate. In these patients, the primary goals of the echocardiographic examination are to assess prosthetic valve function (because significant thrombus may result in stenosis and/or regurgitation) and to exclude other intracardiac sources of thrombus formation (e.g., associated left ventricular systolic dysfunction).

Transesophageal echocardiography provides imaging of atrial structures in more detail and has led to the recognition of other anatomic variants and disease processes that may be associated with systemic embolic events:

■ Patent foramen ovale
■ Interatrial septal aneurysm
■ A swirling pattern of blood flow in the left atrium in the absence of an exogenous "con-

trast" agent (thought to represent flow stasis and often called *spontaneous contrast*)

■ Atherosclerosis in the aorta

A *patent foramen ovale* is present in 25% to 35% of unselected patients at autopsy. During fetal development, incomplete closure of the interatrial septum shunts oxygenated placental blood from the right to left atrium and then to the brain. This potential interatrial communication fuses within the first few days after birth in most individuals. If the flap valve covering the fossa ovalis remains unfused, there usually is no passage of blood across the interatrial septum. The "flap" is functionally closed because left atrial pressure normally exceeds right atrial pressure. However, if right atrial pressure transiently exceeds left atrial pressure (as during a cough or the Valsalva maneuver), or if right atrial pressure chronically exceeds left atrial pressure (e.g., after pulmonary embolization or with chronic lung disease), there can be right-to-left passage of blood (or thrombi) across the interatrial septum.

Echocardiographic demonstration of a patent foramen ovale is possible with color flow Doppler imaging from a transesophageal approach in only about 5% to 10% of patients, with a lesser number detected by transthoracic color Doppler imaging. Detection of a patent foramen is enhanced by intravenous injection of echo contrast material (such as agitated saline solution) providing opacification of the right-sided heart structures. Passage of contrast across the interatrial septum is seen as bright echo contrast in the left atrium within one to three beats of its appearance in the right atrium (Fig. 15–24). It is important to use a view in which the contrast effect does not obscure identification of microbubbles in the left side of the heart. Often the site of origin of the contrast in the left atrium can be identified on frame-by-frame analysis. Using echo contrast, a patent foramen is detectable at rest in approximately 5% of the general population. When maneuvers to transiently increase right atrial pressure are performed simultaneously with contrast injection, the prevalence of detectable patent foramen ovale by contrast transesophageal echocardiography increases to approximately 25%—similar to the incidence at autopsy.

Accurate detection of a patent foramen ovale is more likely on transesophageal imaging due to improved image quality (Fig. 15–25). However, contrast injections still are needed to detect all cases. Passage of very small microbubbles through the pulmonary capillaries can occur; these typically appear in the left atrium via the pulmonary veins late after the appearance of contrast material in the right atrium. The examiner should evaluate whether contrast material

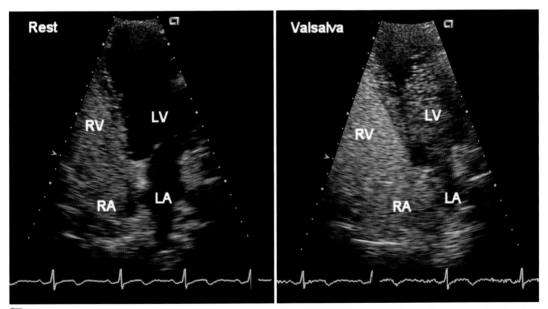

FIGURE 15–24. Patent foramen ovale on transthoracic echocardiography. At rest *(left)*, saline contrast fills the right heart with no evidence of contrast in the left heart. After a second contrast injection during Valsalva maneuver, contrast material is seen in the left atrium and ventricle within three beats of appearance of contrast material in the right heart.

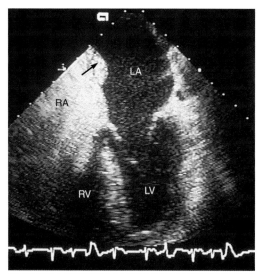

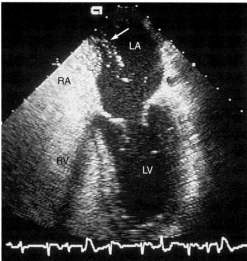

■ **FIGURE 15–25.** Atrial septal aneurysm *(top)* with a patent foramen ovale *(bottom)* demonstrated on transesophageal echocardiography in a four-chamber view after injection of agitated saline solution in peripheral vein. Small microbubbles *(arrow)* are seen traversing the defect from the opacified right into the unopacified left atrium.

in the left atrium detected on transesophageal imaging passed across the interatrial septum or reflects transpulmonary passage. With an atrial septal defect or patent foramen ovale, contrast material appears in the left atrium within three beats of its appearance in the right heart. With transpulmonary passage, contrast material is seen in the left heart after more than three beats.

In young patients (<45 years) with transient ischemic attacks or cerebrovascular events, a higher incidence of patent foramen ovale is found

than in the general population, suggesting that passage of thrombi across the atrial septum may be a significant cause of systemic embolic events in these patients. This diagnosis is most secure in a patient with a patent foramen ovale when a peripheral venous source of thrombi is also identified. Some centers advocate closure of a patent foramen ovale in a patient with a systemic embolic event. Intracardiac or transesophageal echocardiography may be used to monitor percutaneous device closure of patent foramen ovales or atrial septal defects (Fig. 15–26).

An *interatrial septal aneurysm* is defined as a transient bulging of the fossa ovalis region of the interatrial septum (total excursion from the septal plane) greater than 15 mm in the absence of chronically elevated left or right atrial pressure (Fig. 15–27). Septal aneurysms are associated with a high likelihood (up to 90%) of associated fenestration. Until recently, the diagnosis rarely was made from transthoracic echo imaging due to suboptimal image quality, and this finding was thought to be of little clinical significance. The excellent views of the interatrial septum on transesophageal echocardiography have resulted in an increasing recognition of this anatomic variant. Several investigators have suggested a possible relationship between the presence of an atrial septal aneurysm and an increased risk of systemic embolic events.

"*Spontaneous*" *contrast* is seen in the left atrium when there is stasis of blood flow. It is seen more often on transesophageal than transthoracic imaging due to the higher transducer frequency and the closer proximity of the left atrium when interrogated from the esophagus but can be seen on transthoracic imaging in some patients. Spontaneous contrast is associated with left atrial enlargement and left atrial thrombus formation, and it may be a marker for a "prethrombotic" state when definite atrial thrombi are not seen. In extreme cases of spontaneous contrast in mitral stenosis patients, the jet of diastolic blood flow across the stenotic mitral orifice can be seen on 2D imaging due to the contrast effect.

Spontaneous contrast can be seen in the left ventricle when there is stasis of blood flow, such as in the region of an apical aneurysm. Spontaneous contrast also is observed frequently in patients with mechanical prosthetic valves. Here the mechanism of spontaneous contrast formation may be different, relating to the mechanical impact of the valve occluder during closure resulting in microcavitation or liberation of gas from solution. Of course, patients with mitral prosthetic valves also may have stasis of blood flow in the left atrium if long-standing disease

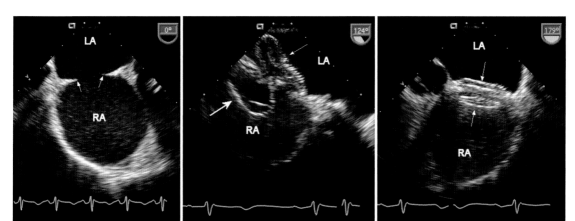

■ **FIGURE 15–26.** Transesophageal echocardiography during placement of a percutaneous atrial septal defect closure device shows: (1) the secundum atrial septal defect *(left)*, (2) the device across the defect with the left atrial side being pulled into position *(arrow)* and the right atrial side being deployed *(middle)*, and (3) closure of the defect with full deployment of both the left and right atrial sides of the device *(right)*.

has resulted in left atrial enlargement and atrial fibrillation.

Indications for Echocardiography in Patients with Systemic Embolic Events

Current understanding of potential cardiac etiologies for systemic embolism is incomplete, and there is considerable controversy as to the indications for transthoracic and transesophageal echocardiography in patients with suspected systemic embolic events. In patients with embolic events, the prevalence of patent foramen ovale is about 30%, compared to a prevalence of 10% in control subjects. Aortic atheromas (see Chapter 16) are seen in 20% of patients with embolic events, compared to 4% of control subjects. Other echocardiographic findings in patients with embolic events include left atrial thrombus in approximately 9%, spontaneous con-

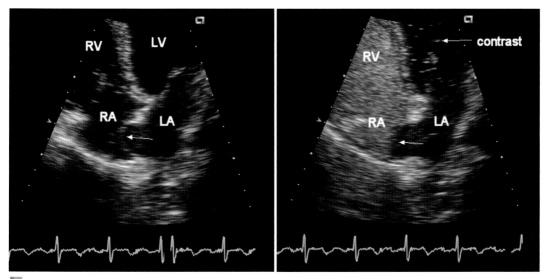

■ **FIGURE 15–27.** Incidental finding of an atrial septal aneurysm *(arrow)* in an elderly patient seen in a transthoracic apical four-chamber view *(left)*. Peripheral venous injection of agitated saline to provide a contrast effect *(right)* shows opacification of the right heart with a few microbubbles seen in the left heart, consistent with a fenestration in the atrial septal aneurysm.

trast in approximately 17%, and atrial septal aneurysm in 13%. The prevalence of thse findings is highest in patients with cryptogenic stroke (e.g., no obvious primary cerebrovascular disease or other etiology). The potential cause-and-effect relationship between some of these echocardiographic findings and clinical embolic events remains controversial as discussed in the Suggested Reading section.

Current ACC/AHA guidelines recommend echocardiography in patients with neurologic or other vascular occlusive events:

■ when there is abrupt occlusion of a major peripheral or visceral artery in patients of any age,

■ in younger patients (<45 years) with a cerebrovascular embolic event,

■ in older patients with a neurologic event without other evidence of cerebrovascular disease, and

■ in patients in whom the clinical therapeutic decision would be altered based on the echocardiographic results.

The use of echocardiography in older patients with cerebrovascular disease of questionable significance or with other evident causes for the cerebrovascular event remains controversial. If transthoracic studies are unrevealing, transesophageal imaging should be performed, given its higher sensitivity for diagnosis of a patent foramen ovale, left atrial thrombus, interatrial septal aneurysm, valvular vegetation, and small intracardiac tumors.

SUGGESTED READING

General Reviews

1. Waller BF (ed): Pathology of the Heart and Great Vessels. New York: Churchill-Livingstone, 1988.
   Multiauthor textbook of cardiac pathology in the current era emphasizing surgical findings. Chapters are included on prosthetic valve dysfunction, endomyocardial biopsy, and diseases of the great vessels, as well as valvular heart disease and cardiac tumors.

2. Becker AE, Anderson RH: Cardiac Pathology: An Integrated Text and Colour Atlas. New York: Raven Press, 1982.
   An atlas of cardiac pathology with excellent illustrations and concise descriptions.

3. Chen EW, Redberg RF: Echocardiographic evaluation of the patient with a systemic embolic event. In: Otto CM (ed): The Practice of Clinical Echocardiography, 2nd ed. Philadelphia: WB Saunders, 2002, pp 806–828.
   Review of role of echocardiography in management of patients with systemic embolic events. Topics include left atrial thrombus, spon-

taneous echo contrast, Chiari's network, mitral valve strands, intracardiac tumors, papillary fibroelastomas, thoracic aortic debris, atrial septal aneurysm, and patent foramen ovale. Includes systematic review of the literature, examples of transthoracic and transesophageal findings, and 204 references.

Cardiac Tumors

4. Salcedo EE, Cohen GI, White RD, Davison MB: Cardiac tumors: Diagnosis and management. Curr Prob Cardiol 17:75–137, 1992.
   Review of the clinical aspects of diagnosis and management of cardiac tumors; 174 references.

5. Hancock EW: Neoplastic pericardial disease. Clin Cardiol 8:673–682, 1990.
   Review article focusing on the presentation and management of malignant pericardial disease; 43 references.

6. Abraham KP, Reddy V, Gattuso P: Neoplasms metastatic to the heart: Review of 3314 consecutive autopsies. Am J Cardiovasc Pathol 3:195–198, 1990.
   Autopsy study (n = 3314) with malignant disease in 24% (n = 806) and cardiac involvement in 12% of these cases (n = 95). Analysis of frequency of primary tumors. Used as the source of data for Table 15–2.

7. Klatt EC, Heitz DR: Cardiac metastases. Cancer 65:1456–1459, 1990.
   A large autopsy series of patients with a malignancy (n = 1029) with a rate of cardiac involvement of 11%. In this study, the lung was the most common primary tumor site (36%). More than 75% of metastatic cardiac disease involved the epicardium, and 34% of such patients had a pericardial effusion.

8. Klarich KW, Enriquez-Sarano M, Gura GM, et al: Papillary fibroelastoma: Echocardiographic characteristics for diagnosis and pathologic correlation. J Am Coll Cardiol 30:784–790, 1997.
   At the Mayo Clinic, 54 patients with papillary fibroelastomas seen on echocardiography were identified over a 15-year period. Pathologic confirmation of the diagnosis was available in 17 patients. On echocardiography, papillary fibroelastomas typically were small (about 1 cm in diameter on average), pedunculated, mobile masses attached to valves (60%) or other endocardial surfaces (40%). Clinically, valve dysfunction was rare and most patients were asymptomatic. Overall, 12 of 54 (22%) patients had either a history of or a subsequent embolic neurologic event.

Left Ventricular Thrombi

9. Stratton JR, Lighty GW Jr, Pearlman AS, Ritchie JL: Detection of left ventricular thrombus by two-dimensional echocardiography: Sensitivity, specificity, and causes of uncertainty. Circulation 66:156–165, 1982.
   In 78 patients with surgical, autopsy, or indium-111 platelet imaging evidence of left ventricular thrombus, the 2D transthoracic echo result was positive or equivocal in 21 of the 22 patients with a thrombus (sensitivity 95%) and was negative in 48 of 56 without a thrombus (specificity 86%). A definitely positive echo study had a positive predictive value of only 29%.

10. Visser CA, Kan G, Meltzer RS, et al: Embolic potential of left ventricular thrombus after myocardial infarction: A two-dimensional echocardiographic study of 119 patients. J Am Coll Cardiol 5:1276–1280, 1985.

In 119 patients with acute myocardial infarction (98 anterior), systemic embolization occurred in 26 patients (22%). Embolization was more likely with protrusion or free mobility of the thrombus.

Left Atrial Thrombi

11. Shrestha NK, Moreno FL, Narciso FV, et al: Two-dimensional echocardiographic detection of intra-atrial masses. Am J Cardiol 48:954–960, 1981.

    One of the few studies comparing detection of left atrial thrombi by transthoracic echo with surgical results. Of the 51 patients with left atrial thrombus at surgery, lesions in 30 were detected by 2D echo (sensitivity 59%). Of the 242 patients without thrombus at surgery, in 239 the 2D echo did not show a thrombus (3 false-positive results, specificity 99%).

12. Herzog CA, Bass D, Kane M, Asinger R: Two-dimensional echocardiographic imaging of left atrial appendage thrombi. J Am Coll Cardiol 3:1340–1344, 1984.

    Description of visualization of the left atrial appendage on transthoracic imaging in the parasternal short-axis view by slight superiomedial angulation of the transducer.

Management of Atrial Fibrillation

13. Tolat AV, Manning WJ: The role of echocardiography in atrial fibrillation and flutter. In: Otto CM (ed): The Practice of Clinical Echocardiography, 2nd ed. Philadelphia: WB Saunders, 2002, pp 829–844.

    Review of the literature on left atrial thrombus formation and the risk of embolic events with cardioversion. Summarizes the clinical approach to the use of echocardiography in management of patients with atrial fibrillation of prolonged or unknown duration. 110 references.

14. Manning WJ, Silberman DI, Gordon SPF, et al: Cardioversion from atrial fibrillation without prolonged anticoagulation with the use of transesophageal echocardiography to exclude the presence of atrial thrombi. N Engl J Med 328:750–755, 1993.

    Transesophageal echocardiography was performed in 119 patients with atrial fibrillation longer than 2 days in duration, who were not receiving long-term anticoagulant therapy and had no contraindications to the transesophageal procedure. Left atrial thrombi were identified in 12 (13%) patients. In the 78 patients without detectable atrial thrombi and successful conversion to sinus rhythm, none had an embolic event. Most of these patients received short-term heparin therapy before cardioversion and warfarin for 1 month after cardioversion.

15. Zabalgoitia M, Halperin JL, Pearce LA, et al: Transesophageal echocardiographic correlates of clinical risk of thromboembolism in nonvalvular atrial fibrillation. J Am Coll Cardiol 31:1622–1666, 1998.

    Clinical factors associated with increased risk of thromboembolism in nonvalvular atrial fibrillation included women older than 75 years, hypertension, congestive heart failure, and a history of prior thromboembolism. Features on transesophageal echocardiography associated with an increased thromboembolic risk included appendage thrombi, dense spontaneous echo contrast in the left atrium, an appendage peak flow velocity less than 20 cm/s, and complex aortic plaque.

16. Goldman ME, Pearce LA, Hart RG, et al: Pathophysioloigc correlates of thromboembolism in nonvalvular atrial fibrillation: I. Reduced flow velocity in the left atrial appendage (The Stroke Prevention in Atrial Fibrillation [SPAF-III] study). J Am Soc Echocardiogr 12:1080–1087, 1999.

    In 721 patients with nonvalvular atrial fibrillation, an atrial appendage emptying flow velocity less than 20 cm/s was associated with dense spontaneous left atrial contrast, atrial appendage thrombus, and subsequent embolic events. Clinical predictors of a low atrial appendage emptying velocity include age, blood pressure, sustained atrial fibrillation, ischemic heart disease, and left atrial size.

17. Asinger RW, Koehler J, Pearce LA, et al: Pathophysioloigc correlates of thromboembolism in nonvalvular atrial fibrillation: II. Dense spontaneous echocardiographic contrast (The Stroke Prevention in Atrial Fibrillation [SPAF-III] study). J Am Soc Echocardiogr 12:1088–1096, 1999.

    Spontaneous left atrial echo contrast was present on transesophageal imaging in 55% of 772 patients with nonvalvular atrial fibrillation, and was dense in 13%. Multivariate predictors of dense spontaneous contrast were age, atrial appendage flow velocity, left atrial size, aortic atheroma, and a plasma fibrinogen level greater than 350 mg/dL.

18. Weigner MJ, Thomas LR, Patel U, et al: Early cardioversion of atrial fibrillation facilitated by transesophageal echocardiography: short-term safety and impact on maintenance of sinus rhythm at 1 year. Am J Med 11:684–702, 2001.

    In 539 patients with atrial fibrillation of at least 2 days (or unknown), transesophageal echocardiography demonstrated atrial thrombi in 13%. Early cardioversion in those without atrial thrombus was associated with a lower recurrence rate of atrial fibrillation at 1 year.

19. Hart RG, Halperin JL, Pearce LA, et al., for the Stroke Prevention in Atrial Fibrillation Investigators: Lessons from the Stroke Prevention in Atrial Fibrillation Trials. Ann Intern Med 138:831–838, 2003.

    Summary of the three Stroke Prevention in Atrial Fibrillation (SPAF) trials with treatment recommendations. The risk of stroke with aspirin therapy depends on clinical risk factors: about 7% per year in high-risk patients (previous embolic event, systolic blood pressure >160 mm Hg, heart failure, and women >75 years), 2% to 4% per year in moderate-risk patients (hypertension but no high-risk features), and in less than 2% per year low-risk patients (no hypertension or high-risk features).

Cardiac Source of Embolus

20. Pearson AC, Labovitz AJ, Tatineni S, Gomez CR: Superiority of transesophageal echocardiography in detecting cardiac source of embolism in patients with cerebral ischemia of uncertain etiology. J Am Coll Cardiol 17:66–72, 1991.

    In 79 patients with unexplained cerebrovascular events, transthoracic echocardiography detected a potential cardiac source of embolus in only 15% compared with 57% by transesophageal echocardiography. Abnormalities detected included atrial septal aneurysms with a patent foramen ovale (9), left atrial thrombus or tumor (6), and left atrial "spontaneous" contrast (13).

21. Fatkin D, Kelly RP, Feneley MP: Relations between left atrial appendage blood flow velocity, spontaneous

echocardiography contrast and thromboembolic risk in vivo. J Am Coll Cardiol 23:961–969, 1994.

In 140 patients with atrial fibrillation, left atrial spontaneous contrast was present in 78 (56%) patients and left atrial thrombus was present in 15 (11%) patients. On multivariate analysis, spontaneous echo contrast was the only significant predictor for the presence of thrombus. Left atrial appendage velocity was negatively associated with the degree of spontaneous contrast, and an appendage velocity less than 35 cm/s was associated with a 30 times higher risk of spontaneous contrast.

22. De Castro S, Cartoni D, Fiorelli M, et al: Morphological and functional characteristics of patent foramen ovale and their embolic implications. Stroke 31:2407–2413, 2000.

In 350 patients with an acute ischemic stroke or transient ischemic attack, a patent foramen ovale (PFO) was identified on transesophageal echocardiography in 29%. Compared to subjects with a PFO without a history of embolism, PFO patients with a cerebral embolic event more often had a right to left shunt at rest and increased mobility of the atrial septum.

23. Homma S, Sacco RL, Di Tullio MR, et al., for the PFO in Cryptogenic Stroke Study (PICSS) Investigators: Effect of medical treatment in stroke patients with patent foramen ovale: patent foramen ovale in cryptogenic stroke study. Circulation 105:2625–2631, 2002.

In a multicenter randomized trial, 630 stroke patients were randomized to treatment with aspirin or warfarin after evaluation by transesophageal echocardiography. A patent foramen ovale (PFO) was present in 34% but there was no difference in clinical events comparing those with and without a PFO, in those with large versus small PFOs, or PFOs associated with an atrial septal aneurysm. In patients with PFO, there was no difference in clinical outcomes in those treated with aspirin versus warfarin.

24. Natanzon A, Goldman ME: Patent foramen ovale: anatomy versus pathophysiology–which determines stroke risk? J Am Soc Echocardiogr 16:71–76, 2003.

In a retrospective study of 78 patients with a PFO detected on TEE, patients with a clinical embolic event (compared to those without) had greater contrast shunting from right to left and had less overlap between the septum primum and septum secundum (7.5 ± 3.4 mm vs 9.9 ± 6.0 mm, P = 0.26). There was no difference in the size of the separation between the septum primum and secundum or in the presence of atrial septal aneurysm. Evidence for elevation of left atrial pressure was more common in those without an embolic event raising the possibility that hemodynamics, not anatomy, determines stroke risk in patients with a PFO.

25. Halperin JL, Fuster V: Patent foramen ovale and recurrent stroke: Another paradoxical twist. Circulation 105:2580–2582, 2002.

Editorial review of the potential association between patent foramen ovale and cerebrovascular events with discussion of clinical implications.

26. Pearson AC, Nagelhout D, Castello R, et al: Atrial septal aneurysm and stroke: A transesophageal echocardiographic study. J Am Coll Cardiol 18:1223–1229, 1991.

In 410 patients undergoing transesophageal echocardiography, an atrial septal aneurysm (defined as a base width >1.5 cm with >1.1 cm total excursion) was found in 32 (8%) patients. Atrial septal aneurysm was diagnosed more frequently in patients with stroke (15% vs 4%; P < .05).

27. Burger AJ, Sherman HB, Charlamb MJ: Low incidence of embolic strokes with atrial septal aneurysms; a prospective long-term study. Am Heart J 139:149–152, 2000.

In a consecutive series of 846 patients undergoing cardiac surgery, 42 (5%) had an atrial septal aneurysm on intraoperative TEE. There were no embolic events as a mean follow-up of 5.8 years suggesting a low risk of embolic events in patients with atrial septal aneurysms.

28. Schneider B, Hofmann T, Justen MH, Meinertz T: Chiari's network: Normal anatomic variant or risk factor for arterial embolic events? J Am Coll Cardiol 26: 203–210, 1995.

A Chiari network was present on 29 of 1436 (2%) of consecutive transesophageal echocardiographic studies. The presence of a Chiari network was associated with a patent foramen ovale in 83%, evidence for right-to-left shunting in 55%, and atrial septal aneurysm in 24% of patients.

29. Roldan CA, Shively BK, Crawford MH: Valve excrescences: Prevalence, evolution and risk for cardioembolism. J Am Coll Cardiol 30:1308–1314, 1997.

Valve excrescences (thin, elongated, mobile structures attached near the leaflet closure line) are seen in approximately 40% of normal individuals on transesophageal echocardiography and do not appear to be associated with an increased risk of thromboembolism.

Aortic Atheroma

30. Karalis DG, Chandrasekaran K, Victor MF, et al: Recognition and embolic potential of intraaortic atherosclerotic debris. J Am Coll Cardiol 17:73–78, 1991.

In 556 patients undergoing transesophageal echocardiography, intraaortic atherosclerotic debris was identified in 7%. The incidence of embolism was higher with pedunculated and mobile versus layered and immobile debris (8 of 11 vs 3 of 25; P < .002).

31. Katz ES, Tunick PA, Rusinek H, et al: Protruding aortic atheromas predict stroke in elderly patients undergoing cardiopulmonary bypass: Experience with intraoperative transesophageal echocardiography. J Am Coll Cardiol 20:70–77, 1992.

Protruding atheromas were identified in 23 of 130 (18%) of patients undergoing transesophageal echocardiography. Strokes occurred in 3 of 12 patients with mobile atheroma versus 2 of 118 without a mobile atheroma (P = .001).

32. Tunick PA, Rosenzweig BP, Katz ES, et al: High risk for vascular events in patients with protruding aortic atheromas: A prospective study. J Am Coll Cardiol 23:1085–1090, 1994.

Of 521 consecutive patients undergoing transesophageal echocardiography, 42 had protruding atheromas and no other potential source of emboli. Compared with 42 age- and gender-matched control subjects, multivariate analysis identified protruding atheromas as the only independent predictor of subsequent vascular events (odds ratio 4.3; 95% confidence intervals 1.2 to 15).

33. Vaduganathan P, Ewton A, Nagueh SF, et al: Pathologic correlates of aortic plaques, thrombi and mobile "aortic

debris" imaged in vivo with transesophageal echocardiography. J Am Coll Cardiol 30:357–363, 1997.

The echocardiographic appearance of aortic plaques was compared with histologic examination in 31 patients undergoing aortic aneurysm or dissection repair. Agreement between histologic and echocardiographic grading of lesion severity was high (73%); the major limitation of ultrasound was its inability to detect superficial ulcerations. Transesophageal echocardiography had a sensitivity of 91% and specificity of 90% for detection of thrombus associated with the atheroma.

The Echo Exam *Cardiac Masses and Source of Embolus*

Structures That May Be Mistaken for an Abnormal Cardiac Mass

Left atrium	Dilated coronary sinus (persistent left superior vena cava)
	Raphe between left superior pulmonary vein and left atrial appendage
	Atrial suture line after cardiac transplant
	Beam-width artifact from calcified aortic valve, aortic valve prosthesis, or other echogenic target adjacent to the atrium
	Interatrial septal aneurysm
Right atrium	Crista terminalis
	Chiari network (Eustachian valve remnants)
	Lipomatous hypertrophy of the interatrial septum
	Trabeculation of right atrial appendage
	Atrial suture line after cardiac transplant
	Pacer wire, Swan-Ganz catheter, or central venous line
Left ventricle	Papillary muscles
	Left ventricular web (aberrant chordae)
	Prominent apical trabeculations
	Prominent mitral annular calcification
Right ventricle	Moderator band
	Papillary muscles
	Swan-Ganz catheter or pacer wire
Aortic valve	Nodules of Arantius
	Lambl's excrescences
	Base of valve leaflet seen *en face* in diastole
Mitral valve	Redundant chordae
	Myxomatous mitral valve tissue
Pulmonary artery	Left atrial appendage (just caudal to pulmonary artery)
Pericardium	Epicardial adipose tissue
	Fibrinous debris in a chronic organized pericardial effusion

Distinguishing Characteristics of Intracardiac Masses

Characteristic	Thrombus	Tumor	Vegetation
Location	LA (especially when enlarged or associated with MV disease)	LA (myxoma) Myocardium Pericardium Valves	Usually valvular Occasionally on ventricular wall or Chiari network
	LV (in setting of reduced systolic function or segmental wall abnormalities)		
Appearance	Usually discrete and somewhat spherical in shape *or* laminated against LV apex or LA wall	Various: may be circumscribed or may be irregular	Irregular shape, attached to the proximal (upstream) side of the valve with motion independent from the valve
Associated findings	Underlying etiology usually evident	Intracardiac obstruction depending on site of tumor	Valvular regurgitation usually present
	LV systolic dysfunction or segmental wall motion abnormalities (exception: eosinophilic heart disease)	Fevers, systemic signs of endocarditis, positive blood cultures	
	MV disease with LA enlargement		

LA, left atrium; MV, mitral valve; LV, left ventricle.

DISEASES OF THE GREAT VESSELS

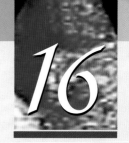

16

Basic Principles

Echocardiographic Approach
  Transthoracic Imaging of the Aorta
    Two-dimensional and Doppler
      Echocardiography
    Limitations of Transthoracic Imaging of the
      Aorta
  Transesophageal Imaging
    Two-dimensional Echocardiography
    Doppler Flows

Clinical Utility
  Chronic Aortic Dilation
  Aortic Dissection
    Transthoracic Imaging
    Transesophageal Imaging
    Alternate Approaches

Sinus of Valsalva Aneurysm
Preoperative and Postoperative Evaluation of
  Aortic Disease
  Preoperative Evaluation
  Residual Dissection Flaps
  Aortic Pseudoaneurysms
Atherosclerotic Aortic Disease
  Aortic Atherosclerosis as a Potential Source
    of Embolus
  Aortic Atherosclerosis as a Marker of
    Coronary Artery Disease
Pulmonary Artery Abnormalities

Limitations/Alternate Approaches

Suggested Reading

Echo Exam

Echocardiographic evaluation of the aorta and main pulmonary artery is a routine part of the standard echocardiographic examination. For descriptive purposes, the aorta is divided into segments, beginning at the aortic valve, including the

- sinuses of Valsalva,
- ascending aorta,
- aortic arch,
- descending thoracic, and
- proximal abdominal aorta.

Evaluation of the "proximal aorta," including the

- aortic annulus,
- sinuses of Valsalva,
- sinotubular junction, and
- proximal ascending aorta,

is a standard component of every echocardiographic examination. In addition, further evaluation of the ascending aorta, arch, and descending aorta can be performed when disease is suspected clinically. Transthoracic images often are suboptimal due to overlying or adjacent air-filled structures, so transesophageal imaging greatly enhances the diagnostic utility of echocardiography for diseases of the aorta.

BASIC PRINCIPLES

Aortic abnormalities include

- dilation,
- aneurysm,

- dissection,
- sinus of Valsalva aneurysm, and
- atherosclerosis.

The most common abnormality of the aorta is *dilation*, or an increase in diameter greater than expected for age and body size. Dilation of the ascending aorta occurs in a variety of diseases. Most cases of ascending aortic dilation are due to hypertension, atherosclerosis, cystic medial necrosis, or are poststenotic in etiology. In addition, proximal aorta dilation is seen in collagen vascular and inflammatory disorders such as Marfan syndrome, rheumatoid arthritis, systemic lupus erythematosus, and Reiter syndrome. With poststenotic dilation or with dilation due to hypertension or atherosclerosis, the contours of the sinuses of Valsalva and the normal narrowing at the sinotubular junction typically are preserved. In contrast, Marfan syndrome is characterized by effacement of the sinotubular junction and enlargement of the sinuses of Valsalva, as well as dilation of the ascending aorta, resulting in a "water balloon" appearance of the proximal aorta (Fig. 16–1).

When aortic dilation is severe, the term *aneurysm* is used. Aneurysms can involve one or more segments of the aorta (ascending, arch, descending) and may be tubular or saccular in configuration. Aortic aneurysms most often are due to cystic medial necrosis, Marfan syndrome, hypertension, atherosclerosis, or collagen-vascular

431

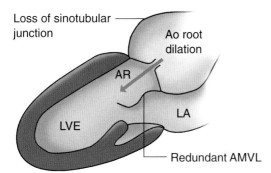

FIGURE 16-1. Schematic diagram of the typical 2D echo findings in Marfan syndrome as seen in a long-axis view. The proximal aorta is markedly dilated with effacement of the sinotubular junction. Aortic annular dilation results in inadequate aortic leaflet apposition with a central jet of aortic regurgitation (AR) and consequent left ventricular enlargement (LVE). Often the anterior mitral leaflet (AMVL) is long and redundant.

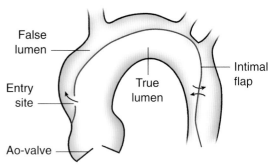

FIGURE 16-2. Schematic diagram of an aortic dissection showing an entry site above the sinotubular junction into a false lumen. In real time, the intimal flap shows rapid undulating motion, independent of the cardiac cycle. As indicated by the arrows across the intimal flap in the descending aorta, multiple flow communications between the true and false lumens may be seen with color flow imaging.

or inflammatory diseases. Aneurysms also may be seen in tertiary syphilis (with a characteristic pattern of calcification), aortic arteritis (such as Takayasu arteritis), and as a result of blunt or penetrating chest trauma. Aortic aneurysms are prone to rupture, so prophylactic repair often is recommended.

An *aortic dissection* is a life-threatening situation in which an intimal tear in the aortic wall allows passage of blood into a "false" channel between the intima and the media (Fig. 16-2). This false channel may be localized or may propagate downstream, often in a spiral fashion, due to the pressure of blood flow in the channel. Complications related to the false lumen include

■ expansion with compression of the true aortic lumen (which supplies major branch vessels),
■ propagation down major branch vessels,
■ thrombosis, or
■ rupture.

An accurate, rapid diagnosis of the presence or absence of aortic dissection and the site of the entry tear is crucial in the treatment of patients with suspected dissection.

There is an increased risk of aortic dissection in patients with aortic valve disease, with a risk approximately five times normal in individuals with a congenital bicuspid or unicuspid aortic valve. Dissection also is more likely in patients with a preexisting aneurysm, although dissection can occur in the absence of dilation in patients with Marfan syndrome. The most prevalent risk factor for aortic dissection is chronic hypertension.

Sinus of Valsalva aneurysms (Fig. 16-3) may be congenital or may be due to infection, Marfan syndrome, or previous surgical procedures. A sinus of Valsalva aneurysm protrudes into adjacent chambers and may be associated with a fistula. Specifically, an aneurysm of the right coronary sinus protrudes into the right ventricular outflow tract, the left coronary sinus into the left atrium, and the noncoronary sinus into the right atrium.

Atherosclerosis of the aorta may lead to dilation, aneurysm, or dissection. In addition, the presence of atheroma may be important as a marker

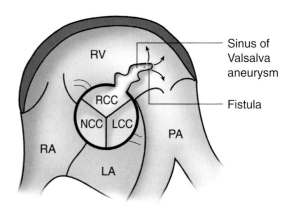

FIGURE 16-3. Schematic diagram of a congenital sinus of Valsalva aneurysm. A long "wind sock"–like membranous outpouching of the right coronary cusp (RCC) protrudes into the right ventricular (RV) outflow tract. If there are fenestrations in the aneurysm, an aortic-to-right ventricular fistula is seen. Note that an aneurysm of the left coronary cusp (LCC) would protrude into the left atrium (LA), whereas an aneurysm of the right coronary cusp (RCC) would protrude into the right atrium (RA).

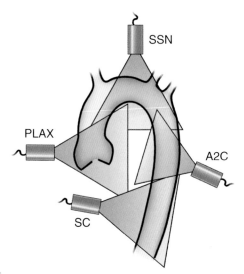

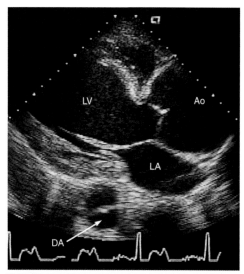

FIGURE 16–4. The use of several acoustic windows for complete evaluation of the aorta from a transcutaneous approach is shown. From a parasternal long-axis (PLAX) window, the sinuses and a segment of the ascending aorta are seen. From the suprasternal notch (SSN) window, the arch and proximal descending thoracic aorta are seen; from a posteriorly angulated apical two-chamber (A2C) approach, the mid-segment of the descending thoracic aorta is seen; and from a subcostal (SC) approach, the distal thoracic and proximal abdominal aortae are seen. In some individuals, the segment of ascending aorta between the standard PLAX and SSN views can be imaged from a high parasternal position. However, in other patients, this segment of the aorta is "missed" on transthoracic imaging.

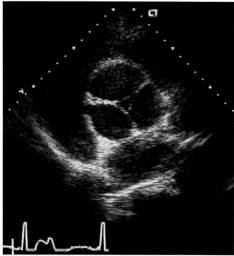

for coexisting coronary artery disease and as a potential source of embolic cerebrovascular events.

ECHOCARDIOGRAPHIC APPROACH

Transthoracic Imaging of the Aorta

Two-dimensional and Doppler Echocardiography

On transthoracic imaging, the *proximal ascending aorta* is seen in parasternal long- and short-axis views (Fig. 16–4). Depending on ultrasound penetration, images of additional segments of the ascending aorta may be obtained by moving the transducer cephalad one or more interspaces. Image quality is enhanced by positioning the patient in a steep left lateral decubitus position, bringing the aorta in contact with the anterior chest wall (Figs. 16–5 and 16–6). Doppler interrogation of the ascending aorta from the parasternal approach is limited to qualitative evaluation of the flow pattern in the proximal aorta and assessment of aortic regurgitation severity (if present) given the nonparallel intercept angle from this

FIGURE 16–5. Parasternal long-axis view in a patient with Marfan syndrome showing dilated sinuses with effacement of the sinotubular junction and a dissection flap in the descending thoracic aorta seen posterior to the left atrium *(arrow; top)*. In short axis the stretched trileaflet valve shows a small central regurgitant orifice *(bottom)*.

position. The ascending aorta also may be imaged from the apical approach in an anteriorly angulated four-chamber view and in an apical long-axis view. While two-dimensional (2D) image quality may be limited at the depth of the ascending aorta from the apical approach, this view does allow a parallel intercept angle between the Doppler beam and the direction of blood flow. In some individuals, images of the ascending aorta can be obtained from the subcostal approach.

The *aortic arch* is imaged from a suprasternal notch or supraclavicular approach with the patient

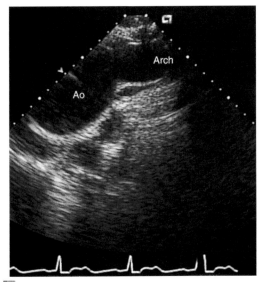

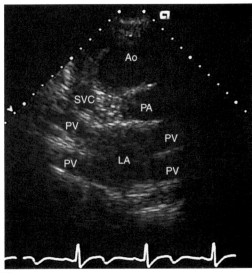

FIGURE 16–6. A long-axis view of the ascending aorta and arch obtained from a right suprasternal notch window in the patient with Marfan syndrome shown in Figure 16–5 shows that the aortic dilation extends only to the proximal segment of the arch.

FIGURE 16–8. Short-axis suprasternal notch view in a normal individual showing the aortic arch (Ao), pulmonary artery (PA), superior vena cava (SVC), left atrium (LA), and four pulmonary veins (PV).

in a supine position with the neck extended. Both longitudinal (Fig. 16–7) and transverse (Fig. 16–8) views of the arch are obtainable in nearly all individuals. Usually only a short segment of the ascending aorta is visible from the suprasternal notch window, but this is variable between patients. Also note that the descending

aorta appears to taper due to an oblique image plane with respect to its curvature (i.e., the descending aorta is only partially in the image plane).

Pulsed or continuous-wave Doppler recordings of descending aortic flow from the suprasternal notch show systolic flow away from the trans-

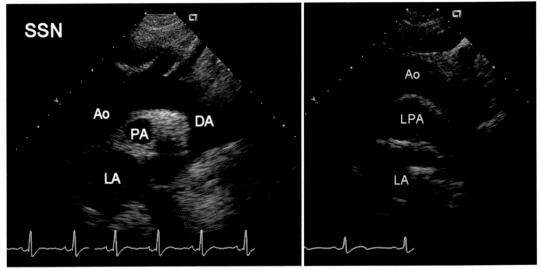

FIGURE 16–7. Suprasternal notch view in the long-axis *(left)* of the aorta in a normal individual showing the ascending aorta (Ao), arch, and descending aorta (DA) with the right pulmonary artery (PA) in short axis and the left atrium (LA) inferiorly. With slight lateral roation and angulation, the left pulmonary artery (LPA) can be depicted *(right)*.

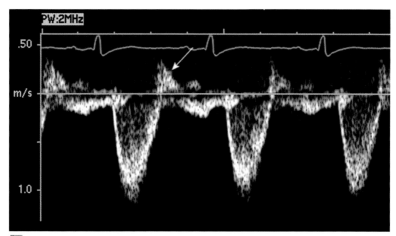

■ FIGURE 16–9. Normal pulsed Doppler recording of flow in the descending thoracic aorta from a suprasternal notch long-axis view. Antegrade flow in systole has a maximum velocity of 1.1 m/s with a normal systolic ejection curve. In diastole, there is brief early diastolic flow reversal, followed by low-velocity antegrade flow in middiastole and absence of flow (or low-velocity reversal) in end-diastole.

ducer at a velocity of approximately 1 m/s. Normal flow in the descending aortic shows

- brief, low-velocity, early diastolic flow reversal;
- low-velocity antegrade flow in mid-diastole; and
- low-velocity flow reversal at end-diastole.

The use of low wall filter settings is needed to appreciate this normal flow pattern (Fig. 16–9).

Although 2D imaging of the ascending aorta is suboptimal from the suprasternal approach, high-quality Doppler flow signals may be obtained because the Doppler beam is aligned parallel to flow. Antegrade flow toward the transducer in systole is seen, the reciprocal of the ascending aortic flow signal recorded from the apex.

The *descending thoracic aorta* is seen in cross section posterior to the left atrium in the parasternal long-axis view. A longitudinal section of this segment of the descending aorta may be obtained by clockwise rotation and lateral angulation of the transducer. From the suprasternal notch approach, a small portion of the descending thoracic aorta is seen. From the apical two-chamber view, a longitudinal section of a segment of the descending aorta is seen by lateral angulation and clockwise rotation of the transducer (Fig. 16–10). Doppler investigation of descending thoracic aortic flow is most easily performed from the suprasternal notch long-axis view. Flow abnormalities may be related to aortic disease (e.g., coarctation), shunts (e.g., patent ductus arteriosus), or aortic valve disease (e.g., regurgitation).

From the subcostal approach, the *distal thoracic* and *proximal abdominal aorta* is seen as it traverses

the diaphragm. From this approach, the angle between the transducer and the aorta allows Doppler interrogation of antegrade flow (Figs. 16–11 and 16–12).

Thus, by combining images from multiple acoustic windows, visualization of much of the ascending aorta, arch, and descending thoracic aorta is possible using transthoracic echocardiography.

In patients with a left pleural effusion, images of the aorta can be obtained by imaging through the fluid from the left posterior chest (paraspinal) with the patient in a right lateral decubitus position (Fig. 16–13).

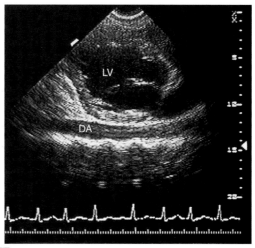

■ FIGURE 16–10. Posteriorly angulated apical two-chamber view showing the descending thoracic aorta (DA) along its long axis in the patient with Marfan syndrome.

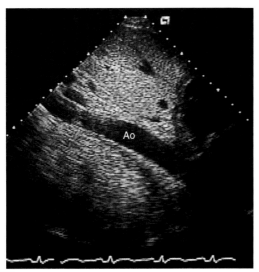

■ **FIGURE 16–11.** Subcostal view of the distal thoracic and proximal abdominal aorta. Although a nonparallel intercept angle from this window limits the quantitative velocity data, velocity recordings are helpful for evaluation of blood flow patterns.

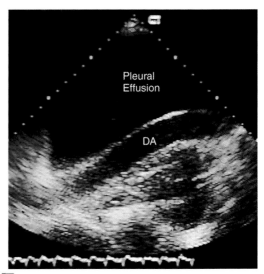

■ **FIGURE 16–13.** Descending thoracic aorta (DA) recorded through a large left pleural effusion with the patient lying on his left side and transducer positioned on the left posterior chest wall.

Limitations of Transthoracic Imaging of the Aorta

The major limitations of the transthoracic approach to ultrasound evaluation of the aorta are acoustic access and image quality. In many individuals, acoustic access is suboptimal or minimal from one or more of the windows needed for full evaluation of the aorta, leaving "gaps" in the echocardiographic examination. Even when

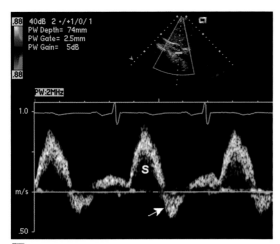

■ **FIGURE 16–12.** Normal flow in the proximal abdominal aorta recorded with pulsed Doppler from a subcostal window. Normal antegrade flow in systole (S) toward the transducer is followed by brief early diastolic flow reversal *(arrow)*.

acoustic access is adequate, image quality often is poor due to beam width at the depth of the aorta–particularly the descending thoracic aorta from apical and parasternal windows. Beam-width artifact, noise, and poor lateral resolution make differentiation of intraluminal defects from artifacts difficult. Because of these limitations, there has been increasing enthusiasm for transesophageal echocardiography in patients with suspected aortic disease.

Transesophageal Imaging

Two-dimensional Echocardiography

The aortic valve, *sinuses of Valsalva,* and *ascending aorta* are seen in an oblique image plane with the transducer at 0° rotation from a high esophageal probe position. A short-axis view at the aortic valve level is obtained by rotating the image plane to approximately 45°, with a short-axis view of the proximal few centimeters of the ascending aorta obtained by slight withdrawal of the probe in the esophagus. In the short-axis plane, evaluation of more distal segments of the ascending aorta is obscured by the position of the air-filled trachea between the esophagus (and transducer) and the ascending aorta. However, by rotating the image plane to approximately 120°, a long-axis view of the aortic valve, sinus of Valsalva, and ascending aorta can be obtained in most patients (Fig. 16–14). More cephalad segments of the ascending aorta may be seen by slowly moving the transducer to a higher esophageal position.

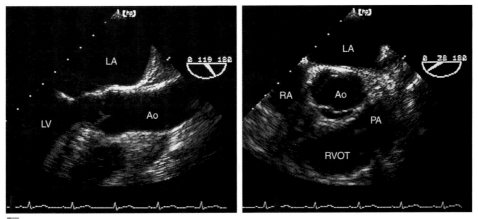

■ **FIGURE 16–14.** Normal ascending aorta seen on transesophageal imaging in long-axis *(left)* and short-axis *(right)* views using a multiplane probe to align the image plane appropriately relative to the aortic long axis.

The *aortic arch* is best imaged from a high esophageal position. Starting with a short-axis view of the descending thoracic aorta, the probe is withdrawn to the level of the arch and then the entire probe is turned toward the patient's right and angulated inferiorly to obtain a long-axis view of the arch. In some patients, images of the aortic arch may be suboptimal due to the positions of the trachea and bronchi. In many cases, transthoracic suprasternal notch views of the arch provide superior image quality.

The *descending thoracic* and *proximal abdominal aorta* are well seen by the transesophageal approach. The descending thoracic aorta lies immediately lateral and slightly posterior to the esophagus so that posterior rotation of the probe provides excellent images in either a cross-sectional (transverse plane at 0°) or long-axis (at 90° to 120°) view (Figs. 16–15 and 16–16). Slight turning of the transesophageal probe is needed at different levels as the aorta curves relative to the esophagus. From a transgastric position, the proximal abdominal aorta is seen posterior to the stomach. Many examiners prefer to examine the length of the aorta in sequential cross-sectional views as the probe is slowly withdrawn from the stomach and esophagus, with imaging of the aortic arch just before probe removal. Any areas of abnormality are then examined in both long- and short-axis views.

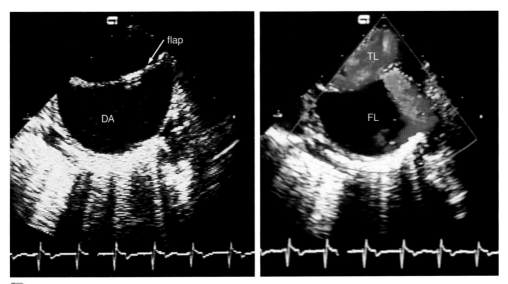

■ **FIGURE 16–15.** On transesophageal imaging, a 2D view *(left)* of the descending thoracic aorta shows a dissection flap *(arrow)*, with flow between the true (TL) and false lumens (FL) seen on color flow imaging *(right)*.

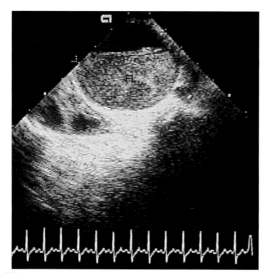

▌ **FIGURE 16–16.** Transesophageal imaging in another patient with an aortic dissection shows prominent spontaneous contrast in the false lumen (FL) due to low flow.

Doppler Flows

Color flow imaging of the aorta shows the normal antegrade flow pattern in the ascending aorta and arch. For the descending aorta, the ultrasound beam is nearly perpendicular to the direction of blood flow. In addition, normal flow shows a hemicylindrical swirling pattern so that normal flow appears red in one half and blue in the other half of a cross-sectional view of descending aorta. Given the constraints of the probe position, alignment of the Doppler beam parallel to aortic flow is difficult from a transesophageal approach. It may be possible to obtain ascending aortic flow from a transgastric "apical" view, but underesti-

mation of flow velocity due to a nonparallel intercept angle should be considered. Quantitative evaluation of aortic flow velocity from other transgastric or transesophageal views rarely is feasible. Aortic flow signals preferably are recorded from a transthoracic approach.

CLINICAL UTILITY

Chronic Aortic Dilation

Aortic dilation often is first recognized on the chest radiograph (Fig. 16–17) or on an echocardiographic examination requested for other reasons. In specific clinical settings, such as Marfan syndrome, aortic dilation is an expected consequence of a systemic disease. In these cases, echocardiography is requested to assess the presence and degree of aortic abnormality.

Measurements of aortic diameter on echocardiography are accurate and reproducible when care is taken to obtain a true short-axis dimension (nonoblique), gain settings are appropriate, and standard measurement conventions (leading edge to leading edge) are used. In patients with aortic dilation, it is important to measure aortic diameter at several locations and to specify the measurement sites. Typical measurements include

- the aortic annulus (the site used for left ventricular outflow tract diameter measurement),
- the aortic leaflet tip level (the standard position of an M-mode of the aortic valve),
- the sinotubular junction,
- the ascending aorta,
- the aortic arch, and
- the descending thoracic aorta (Fig. 16–18).

While all these measurements are not needed in every patient, quantitative evaluation of the

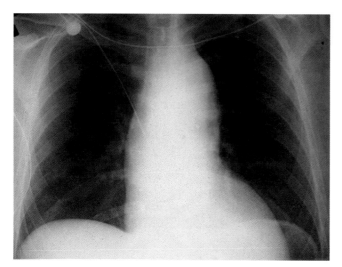

▌ **FIGURE 16–17.** Chest radiography showing a dilated ascending aorta and wide mediastinum, raising the diagnostic possibility of aortic dissection, which was present in this 36-year-old man with congenital aortic stenosis and acute onset of chest pain.

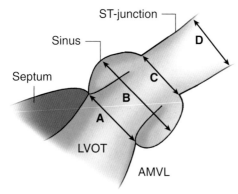

FIGURE 16–18. Schematic diagram of the sinuses and ascending aorta showing the possible measurement sites for "aortic" diameter. Left ventricular outflow tract (LVOT) diameter (A) is used for transaortic stroke volume calculations in the continuity equation. The aortic leaflet tips (B) in systole define the usual site for M-mode measurements and usually indicate maximum diameter of the sinuses of Valsalva. The sinotubular (ST) junction typically is the narrowest segment of the ascending aorta (C), with variable degrees of dilation in the ascending aorta itself (D). The site of measurement should be specified in the echocardiographic report. The term *aortic root* is nonspecific and should be avoided.

extent and severity of aortic dilation is extremely useful in follow-up and treatment of patients with chronic, progressive aortic dilation. With discrete aneurysms, maximum diameter and length also are measured.

Sequential transthoracic studies of the degree of aortic dilation are used to observe patients with Marfan syndrome. Prophylactic ascending aorta and valve replacement may be recommended when the degree of ascending aortic dilation reaches a critical range (some authorities suggest a value between 50 and 60 mm maximum diameter). For other etiologies of aortic dilation, sequential studies also may be used to assess whether the dilation is progressive or stable over time. Transesophageal evaluation of chronic aortic dilation is reserved for patients with inadequate transthoracic images.

Aortic Dissection

Transthoracic Imaging

EVALUATION OF THE AORTA. A transthoracic echocardiographic examination for aortic dissection includes evaluation of the

- ascending aorta from the standard and high parasternal windows,
- aortic arch from the suprasternal notch window,

- descending aorta from parasternal and apical windows, and
- proximal abdominal aorta from a subcostal approach.

When a left pleural effusion is present, the descending thoracic aorta can be imaged through the effusion with the transducer positioned on the left posterior chest wall.

The echocardiographic diagnosis of aortic dissection (Fig. 16–19) is most secure when there is

- a dilated aortic lumen;
- a linear, mobile echogenic structure with a pattern of motion different than the aortic wall; and
- different color Doppler flow patterns in the true and false lumen.

When a definite, undulating intimal flap is seen, the specificity of transthoracic echocardiography for diagnosis of dissection is high (Table 16–1). However, beam-width artifact and reverberations can be mistaken for intraluminal structures by an inexperienced observer, resulting in a specificity of less than 100%, particularly when the images are not "classic" or image quality is suboptimal.

Conversely, the sensitivity of transthoracic echocardiography for aortic dissection is quite low (i.e., the inability to demonstrate an internal flap does not reliably exclude the diagnosis). This low sensitivity is due to poor image quality, particularly of the segment of ascending aorta between the sinotubular junction and the aortic arch, and the poor far-field resolution of the descending thoracic aorta from the transthoracic approach.

COMPLICATIONS OF AORTIC DISSECTION. Indirect signs of aortic dissection on transthoracic imaging (Fig. 16–20) include

- aortic dilation,
- the presence of aortic regurgitation, or
- evidence of other complications of aortic dissection, including
  - a regional wall motion abnormality (usually due to right coronary artery occlusion), and
  - pericardial effusion.

While the presence of these abnormalities does not confirm the diagnosis (because there are many other etiologies for these findings), their presence or absence may weight the clinical evidence toward or away from a diagnosis of dissection. Complications of aortic dissection can be recognized on echocardiography and have important clinical implications both for diagnosis and therapy. Aortic regurgitation is nearly always present. Chronic regurgitation is due to aortic dilation and/or associated anatomic valve abnormalities. Acute regurgitation (often superimposed

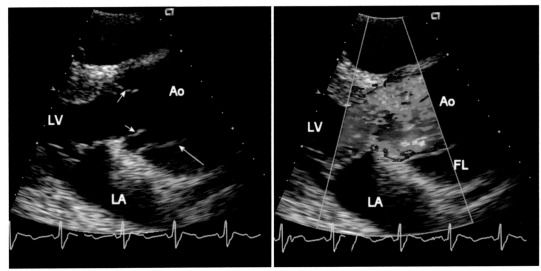

FIGURE 16–19. Transthoracic parasternal long-axis view *(left)* shows a dilated ascending aorta with a linear echo *(long arrow)* posterior to the aortic valve leaflets *(small arrows)*, which showed motion independent of the aortic walls consistent with a dissection flap. Color flow Doppler *(right)* shows flow only in the true lumen, with no flow seen in the false lumen (FL) in this view.

on chronic) is due to further aortic dilation or to inadequate leaflet support due to retrograde extension of the dissection. In extreme cases, a flail aortic leaflet is seen.

Coronary artery ostial occlusion can occur as a result of the dissection flap separating the coronary artery from normal blood flow or by compression of the vessel. The resultant wall motion abnormalities—inferior for right coronary obstruction, anterolateral for left main obstruction—are easily recognized on echocardiography. The diagnostic difficulty in this situation is recognizing that

TABLE 16–1

Diagnosis of Aortic Dissection

First Author/ Year	N	Approach	Sensitivity	Specificity	Standard of Reference
Victor/1981	42	TTE	80% (12/15)	96% (26/27)	Angiography
Erbel/1987	21	TTE	29% (6/21)	(All had dissection)	Surgery or angiography
		TEE	100% (21/21)		
Hashimoto/1989	22	TTE	71% (15/21)	(All had dissection)	Angiography (17) and/or surgery (12)
		TEE	100% (22/22)		
		CT	100% (8/8)		
Ballal/1991	61	TEE	97% (33/34)	100% (27/27)	Angiography, surgery, or autopsy
		CT	67% (16/24)	100% (7/7)	
Nienaber/1992	53	TTE	83% (26/31)	63% (14/22)	Surgery, autopsy, or angiography
		TEE	100% (31/31)	66% (15/22)	
		MRI	100% (31/31)	100% (22/22)	
Nienaber/1993	110	TTE	59% (37/62)	83% (39/48)	Surgery (62), autopsy (7), and/or angiography (64)
		TEE	98% (43/44)	98% (25/26)	
		MRI	98% (58/59)	87% (27/31)	
		CT	94% (45/48)	83% (38/46)	

TTE, transthoracic echocardiography; TEE, transesophageal echocardiography; CT, computed tomography; MRI, magnetic resonance imaging.
Data from Victor et al: Am J Cardiol 48:1155–1159, 1981; Erbel et al: Br Heart J 58:45–51, 1987; Hashimoto et al: J Am Coll Cardiol 14:1253–1262, 1989; Ballal et al: Circulation 84:1903–1914, 1991; Neinaber et al: Circulation 85:434–447, 1992; Neinaber et al: N Engl J Med 328:1–9, 1993.

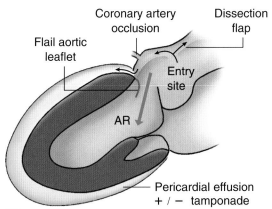

FIGURE 16–20. Potential complications of dissection of the ascending aorta are shown schematically. If the dissection proceeds retrograde (as well as antegrade) from the entry site, the false lumen can cause (1) occlusion in the coronary artery ostium with resultant myocardial infarction, (2) loss of support of an aortic leaflet with consequent severe aortic regurgitation (AR), or (3) rupture into the pericardium, which may result in tamponade physiology.

the wall motion abnormalities are a secondary event due to aortic dissection rather than the primary event (e.g., acute myocardial infarction due to coronary thrombosis).

Distal vessel obstructions rarely will be recognized during the cardiac ultrasound examination. However, the possibility of aortic dissection should be considered in patients with distal vessel obstructions referred for echocardiography to "rule out" a cardiac source of embolus. The correct diagnosis of distal vessel obstruction due to a dissection flap (rather than an embolus) may be made by the astute echocardiographer.

Aortic dissections can rupture in one of several ways. *External* rupture into the mediastinum or pleural space often results in exsanguination with acute hemodynamic collapse. If the rupture *thromboses,* the patient may exhibit a mediastinal hematoma and/or pleural effusion (more often left than right). Alternatively, the dissection can rupture at the aortic annulus into the pericardial space. Again, uncontrolled rupture leads to an acute pericardial effusion with tamponade and rapid hemodynamic collapse. However, a partial rupture or a leak may result in a smaller pericardial effusion. Obviously, the presence of any amount of pericardial fluid in a patient with an aortic dissection is an alarming sign and should prompt rapid intervention.

ECHOCARDIOGRAPHIC DIFFERENTIAL DIAGNOSIS. In most cases where transthoracic echocardiography is requested to "rule out" aortic dissection, the differential diagnosis is broad, with aortic dissection being one of many (and often

the least likely) possible diagnoses. Thus, if the echocardiographic appearance of the aorta is normal, echocardiographic examination for other possible etiologies of chest pain is needed, including

- coronary artery disease (e.g., wall motion abnormalities),
- valvular disease (e.g., aortic stenosis),
- pulmonary embolus, and
- pericarditis.

When the clinical suspicion of aortic dissection is low to intermediate, a normal aorta on echocardiography further decreases the posttest likelihood of disease, so other diagnoses might be pursued. However, when the clinical suspicion is moderate to high, a "negative" transthoracic echocardiogram does *not* substantially decrease the posttest likelihood of disease, so prompt further evaluation is needed. In fact, when the clinical suspicion is high, many clinicians would argue that transthoracic echocardiography is inappropriate; either transesophageal echocardiography, magnetic resonance imaging, computed tomography, or angiographic evaluation should be performed promptly.

Transesophageal Imaging

Transesophageal images of the aorta are far superior to transthoracic images in most patients because of (1) the shorter distance between the transducer and aorta, (2) the use of a higher frequency transducer, and (3) better ultrasound tissue penetration (higher signal-to-noise ratio). The descending thoracic aorta can be examined in its entirety from the diaphragm to the arch in both long- and short-axis planes.

Features of aortic dissection seen on transesophageal imaging include any combination of

- a dissection flap that appears as a linear, bright echogenic structure in the aortic lumen with erratic motion compared with normal systolic pulsations (Fig. 16–21);
- color Doppler evidence of blood flow in both the true (bounded by endothelium) lumen and false (bounded by media) lumen;
- the entry site into the false lumen;
- other communications between the two channels;
- thrombosis of the false lumen; or
- a hematoma in the wall of the aorta (instead of an initial flap).

An aortic wall hematoma has the same clinical implications as a classic intimal flap so that careful evaluation for this possibility is needed. This area of hematoma appears as an echogenic mass

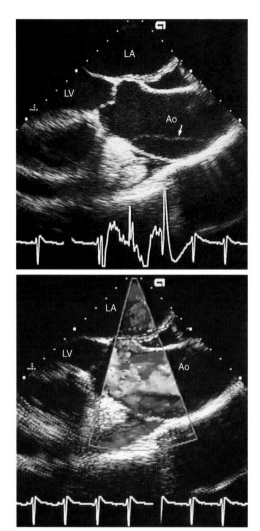

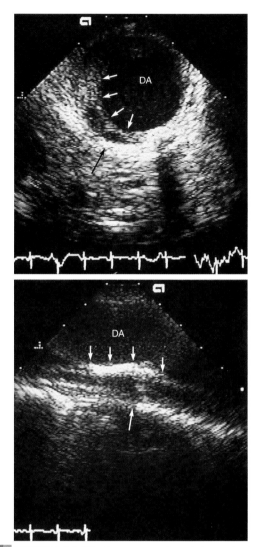

FIGURE 16–21. Transesophageal echocardiography showing a typical ascending aortic dissection in a long-axis view *(top)*. Color flow imaging shows flow in both the true and false lumen *(bottom)*.

FIGURE 16–22. In a transesophageal short-axis view of the descending thoracic aorta (DA), a "thick" or double-walled appearance is seen *(top)*, suggestive of an intramural hematoma. In a long-axis view, the atherosclerotic plaque *(small arrows)* is "lifted" off the posterior aortic wall *(large arrow)*. This patient was treated medically and has done well.

adjacent to the aortic lumen and bounded by the bright adventitial echo signal (Figs. 16–22 and 16–23).

The proximal segment of the ascending aorta is seen on transesophageal imaging in the short-axis plane at the aortic valve level. However, evaluation of the ascending aorta depends on use of a long-axis view. Evaluation of the ascending aorta is particularly important because the decision between emergency surgical intervention and medical therapy hinges on whether the dissection originates in (or involves) the ascending aorta. Note that even a localized dissection flap in the ascending aorta carries a grim prognosis and warrants surgical treatment. Again, color flow imaging may further define the entry site and demonstrate flow in true and false lumens.

The sensitivity of transesophageal echocardiography for the diagnosis of aortic dissection is high (>97%; see Table 16–1). Although specificity also is high, it is less than 100% due to misinterpretation of ultrasound artifacts, such as reverberations, beam-width artifacts, and oblique imaging planes. Careful evaluation from multiple views with adjustment of instrument settings helps avoid these false-positive diagnoses.

Alternate Approaches

Several centers have suggested that transesophageal echocardiography is the procedure of choice for evaluation of acute aortic dissections

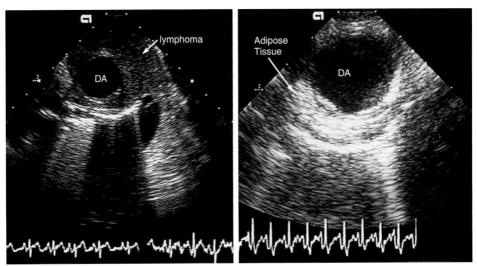

■ **FIGURE 16–23.** Potential false-positive echocardiographic findings with transesophageal imaging in two patients with no clinical evidence of aortic disease. On the *left*, lymphoma is seen surrounding the descending thoracic aorta. On the *right*, prominent paraaortic adipose tissue is seen.

given its high sensitivity/specificity plus the ability to perform the study quickly at the patient's bedside (Table 16–2). However, there are several accurate alternate techniques (Figs. 16–24 to 16–26) available for evaluation of possible acute aortic dissection including

■ rapid spiral chest computed tomography (CT),
■ magnetic resonance imaging (MRI), and
■ contrast angiography.

The choice of a particular procedure in an individual patient depends not only on availability of these tests but also on the differential diagnosis in the individual patient. Contrast angiography may be most appropriate when acute myocardial infarction is a likely diagnosis, since evaluation (and treatment) of coronary artery obstruction can be performed quickly if dissection is not present. Wide-angle tomographic imaging procedures (CT, MRI) may be most helpful in cases in which the differential diagnosis includes mediastinal tumor. Both CT and MRI approaches also allow three-dimensional (3D) visualization of the aorta, which may be helpful in clinical decision making. Echocardiography has the advantage of allowing evaluation of aortic valve anatomy and function, overall and regional left ventricular systolic function, and the presence and significance of a pericardial effusion.

Alternatively, the choice of imaging procedures may be driven by the specific additional information needed in an individual patient. Examples include distal vessel anatomy (angiography), adjacent mediastinal disease (CT or MRI), or valvular function (echocardiography).

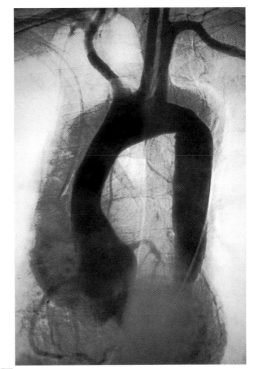

■ **FIGURE 16–24.** Subtraction contrast angiogram shows an aortic dissection extending from the aortic valve level to the proximal descending thoracic aorta. The true lumen is more densely opacified than the false lumen.

Sinus of Valsalva Aneurysm

A sinus of Valsalva aneurysm can be due to

■ congenital disease,
■ acute infection (e.g. endocarditis), or
■ an inflammatory process.

TABLE 16–2		
Diagnostic Imaging Procedures in Aortic Disease		
Procedure	**Advantages**	**Disadvantages**
Transthoracic echocardiography	Portable, rapid Inexpensive Evaluation of LV function Evaluation of aortic valve function Evaluation of pericardial effusion	Moderate sensitivity/specificity due to poor acoustic access and suboptimal image resolution
Transesophageal echocardiography	High sensitivity/specificity Portable, rapid Evaluation of LV fx, valve fx, PE Can assess proximal coronary arteries	Some risks (esp. if esophageal disease is present) Cannot evaluate distal coronary arteries
Chest computed tomography	High sensitivity/specificity Wide field of view	Site of intimal tear not well defined Not portable Ionizing radiation Little data on LV, aortic valve Cannot evaluate coronary involvement
Magnetic resonance imaging	High sensitivity/specificity Wide field of view Evaluation of pericardial effusion	High cost, not portable, limited availability Limited evaluation of valvular and ventricular function Cannot evaluate coronary involvement
Contrast aortography	High sensitivity/specificity Branch vessel anatomy Evaluation of AR Can assess and intervene for coronary artery disease	Expensive, invasive Ionizing radiation Limited availability Not portable No evaluation for pericardial effusion

LV, Left ventricle; fx, function; PE, pericardial effusion; AR, aortic regurgitation.

Echocardiographically, a dilated and distorted sinus of Valsalva is seen both in long- and short-axis views at the aortic valve level either from a transesophageal or transthoracic approach. A congenital aneurysm often is complex in shape with a "wind sock" appearance of a mass of irregular, mobile echos protruding from the aortic sinus into adjacent cardiac structures (Fig. 16–27). If the aneurysm is not fenestrated, Doppler flow examination is unremarkable. More commonly, multiple fenestrations are present, with high-velocity turbulent flow from the high-pressure aorta to the low-pressure adjacent chambers detectable by continuous-wave, pulsed wave, and color flow Doppler techniques. Note that infection of a previously competent congenital sinus of Valsalva

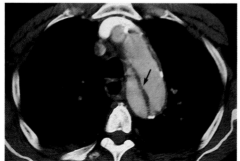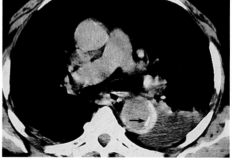

■ **FIGURE 16–25.** On chest CT, a clear dissection flap *(arrow)* is seen in the aortic arch *(left)*. In a second patient, an atypical dissection is seen with displacement of intimal calcification *(arrow)* by an intramural thrombus in the descending thoracic aorta *(right)*.

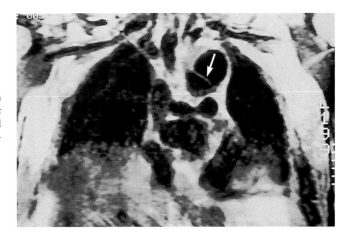

FIGURE 16–26. In a 61-year-old man with cystic medial necrosis and previous ascending aortic dissection and graft placement, MRI in the coronal plane shows persistent dilation and a chronic dissection flap *(arrow)* in the aortic arch.

aneurysm may result in flow across a necrotic area of infection.

Acquired sinus of Valsalva aneurysms tend to be less irregular in shape. The dilation of the sinuses that occurs in Marfan syndrome symmetrically involves all three sinuses with a rounded, smooth pattern of dilation. Because of persistent sinus of Valsalva dilation in patients with Marfan syndrome, replacements of the ascending aorta are performed with a composite valve and graft (with reimplantation of the coronaries) to avoid sinus dilation and rupture with separate replacements of the aorta. A sinus of Valsalva aneurysm due to endocarditis tends to result in a more spherical, but still irregular-appearing

dilation of the sinus (Fig. 16–28). Again, the aneurysm protrudes and may rupture into adjacent cardiac structures depending on which sinus is involved.

Preoperative and Postoperative Evaluation of Aortic Disease

Preoperative Evaluation

In some cases, the suspicion of aortic dissection is so high that transesophageal echocardiographic examination may be performed initially in the operating room with the patient anesthetized and undergoing preparation for surgery. In these cases, the echocardiographer aims to rapidly

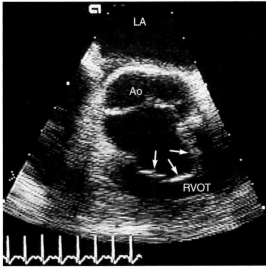

FIGURE 16–27. Congenital sinus of Valsalva aneurysm of the right coronary cusp *(arrows)* protruding into the right ventricular outflow tract on a transesophageal short-axis view.

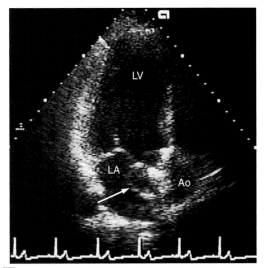

FIGURE 16–28. Acquired sinus of Valsalva aneurysm *(arrow)* after aortic valve replacement in an apical long-axis view protruding into the left atrium.

confirm or exclude the suspected diagnosis. If a dissection is present, evaluation of the entry site and extent of dissection is helpful in planning the surgical approach. Recognition of complications such as aortic regurgitation, coronary ostial occlusion, or pericardial effusion also may affect acute patient treatment.

Residual Dissection Flaps

Transesophageal echocardiography may be used intraoperatively to assess for residual dissection following surgical repair. A residual dissection flap, with flow in both true and false lumens, persists in most patients (possibly as many as 70% to 80%) following emergency surgery for acute dissection. The usual operative procedure is to close the entry site by replacing a segment of the involved aorta with a prosthetic graft. At the distal graft anastomosis, the flap may persist. Often this persistence is intentional because some branch vessels may be supplied by the false lumen and other vessels by the true lumen. Thus the finding of a dissection flap in the aortic arch or descending aorta of a patient with a previous ascending aortic dissection and graft repair may represent stable residual disease or a second acute process. These conditions are differentiated by comparison with previous imaging studies (when available) and careful clinical evaluation. Some investigators have suggested that persistence of an intimal flap and flow in the false lumen are poor prognostic signs.

In patients with ascending aortic grafts, echocardiographic follow-up is warranted to assess for late complications. In patients with a valved conduit, a baseline study is indicated postoperatively to allow comparison with future studies in terms of prosthetic valve function (see Chapter 13). The prosthetic aortic graft itself appears as an echodense, cylindrical structure with a uniform diameter (Fig. 16–29). Although most surgeons now resect the native diseased aorta, in the past, the native aorta often was "wrapped around" the prosthetic graft resulting in irregular areas of thickening anterior and posterior to the graft on echocardiography. Even with resection of the native aortic segment, postoperative periaortic scar tissue may be prominent. The coronary arteries retain their normal insertions if a segment of the native aorta has been preserved. In these cases, careful examination for dilation of the remaining aortic tissue and the sinuses of Valsalva is needed. When the graft extends to the aortic valve level, the right and left coronary ostia are reimplanted into the graft along with a small "button" of native aortic tissue. Dilation or loss of structural integrity of this aortic tissue or dehiscence of the coronary reimplantation suture line results in myocardial

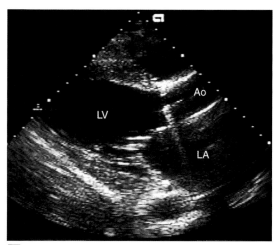

FIGURE 16–29. Composite ascending aortic graft and valve replacement postoperatively in a patient with Marfan syndrome.

infarction due to disruption of coronary blood flow. In addition, this complication can lead to aortic rupture or pseudoaneurysm formation.

Aortic Pseudoaneurysms

A pseudoaneurysm, escape of blood from the graft lumen into an area contained by surrounding scar tissue or the native aorta, can occur at the proximal or the distal graft anastomoses to the aorta or at the coronary reimplantation sites. Rarer instances of rupture of the graft material itself have been reported. A pseudoaneurysm appears as an echolucent area adjacent to the aortic graft (Fig. 16–30). Flow into this region can be demonstrated with color flow imaging, although a transesophageal study often is necessary for adequate image quality. The pseudoaneurysm may rupture into the mediastinum or pleural spaces (both of which are likely to be fatal) or back across the aortic annulus into the left ventricle. This pseudoaortic regurgitation consists of flow from the pseudoaneurysm into the left ventricle in diastole, with flow from the left ventricle into the pseudoaneurysm in systole. The characteristics of this flow signal on pulsed and continuous-wave Doppler are similar to those of transvalvular aortic regurgitation. Color flow imaging shows the flow around, rather than through, the prosthetic aortic valve.

Atherosclerotic Aortic Disease

Aortic Atherosclerosis as a Potential Source of Embolus

The excellent-quality images of the aorta obtained by transesophageal echocardiography have led

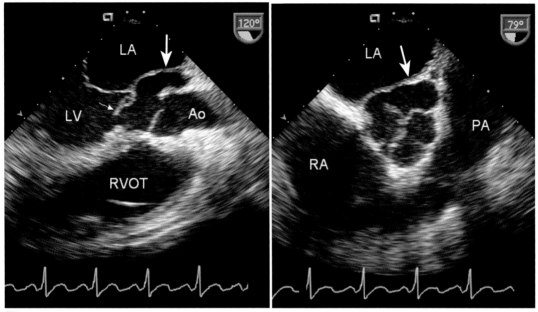

■ **FIGURE 16–30.** Echocardiography was requested for evaluation of cardiogenic shock in a 32-year-old man with *Pseudomonas* endocarditis. Transesophageal imaging in a long-axis view *(left)* shows a flail noncoronary leaflet of the aortic valve *(small arrow)* in association with disruption of the posterior aortic sinus of Valsalva, resulting in a psuedoanerysm *(large arrow)* between the aorta and left atrium. The normal right coronary cusp of the aortic valve is seen in a closed position. On color Doppler, flow into and out of the psudeoanerysm from the aorta and severe aortic regurgitation were seen. The short-axis view *(right)* at the level of communication between the aorta and pseudoaneurysm *(arrow)* shows the distorted appearance of the aortic valve and sinuses.

to the observation of extensive atherosclerotic plaque in many individuals, with mobile thrombus attached to the atheroma in some cases. These observations have generated the hypothesis that atherosclerosis of the ascending aorta and arch may serve as a nidus for embolic material, resulting in cerebrovascular events (see Suggested Readings 30 to 33 in Chapter 15). These areas of atherosclerosis rarely are seen on transthoracic imaging due to poor image quality related to acoustic access, the depth of the aorta from the transthoracic approach, and the use of a lower frequency transducer. Echocardiographic evaluation of the extent and severity of atheroma correlates well with histologic examination, and transesophageal echocardiography is both sensitive and specific for detection of atheroma-related thrombus formation.

Aortic Atherosclerosis as a Marker of Coronary Artery Disease

The presence of detectable atherosclerotic plaques in the descending aorta on transesophageal echocardiography (Fig. 16–31) indicates the presence of atherosclerosis and thus is a marker of coronary artery disease with a sensitivity of 90%. Conversely, the absence of detectable atherosclerosis in the descending thoracic aorta suggests that significant coronary artery disease is not present with a specificity of 90%.

Pulmonary Artery Abnormalities

Most abnormalities of the pulmonary artery are congenital, including poststenotic dilation, branch pulmonary artery stenosis, and an abnormal position of the pulmonary artery, as in transposition of the great vessels. However, the pulmonary artery may be involved by systemic diseases that affect the aorta, such as Takayasu arteritis. Pulmonary artery dissection is rare but has been reported in patients with chronic pulmonary hypertension.

The finding of a dilated pulmonary artery raises the possibility of

■ right-sided volume overload (e.g., atrial septal defect),
■ pulmonary hypertension, or
■ idiopathic dilation of the pulmonary artery.

The finding of a dilated main pulmonary artery mandates a careful evaluation for right-sided pressure or volume overload. Idiopathic dilation of the pulmonary artery is a rare diagno-

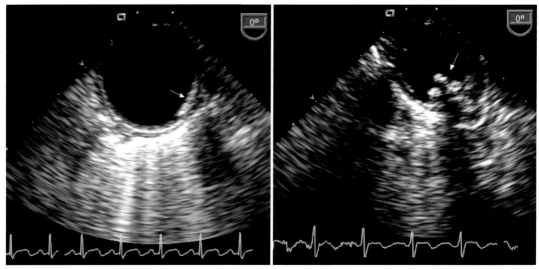

■ FIGURE 16–31. Transesophageal short-axis view of the descending thoracic aorta *(left)* showing a laminar atherosclerotic plaque *(arrow)* with shadowing suggesting calcfication. In a different patient *(right)*, a larger atherosclerotic plaque with protruding thrombus *(arrow)* and severe shadowing is seen.

sis and should only be considered if there is no other cause for pulmonary artery dilation.

The pulmonary artery can be depicted on transthoracic echocardiography in a parasternal short-axis view at the aortic valve level or in a right ventricular outflow view. In adults, it may be difficult to visualize the anterior pulmonary artery wall due to overlying lung tissue. In younger patients, the pulmonary artery can be demonstrated from the anteriorly angulated apical four-chamber view by further anterior angulation. The subcostal short-axis view allows an alternate approach to depict the pulmonary artery in most patients. From the suprasternal notch window, the right pulmonary artery is seen in cross section in the long-axis view of the aortic arch (see Fig. 16–7) and in its long axis in the orthogonal view (see Fig. 16–8). The left pulmonary artery can be imaged by slight lateral angulation and posterior rotation from the standard long-axis suprasternal notch view.

Transesophageal images of the pulmonary artery can be obtained in a 0° image plane by slowly withdrawing the probe to an esophageal level superior to the left atrium. This view shows the long axis of the pulmonary artery and its bifurcation, but may not be obtained in all patients due to interposition of the air-filled bronchus (Fig. 16–32). The pulmonary artery also can be imaged in the 90° plane (analogous to the transthoracic right ventricular outflow view) by turning the transducer to the patient's right from the left ventricular long-axis view. However, image quality

may be suboptimal due to the distance of the pulmonary artery from the transducer in this view.

Alternate approaches to evaluation of the pulmonary artery include computed tomographic or magnetic resonance image scanning and contrast angiography. Evaluation for pulmonary emoblism typically includes a radionuclide ventilation/perfusion scan.

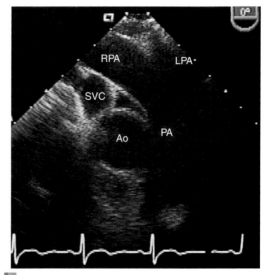

■ FIGURE 16–32. Transesophageal view of the pulmonary artery from a high esophageal position in the 0° image plane orientation. This view cannot be obtained in all patients due to interposition of the air-filled bronchus.

LIMITATIONS/ALTERNATE APPROACHES

The major limitations of echocardiographic evaluation of diseases of the great vessels are acoustic access and image quality. From the transthoracic approach, images of each segment of the aorta can be obtained, but image quality depends on the body habitus of the patient, the skill of the sonographer, and careful attention to the technical details of image acquisition. Interpretation of the images obtained must consider the likelihood of false-positive findings from beam-width artifacts, reverberations, and oblique image planes, as well as false-negative findings due to limited acoustic access and poor resolution.

Transesophageal imaging obviates many of these limitations by providing optimal acoustic access and excellent resolution. However, reverberations, beam-width artifacts, and oblique image planes still can result in apparent intraluminal "abnormalities," particularly in the ascending aorta, that in fact represent ultrasound artifacts. Use of a biplane or multiplane probe is essential, because the ascending aorta is depicted only at its base using the transverse image plane (single-plane probe). Even with a multiplane probe, a few centimeters of the ascending aorta at its junction with the arch may not be adequately demonstrated due to the interposed air-filled bronchial tree. Images of the ascending aorta are of particular importance in suspected aortic dissection because the entry site (ascending or descending aorta), rather than the simple presence or absence of disease, determines therapy.

Alternate approaches provide excellent quality images of the aorta with sensitivities and specificities for diagnosis of aortic dissection at least comparable with those of transesophageal echocardiography. Chest computed tomography can be used to evaluate aortic disease with the advantages of a wide field of view, high accuracy, and wide availability. Disadvantages include the use of ionizing radiation and the nonportable nature of the study. Chest CT may identify associated pericardial effusion but is of limited value in evaluation of left ventricular or aortic valve function. Three-dimensional reconstructions of CT scans (Fig. 16–33) enhance the abilty to relate anatomic findings to each other.

Magnetic resonance imaging of the aorta has the advantages of high resolution, high diagnostic accuracy, wide field of view, and the ability to orient the images along the long axis of the aorta.

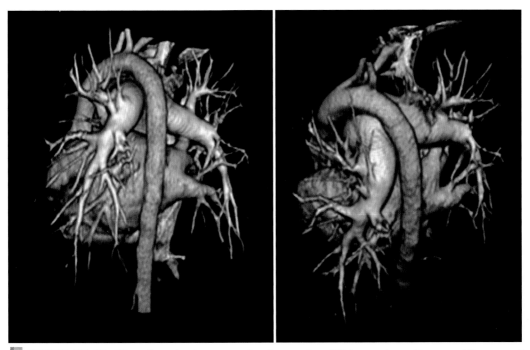

■ **FIGURE 16–33.** Three-dimensional reconstruction from a chest CT in a patient with congentially corrected transposition of the great vessels and severe pulmonary artery dilation. The 3D views show the anatomy and relationships of the great vessels in detail and the image can be rotated, as illustrated, to depict different aspects of the great vessels.

As with chest CT, MRI equipment is not portable. In addition, it is not as widely available, is expensive, and provides limited data on ventricular and valvular function in routine clinical use. However, both chest CT and MRI can provide data on branch vessel involvement, information that rarely is obtainable with echocardiography.

Contrast aortography allows accurate diagnosis of aortic disease, including aortic dissection, and may be the initial diagnostic procedure if the possibility of coronary artery disease is high on the differential diagnosis. Aortography allows evaluation of the degree of aortic regurgitation, involvement of branch vessels, and (by separate contrast injection) left ventricular systolic function. Cardiac catheterization, with contrast aortography, is the only diagnostic procedure that provides detailed coronary anatomy and allows rapid intervention if coronary artery obstruction is present. Disadvantages of contrast aortography are that it is not portable, uses ionizing radiation, is invasive, and is expensive.

Again, the choice of imaging procedures in a patient with suspected aortic disease depends largely in the differential diagnosis, the specific data needed in that patient, and procedure availability.

SUGGESTED READING
Aortic Dissection

1. Ryan EW, Bolger AF: Aortic dissection and trauma: Value and limitations of echocardiography. In: Otto CM (ed): The Practice of Clinical Echocardiography, 2nd ed. Philadelphia: WB Saunders, 2002, pp 46–63.
   Review of the pathophysiologic and clinical presentation of aortic dissection and the role of echocardiography both for the initial diagnosis, management at the time of surgery, and long-term follow-up; 130 references.

2. Willens HJ, Kessler KM: Transesophageal echocardiography in the diagnosis of diseases of the thoracic aorta: Part 1. Aortic dissection, aortic intramural hematoma, and penetrating atherosclerotic ulcer of the aorta. Chest 116:1772–1779, 1999.
   Concise and easy to read review of the TEE diagnosis of aortic dissection and intramural hematoma with self-assessment questions, review of the literature, case examples, and 44 references.

3. Nienaber CA, Eagle KA: Aortic dissection: New frontiers in diagnosis and management. Part I: From etiology to diagnostic strategies. Circulation 108:628–635, 2003. Part II: Therapeutic management and follow-up. Circulation 108:772–778, 2003.
   Review of etiology, classification, natural history, diagnosis, medical and surgical management of aortic dissection. Essential reading.

4. Fedak PW, Verma S, David TE, et al: Clinical and pathophysiological implications of a bicuspid aortic valve. Circulation 106:900–904, 2002.
   A bicuspid aortic valve is associated with aortic dilation in over 50% of patients and is associated with an increased risk of aortic dissection.

5. Cigarroa JE, Isselbacher EM, DeSanctis RW, Eagle KA: Diagnostic imaging in the evaluation of suspected aortic dissection. Old standards and new directions. N Engl J Med 328:35–43, 1993.
   Excellent review, with examples of diagnostic imaging procedures for aortic dissection, including aortography, computed tomographic scanning, magnetic resonance imaging, and echocardiography. Discusses the choice of imaging procedure in patients with suspected aortic dissection.

6. Nienaber CA, Spielmann RP, von Kodolitsch Y, et al: Diagnosis of thoracic aortic dissection. Magnetic resonance imaging versus transesophageal echocardiography. Circulation 85:434–447, 1992.
   Comparison of magnetic resonance imaging and transesophageal echocardiography in suspected aortic dissection. False-positive results on transesophageal echocardiography were related to reverberations, extensive plaque formation, and previous periaortic trauma. Magnetic resonance imaging was helpful in resolving these false-positive echocardiographic findings.

7. Nienaber CA, von Kodolitsch Y, Nicolas V, et al: The diagnosis of thoracic aortic dissection by noninvasive imaging procedures. N Engl J Med 328:1–9, 1993.
   Further extension of the authors' study (Suggested Reading 6), including computed tomography, magnetic resonance imaging, transthoracic echocardiography, and transesophageal echocardiography diagnosis of aortic dissection. Again, the specificity of transesophageal echocardiography was lowest (86%) for the ascending aorta due to echo reverberation and atherosclerotic plaque. Magnetic resonance imaging and transesophageal echocardiography had the highest overall predictive value, and neither computed tomography nor aortography provided further significant information in the patients in this series. The authors advocate that transthoracic echocardiography should be followed by either MRI or transesophageal echocardiography to provide a definitive diagnosis before surgical intervention.

8. Chan K-L: Usefulness of transesophageal echocardiography in the diagnosis of conditions mimicking aortic dissection. Am Heart J 122:495–504, 1991.
   In 22 patients with suspected (but absent) aortic dissection, ischemic disease was present in 5. Of the remaining 17 patients, transesophageal echocardiography demonstrated aortic disease in 16 patients with dilation in 10 (63%), atheromas in 7 (41%) (5 also had dilation), an extrinsic aortic mass in 2, a posttraumatic clot in the descending aorta in 1, and an anastomotic leak at a coronary reimplantation site in 1 patient. Thus, transesophageal echocardiography provided valuable clinical data, even when aortic dissection was excluded.

9. Erbel R, Oelert H, Meyer J, et al., for the European Cooperative Study Group on Echocardiography: Effect of medical and surgical therapy on aortic dissection evaluated by transesophageal echocardiography: Implications for prognosis and therapy. Circulation 87:1604–1615, 1993.
   Of 168 patients treated for acute aortic dissection, a persistent patent false lumen was seen at follow-up in 93% (28 of 30) after surgery for ascending aortic dissection that extended into the descending aorta but in only 11% (2 of 18) with dissection confined to the ascending aorta. The authors propose that thrombus formation in the

false lumen is a good prognostic sign, which is associated with a lower rate of complications and reoperation.

10. Dohmen G, Kuroczynski W, Dahm M, et al: Value of echocardiography in patient follow-up after surgically corrected type A aortic dissection. Thorac Cardiovasc Surg 49:343–348, 2001.

Residual abnormalities and complications were common after aortic dissection repair with more than mild aortic regurgitation in 25%, a distal aneurysm greater than 5 cm in diameter in 33%, a residual distal dissection flap in 81%, and a new proximal aortic dissection in 10%. Transesophageal echocardiography was optimal for evaluation of flow patterns and entry sites whereas CT and MRI were better for visualization of aortic arch pathology.

11. Hagan PG, Nienaber CA, Isselbacher EM, et al: The International Registry of Acute Aortic Dissection (IRAD): New insights into an old disease. JAMA 283:897–903, 2000.

In a registry of 464 patients with acute aortic dissection (62% ascending), the most common initial symptom was sharp chest pain. Physical findings of aortic regurgitation were present in only 32%, only 15% had a pulse deficit, and the chest radiograph was normal in 12%. Hospital mortality for a type A (ascending) dissection was 26% with surgery and 58% with medical therapy. For type B (descending) dissection, mortality was 11% with medical therapy.

12. Moore AG, Eagle KA, Bruckman D, et al: Choice of computed tomography, transesophageal echocardiography, magnetic resonance imaging, and aortography in acute aortic dissection: International Registry of Acute Aortic Dissection (IRAD). Am J Cardiol 89:1235–1238, 2002.

In a registry of 628 patients with acute aortic dissection, the first choice of imaging test was chest CT in 63%, echocardiography in 32%, aortography in 4%, and MRI in 1%. However, two-thirds of patients had more than one imaging study with transesophageal echocardiography performed in 58% of those with a second study. Sensitivity of transesophageal echocardiography for the diagnosis of ascending dissection was 90%, compared to 93% for CT.

13. Movsowitz HD, Levine RA, Hilgenberg AD, et al: Transesophageal echocardiographic description of the mechanisms of aortic regurgitation in acute type A aortic dissection: implications for aortic valve repair. J Am Coll Cardiol 36:884–890, 2000.

In 50 consecutive patients undergoing ascending aortic dissection repair, significant aortic regurgitation was present in 44%. Mechanisms of aortic regurgitation in patients with intrinsically normal leaflets included proximal aortic dilation with leaflet tethering, leaflet prolapse, and dissection flap prolapse through the aortic orifice. Identification of the mechanism of aortic regurgitation can assist the surgeon in optimizing the surgical procedure.

Aortic Intramural Hemorrhage

14. Mohr-Kahaly S, Erbel R, Kearney P, et al: Aortic intramural hemorrhage visualized by transesophageal echocardiography: Findings and prognostic implications. J Am Coll Cardiol 23:658–664, 1994.

Localized intramural hemorrhage results in a layered appearance of the aorta on transesophageal imaging. This variant of aortic dissection was seen in 15 of 114 patients. The length of the intramural hematoma ranged from 3 to 20 cm with a thickness of 0.7 to 3 cm. At 11-month follow-up, the mortality rate was 53% (8 of

15)–five (33%) patients had classic aortic dissection, four (27%) had aortic rupture, and five (33%) became asymptomatic with medical therapy.*

15. Keren A, Kim CB, Hu BS, et al: Accuracy of biplane and multiplane transesophageal echocardiography in diagnosis of typical acute aortic dissection and intramural hematoma. J Am Coll Cardiol 28:627–636, 1996.

In a consecutive series of 112 patients undergoing transesophageal echocardiography for suspected aortic dissection, echocardiographic findings were compared to findings at surgery or autopsy. The sensitivity of transesophageal echocardiography for the presence of aortic dissection was 98% with a specificity of 95%. The sensitivity of transesophageal echocardiography for detection of intramural hematoma was 90% with a specificity of 99%. Echocardiography also was highly accurate for detection of associated aortic regurgitation and pericardial tamponade.

16. Pepi M, Campodonico J, Galli C, et al: Rapid diagnosis and management of thoracic aortic dissection and intramural haematoma: A prospective study of advantages of multiplane vs. biplane transoesophageal echocardiography. 1:72–79, 2000.

The accuracy of multiplane TEE for detection of aortic dissection or intramural hematoma is high and this approach also allows evaluation of the entry site, coronary artery involvement, aortic regurgitation, and pericardial effusion.

Aortic Pseudoaneurysms

17. Zoghbi WA: Echocardiographic recognition of unusual complications after surgery on the great vessels and cardiac valves. In: Otto CM (ed): The Practice of Clinical Echocardiography, 2nd ed. Philadelphia: WB Saunders, 2002, pp 551–570.

Review and discussion of complications after aortic surgery including pseudoaneurysms of composite aortic grafts and complications after composite valve and proximal aortic replacement. Excellent illustrations of the surgical techniques and echocardiographic findings.

18. Barbetseas J, Crawford ES, Sail HJ, et al: Doppler echocardiographic evaluation of pseudoaneurysms complicating composite grafts of the ascending aorta. Circulation 85:212–222, 1992.

Description of the echocardiographic appearance of pseudoaneurysm formation after ascending aortic graft surgery in eight cases. Periannular and coronary artery dehiscences were detected by echocardiography using both 2D imaging (transthoracic or transesophageal or both) and Doppler flow studies.

Marfan Syndrome

19. Pyeritz RE, McKusick VA: The Marfan syndrome: Diagnosis and management. N Engl J Med 300:772–777, 1979.

Concise review article on the clinical manifestations of Marfan syndrome. Nearly all patients with Marfan syndrome have (or develop) proximal aortic dilation as seen on echocardiography. Annual echocardiographic examination is advocated.

20. Roman MJ, Devereux RB, Kramer-Fox R, O'Loughin J: Two-dimensional echocardiographic aortic root dimensions in normal children and adults. Am J Cardiol 64:507–512, 1989.

Aortic sinuses dimensions can be normalized for the expected value for age and body size as:

Children (<18 years): Predicted sinus dimension = 1.02 + (0.98 BSA)

Adults (age 18–40 years): Predicted sinus dimension = 0.97 + (1.12 BSA)

Adults (>40 years): Predicted sinus dimension = 1.92 + (0.74 BSA)

Where BSA = body surface area in m²

21. Simpson IA, de Belder MA, Treasure T, et al: Cardiovascular manifestations of Marfan's syndrome: Improved evaluation by transesophageal echocardiography. Br Heart J 69:104–108, 1993.

     Transesophageal echocardiography studies in 11 patients with Marfan syndrome, suspected aortic dissection, and inadequate transthoracic echocardiography images revealed evidence for dissection in six subjects with surgical confirmation in all six cases.

22. Shores J, Berger KR, Murphy EA, Pyeritz RE: Progression of aortic dilatation and the benefit of long-term beta-adrenergic blockade in Marfan's syndrome. N Engl J Med 330:1335–1341, 1994.

     Echocardiography was used to follow the rate of proximal aortic dilation in 70 patients with Marfan syndrome in a randomized trial of beta-blockade therapy. Maximal measured aortic diameter was divided by the predicted diameter for the patient age, height, and weight. This "aortic ratio" was comparable both between patients and in the same patient during growth of the body. The rate of progression, measured as the slope of the aortic ratio regression line, was significantly lower in the treatment group compared with control subjects (P < .001).

23. Legget ME, Unger TA, O'Sullivan CK, et al: Aortic root complications in Marfan's syndrome: Identification of a lower risk group. Heart 75:389–395, 1996.

     Echocardiography was used to follow disease progression in 89 patients with Marfan syndrome. To compare proximal aortic dimensions as patients aged, the normalized root ratio was used as a measure of disease progression. A ratio of actual to predicted aortic dimension 1.3 or greater predicted an increased likelihood of ascending aortic dissection. An increase in the aortic ratio ≥5% also predicted a poor clinical outcome.

24. Alizad A, Seward JB: Echocardiographic features of genetic diseases: Part 4. Connective tissue. J Am Soc Echocardiogr 13:325–330, 2000.

     Review with illustrations of echocardiographic and clinical findings in Ehlers-Danlos and Marfan syndrome.

25. Pyeritz RE: The Marfan syndrome. Ann Rev Med 51:481–521, 2000.

     Detailed review of all aspects of the Marfan syndrome by a leader in this field; 131 references.

Aortic Atheroma

26. Fazio GP, Redberg RF, Winslow T, Schiller NB: Transesophageal echocardiographically detected atherosclerotic aortic plaque is a marker for coronary artery disease. J Am Coll Cardiol 21:144–150, 1993.

     In 61 patients (31 females) with previous coronary angiography, transesophageal echocardiography showed atherosclerotic plaque in the descending thoracic aorta in 37 of 41 (sensitivity 90%) with documented coronary artery disease (>50% left main or >70% left anterior descending artery, right coronary artery, or circumflex). Of the 20 patients without significant coronary disease, 18 (specificity 90%) had no evidence for atherosclerosis in the descending aorta on transesophageal echocardiography.

27. Willens HJ, Kessler KM: Transesophageal echocardiography in the diagnosis of diseases of the thoracic aorta: Part II–Atherosclerotic and traumatic diseases of the aorta. Chest 117:233–243, 2000.

     Review of the role of transesophageal echocardiography in detection of aortic atherosclerosis and the clinical implications of this finding; 72 references.

28. Aman M, Amanullah MD, Bradley J, et al: Usefulness of complex atherosclerotic plaque in the ascending aorta and arch for predicting cardiovascular events. Am J Cardiol 89:1423–1426, 2002.

     In 127 consecutive patients undergoing transesophageal echocardiography for various reasons with prospective follow-up at 1 year, a complex plaque (≥4 mm in thickness or any plaque with mobile components) was present in 45% and noncomplex plaque in 55%. The primary clinical outcome, death, or a cerebral embolic event, occurred in 15% and a secondary clinical endpoint, carotid endarterectomy or coronary revascularization, occurred in 20%. The rate of endpoints was 60% in those with complex plaque compared to 16% in those with noncomplex plaque (P < .001) and complex plaque was a predictor of outcome on multivariate analysis.

Traumatic Aortic Rupture

29. Smith MD, Cassidy JM, Souther S, et al: Transesophageal echocardiography in the diagnosis of traumatic rupture of the aorta. N Engl J Med 332:356–362, 1995.

     Transesophageal echocardiography was attempted in 101 patients with possible aortic trauma and was successful in 93 patients. Aortic rupture was diagnosed on transesophageal images in 11 (12%) studies with confirmation by aortography, surgery, or autopsy showing a sensitivity of 100% and a specificity of 98% (one false-positive result). The typical appearance of aortic trauma on transesophageal echocardiography is a mobile 2- to 3-cm intraluminal flap or mass just distal to the junction of the aortic arch and descending thoracic aorta.

30. Vignon P, Gueret P, Vedrinne JM, et al: Role of transesophageal echocardiography in the diagnosis and management of traumatic aortic disruption. Circulation 92:2959–2968, 1995.

     In 32 consecutive trauma patients with suspected traumatic disruption of the aorta, two distinct echocardiographic patterns were seen: subadventitial traumatic disruption in 10 patients and traumatic intimal flaps in three patients. The remaining 18 patients had a normal echo and angiogram. Transesophageal echocardiography had a sensitivity of 91% and a specificity of 100% for diagnosis of subadventitial traumatic disruption compared to confirmation by aortography, surgery, or autopsy. Disruption can be recognized on transesophageal echocardiography by the presence of a thick flap (the disrupted aortic wall) that traverses the lumen at the level of the aortic isthmus, an irregular appearance to aortic wall due to pseudoaneurysm formation, and similar flow patterns on both sides of the disrupted aortic wall.

31. Pretre R, Chilcott M: Blunt trauma to the heart and great vessels. N Engl J Med 336:626–632, 1997.

     Review of cardiac trauma including types and mechanisms of injury, diagnosis, and management. The most common injury due to blunt trauma to the chest wall is thoracic aortic disruption at the aortic isthmus (just beyond the left subclavian artery).

The Echo Exam *Diseases of the Great Vessels*

Examination of the Aorta

Aortic Segment	Modality	View	Recording	Limitations
Proximal aorta	TTE	Parasternal long axis	Images of sinuses of Valsalva, aortic annulus, and sinotubular junction	Shadowing of posterior aorta
	TEE	High esophageal long axis	Standard long-axis plane by rotating to about 120–130°	
Ascending	TTE	Parasternal long axis	Move transducer superiorly to image sinotubular junction and ascending aorta	Only limited segments visualized, variable between patients
	TTE Doppler	Apical	LVOT and ascending aorta flow recorded with pulsed or CW Doppler from an anteriorly angulated four-chamber view	Velocity underestimation if the angle between the Doppler beam and flow is not parallel
	TEE	High esophageal long axis	From long-axis view, move transducer superiorly to image ascending aorta	The distal ascending aorta may not be visualized
Arch	TTE	Suprasternal	Long- and short-axis views of aortic arch	Descending aorta appears to taper as it leaves the image plane
	TEE	High esophageal	From the short-axis view of the initial segment of the descending thoracic aorta, turn the probe toward the patient's right side and angulate inferiorly	View not obtained in all patients. The aortic segment at the junction of the ascending aorta and arch may not be visualized
Descending thoracic	TTE	Parastenal and modified apical views	Rotate from long-axis view to image thoracic aorta in long axis posterior to left ventricle From apical two-chamber view, use lateral angulation and clockwise rotation to image aorta	Depth of thoracic aorta on TTE limits image qualtiy. TEE usually needed for diagnosis
	TTE Doppler	Suprasternal	Descending aorta flow recorded with pulsed Doppler from SSN view	Low wall filters needed to evaluate for holodiastolic flow reversal
Proximal abdominal	TTE	Subcostal	Long axis of proximal abdominal aorta	Only the proximal segement is visualized
	TTE Doppler	Transgastric	Proximal abdominal aorta flow recorded with pulsed Doppler	Low wall filters needed to evaluate for holodiastolic flow reversal
	TEE	Transgastric	From the transgastric position, portions of the abdominal aorta may be seen posteriorly	Does not allow evaluation of entire abdominal aorta

Aortic Dissection

Dissection flap In aortic lumen
                     Independent motion
                     True and false lumen
                     Entry sites
                     Thrombosis of false lumen
Intramural hematoma
Indirect findings Aortic dilation
                     Aortic regugitation
                     Coronary ostial involvement
                     Pericardial effusion

Sinus of Valsalva Aneurysm

Congenital Complex shape
                Protrusion into RVOT
                Fenestrations
Acquired Infection or inflammation
                Symetric shape
                Communication with aorta
                Potential for rupture

Aortic Atheroma

Complex (≥4 mm or mobile)
Associated with
    Coronary artery disease
    Cerebroembolic events

Complications of Thoracic Aortic Dissection

Aortic valve regurgitation
    Due to aortic dilation
    Due to leaflet flail
Coronary artery occlusion due to dissection at the orifice
    Ventricular fibrillation
    Acute myocardial infarction
Distal vessel obstruction or occlusion
    Carotid (stroke)
    Subclavian (upper limb ischemia)
Aortic rupture
    Into the pericardium
        Pericardial effusion
        Pericardial tamponade
    Into the mediastinum
    Into the pleural space
        Pleural effusion
        Exsanguination

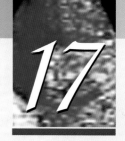

THE ADULT WITH CONGENITAL HEART DISEASE

Echocardiographic Approach
  Congenital Stenotic Lesions
  Congenital Regurgitant Lesions
  Abnormal Intracardiac Communications
    (Shunts)
  Abnormal Chamber and Great Vessel
    Connections

Congenital Defects Seen in Adults with or without Previous Cardiac Surgery
  Congenital Aortic Valve Abnormalities
  Congenital Obstructions to Right Ventricular
    Outflow
  Congenital Abnormalities of the Aorta
    Aortic Coarctation
    Marfan Syndrome
    Sinus of Valsalva Aneurysm
  Coronary Arteriovenous Fistula
  Congenital Regurgitant Lesions
    Ebstein Anomaly of the Tricuspid Valve
    Myxomatous Mitral Valve Disease
  Atrial Septal Defects
    Anatomy
    Imaging
    Doppler Examination
    Contrast Echocardiography
    After Atrial Septal Defect Repair

Ventricular Septal Defects
  Anatomy
  Imaging
  Doppler Findings
Patent Ductus Arteriosus
Ventricular Inversion
"Incidental" Congenital Anomalies
Other Congenital Cardiac Diseases
  Presenting in Adults

Adult Congenital Heart Disease with Prior Surgical Procedures
  Classification of Types of Procedures
  Tetralogy of Fallot
  Transposition of the Great Arteries
  Tricuspid Atresia
  Truncus Arteriosus

Limitations of Echocardiography/Alternate Approaches
  Calculations of Shunt Ratios
  Imaging
  Intracardiac Hemodynamics
  Integrating the Diagnostic Approach

Suggested Reading

Echo Exam

T here are two basic categories of congenital heart disease in adults:

- The initial clinical presentation of previously undiagnosed and untreated congenital defects
- Survival into adulthood of patients with known congenital heart disease and previous surgical procedures

In adult patients with no previous diagnosis of heart disease, a congenital defect often is not considered as a potential cause of symptoms, and thus the initial diagnosis may be made at the echocardiographic examination. In these patients, the diagnostic challenge is to recognize and correctly evaluate the congenital abnormality. In patients with known congenital disease and previous surgical procedures, the diagnostic challenge for the echocardiographer is to identify the postoperative anatomy and assess the physiologic consequences of residual defects in each patient. With "corrective" surgery, as well as with "palliative" procedures, many patients have significant residual or progressive abnormalities.

Both these challenges can be met by a logical and methodical approach to the echocardiographic examination with application of the basic principles of ultrasound imaging and Doppler data described throughout this text. Unusual imaging planes and careful integration of imaging and Doppler data may be needed for complete assessment of congenital heart disease. In addition, the physician and sonographer must have a thorough understanding of the three-dimensional (3D) anatomic relationships for each type of congenital defect.

Obviously, a comprehensive discussion of the echocardiographic findings in adult congenital heart disease is beyond the scope of this text. Instead, an overview of the echocardiographic approach to these patients and examples of the more common abnormalities will be presented. The reader is referred to the specialized references listed at the end of the chapter for more detailed information.

ECHOCARDIOGRAPHIC APPROACH

Congenital heart disease in adults can be grouped into several categories (Table 17–1):

- Stenotic lesions
- Regurgitant lesions
- Intracardiac shunts
- Abnormal connections
- Combinations or complex congenital disease

Congenital Stenotic Lesions

Congenital stenotic lesions are common, including obstruction to right or left ventricular outflow (either subvalvular, valvular, or supravalvular), obstruction to left ventricular inflow (congenital mitral stenosis, cor triatriatum), and narrowings in the great vessels (aortic coarctation, branch pulmonary artery stenosis).

The anatomy of a congenital stenotic lesion is specific for each condition (as discussed subsequently), although, in adult patients, images of the stenotic region may be suboptimal. The physiology and fluid dynamics of congenital stenosis are identical to those seen in acquired disease. There is laminar, normal-velocity flow upstream and a flow disturbance downstream from the narrowing. In the narrowed region itself, a high-velocity laminar jet of flow is present, with velocity (V, in m/s) related to the pressure difference (ΔP, in mm Hg) across the narrowing as stated in the simplified Bernoulli equation:

$$\Delta P = 4V^2$$

When a parallel intercept angle can be obtained between the jet and the ultrasound beam, quantitative data on stenosis severity and intracardiac hemodynamics can be derived. For example, if the maximum velocity across a subpulmonic stenosis is 4.5 m/s, then the maximum right ventricular to pulmonary artery systolic pressure difference is approximately 80 mm Hg. Quantitative evaluation of stenosis severity for a congenitally stenotic lesion includes calculation of maximum and mean pressure gradients as for acquired valve stenosis. Similarly, when possible, valve area calculations are performed either using the continuity equation (aortic valve) or the pressure half-time method (mitral valve).

Several significant differences between congenital and acquired stenosis should be noted. First, congenital stenosis of ventricular outflow, for both right and left ventricles, may involve the subvalvular or supravalvular region rather than (or in addition to) stenosis of the valve itself. Careful evaluation with conventional pulsed Doppler or color flow imaging to identify the poststenotic flow disturbance is helpful in determining the exact site of obstruction. Second, when serial stenoses are present, quantitation of the contribution of each level of obstruction to the overall degree of stenosis can be difficult using Doppler echo methods. Third, the proximal flow pattern in congenital stenosis often is characterized by a greater increase in velocity due to anatomic tapering of the proximal flow region (e.g., in aortic coarctation or in the congenitally stenotic pulmonic valve). In these situations, accurate pressure gradient calculations should include the proximal velocity (V_{prox}) as well as the jet velocity (V_{jet}) in the Bernoulli equation:

$$\Delta P = 4(V_{jet}^2 - V_{prox}^2)$$

Otherwise, evaluation of congenital stenosis is similar to evaluation of acquired stenosis in adults, and the methods described in detail in Chapter 11 can be applied in this patient group.

Congenital Regurgitant Lesions

Careful imaging of a congenitally regurgitant valve may reveal the specific mechanism of regurgitation in that patient. For the atrioventricular valves, particular attention is focused on the number and position of papillary muscles; the chordal attachments (especially aberrant ones); leaflet size, shape, thickness, redundancy, and motion; and annulus size and shape. Malformations can include myxomatous changes of the leaflets, abnormal leaflet position (Ebstein anomaly), and abnormal chordal attachments (atrioventricular canal defect). The semilunar valves may be regurgitant due to great vessel dilation or a leaflet fenestration.

The physiology of congenital regurgitation is no different from that of acquired regurgitation. There is a flow disturbance in the chamber receiving the regurgitant flow with progressive dilation (and eventual dysfunction) of the volume-overloaded cardiac chambers. Evaluation of congenital regurgitation is similar to evaluation of acquired regurgitation, as detailed in Chapter 12.

Abnormal Intracardiac Communications (Shunts)

An abnormal intracardiac communication is characterized by blood flow across the defect, with the direction, timing, and volume of flow determined by the size of the orifice, the pressure gradient across the defect, and the relative resistance to flow of the vascular beds on each side of the defect. If left-sided heart pressures exceed right-sided pressures (pulmonary vascular resistance is low), left-to-right flow across the defect predominates. Small degrees of right-to-left shunting may be present briefly during the cardiac cycle, because right-sided pressures may transiently exceed left-sided pressures.

With conventional pulsed Doppler ultrasound or with color flow imaging, a flow disturbance is found downstream from the defect: on the right side of the interventricular septum for a ventricular septal defect, in the right atrium for an atrial septal defect, and in the pulmonary artery for a patent ductus arteriosus.

Analogous to a stenotic or regurgitant orifice, the velocity of blood flow through the shunt orifice is related to the pressure gradient across the defect, as stated in the Bernoulli equation. Thus a small ventricular septal defect results in a high-velocity systolic flow signal (approximately 5 m/s), because left ventricular systolic pressure greatly exceeds right ventricular systolic pressure (by approximately 100 mm Hg). Conversely, flow across an atrial septal defect typically is low in velocity because only a modest left atrial to right atrial pressure difference is present.

A left-to-right intracardiac shunt imposes a chronic volume overload on the receiving chamber(s) with consequent dilation of the affected chamber(s). With an atrial septal defect, both right atrial and right ventricular dilation, along with paradoxical septal motion, are seen. With a patent ductus arteriosus, the volume overload is imposed on the left atrium and left ventricle. Although it might seem that a ventricular septal defect would cause right ventricular volume overload, in fact, right ventricular size usually is normal because the left ventricle effectively ejects the shunt flow across the defect directly into the pulmonary artery in systole. Instead, left atrial and left ventricular dilation are seen, because these chambers receive the increased pulmonary blood flow as it returns to the left side of the heart via the pulmonary veins.

The volume of blood flow (Q) across an intracardiac shunt—the ratio of pulmonary to systemic blood flow (Q_p:Q_s)—can be determined by Doppler echo measurements of stroke volume at two intracardiac sites (Fig. 17–1). In the case of an atrial septal defect, transpulmonic volume flow (Q_p) is calculated from pulmonary artery (PA) cross-sectional area (CSA) and velocity-time integral (VTI), while systemic volume flow (Q_s) is calculated from measurements of left ventricular outflow tract (LVOT) cross-sectional area and velocity-time integral:

Shunt ratio

$$Q_p = \text{CSA}_{\text{PA}} \times \text{VTI}_{\text{PA}}$$

$$Q_s = \text{CSA}_{\text{LVOT}} \times \text{VTI}_{\text{LVOT}}$$

so that

$$Q_p:Q_s = \frac{\text{CSA}_{\text{PA}} \times \text{VTI}_{\text{PA}}}{\text{CSA}_{\text{LVOT}} \times \text{VTI}_{\text{LVOT}}}$$

This approach is accurate when two-dimensional (2D) images are of adequate quality for precise diameter measurements (for calculation of a circular cross-sectional area) and when Doppler velocity data are recorded at a parallel intercept angle to flow. Potential errors in estimation of the Q_p:Q_s ratio may arise as for any Doppler echo stroke volume measurement (see Chapter 6).

With significant left-to-right shunting, pulmonary pressures become elevated, and irreversible pulmonary hypertension may develop over time. When pulmonary vascular resistance equals or exceeds systemic vascular resistance, the direction of shunt flow reverses, resulting in decreased systemic oxygen saturation and cyanosis. Irreversible pulmonary hypertension with equalization of pulmonary and systemic pressures due to an intracardiac shunt is known as *Eisenmenger's physiology*. This phenomenon can occur in infancy, particularly with a large ventricular septal defect, but also can occur later in life when the pulmonary-to-systemic shunt ratio chronically exceeds 2:1.

Abnormal Chamber and Great Vessel Connections

Echocardiographic diagnosis is more difficult when there are abnormal connections between the atrium and the ventricles and/or between the ventricles and great vessels. In adults, poor acoustic access may further compromise the examination. However, with a systematic approach, a correct anatomic evaluation usually is possible.

Because the position of the heart in the chest may be abnormal, the echocardiographer cannot rely on the intrathoracic position of the chambers for correct identification of cardiac anatomy. In *dextrocardia*, the heart is located in the right hemithorax with the apex in the right midclavicular line. With *situs inversus*, there is right-to-left reversal of thoracic and abdominal viscera. *Dextroversion* is a rightward shift in the cardiac apex without mirror-image inversion.

The first step in a systematic examination of complex congenital heart disease is determination of atrial situs. The inferior vena cava nearly

TABLE 17–1

Common Unoperated Congenital Heart Disease Seen in Adults

Congenital Defect	2D Echo Findings	Doppler Findings
Bicuspid aortic valve	Bicuspid valve identified in systole (raphe seen in diastole)	Mild stenosis and/or regurgitation
Unicuspid aortic valve	Abnormal, deformed aortic valve with systolic doming; sometimes the unicuspid orifice can be imaged	Aortic stenosis (may be severe) and/or aortic regurgitation
Subaortic membrane	Membrane from anterior MV leaflet to ventricular septum; TEE may be needed for visualization	High-velocity signal just proximal to aortic valve; AR due to nonsupport of aortic annulus or to a "jet lesion"
Pulmonic stenosis	Thickened pulmonic valve leaflets with systolic doming, increased *a* wave on pulmonic M-mode	Mild pulmonic stenosis (more severe stenosis is recognized and treated in childhood)
Aortic coarctation	Coarctation may not be easy to visualize since descending thoracic aorta goes out of the image plane from SSN; associated with bicuspid aortic valve; highly pulsatile aortic root and akinetic abdominal aorta	High-velocity systolic flow in descending thoracic aorta with extension of flow into diastole with severe obstruction; nonparallel intercept angle limits quantitation of severity in unoperated patients
Marfan syndrome	Dilated aortic root with loss of the sinotubular junction; elongated, redundant anterior MV leaflet; dilation of ascending aorta, arch, and descending aorta may be present	Aortic regurgitation
Sinus of Valsalva aneurysm	Dilated, thin sinus with "wind sock" type of projection into adjacent cardiac structures depending on sinus involved	May have fistula from aorta into RA, LA, RV, or LV depending on cusp involved
Coronary AV fistula	May not be able to visualize fistula, but coronary sinus may be dilated; proximal coronary artery may be dilated	Disturbed flow in coronary sinus or in abnormal epicardial echolucent structures
Ebstein anomaly	Septal tricuspid valve leaflet is adherent to RV wall, appearing "apically displaced"; apparent RA enlargement (part of anatomic RV is physiologically part of RA); associated with WPW and with right-to-left atrial shunt	Tricuspid regurgitation
Myxomatous mitral valve disease	Thick, redundant, prolapsing mitral valve leaflets; LV and LA enlargement depending on severity of MR; tricuspid and aortic valves also may be affected; can be seen in syndrome of polyvalvular dysplasia	Mitral regurgitation

	Two-dimensional findings	Doppler/contrast findings
Atrial septal defects	Right ventricular and right atrial volume overload with RVE, RAE, and paradoxical ventricular septal motion	$Q_p:Q_s$ can be calculated from Doppler stroke volume measurements in LVOT (or Ao) versus PA
	Secundum ASD: Absence of interatrial septum in fossa ovalis region best seen on subcostal or parasternal four-chamber view	Color flow imaging of left-to-right flow across interatrial septum; IV echo contrast shows some right-to-left shunting
	Primum ASD: Defect in IAS adjacent to central fibrous body; associated with atrioventricular valve abnormalities (cleft anterior MV leaflet)	Color flow imaging of left-to-right flow across interatrial septum; may have associated mitral regurgitation
	Sinus venosus ASD: Defect at SVC-RA junction (may be associated with anomalous PVR); TEE helpful for imaging defect; suspect when $Q_p:Q_s$ is elevated without clear evidence of secundum or primum ASD	TEE to visualize site of defect and left-to-right flow with color imaging
Partial anomalous pulmonary venous return	RVE, RAE, and paradoxical septal motion reflecting right-sided volume overload (may be associated with ASD)	Suspect when $Q_p:Q_s$ >1 with no evidence for flow across interatrial septum
Ventricular septal defects	*Small VSD:* Membranous, muscular, or outflow defects may be difficult to image: membranous defects may be partially or completely closed (ventricular septal aneurysm) by the septal leaflet of the tricuspid valve	High-velocity jet from left to right in systole with pulsed or CW Doppler; color flow imaging shows flow disturbance on right ventricular side of the defect; normal PA pressures
	Eisenmenger VSD: Large defect, often membranous or subaortic, with equal size and wall thickness of IV and RV	Low-velocity bidirectional flow across the ventricular defect; severe pulmonary hypertension
Patent ductus arteriosus	Mild LV and LA enlargement; duct itself rarely visualized in adults	Diastolic flow reversal in the pulmonary artery (typically along the anterior PA wall); diastolic flow reversal in the descending thoracic aorta
Ventricular inversion (corrected transposition)	RV-LV reversal; pattern of blood flow is physiologic: RA to LV to PA; LA to RV to Ao	Normal physiology in absence of associated defects; Doppler findings of pulmonic stenosis, VSD, atrioventricular valve regurgitation when present
	Associated defects are common, including pulmonic stenosis, VSD, heart block, and Ebstein's type anomaly of the inverted tricuspid valve with systemic atrioventricular valve regurgitation	
Persistent left SVC	Dilated coronary sinus; absence of innominate vein on SSN view; small right SVC	Contrast injection from left arm opacifies coronary sinus first, then right atrium
Hypertrophic cardiomyopathy	Asymmetrically hypertrophied LV with several patterns of involvement; 2D and M-mode signs of dynamic LVOT obstruction	Dynamic LVOT obstruction; mitral regurgitation; diastolic LV dysfunction
Tetralogy of Fallot	Large, overriding aorta; VSD: subvalvular or valvular pulmonic stenosis	High-velocity flow in RVOT and/or across pulmonic valve; bidirectional flow across VSD

AR, aortic regurgitation; ASD, atrial septal defect; IAS, interatrial septum; LA, left atrium; LVOT, left ventricular outflow tract; LV, left ventricle; MV, mitral valve; PA, pulmonary artery; PDA, patent ductus arteriosus; PVR, pulmonary venous return; RA, right atrium; RAE, right atrial enlargement; RV, right ventricle; RVE, right ventricular enlargement; RVOT, right ventricular outflow tract; SSN, suprasternal notch; SVC, superior vena cava; TEE, transesophageal echocardiography; TGA, transposition of the great arteries; TOF, tetralogy of Fallot; VSD, ventricular septal defect; WPW, Wolff-Parkinson-White (pre-excitation) syndrome.

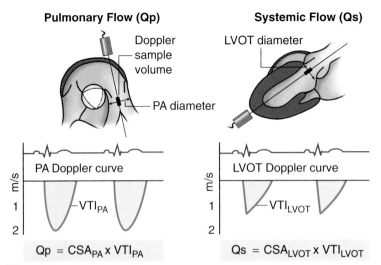

FIGURE 17–1. Schematic diagram of Doppler echo shunt ratio calculation. Pulmonary flow (Q_p) is calculated from transpulmonic stroke volume calculation using pulmonary artery (PA) diameter measured at the site of the Doppler sample position and the velocity-time integral (VTI) of pulmonary artery flow. A circular cross-sectional area (CSA) is assumed. Similarly, systemic flow (Q_s) is calculated from left ventricular outflow tract (LVOT) diameter and the velocity-time integral of left ventricular outflow tract.

always drains into the right atrium, allowing correct identification of this chamber by imaging the inferior vena cava from a subcostal approach and following it into the right atrium. Thus, the subcostal window often is a useful starting point for examination of a patient with complex congenital heart disease. The left atrium, then, is the "other" atrial chamber, because although the pulmonary veins normally drain into the left atrium, this is not always the case (e.g., partial or total anomalous pulmonary venous return).

The anatomic right and left ventricles can be distinguished from each other by several features. The anatomic right ventricle has

- prominent trabeculation,
- a moderator band,
- an infundibular region,
- a more apical atrioventricular annulus than the left ventricle, and
- a tricuspid valve.

Fibrous continuity of the anterior mitral valve leaflet and the aortic valve occurs only with a normally related left ventricle and aortic root. When the anatomic right ventricle connects to the aortic root, a band of myocardium is seen between the base of the atrioventricular valve leaflet and the great vessel. The atrioventricular valves develop with the appropriate anatomic ventricle, so identification of the mitral valve is another feature that differentiates the left from the right ventricle. Caution is needed if a cleft anterior mitral valve leaflet is present because it may superficially resemble the tricuspid valve. In addition to the number of atrioventricular valve leaflets, the relative positions of the atrioventricular valve annuli are helpful, since the tricuspid valve annulus lies slightly closer to the apex than the mitral valve annulus. Note that ventricular size, shape, and/or wall thickness do not distinguish the two ventricles, because congenital lesions can result in dilation and hypertrophy of either chamber.

After identifying the atrium and ventricles, attention is directed toward the great vessels. The aortic root is best identified by following the vessel downstream to image the arch and head and neck vessels. Origins of the coronary arteries also may be seen, but anomalous origin of the coronary arteries from the pulmonary artery must be considered. The pulmonary artery is identified by its bifurcation into right and left branches.

The position of the great vessels within the thorax and relative to each other often is altered in congenital disease. Normally, the pulmonary artery lies anterior and slightly medial to the aortic root at its origin and then courses posteriorly and laterally, with the right pulmonary artery lying posterior to the ascending aorta. The aortic annulus normally lies posterior to the right ventricular outflow tract, with the aortic root extending medially and anteriorly before turning posterolaterally to form the aortic arch. The normal relationship of the aortic and pulmonic valve planes is approximately perpendicular to each other, with the pulmonary valve slightly more superior within the chest than the aortic

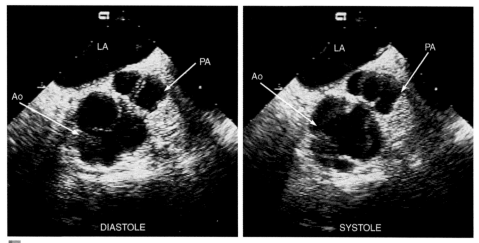

FIGURE 17-2. Transposed great arteries seen on a transesophageal view with an anterior aorta and a smaller posterior pulmonary artery with a bicuspid valve in a 42-year-old with congenital transposition of the great arteries, pulmonic stenosis, and a ventricular septal defect.

valve. With transpositions of the great vessels, these relationships are altered so that the semilunar valves lie in the same tomographic plane, and the aorta and pulmonary artery lie parallel to each other instead of in their normal "crisscross" positions (Fig. 17–2). If the aorta is located anterior and to the left, L (for levo) transposition is present. An anterior and medial (rightward) aorta is termed D (for dextro) transposition.

Most patients with abnormal connections between the cardiac chambers and great vessels have associated abnormalities that require echocardiographic evaluation. These include intracardiac shunts, stenotic and regurgitant lesions, pulmonary hypertension, and ventricular dysfunction. The echocardiographic examination in these patients is facilitated by the following:

- Knowledge of the clinical history, including previous surgical procedures and diagnostic tests
- Formulation of specific clinical questions to be answered by the echocardiographic examination

During the examination, the physician and sonographer work together in

- identifying the cardiac chambers, great vessels, and their connections;
- identifying associated defects, and evaluating the physiologic consequences of each defect with appropriate Doppler modalities; and
- identifying which clinical questions remain unanswered at the end of examination, and proposing appropriate alternate diagnostic tests that can provide answers to these questions.

CONGENITAL DEFECTS SEEN IN ADULTS WITH OR WITHOUT PREVIOUS CARDIAC SURGERY

Congenital Aortic Valve Abnormalities

Although a congenital bicuspid aortic valve is the most common type of congenital heart disease (reported to occur in 1% to 2% of the general population), the bicuspid valve often is functionally normal until about age 50 to 60 years, when superimposed fibrocalcific changes lead to aortic valve stenosis. Significant regurgitation of a congenital bicuspid valve occurs somewhat less commonly but presents in young adulthood with a diastolic murmur and symptoms of exercise intolerance.

The presentation of significant left ventricular outflow obstruction in a young adult should prompt consideration of abnormalities other than a bicuspid valve—specifically a unicuspid aortic valve, a subaortic membrane, or hypertrophic cardiomyopathy. A unicuspid aortic valve will appear as a thickened, deformed valve with systolic bowing of the valve on ultrasound imaging. A high parasternal short-axis view may show the eccentric unicuspid opening in systole, even allowing planimetry of the valve orifice. Doppler echocardiography can be used to determine the transvalvular gradient and valve area as for any type of aortic valve stenosis. Restenosis of the aortic valve in patients who previously underwent surgical valvotomy in childhood or adolescence is common. Restenosis occurs in up to 40% of patients a mean of 13 years after open surgical valvotomy.

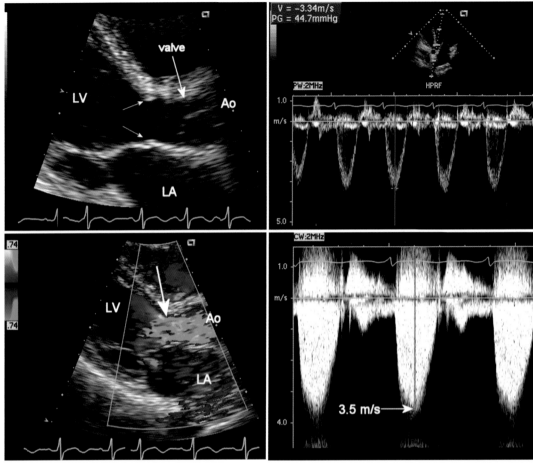

■ **FIGURE 17-3.** Parasternal long-axis 2D view *(top left)* in a patient with a systolic murmur showing a subtle ridge *(arrows)* in the left ventricular outflow tract. Color Doppler *(bottom left)* shows an increase flow velocity in this region suggesting the possibilty of a subaortic membrane *(arrow)*. High PRF Doppler *(top right)* shows an increase velocity to at least 3.3 m/s at this location and continuous-wave Doppler shows a maximum outflow velocity of 3.5 m/s *(bottom right)*.

Congenital subaortic obstruction can range anatomically from a muscular ridge to a thin membrane (Figs. 17–3 and 17–4). Although typically located 1 to 1.5 cm apically from the aortic valve plane, the membrane may be located immediately adjacent to the aortic valve. In either case, a subaortic membrane can be difficult to see in adults due to poor acoustic access. The possibility of a subaortic membrane should be considered when high-velocity flow is recorded in the left ventricular outflow tract, but the aortic valve leaflets appear normal. Transesophageal echocardiography may allow direct imaging of the subaortic membrane, especially if multiple image planes are used to identify this thin structure. Conventional pulsed Doppler, high-pulse-repetition-frequency Doppler, and color flow imaging can be helpful from either transthoracic or transesophageal approaches in demonstrating that, in contrast to

valvular aortic stenosis, the increase in antegrade velocity and poststenotic flow disturbance occur on the left ventricular side of the aortic valve, indicating that subaortic obstruction is present. Coexisting aortic regurgitation may be present due to chronic exposure of the aortic valve leaflets to the high-velocity subaortic flow, resulting in a "jet lesion" on the aortic valve, or (rarely) due to fibrous attachments from the subaortic membrane to the aortic valve leaflets.

Congenital Obstructions to Right Ventricular Outflow

Right ventricular outflow obstruction may be subvalvular (in the muscular outflow tract), valvular, or supravalvular (either in the main pulmonary artery or its major branches). Pulmonic stenosis can occur as an isolated anomaly but more often is part of a complex of abnormalities (for example,

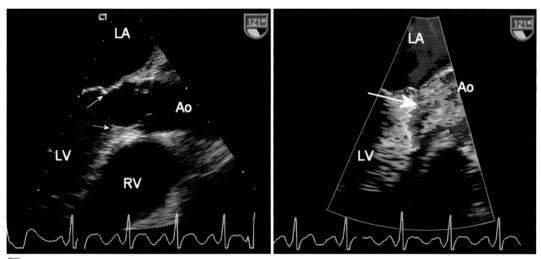

FIGURE 17–4. Transesophageal echocardiography in the same patient as in Figure 17–3 shows the subaortic membrane more clearly *(arrows)* in a long-axis view *(left)* with the flow disturbance demonstrated proximal to the aortic valve *(arrow)* on color Doppler *(right)*.

tetralogy of Fallot) or is associated with other abnormalities (for example, ventricular inversion).

The level of outflow obstruction can be determined using pulsed Doppler and color flow to identify the anatomic site at which the flow velocity increases and the poststenotic flow disturbance appears. The obstruction itself may be depicted on 2D echocardiography as a muscular subpulmonic ridge; as deformed, doming pulmonic valve leaflets; or as a narrowing in the pulmonary artery. If significant obstruction is present, compensatory right ventricular hypertrophy typically is seen.

The degree of obstruction can be measured by Doppler ultrasound using the Bernoulli equation (Fig. 17–5) with the proviso that only an estimate of the total obstruction may be possible if serial stenoses are present. Note that in the presence of pulmonic stenosis, the tricuspid regurgitant jet velocity remains an accurate reflection of the right ventricular to right atrial systolic pressure difference but no longer indicates pulmonary artery systolic pressure. Instead, pulmonary artery systolic pressure (PAP) can be estimated by (1) calculation of the right ventricular systolic pressure by adding the right ventricular to right atrial gradient (ΔP_{RV-RA} calculated from the tricuspid regurgitant jet) to an estimate of right atrial pressure (P_{RA}) and then (2) subtracting the right ventricular to pulmonary artery gradient (ΔP_{RV-PA}) calculated from the pulmonic stenosis jet:

$$PAP = (\Delta P_{RV-RA} + P_{RA}) - \Delta P_{RV-PA}$$

The end-diastolic velocity in the pulmonic regurgitation jet also may give useful data on pulmonary artery pressures because it reflects the diastolic pressure difference between the pulmonary artery and the right ventricle (high in patients with pulmonary hypertension, low in patients with pulmonic stenosis, and normal pulmonary artery diastolic pressures).

Congenital Abnormalities of the Aorta

Aortic Coarctation

A congenital narrowing in the proximal descending thoracic aorta most often is located just upstream from the entry site of the ductus arteriosus. Less often, postductal coarctation is seen. The coarctation may be relatively discrete, with involvement of only a short segment of the aorta, or may be a long, tubular narrowing. Imaging of the coarctation site is difficult from transthoracic or suprasternal notch windows in adults. From the suprasternal notch approach, the descending thoracic aorta has a tapering appearance, even in normal individuals, due to the oblique tomographic view of the descending aorta obtained as the descending aorta leaves the image plane. Adults with previous surgical repair of a coarctation may present with restenosis, depending on the specific surgical procedure used and the patient's age at the time of repair. For both operated and unoperated coarctations, transesophageal imaging with a long-axis view of the descending aorta may be helpful.

Doppler examination shows an increased velocity across the coarctation and, if the obstruc-

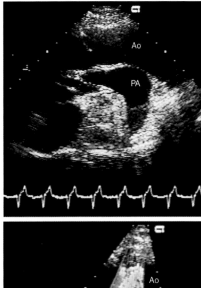

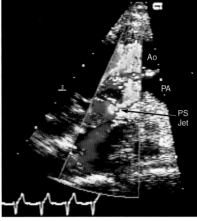

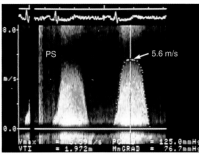

■ **FIGURE 17–5.** Two-dimensional parasternal long-axis view *(top)* of the same patient as in Figure 17–2 showing the transposed great vessels. Color flow imaging *(middle)* shows an eccentric jet with proximal acceleration across the stenotic bicuspid pulmonic valve. Note the proximal isovelocity surface area. Continuous-wave Doppler from a high right parasternal position *(bottom)* shows a maximum velocity of 5.6 m/s consistent with a maximum pulmonic stenosis (PS) pressure gradient of 125 mm Hg.

tion is severe, persistent antegrade flow into diastole (Fig. 17–6). If elevated, the proximal velocity should be included in the Bernoulli equation for pressure gradient estimation. The jet direction in an unoperated coarctation may be very eccentric, so it rarely is possible to achieve a parallel align-

ment between the ultrasound beam and jet direction, leading to underestimation of the severity of obstruction. In restenosis of a previously operated coarctation, the jet orientation tends to be more symmetrical, and a parallel intercept angle with correct estimation of the pressure gradient is more likely. In either case, other clinical methods for assessing severity of the coarctation are available (e.g., upper versus lower extremity blood pressure).

Marfan Syndrome

Marfan syndrome is inherited in an autosomal dominant pattern with variable penetrance. It is characterized by a specific, but variable, gene defect coding for fibrillin, a component of microfibrils (a key structure in elastic fibers), resulting in musculoskeletal, ocular, and cardiovascular manifestations. Cardiovascular abnormalities of Marfan syndrome include dilation, aneurysm formation, and rupture of peripheral arteries, an abnormally redundant anterior mitral valve leaflet, and most important, dilation and dissection of the aorta. Echocardiography may be helpful in confirming or excluding a diagnosis of Marfan syndrome in patients with a suspected diagnosis. Examination also is indicated to screen first-degree relatives of an affected individual.

Characteristic echocardiographic findings include dilation of the aortic annulus, aortic root, sinuses of Valsalva, and ascending aorta with loss of a clearly defined sinotubular junction (see Chapter 16). Aortic annular dilation results in aortic regurgitation and consequent left ventricular volume overload. Aortic dissection occurs frequently and can occur even when aortic dilation is not severe. With an aortic root diameter of more than 50 to 55 mm, the risk of spontaneous rupture is high, so many clinicians recommend periodic echocardiographic examination with prophylactic aortic root replacement with a valved aortic conduit when ascending aortic diameter exceeds this limit.

Sinus of Valsalva Aneurysm

A congenital aneurysm of the aortic sinuses of Valsalva appears as a thin, dilated area that projects into adjacent cardiac structures, often with a fistulous communication depending on which sinus is involved. On echocardiographic imaging, a congenital aneurysm often has a "wind sock" appearance with a long, convoluted, mobile sac of tissue extending from the aortic sinus into adjacent cardiac structures (see Fig. 16–3). This appearance contrasts with the more symmetrical dilation seen in aneurysms due to endocarditis. An aneurysm of the noncoronary sinus projects into the right

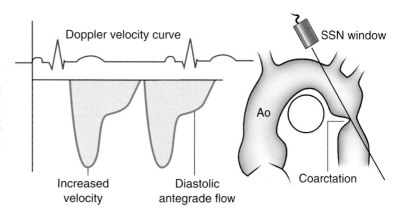

FIGURE 17–6. Aortic coarctation. From a suprasternal notch (SSN) window, continuous-wave Doppler of the coarctation shows an increased velocity in systole with persistent antegrade flow into diastole. Imaging of the coarctation often is suboptimal in adults.

atrium, the left coronary cusp into the left atrium, and the right coronary cusp into the right ventricular outflow tract. If a fistula is present, pulsed and color Doppler flow imaging demonstrate a left-to-right shunt with a flow disturbance in the receiving chamber. Continuous-wave Doppler shows a high-velocity systolic and diastolic flow signal.

Coronary Arteriovenous Fistula

A coronary arteriovenous fistula is a rare congenital anomaly that may present in young adults as a continuous murmur. Abnormal communication from a coronary artery to the coronary sinus or right atrium has been described. A coronary arteriovenous fistula is recognized echocardiographically as an abnormal area of dilation with diastolic or continuous flow plus a flow disturbance at the site of entry into the cardiac chamber (Fig. 17–7).

Other coronary artery abnormalities may be diagnosed on echocardiography, particularly when transthoracic or transesophageal images are of high quality, allowing identification of the proximal coronary arteries, such as the origin of the circumflex coronary artery from the right sinus of Valsalva, the origin of the right coronary artery from the left sinus of Valsalva, or the origin of the left main coronary from the right sinus of Valsalva. An anomalous coronary artery arising from the pulmonary artery rarely is diagnosed initially in adulthood because the resulting myocardial ischemia leads to significant clinical manifestations at a younger age.

Congenital Regurgitant Lesions

Ebstein Anomaly of the Tricuspid Valve

Ebstein anomaly is characterized by adherence of the basal segments of one (most often the septal) or more of the leaflets of the tricuspid valve to the right ventricular endocardium, resulting in the appearance of apical displacement of the tricuspid valve attachment (Fig. 17–8). In Ebstein anomaly, the distance between the tricuspid and mitral annulus exceeds the normal 10-mm difference. In severe cases, the tricuspid valve may be displaced nearly to the right ventricular apex. In addition, the tricuspid valve leaflets are thickened and malformed. Functionally, tricuspid regurgitation nearly always is present and may be severe. Typically, there is no antegrade obstruction to right ventricular diastolic filling (Fig. 17–9).

Owing to the apical displacement of the tricuspid leaflet insertion, a portion of the anatomic right ventricle physiologically serves as part of the right atrium. This "atrialized" ventricle adds to the appearance of right atrial enlargement, which is augmented by chronic atrial volume overload from tricuspid regurgitation. Ebstein anomaly may be seen as an isolated anatomic defect or may be associated with an aberrant atrioventricular conduction bypass tract (Wolff-Parkinson-White syndrome), an atrial septal defect, or other congenital anomalies (e.g., ventricular inversion). Ebstein anomaly of the anatomic tricuspid valve in a patient with ventricular inversion results in systemic atrioventricular valve regurgitation and chronic volume overload of the systemic ventricle.

Myxomatous Mitral Valve Disease

Like a bicuspid aortic valve, myxomatous mitral valve disease may be silent clinically until late in life, when progressive leaflet changes result in significant mitral regurgitation and symptom onset (see Chapter 12). The thickened, redundant mitral valve leaflets of myxomatous disease may result in slowly increasing severity of chronic mitral regurgitation with progressive volume overload of the left ventricle and atrium. Alternatively, chordal rupture can result in acute mitral regurgitation with abrupt symptom onset. Myxomatous involvement of tricuspid and, less often, aortic valves also may be present.

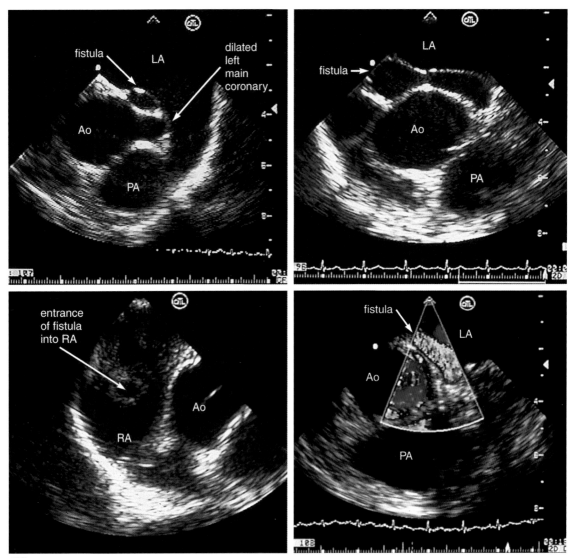

■ FIGURE 17-7. Coronary arteriovenous fistula from the left main coronary artery to the right atrium in a 20-year-old woman with a continuous murmur on auscultation. Transthoracic echocardiography showed an abnormal flow pattern in the right atrium. Transesophageal imaging showed a dilated left main coronary artery *(top left)* with a tortuous channel *(top right)* leading to an entrance in the right atrium *(bottom left)*. Color flow imaging shows disturbed systolic and diastolic flow in the fistula *(bottom right)*.

Atrial Septal Defects

Anatomy

There are three basic anatomic types of atrial septal defect (Fig. 17–10). The most common is a secundum defect, in which the central section of the atrial septum (the fossa ovalis) is absent due to failure of the secundum atrial septum to cover the foramen secundum during development.

A primum atrial septal defect is absence of the section of the interatrial septum adjacent to the central fibrous body. Developmentally, there is abnormal formation of the septum primum with failure of closure of the foramen primum. Primum defects often are associated with abnormalities of the atrioventricular valves, especially a cleft anterior mitral leaflet. A cleft anterior leaflet can be seen in parasternal short-axis and long-axis views, demonstrating the cleft with differing motion of the medial and lateral segments of the anterior leaflet (Fig. 17–11). In the long-axis view, lateral to medial angulation of the image plane shows the differing patterns of leaflet motion. The cleft mitral valve may be competent if adequate apposition of the edges of the cleft occurs in systole or may result in mitral regurgitation if

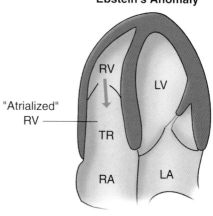

Ebstein's Anomaly

■ **FIGURE 17–8.** Schematic diagram of Ebstein anomaly showing apical displacement of the tricuspid valve, and "atrialization" of the base of the right ventricle. Tricuspid regurgitation with right ventricular and right atrial enlargement typically is present.

closure is functionally inadequate. In a more severe developmental abnormality–atrioventricular canal defect–the entire central fibrous body is absent, resulting in a primum atrial septal defect, a ventricular septal defect, and abnormalities of the atrioventricular valves.

The third type of atrial septal defect is the sinus venosus defect. This abnormal communication between right and left atrium is located near the junction of either the superior or inferior vena cava and the right atrium. Developmentally, it is related to abnormal fusion between the embryologic sinus venosus and the atrium. A sinus venosus defect may be associated with partial anomalous pulmonary venous return. Partial

anomalous pulmonary venous return also may be seen as an isolated defect and may not present until adulthood. The anomalous veins can drain directly into the right atrium or into the superior or inferior vena cava.

Imaging

Ultrasound imaging of an atrial septal defect is most reliable from a subcostal approach so that the ultrasound beam is perpendicular to the plane of the interatrial septum. From apical or parasternal windows, apparent loss of signal from the atrial septum may be due to a parallel alignment between the ultrasound beam and the structures

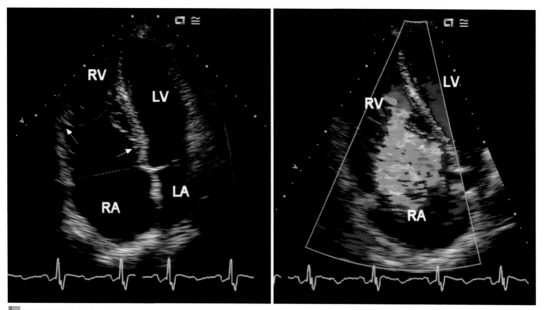

■ **FIGURE 17–9.** Apical four-chamber view *(left)* of an adult with Ebstein anomaly showing the apically displaced tricuspid valve *(arrow)*, compared to the tricuspid annulus *(dashed line)*, with right ventricular and right atrial enlargement. Color flow Doppler *(right)* shows severe tricuspid regurgitation.

Secundum ASD

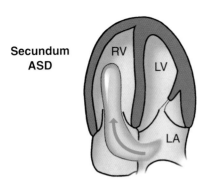

Primum ASD

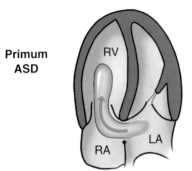

Sinus Venosus ASD

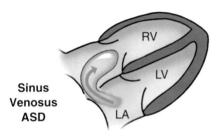

FIGURE 17–10. Schematic of primum, secundum, and sinus venosus atrial septal defects (ASDs). A secundum atrial septal defect is seen in the midsection of the atrial septum with prominent left-to-right flow on color imaging *(stippled area)*. Paradoxical septal motion and right ventricular and right atrial enlargement are present when the shunt is significant. A primum atrial septal defect is located near the atrioventricular connection and may be associated with abnormalities of the atrioventricular valves. A sinus venosus atrial septal defect is located at the base. Imaging of a sinus venosus defect may be difficult on transthoracic views but sometimes can be demonstrated from a subcostal approach.

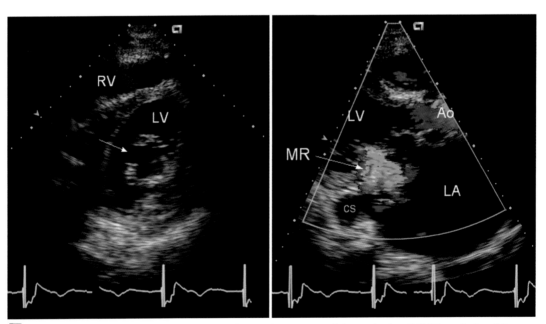

FIGURE 17–11. Cleft anterior mitral valve leaflet seen in a parasternal short-axis view *(left)*. Discontinuity of the anterior leaflet is seen *(arrow)*. On color flow imaging in a long-axis view *(right)*, an eccentric regurgitant jet with proximal acceleration is present.

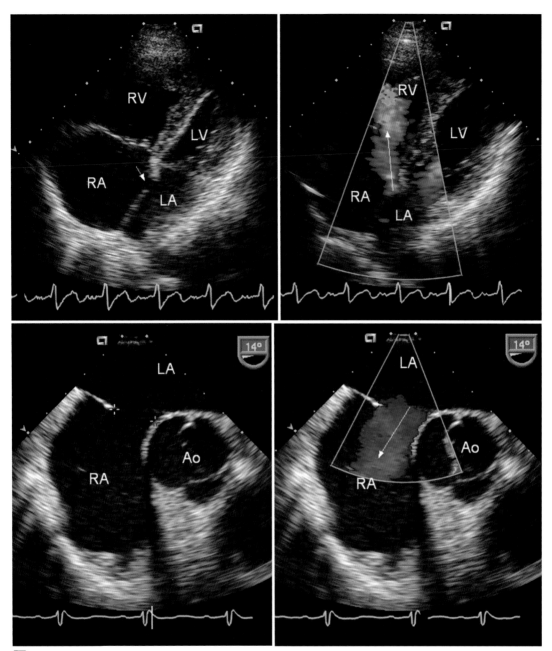

■ **FIGURE 17–12.** A secundum atrial septal defect is seen on transthoracic imaging *(top)* in a foreshortened apical four-chamber view *(arrow)* in association with marked right atrial and ventricular enlargement due to the left to right shunt seen on color flow imaging *(top right)*. Transesophageal imaging allows more precise localizaion and measurement of the septal defect *(bottom)*. Left to right flow across the defect is low velocity, as the pressure difference is small, so a uniform color signal is seen.

of interest (i.e., no ultrasound is reflected back to the transducer).

Secundum atrial septal defects are seen in the central portion of the atrial septum (Fig. 17–12), and primum defects (Fig. 17–13 and 17–14) are seen adjacent to the annuli of the atrioventricular valves. Imaging of a sinus venosus defect may not

be possible on a transthoracic study. However, because the defect is located in the superior and posterior aspects of the interatrial septum, a sub-costal approach can visualize the defect in some patients. Transthoracic echocardiography from a subcostal approach has a sensitivity of 89% for detection of a secundum atrial septal defect and

AV-Canal

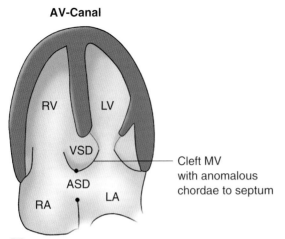

■ **FIGURE 17–13.** Schematic of an atrioventricular canal defect in a four-chamber view.

100% for a primum defect, but only 44% for a sinus venosus defect. Sinus venosus defects are well depicted from the transesophageal approach (Figs. 17–15 to 17–17).

If an atrial septal defect is associated with a significant left-to-right shunt (Fig. 17–18), right atrial enlargement, right ventricular enlargement, and paradoxical septal motion consistent with right-sided volume overload (Fig. 17–19) are uniformly present. In fact, evidence for right-sided heart volume overload often is the first abnormality noted during the echocardiographic examination. When evidence for right-sided heart volume overload is present in the absence of a visualized atrial septal defect or other definable cause for volume overload (e.g., tricuspid regurgitation), transesophageal imaging should be performed to evaluate for the possibility of a sinus venosus defect or partial anomalous pulmonary venous return.

Doppler Examination

Color flow imaging often allows reliable identification of the atrial septal defect flow based on the spatial distribution of the flow disturbance from the left to right atrium. However, multiple tomographic image planes are needed for correct identification of the origin of the flow signal. In some cases, the diastolic/systolic low-velocity flow signal across the atrial septal defect can be difficult to distinguish from other venous flow signals in the right atrium. Care must be taken to avoid mistaking superior vena cava flow into the right atrium, which often streams along the interatrial septum, for atrial septal defect flow. This appearance can be particularly misleading in high-volume flow states, such as pregnancy. Occasionally, a tricuspid regurgitant jet directed along the interatrial septum results in a confusing flow pattern, as well.

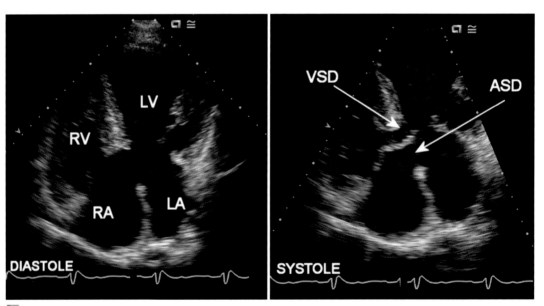

■ **FIGURE 17–14.** Ostium primum atrial septal defect with an accompanying ventricular septal defect, i.e. an atrioventricular canal. In an apical four-chamber view in diastole *(left)*, the communication between all four chambers is seen with the mitral and tricuspid valves open. In systole *(right)*, the atrioventricular valves are closed with the ventricular and atrial septal defects seen. These findings are consistent with Eisenmenger's physiology unless severe pulmonic stenosis is present.

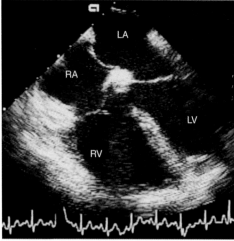

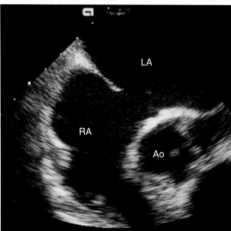

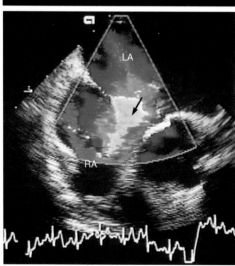

FIGURE 17-15. Transesophageal echocardiographic demonstration of an atrial septal defect in a 53-year-old woman. In a standard four-chamber view, the septum appears intact *(top)*. However, with slight anterior angulation, a defect is seen adjacent to the aortic root *(middle)* with color flow showing left-to-right flow across the defect *(bottom)*.

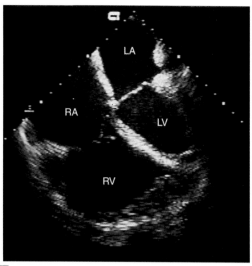

FIGURE 17-16. Sinus venosus atrial septal defect in a 74-year-old man. Although the transesophageal four-chamber view shows marked volume overload of the right side of the heart, the atrial septum appears intact in this view.

The subcostal window is optimal for color imaging of flow across the atrial septal defect, since the direction of flow is parallel to the ultrasound beam. Color flow imaging from other windows (including parasternal and apical) also is helpful, because it is the location and timing of the flow disturbance—rather than the absolute velocity of flow—that are diagnostic of the defect in the atrial septum. Color flow imaging shows a broad flowstream from left to right atrium in both diastole and systole with a more prominent diastolic component. With large shunts, the flow across the atrial septum extends across the open tricuspid valve into the right ventricle in diastole. Proximal flow acceleration on the left atrial side of the septum usually is evident.

Transesophageal echocardiography is helpful for further definition of the site and size of an atrial septal defect if transthoracic images are suboptimal. In addition, transesophageal imaging usually is needed when a sinus venosus defect or partial anomalous pulmonary venous return is suspected. Using a biplane or multiplane approach, 2D and color flow imaging will identify the abnormal defect and flow communication in the superior aspect of the posterior portion of the interatrial septum. Small secundum defects also are most likely to be detected from a transesophageal approach. The severity of left-to-right shunting across the atrial septal defect can be measured as described previously (Fig. 17–20).

Contrast Echocardiography

In a patient with a primum or secundum atrial septal defect, peripheral venous injection of echo

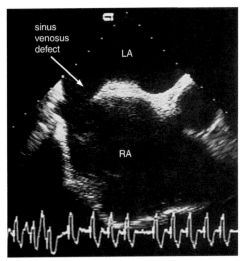

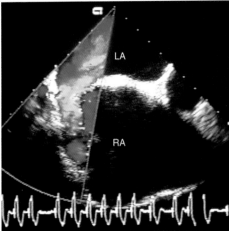

FIGURE 17–17. In the same patient as in Figure 17–16, the region of the atrial septum just inferior to the superior vena cava is absent *(top)*, and color flow demonstrates left-to-right flow across this defect *(bottom)*.

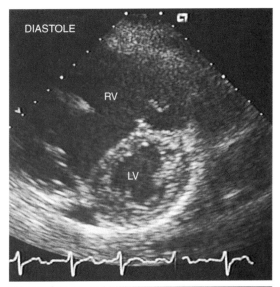

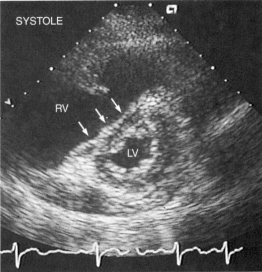

FIGURE 17–18. Right ventricular enlargement due to a secundum atrial septal defect in a 65-year-old woman with new-onset atrial fibrillation seen in a parasternal short-axis view in diastole *(top)* and in systole *(bottom)*.

contrast material shows passage of microbubbles across the interatrial septum, even when the shunt is predominantly left to right in direction. The explanation for this observation is that right atrial pressure transiently and briefly exceeds left atrial pressure, allowing passage of a small volume of blood from right to left. This small volume can be depicted when contrast echoes from the right atrium appear in the left atrium. Dense contrast in the right atrium also allows demonstration of a "negative" contrast jet across the atrial septal defect; that is, the blood flow from the left atrium into the right atrium will appear as an area with no echo contrast.

Contrast echo studies are rarely needed for diagnosis of an atrial septal defect when typical

2D echo, Doppler, and color flow imaging findings are present. The principle of using echo contrast to identify very small degrees of right-to-left shunting can be used to detect a patent foramen ovale as a potential etiology for a systemic embolic event (see Chapter 15).

After Atrial Septal Defect Repair

With a prior atrial septal defect repair, there may be mild residual right ventricular and right atrial dilatation. More than mild persistent dilation should prompt a search for a

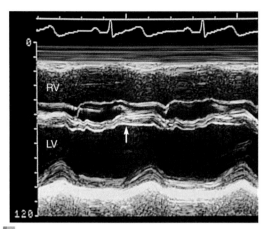

FIGURE 17–19. Paradoxical septal motion (note anterior motion in systole) and right ventricular enlargement on M-mode in a 21-year-old woman with an atrial septal defect.

residual defect or a leak around the patch repair.

Ventricular Septal Defects

Anatomy

There are four anatomically different types of ventricular septal defects (Fig. 17–21). The most common type is a membranous defect located in the region of the membranous septum immediately inferomedial to the aortic valve and lateral to the septal leaflet of the tricuspid valve. Small membranous ventricular septal defects may close spontaneously during childhood by approximation of the tricuspid valve septal leaflet across the defect. A completely closed defect may be undetectable in adulthood, or a residual anatomic abnormality—a ventricular septal aneurysm—may be visualized at the closure site without evidence

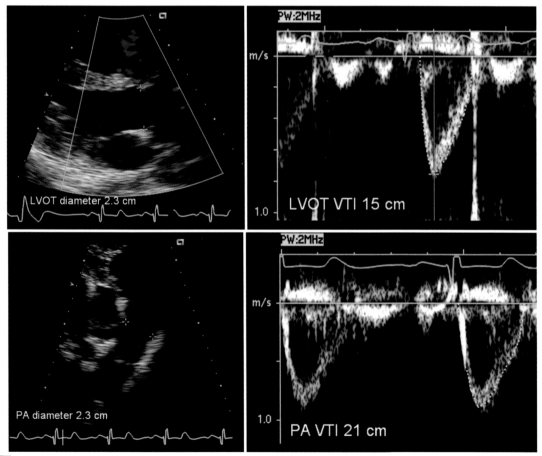

FIGURE 17–20. Calculation of the shunt ratio in a patient with an atrial septal defect. Systemic flow (Q_s) is calculated from the left ventricular outflow tract diameter (2.2 cm) and Doppler velocity time integral (VTI 15 cm) *(top)*, while pulmonary blood flow is calculated from the pulmonary artery diameter (2.3 cm) and Doppler velcoity time integral (VTI 21 cm) *(bottom)*. In this example, Q_p is 87 and Q_s is 57 mL so that $Q_p : Q_s$ is only 1.5, a value of borderline significance.

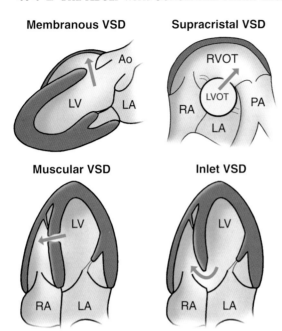

FIGURE 17–21. Schematic of types of ventricular septal defects (VSDs). A membranous VSD is seen in a medially angulated parasternal long-axis view, immediately adjacent to the aortic valve. A supracristal VSD is seen well in a short-axis view just below the aortic valve with flow from the left ventricular outflow tract (LVOT) into the outflow region of the right ventricle. A muscular VSD can be located anywhere in the muscular portion of the ventricular septum and may be multiple. An inlet VSD is seen in the apical four-chamber view and may be associated with an atrioventricular canal defect.

of blood flow from the left to the right ventricle. Incomplete closure leads to a persistent, albeit smaller, ventricular septal defect, which may be difficult to distinguish from septal aneurysm on 2D imaging. However, color flow and continuous-wave Doppler show typical evidence for an abnormal flow communication between the left and right ventricle even when the defect is small.

Muscular ventricular septal defects occur at any location in the muscular portion of the septum and may be multiple. When small, imaging the defect may not be possible with a tomographic imaging technique (such as echocardiography) even when multiple image planes are examined. Again, Doppler data are diagnostic in this situation.

Inlet ventricular septal defects are the result of failure of complete formation of the central fibrous body. This defect is located inferior to the aortic valve plane, adjacent to the mitral and tricuspid valve annuli. Inlet defects often are associated with other anomalies of the central fibrous body such as a primum atrial septal defect, atrioventricular valve abnormalities, or a complete atrioventricular canal defect.

Supracristal ventricular septal defects are located in the right ventricular outflow portion of the septum (above the crista ventricularis), lateral and just inferior to the aortic valve. These defects are rarely initially diagnosed in adulthood.

Imaging

As noted, while large defects may be visualized easily with 2D echocardiography, small defects may be very difficult to demonstrate. Membranous defects are imaged best in a parasternal long-axis view angulated slightly medially (Figs. 17–22 to 17–24). In the short-axis view just below the aortic valve level, the defect is seen in a 10-o'clock position inferior to the right coronary cusp of the aortic valve and adjacent to the septal leaflet of the tricuspid valve. In this view, a supracristal defect is located at the 2-o'clock position, inferior to the left coronary leaflet of the aortic valve and adjacent to the pulmonic valve. A supracristal defect is imaged in the long-axis plane by lateral angulation of the transducer from the standard long-axis view. Muscular ventricular septal defects may be seen in sequential basal-to-apical short-axis views of the left ventricle or in the apical four-chamber view. Inlet defects are best imaged in the apical four-chamber view or from the parasternal window in a short-axis view at the mitral valve level.

With a ventricular septal defect and a left-to-right shunt, dilation of the left ventricle and left atrium is seen due to volume overload of these chambers. Right ventricular size usually is normal, since the systolic flow across the defect is ejected directly into the pulmonary artery. Left ventricular systolic function typically is preserved because the shunt flow is ejected into the low-impedance pulmonary vascular bed. With large shunts, pulmonary vascular hypertension supervenes, resulting in Eisenmenger's physiology with right ventricular hypertrophy and dilation (Fig. 17–25).

Doppler Findings

Pulsed or color Doppler flow imaging shows a flow disturbance on the right side of the ventricular septum (with a left-to-right shunt). The presence and location of this flow disturbance are diagnostic even in the absence of a demonstrable defect on 2D imaging. The flow disturbance is detectable in the defect itself with proximal acceleration on the left side of the septum, immediately adjacent to the defect. Conventional pulsed Doppler ultrasound has a sensitivity of 90% and a specificity of 98% for detection of a ventricular septal defect. The sensitivity of color flow imaging probably is even greater.

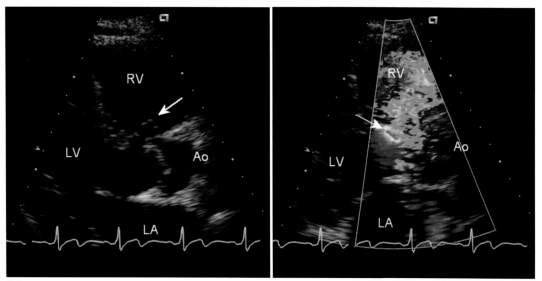

■ **FIGURE 17–22.** Small membranous ventricular septal defect with associated ventricular septal aneurysm *(arrow)* seen in a medially angulated parasternal long-axis view *(left)* in a 21-year-old man. Color flow Doppler in the same view *(right)* shows acceleration of flow in the orifice with a systolic flow disturbance in the right ventricular outflow tract.

Continuous-wave Doppler ultrasound shows a high-velocity left-to-right signal, with the shape of the velocity curve similar to that of mitral regurgitation, as determined by the instantaneous left ventricular to right ventricular pressure differences. In diastole, left-to-right shunting persists at a lower velocity (proportional to the diastolic left ventricular to right ventricular pressure differences) with the shape of the time-velocity curve similar to that of mitral stenosis. Brief reversal of flow may be, but is not always, present during isovolumic relaxation and contraction phases. Both the diastolic flow and brief reversals during the isovolumic periods are low velocity and thus may not be appreciated except at low high-pass filter settings on the Doppler spectral recording. Because this reversal of flow may not occur, intravenous injection of echo contrast material is less

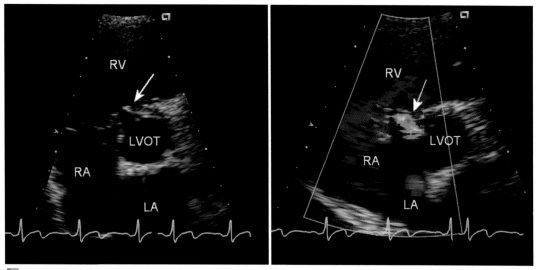

■ **FIGURE 17–23.** In the same patient as in Figure 17–22, the parasternal short-axis view *(left)* shows the ventricular septal aneurysm and defect *(arrow)* just inferior to the right coronary sinus of Valsalva at the 10-o'clock position of the left ventricular outflow tract (LVOT). Color Doppler *(right)* demonstrates left-to-right systolic flow across this defect.

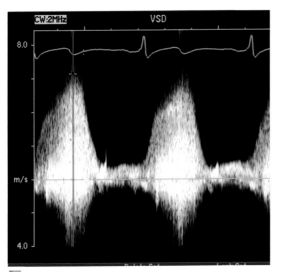

■ **FIGURE 17–24.** Continuous-wave Doppler of the small ventricular septal defect shown in Figures 17–22 and 17–23 from a parasternal window, demonstrates a high velocity (6 m/s) signal toward the transducer (with some channel cross-talk) corresponding to the high pressure difference between the left and right ventricles in systole. Because LV diastolic pressure is slightly higher than RV diastolic pressure, low velocity flow from left to right also is seen in diastole.

sensitive for detection of an intracardiac shunt at the ventricular level than at the atrial level.

Calculation of a pulmonic-to-systemic shunt ratio rarely is needed in adults with ventricular septal defects because either (1) the defect is small with a small volume of left-to-right shunt, or (2) a large defect with a significant shunt in childhood now has resulted in Eisenmenger's physiology with equalization of right and left ventricular pressures. If calculation of a shunt ratio is needed, systemic flow can be calculated in the aorta, and pulmonary flow can be calculated either in the pulmonary artery (if not disturbed by the septal defect flow) or across the mitral valve (pulmonary venous return).

Patent Ductus Arteriosus

A patent ductus arteriosus often is difficult to image in adults because of limited acoustic access. However, the chronic volume overload of the left atrium and left ventricle is manifested as dilation of these chambers. Left-to-right flow through the ductus can be detected with either conventional pulsed or color Doppler flow imaging using both parasternal short-axis and right ventricular outflow views of the pulmonary artery (Figs. 17–26 and 17–27). Diastolic ductal flow in the pulmonary artery, typically seen along the lateral wall of this vessel, has a sensitivity of 96% and specificity of 100% for diagnosis of a patent ductus

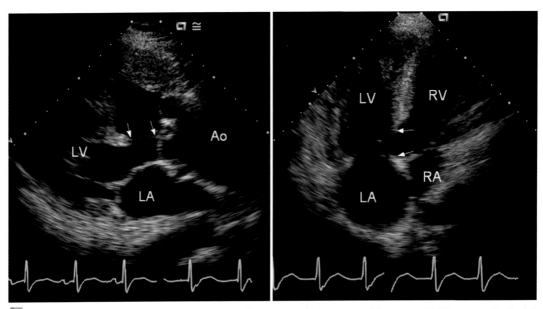

■ **FIGURE 17–25.** Large ventricular septal defect *(between arrows)* in a 26-year-old woman with Eisenmenger's physiology seen in a parasternal long-axis view *(left)* and apical four-chamber view *(right)*. Severe right ventricular hypertrophy is present. Doppler examination will show low-velocity bidirectional flow across the defect due to equalization of right and left ventricular pressures.

Patent Ductus Arteriosus

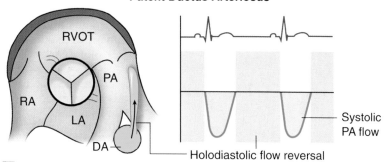

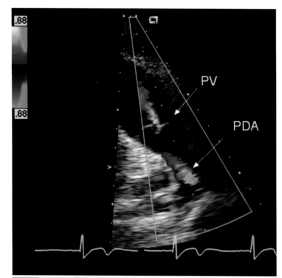

■ FIGURE 17–26. Schematic of a patent ductus arteriosus. Flow *(stippled area and arrow)* from the descending aorta into the pulmonary artery often streams along the lateral wall of the pulmonary artery on color flow imaging. Pulsed or continuous-wave Doppler shows holodiastolic flow reversal in the pulmonary artery. Systolic flow typically is abnormal as well, since aortic pressure exceeds pulmonary artery pressure throughout the cardiac cycle (giving rise to a continuous murmur on auscultation).

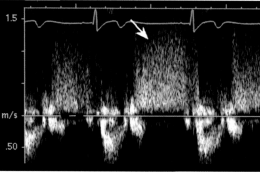

■ FIGURE 17–27. Patent ductus arteriosus (PDA) in a 22-year-old patient referred for an asymtomatic murmur. The parasternal right ventricular outflow view shows the pulmonary artery with a color jet of pulmonic regurgitation at the pulmolnary valve (PV) level and a second color jet in diastole in the pulmonary artery. Pulsed Doppler of the patent ductus flow shows characteristic diastolic flow reversal *(arrow)* extending into early systole. The pulmonic regurgitant signal was shorter with a lower velocity.

arteriosus. Recording of flow in the descending aorta, from a suprasternal notch approach, shows holodiastolic flow reversal due to antegrade flow into the ductus in diastole. This finding must be distinguished from diastolic flow reversal due to aortic regurgitation, because the two conditions may coexist in adult patients.

Ventricular Inversion

Congenitally corrected transposition of the great arteries (TGA) is more clearly designated "ventricular inversion," because the anatomic right ventricle serves as the systemic ventricle, and the anatomic left ventricle serves as the venous ventricle. Physiologically, the pathway of venous and systemic blood flow is normal in uncomplicated ventricular inversion (Fig. 17–28). Systemic venous blood returns to the right atrium, crosses the mitral valve into an anatomic left ventricle, and then is ejected into the pulmonary artery. Pulmonary venous return to the left atrium crosses the tricuspid valve into an anatomic right ventricle and then is ejected into the aorta. In the absence of associated defects, the diagnosis may be made "incidentally" in adulthood (Fig 17–29). However, associated defects are common, including ventricular septal defects, pulmonic stenosis, complete heart block, and Ebstein anomaly of the "inverted" tricuspid valve. Dilation, and eventual systolic dysfunction, of the systemic ventricle is common, although it is unclear whether this is due to the anatomy of the right ventricle being less suited to performing as the systemic ventricle, to inadequate coronary blood flow via the right coronary artery, or to associated systemic atrioventricular valve regurgitation.

On echocardiographic examination, ventricular inversion is recognized by identifying the anatomic ventricles in a side-by-side orientation

Ventricular Inversion

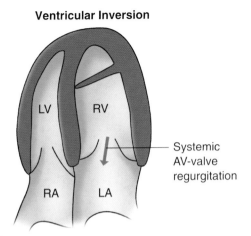

FIGURE 17–28. Schematic of ventricular inversion. With ventricular inversion (or "corrected" transposition of the great arteries), systemic venous blood returns to the right atrium, passes across the mitral valve into an anatomic left ventricle, and exits the left ventricle into the pulmonary artery. Pulmonary venous return into the left atrium is directed across the tricuspid valve into an anatomic right ventricle (with moderate band) and from there into the aorta. Common associated abnormalities are an Ebstein-type malformation of the tricuspid valve resulting in systemic atrioventricular valve regurgitation, pulmonic stenosis, a ventricular septal defect, and complete heart block.

and demonstrating the pathway of blood flow. Associated defects have 2D echo and Doppler findings as described for each abnormality. In addition, the position of the great vessels is abnormal, with the two semilunar valves lying in the same image plane—best seen in parasternal short-axis views—and with the great vessels parallel to each other—best seen in parasternal long-axis views. Typically, the aortic annulus is anterior and to the left of the pulmonic valve. Ventricular inversion also is associated with dextroversion (apex points toward the right), which makes the echocardiographic examination technically more difficult because the cardiac structures lie directly behind the sternum, limiting acoustic access.

"Incidental" Congenital Anomalies

A few congenital anomalies have no known adverse clinical effects but are important in that, if not recognized, they can be mistaken for pathologic conditions and prompt other (possibly harmful) diagnostic tests. A persistent left superior vena cava is seen in a small percentage (0.3% to 0.5%) of otherwise normal individuals and in a higher percentage (3% to 10%) of patients with other congenital heart abnormalities. Since this vein drains into the coronary sinus, dilation of the coronary sinus is seen on parasternal long- and short-axis views and on an apical four-chamber

view angulated posteriorly (see Fig. 15–5). This latter view nicely illustrates the entry of the dilated coronary sinus into the right atrium. The diagnosis can be confirmed (if questions remain) by injection of echo contrast material into the left arm, which will first opacify the coronary sinus and then the right atrium. Injection of echo contrast material into the right arm will opacify only the right atrium. The dilated coronary sinus can protrude into the left atrium, particularly on the parasternal long-axis view, sometimes being mistaken for a left atrial mass.

Idiopathic dilation of the pulmonary artery is another uncommon benign abnormality. The diagnosis is made when the pulmonary artery is enlarged but there is no evidence of pulmonic stenosis (which might result in poststenotic dilation) or other congenital abnormalities.

A Chiari network is a prominent inferior vena cava valve with fibrous extensions to the crista terminalis and/or coronary sinus valve seen in 2% of patients undergoing transesophageal echocardiography. These fibrous connections are fenestrated and lax, forming a "network" which shows rapid chaotic motion during the cardiac cycle. On 2D imaging, the appearance of small, echogenic targets moving rapidly in the right atrium suggests this diagnosis. Although the Chiari network itself is benign, there is a high likelihood of an associated atrial septal aneurysm or patent foramen ovale.

Other Congenital Cardiac Diseases Presenting in Adults

In addition to conditions considered under the category of congenital heart disease, other cardiac diseases in adults are congenital (or genetic) in origin but usually present in adulthood. For example, hypertrophic cardiomyopathy and Marfan syndrome are inherited disorders (see Chapters 9 and 16). Other types of cardiomyopathy may show a familial pattern, suggesting a genetic component. As our knowledge of molecular cardiology expands, other "acquired" diseases may be found to be genetic in origin.

ADULT CONGENITAL HEART DISEASE WITH PRIOR SURGICAL PROCEDURES

Classification of Types of Procedures

Numerous palliative and corrective surgical treatments for congenital heart disease have been developed since the first closure of a patent ductus arteriosus in 1938. These procedures can be grouped in several categories, as indicated in Table 17–2 and as listed here.

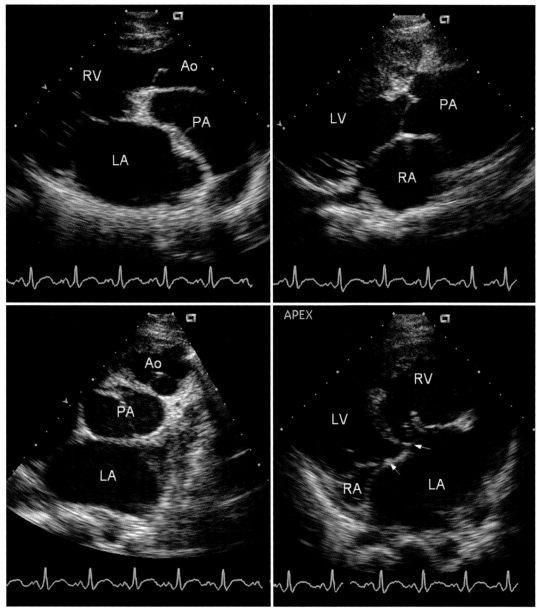

■ **FIGURE 17–29.** In a patient with congentiallly corrected transposition of the great arteries (ventricular inversion), two long-axis images are obtained from a parasternal position with the aorta and pulmonary artery in a side-by-side orientation. The systemic right ventricle and anteriorly located aorta are seen *(upper left)* with the muscular separation between the atrioventricular valve and semilunar valve evident. This anterior great vessel was identified as the aorta by following it superiorly to the arch and head and neck vesels. With slight lateral angulation, a long-axis view of the venous left ventricle and posteriorly located (and dilated) pulmonary artery is seen *(upper right)*. Note the fibrous continuity between the atrioventricular and semilunar valve. In the short-axis view *(lower left)*, the aortic and pulmonic valves are both seen in cross section with the aortic valve located anterior to the pulmonic valve. The apical four-chamber view in the standard display format demonstrates the anatomic right ventricle (RV) on the patient's left, which serves as the systemic ventricle. Note apical displacement of the tricuspid valve septal leaflet compared to the mitral leaflet insertion (arrows). This patient has significant regurgitation of the systemic (anatomic tricupsid) atrioventricular valve resulting in left atrial enlargement.

TABLE 17-2

Common Operations for Congenital Heart Disease Seen in Surviving Adults

Type	Procedure	Description	Defects Treated	Years
Shunts	Blalock-Taussig	Anastomosis of subclavian artery to PA (with or without modification)	Reduced pulmonary blood flow (TOF, TGA, pulmonary atresia, tricuspid atresia)	1945–present
	Blalock-Hanlon	Conduit (subclavian remains intact) Surgical atrial septostomy (largely replaced by percutaneous blade-and-balloon septostomy)	TGA (early palliation), mitral atresia, complex congenital heart disease	1950–early 1980s (occasionally still performed)
	Rashkind balloon	Percutaneous atrial	TGA	1966–present
	Potts	Descending aorta to left PA	Alternate to Blalock	1946–mid-1960s
	Waterston	Ascending aorta to right PA	Alternate to Blalock	1962–present
	Glenn	SVC to divided right PA (bidirectional = SVC to right PA without isolation from left PA)	Tricuspid atresia, pulmonic atresia, constitutes a portion of a hemi-Fontan	1959–present (1985–present)
Closures	Atrial septal defect (ASD)	Primary; patch or percutaneous closure	ASD with Q_p:Q_s 2:1	1954–present
	Ventricular septal defect (VSD)	Primary or patch closure	Isolated VSD or with other anomalies (TOF)	1955–present
	Patent ductus arteriosus (PDA)	Ligation +/– division of PDA (transcatheter technique 1981)	Patent ductus arteriosus	1938–present
	Endocardial cushion defect repair	Closure of ASD and VSD, repair of atrioventricular valve abnormalities (e.g., cleft mitral leaflet)		
PA banding		PA band to decrease PA flow and pressure	Large left-to-right shunts	1952–present
Atrial baffles	Mustard	Dacron or pericardial baffle directs systemic venous return to PA via LV, pulmonary venous return to aorta via RV	TGA (replaced by arterial switch procedures at many centers)	1964–present
	Senning	RA free wall and interatrial septal tissue used for similar baffle	TGA (replaced by arterial switch procedures at many centers)	1959–1964, 1980–present

	Procedure	Description	Indication	Dates
Relief of stenosis	Aortic coarctation repair	Various procedures including end-to-end anastomosis, patch enlargement, Gore-Tex graft; balloon dilation for recoarctation	Aortic coarctation	1944–present Balloon dilation 1983–present
	Pulmonic valvotomy	Brock trans-RV approach; direct surgical repair Balloon dilation	TOF, pulmonic stenosis	1948–1960s 1960s–present
	Aortic valvotomy	Direct surgical valvotomy or percutaneous balloon dilation	Congenital aortic stenosis	1982–present
	Mitral repair	Open commissurotomy	Congenital mitral stenosis	
	Konno procedure	LVOT enlargement by creation of a VSD, which is then patched, plus aortic valve replacement	LV outflow obstruction not amenable to valvotomy	1976–present
Great vessel switch	Jatene procedure	Switch of aortic root and PA trunk, coronaries transposed to neoaorta	TGA	1976 (Brazil) 1988–present
	Fontan procedure	Conduit from RA to PA with prosthetic conduit (+/− valve)	TGA, double-inlet ventricle with pulmonic stenosis, tricuspid atresia	1971–present
Conduits	Rastelli procedure	Valved conduit from RV to transected PA. LV to aorta via VSD and intraventricular patch	TGA + VSD + subvalvular pulmonic stenosis, truncus arteriosus, double-outlet RV	1968–present
	Damus-Kaye Stansel	Supravalvular anastomosis of aorta and PA (functions as aortopulmonary window) to relieve subvalvular stenosis	Irreparable subaortic obstruction with a double-inlet ventricle	1975–present
	Norwood procedure	Ascending aorta enlarged with pulmonary trunk; Fontan from RV to PA (two-stage procedure)	Aortic valve atresia, hypoplastic left heart	1983–present

AR, aortic regurgitation; ASD, atrial septal defect; IAS, interatrial septum; LA, left atrium; LVOT, left ventricular outflow tract; LV, left ventricle; MV, mitral valve; PA, pulmonary artery; PDA, patent ductus arteriosus; PVR, pulmonary venous return; RA, right atrium; RAE, right atrial enlargement; RV, right ventricle; RVE, right ventricular enlargement; RVOT, right ventricular outflow tract; SSN, suprasternal notch; SVC, superior vena cava; TEE, transesophageal echocardiography; TGA, transposition of the great arteries; TOF, tetralogy of Fallot; VSD, ventricular septal defect; WPW, Wolff-Parkinson-White (pre-excitation) syndrome.

- Shunts
- Closures
- Pulmonary banding
- Atrial baffles
- Relief of stenosis
- Great vessel switch
- Conduits

The approximate years during which each procedure was performed are shown to indicate which are likely to be encountered in a patient of a given age and to provide a historical explanation of why a patient may have had a particular procedure.

In conditions with low pulmonary blood flow, such as tetralogy of Fallot, transposition of the great arteries, pulmonary atresia, or tricuspid atresia, an intracardiac shunt is created to increase pulmonary blood flow. Shunts may redirect flow from a systemic artery to a pulmonary artery (Blalock-Taussig, Potts, Waterston), from a systemic vein to the pulmonary artery (Glenn), or at the atrial level (Blalock-Hanlon or balloon atrial septostomy). In some cases, these shunts are removed ("taken down") at the time of subsequent corrective surgery. Complications of surgical shunts include

- inadequate pulmonary blood flow due to kinking or closure of the shunt,
- excessive pulmonary blood flow resulting in pulmonary hypertension, and
- thrombus formation.

Procedures to close congenital intracardiac shunts—atrial septal defects, ventricular septal defects, patient ductus arteriosus—are conceptually straightforward and may be performed by suturing the edges of the defect (primary closure) or by using a pericardial or synthetic patch. The most common long-term complication of a shunt closure is a residual shunt.

Pulmonary banding is a palliative procedure that creates functional pulmonary stenosis to reduce pulmonary blood flow and "protect" the pulmonary vasculature from irreversible pulmonary hypertension. It is performed in patients with a large left-to-right shunt when definitive repair is not possible or must be delayed. If the degree of banding is not adequate, pulmonary hypertension still may ensue. Distal migration of the band can result in unequal right versus left pulmonary artery obstruction.

Atrial baffle procedures for transposition of the great arteries are designed to redirect intraatrial flow so that systemic venous return goes to the pulmonary artery (via the anatomic mitral valve and left ventricle) and pulmonary venous return goes to the aorta (via the anatomic tricuspid valve and right ventricle). The 3D anatomy of these baffles is complex and may be difficult to demonstrate on a transthoracic study due to poor ultrasound penetration at that depth. A transesophageal approach improves image quality, but an experienced examiner and multiple tomographic planes are needed to fully assess the interatrial baffle. Late complications of this procedure include baffle obstruction, baffle leaks, systolic dysfunction of the systemic (anatomic right) ventricle, and arrhythmias. More recently, the great vessel switch procedure has been used to treat patients with transposition. Complications of this procedure are related to reimplantation of the coronary arteries and supravalvular great vessel obstruction at the anastomotic sites.

Procedures to relieve congenital stenotic lesions include aortic coarctation repair; pulmonic, aortic, or mitral valvotomy either with direct surgical inspection or with a percutaneous balloon; and the Konno procedure to relieve left ventricular outflow obstruction. A residual gradient may be present after these procedures, and valvular regurgitation may be induced.

More complex intracardiac repairs that use conduits (with or without valves) include

- the Fontan procedure (right atrial to pulmonary artery),
- the Rastelli procedure,
- the Damus-Kaye-Stansel procedure, and
- the Norwood procedure.

Many patients with a prior Rastelli or Fontan procedure are now being seen as young adults (Figs. 17–30 and 17–31). Complications of the Rastelli procedure include subaortic obstruction in the left ventricular to aortic baffle, obstruction of the right-sided conduit, and residual ventricular septal defects. Evaluation of patients with a Fontan procedure is complicated by the numerous variations of the surgical approach in the method of connecting systemic venous return to the pulmonary artery. These patients often require transesophageal imaging for visualization. Late complications of the Fontan procedure include baffle obstruction, interatrial shunts, and thrombus formation.

When patients with previous surgical procedures for congenital heart disease present for echocardiographic evaluation, more detailed references on congenital heart disease can be helpful in planning, performing, and interpreting the echocardiographic examination. Echocardiographers dealing with these patients should consult these sources (see Suggested Reading).

Tetralogy of Fallot

The three primary characteristics of tetralogy of Fallot (Fig. 17–32) are a

- membranous ventricular septal defect,
- large aorta positioned across the ventricular septal defect ("overriding"), and
- right ventricular outflow obstruction that may be sub-, supra-, or valvular in location.

The fourth feature of this tetralogy is right ventricular hypertrophy secondary to outflow obstruction.

Adults with an untreated tetralogy of Fallot are rarely seen due to the high mortality of this condition without surgical intervention. In adults with a repaired tetralogy of Fallot, the ventricular septal defect patch is evident, the aortic root is enlarged, and some degree of residual right ventricular outflow obstruction may be present (Fig. 17–33). However, the major long-term issue in adults with surgically treated tetralogy of Fallot is late pulmonic regurgitation (Fig 17–34).

Transposition of the Great Arteries

Adults with surgical treatment of TGA undergo echocardiographic evaluation either for routine follow-up examination in the asymptomatic patient or for recurrent cardiac symptoms. Adults with a previous interatrial baffle procedure are most often seen given the more recent introduction of the arterial switch procedure (Fig. 17–35). Echocardiographic evaluation includes identification of the transposed great arteries, correct identification of the two ventricles, evaluation of the blood flow pathway, and evaluation of the intraatrial baffle with transthoracic and transesophageal echocardiography.

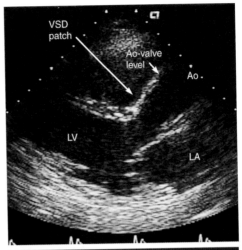

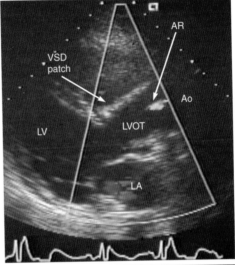

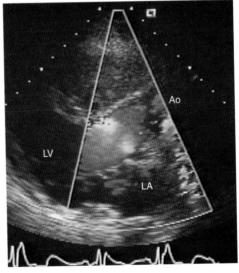

FIGURE 17–30. Parasternal long-axis view in a 26-year-old woman with transposition of the great arteries and a ventricular septal defect with a prior Rastelli repair. The aortic valve *(arrow)* is located superiorly with the ventricular septal defect patch forming an elongated outflow tract *(top)*. A small amount of aortic regurgitation is present in diastole *(middle)*, but there is no evidence of subaortic obstruction in systole *(bottom)*.

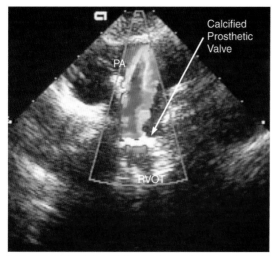

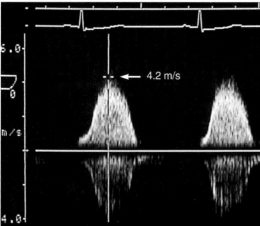

FIGURE 17–31. In a 33-year-old asymptomatic woman with transposition of the great arteries and a prior Rastelli repair, transesophageal imaging shows severe calcification of the prosthetic valve *(arrow)* in the right ventricular to pulmonary artery conduit with a stenotic jet seen on color flow imaging *(top)* with a velocity of 4.2 m/s by continuous-wave Doppler recording *(bottom)*.

Tricuspid Atresia

Evaluation of the adult patient with tricuspid atresia includes assessment of the previous surgical procedures to increase pulmonary blood flow. A complete surgical history is very helpful in directing the echocardiographic examination since the exact location of the conduit and the use of a valved versus nonvalved conduit vary from patient to patient. Systemic arterial or venous shunts to the pulmonary artery may be difficult to demonstrate if image quality is suboptimal, in which case other tomographic imaging procedures or angiography may be needed. If a Fontan conduit or anastomosis from the right atrium to

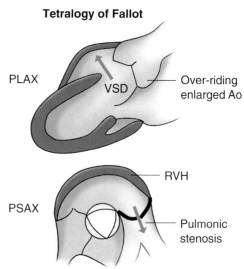

FIGURE 17–32. Schematic of tetralogy of Fallot. Tetralogy of Fallot is characterized by a large ventricular septal defect with an enlarged aorta that spans (or overrides) the defect, pulmonic stenosis (which may be subpulmonic or valvular), and compensatory right ventricular hypertrophy (RVH).

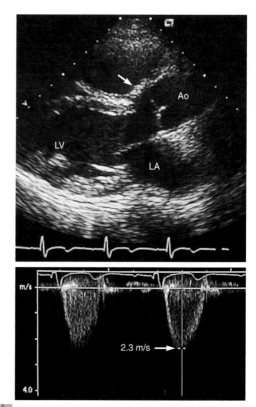

FIGURE 17–33. A 23-year-old woman with repaired tetralogy of Fallot. The overriding aorta and ventricular septal defect patch are seen in the parasternal long-axis view *(top)*. This patient has mild residual pulmonic stenosis (jet velocity 2.3 m/s) after a patch enlargement of the right ventricular outflow tract *(bottom)*.

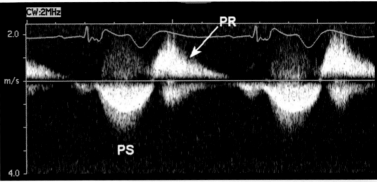

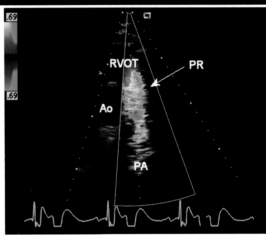

FIGURE 17–34. In a 34-year-old woman with a repaired tetralogy of Fallot, progressive right ventricular enlargement is noted. Evaluation of the pulmonic valve shows severe pulmonic regurgitaion with continuous-wave Doppler *(top)* characterized by a midly increased antegrade velocity (PS) and a dense pulmonic regurgitant signal (PR). Color Doppler *(bottom)* shows flow filling the right ventricular outflow tract in diastole. Because the flow velocity is low, this finding may be missed on real-time viewing of the images, emphasizing the importance of frame-by-frame review when this diagnosis is suspected.

Transposition of the Great Arteries

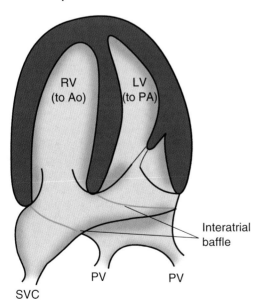

FIGURE 17–35. Schematic of interatrial baffle repair for transposition of the great arteries which directs systemic venous return to the anatomic left ventricle (and then to the pulmonary artery) and pulmonary venous return to the anatomic right ventricle (and then aorta). With this repair, the anatomic right ventricle serves as the systemic ventricle. Adequate visualization of the interatrial baffle usually requires transesophageal imaging in adults.

pulmonary artery is present, it usually can be visualized anteromedially and superiorly to the right atrium (Fig. 17–36).

Truncus Arteriosus

A surgically treated patient with truncus arteriosus will have variable 2D echocardiographic findings depending on the anatomic type of truncus present and the specific repair performed. Again, obtaining a complete surgical history before performing the study is very helpful. The echocardiographic examination then is directed toward the specific clinical question, after demonstrating the basic anatomy and pathway of blood flow in the patient.

LIMITATIONS OF ECHOCARDIOGRAPHY/ ALTERNATE APPROACHES

Calculations of Shunt Ratios

Accurate calculation of shunt ratios by Doppler echocardiography depends on accurate stroke volume determinations at two intracardiac sites. Each of these stroke volume determinations can be affected by several factors, as discussed in Chapter 6. Specifically, both the mean spatial flow

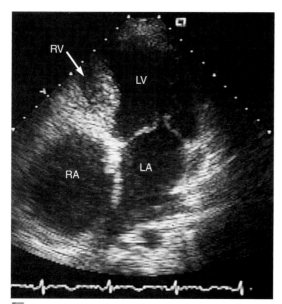

FIGURE 17–36. Tricuspid atresia in a 24-year-old woman with a previous Fontan conduit from the right atrium to the pulmonary artery. The large right atrium, absent tricuspid valve, and small residual right ventricular chamber (connected to the left ventricle via a ventricular septal defect) are seen.

velocity and the cross-sectional area of flow must be measured correctly. Flow at each site is assumed to be laminar with a flat flow velocity profile. Furthermore, accuracy depends on a parallel intercept angle between the direction of blood flow and the ultrasound beam. The cross-sectional area of flow typically is assumed to be circular and is calculated from a 2D echo diameter measurement. Small errors in diameter measurement (which is squared in calculating a circular area) translate into large errors in stroke volume determinations. In adult patients, imaging of the diameter of the pulmonary artery often is difficult and thus is the major source of error in Doppler-derived shunt ratios.

Alternate methods for calculation of pulmonary to systemic shunt ratios include (1) cardiac catheterization with measurement of intracardiac oxygen saturations and total body oxygen consumption, and (2) first-pass radionuclide estimation from the early recirculation pattern of the time-activity curve.

Imaging

Two-dimensional transthoracic echocardiographic imaging in adult patients with congenital heart disease may be limited by poor acoustic access (Table 17–3). Even when image quality is acceptable, evaluation of posterior structures may be limited by lateral resolution at the depth of interest. This can be a problem, particularly in the evaluation of posterior conduits, interatrial baffle repair procedures, sinus venous atrial septal defects, or anomalous pulmonary venous return. Transesophageal echocardiography offers improved image quality, especially of posterior structures, and is a useful adjunct to transthoracic imaging in this patient population.

Evaluation of extracardiac anatomy also is difficult. This limits evaluation of the pulmonary artery branches, systemic arterial or venous shunts to the pulmonary artery, and abnormalities of the ascending aorta and aortic arch. Other tomographic imaging techniques are especially helpful in assessing the position of the cardiac structures in the chest and in evaluating mediastinal abnormalities not accessible by ultrasound. Both chest computed tomography and magnetic resonance imaging can be used, with the advantage of a wide field of view for both techniques. With magnetic resonance imaging, the data can be reformatted, in an orientation based on the long axis of the left ventricle, into standard long- and short-axis views, facilitating identification of abnormal structures.

Other limitations of echocardiography are due to the use of a tomographic approach. For example, coronary anatomy cannot be assessed adequately with tomographic techniques. Angiography, with injection of dye into the coronary arteries, followed by cine- or digital radiographic recording is needed. Another example of potential shortcomings of echocardiography is that multiple ventricular septal defects may be missed unless careful evaluation in numerous tomographic planes is performed. A silhouette technique, such as ventriculography from an angle where the septum forms one of the borders of the ventricular chamber, has a higher reliability for this diagnosis. Limitations of angiography include the risks of contrast dye injection and its cost and invasive nature. Recent improvements in 3D echocardiographic displays may soon provide a clinically useful approach to evaluation of complex congenital heart disease.

Intracardiac Hemodynamics

While the definitive method for assessment of intracardiac hemodynamics remains cardiac catheterization with direct pressure measurement, much indirect information on intracardiac hemodynamics can be derived from the continuous-wave Doppler signal. Pulmonary artery pressure can be approximated by evaluation of pulmonic regurgitation and/or the tricuspid regurgitant jet. Maximum and mean pressure gradients across

TABLE 17-3
Alternate Diagnostic Imaging Procedures in Congenital Heart Disease

Diagnostic Test	Strengths	Weaknesses
Echocardiography (transthoracic, including Doppler)	Detailed 2D anatomy allowing identification of anatomic chambers, valves, and great vessels; blood flow pathway; structural abnormalities Assessment of stenotic and regurgitant lesions by Doppler Detection of intracardiac shunts Assessment of ventricular size and systolic function Estimate of PA pressure Noninvasive, no discomfort	Poor acoustic access limits image quality in some individuals Definition of posterior structures is suboptimal Q_p:Q_s calculation depends on accurate diameter measurements No direct measures of intracardiac pressures Q_p:Q_s calculations
Transesophageal echocardiography	Excellent image quality, especially of posterior structures Detailed Doppler evaluation of pulmonary veins, interatrial septum atrioventricular valves is possible	Anterior cardiac structures now in far field of ultrasound image Apex may not be visualized Oblique image planes limit quantitative measurements of chamber size Some risk of procedure, plus discomfort to patient
Radionuclide ventriculography	Nongeometric accurate EF determination Detection and quantitation of intracardiac shunts using first pass time-activity curve	EF less accurate with irregular rhythms (e.g., atrial fibrillation) With abnormal position of the ventricle, it may be difficult to "isolate" LV for accurate EF calculations Limited anatomic data No evaluation of valve function
Computed tomography	Detailed anatomic images on gated to cardiac cycle Excellent for posterior structures, extracardiac vascular abnormalities, and exact position of cardiac structures in the chest	Limited image quality if not "gated" to cardiac cycle May need intravenous contrast injection Radiation exposure Little physiologic data
Magnetic resonance imaging	Detailed anatomic images on gated to gated cycle Excellent for posterior structures, extracardiac vascular abnormalities, and position related to chest wall Blood has intrinsic "contrast" using different MRI sequences Images can be realigned to cardiac major and minor axes Cine-MRI allow assessment of ventricular function	Tomographic sections at different times in the cardiac cycle Still images provide little data on dynamic cardiac function Research on assessment of valve dysfunction with MRI is in progress Expensive, not portable
Cardiac catheterization	Direct measurement of intracardiac pressures Detection and quantitation of intracardiac shunts Assessment of ventricular size and systolic function Only method that adequately assesses coronary anatomy	Invasive (risks and discomfort) Expensive Requires contrast injection for depiction of structures

EF, ejection fraction; LV, left ventricle; MRI, magnetic resonance imaging; PA, pulmonary artery.

stenotic valves can be measured accurately with Doppler techniques. Inferences about the chronicity of regurgitation and the presence or absence of v waves can be made from the shape of the regurgitant velocity curve. Estimates of left ventricular end-diastolic pressure may be possible based on aortic regurgitant velocity at end-diastole, the pattern of left ventricular diastolic filling, or pulmonary venous flow patterns. However, invasive pressure measurements still are often needed for appropriate clinical decision making in adults with congenital heart disease. In particular, evaluation of pulmonary vascular resistance, which requires invasive data, is an essential factor in patient treatment.

Integrating the Diagnostic Approach

Whichever diagnostic imaging procedure is performed first in an individual patient—be it echocardiography, catheterization, or a magnetic resonance imaging scan—the next step should be to consider the data acquired in terms of both the anatomic and physiologic diagnoses and the certainty that these diagnoses are correct. Then, the remaining important clinical questions should be formulated and the most appropriate study to answer those questions performed next. When this approach is used, the echocardiogram may be the initial test to assess cardiac anatomy and physiology or may be performed only to answer a specific clinical question.

SUGGESTED READING

1. Snider AR: General echocardiographic approach to the adult with suspected congenital heart disease. In: Otto CM (ed): The Practice of Clinical Echocardiography, 2nd ed. Philadelphia: WB Saunders, 2002, pp 845–867.

   A detailed discussion of the echocardiographic approach to segmental analysis of the heart and a review of the echocardiographic features of frequently encountered complex congenital cardiac defects.

2. King ME: Echocardiographic evaluation of the adult with unoperated congenital heart disease. In: Otto CM (ed): The Practice of Clinical Echocardiography, 2nd ed. Philadelphia: WB Saunders, 2002, pp 868–900.

   Advanced discussion of the echocardiographic evaluation of adults with congenital valvular abnormalities, obstructive outflow lesions, septal defects and shunt lesions, coronary fistulas, and complex congenital heart disease. Includes 31 illustrations and 135 references.

3. Child JS: Echocardiographic evaluation of the adult with postoperative congenital heart disease. In: Otto CM (ed): The Practice of Clinical Echocardiography, 2nd ed. Philadelphia: WB Saunders, 2002, pp 901–922.

   Review of echocardiographic findings in adults with previous surgical procedures for congenital heart disease with an emphasis on expected findings and common complications. Topics include general postoperative issues, palliative procedures, corrective procedures for simple lesions (e.g., septal defects) and repair of complex malformations. More than 120 references.

4. Brickner ME, Hillis LD, Lange RA: Congenital heart disease in adults. N Engl J Med 342:256–263, 334–342, 2000.

   Review article (in two parts) with summary of the anatomy, presentation, diagnosis, and management of common types of congenital heart disease in adults. Includes atrial and ventricular septal defects, patent ductus arteriosus, aortic and pulmonic stenosis, aortic coarctation, tetralogy of Fallot, Ebstein anomaly, transposition of the great arteries, and Eisenmenger syndrome. Excellent schematic drawings of each condition and 197 references.

5. Webb GD: Challenges in the care of adult patients with congenital heart disease. Heart 89:465–469, 2003.

   Review of the major management issues in adults with congenital heart disease which will help the echocardiographer understand what aspects of the ultrasound examination are most important for clinical decision making.

6. Sahn DJ, Anderson F: Two-Dimensional Anatomy of the Heart. New York: John Wiley & Sons, 1982.

   Useful reference with comprehensive schematic drawings and echocardiographic images for each type of congenital heart disease.

7. Snider AR, Serwer GA, Ritter SB: Echocardiography in Pediatric Heart Disease, 2nd ed. St. Louis: Mosby, 1997.

   Detailed text with illustrations on the echocardiographic approach to congenital heart disease. Useful reference.

8. Gatzoulis MA, Welsh GD, Daubeney PEF: Adult Congenital Heart Disease: Diagnosis and Management. Edinburgh: Churchill-Livingston, 2003.

   An excellent up-to-date textbook covering all aspects of adult congenital heart disease. An essential reference book for echocardiographers.

9. Perloff JK, Child JS: Congenital Heart Disease in Adults, 2nd ed. Philadelphia: WB Saunders, 1998.

   Comprehensive textbook detailed the survival patterns, medical and surgical therapy, and long-term residua and sequelae after surgical or percutaneous intervention.

10. Emmanouilides GC, Riemenschneider TA, Allen HA, Gutgesell HP (eds): Moss and Adams, Heart Disease in Infants, Children and Adolescents (Including the Fetus and Young Adult), 5th ed. Baltimore: Williams & Wilkins, 1995.

    Comprehensive detailed textbook of pediatric cardiology. Useful reference for descriptions of congenital abnormalities, clinical presentation and management, and surgical procedures.

11. Relier MD, McDonald RW, Gerlis LM, Thornburg KL: Cardiac embryology: Basic review and clinical correlations. J Am Soc Echocardiogr 4:519–531, 1991.

    Brief review of cardiac embryology with correlation with clinical syndromes of congenital heart disease.

12. Hausmann D, Daniel WG, Mugge A, et al: Value of transesophageal color Doppler echocardiography for detection of different types of atrial septal defect in adults. J Am Soc Echocardiogr 5:481–488, 1992.

    In 121 adults with an atrial septal defect, all six ostium primum defects were diagnosed on transthoracic imaging (sensitivity 100%). Of the 97 secundum defects, 95% (54 of 57) of those greater than 5 mm in diameter and 20% (8 of 40) of those less than 5 mm in diameter were detected on transthoracic imaging. All were detected on transesophageal study. A sinus venosus defect was diagnosed in only 9% (1 of 11) on transthoracic and 100% (11 of 11) on trans-

esophageal imaging. Partial anomalous venous return was missed in all 12 cases on transthoracic imaging and correctly identified in 83% (10 of 12) on transesophageal study.

13. Moller JH, Anderson RC: 1000 consecutive children with a cardiac malformation with 26- to 37-year follow-up. Am J Cardiol 70:661–667, 1992.

   In 997 children with congenital heart disease diagnosed 30 to 40 years ago, 712 are alive, with 632 (89%) being asymptomatic without plans for further treatment.

14. Perloff JK (Conference Chairman): 22nd Bethesda Conference. Congenital heart disease after childhood: An expanding patient population. J Am Coll Cardiol 18:311–342, 1991.

   Series of articles describing the outcome, diagnosis, and management of adults with congenital heart disease.

15. O'Fallon WM, Weldman WH (eds): Long-term follow-up of congenital aortic stenosis, pulmonary stenosis, and ventricular septal defect: Report from the Second Joint Study on the Natural History of Congenital Heart Defects (NHS-2). Circulation 87(Suppl 2):I1–I126, 1993.

   Reports of several long-term outcome studies of patients with congenital heart disease.

16. Lundstrom U, Bull C, Wyse RKH, Somerville J: The natural and "unnatural" history of congenitally corrected transposition. Am J Cardiol 65:1222–1229, 1990.

   In 111 patients with congenitally corrected transposition, only 9% had no associated anatomic abnormalities. The most common associated anomalies were a ventricular septal defect in 81%, pulmonary stenosis in 72% (valvular or subvalvular), tricuspid valve abnormalities in 33% (usually Ebstein's anomaly), atrial septal defect in 11%, and a double outlet right ventricle in 11%. The median age of survival was 20 years (range 1 to 58 years) with 46% having undergone intracardiac repair procedures.

17. Horvath KA, Burke RP, Collins JJ, Cohn LH: Surgical treatment of adult atrial septal defect: Early and long-term results. J Am Coll Cardiol 20:1156–1159, 1992.

   Surgical repair of secundum or sinus venosus atrial septal defects was performed in 166 adults (mean age 44 years with 35% ≥50 years old) with an operative mortality of only 1.2% and a 10-year survival rate of 94%. These results emphasize the importance of the echocardiographic recognition of atrial septal defects in adults without a previous diagnosis of congenital heart disease.

18. Driscoll DJ, Offord KP, Feldt RH, et al: Five- to fifteen-year follow-up after Fontan operation. Circulation 85:469–496, 1992.

   The 10-year survival after the Fontan operation in 352 patients (mean age at surgery 11 years, range 1 to 42 years) was 60% with reoperations necessary in 29% of the study group. The primary congenital lesion was tricuspid atresia in 36%, and an univentricular heart in 64%. Detailed outcome measures in these patients including recurrent hospitalization, exercise capacity, arrhythmias, and functional class are reported.

19. Murphy JG, Gersh BJ, Mair DD, et al: Long-term outcome in patients undergoing surgical repair of tetralogy of Fallot. N Engl J Med 329:593–599, 1993.

   The 30-year actuarial survival rate for patients with a repaired tetralogy of Fallot was 90% of the expected survival rate with excellent functional status after surgery. Predictors of a poor outcome were older age (>12 years old) at surgical repair, a previous Waterston or Potts shunt procedure, and a higher postoperative ratio of right-to-left ventricular systolic pressure.

20. Hopkins WE, Waggoner AD: Right and left ventricular area and function determined by two-dimensional echocardiography in adults with the Eisenmenger syndrome from a variety of congenial anomalies. Am J Cardiol 72:90–94, 1993.

   Of 24 adults (age 19 to 45 years) with Eisenmenger's physiology, the 15 patients with a nonrestrictive ventricular septal defect had similar right and left ventricular sizes and preserved right ventricular systolic function. The nine patients without a ventricular septal defect (Eisenmenger's physiology due to patent ductus arteriosus or atrial septal defect) had severe right ventricular dilation and systolic dysfunction. These discordance patterns of ventricular response to differing shunt locations are reflected in the echocardiographic findings in adults with Eisenmenger's syndrome.

21. Celermajer DS, Bull C, Till JA, et al: Ebstein's anomaly: Presentation and outcome from fetus to adult. J Am Coll Cardiol 23:170–176, 1994.

   Of 220 cases of Ebstein anomaly diagnosed over a 33-year period at five London hospitals, 23 (10%) initially presented in adulthood. Symptoms at presentation in these 23 patients were arrhythmias (44%), heart failure (26%), an incidental murmur (13%), or other (17%). Associated defects were uncommon (only 8%) in the adult patients. The severity of Ebstein anomaly was graded using the four-chamber view at end-diastole to calculate the ratio of the area of the right atrium; in addition, atrialized right ventricle compared with the functional right ventricle plus left heart. This severity scale, which ranged from a ratio less than 0.5 (mild) to 1.5 or greater (severe), was a significant predictor of death. Other predictors included fetal presentation and right ventricular outflow tract obstruction.

22. Randolph GR, Hagler DJ, Connolly HM, et al: Intraoperative transesophageal echocardiography during surgery for congenital heart defects. J Thorac Cardiovasc Surg 124:1176–1182, 2002.

   In 1002 patients undergoing surgery for congenital heart disease (age range 2 days to 85 years), intraoperative transesophageal echocardiography affected clinical management in 14% of cases. Although intraoperative transesophageal echocardiography is recommended for all congenital heart surgery, the most impact was seen with valve repairs and complex outflow tract reconstructions.

23. Masani ND: Transesophageal echocardiography in adult congenital heart disease. Heart 86(Suppl II):II30–II40, 2001.

   Detailed review of a general approach to transesophageal echocardiography in congenital heart disease along with typical findings. Excellent illustrations and summary tables.

24. Sahn DJ, Vick GW III: Review of new techniques in echocardiography and magnetic resonance imaging as applied to patients with congenital heart disease. Heart 86(Suppl II):II41–II53, 2001.

   Readable and profusely illustrated review of both newer echocardiography approaches and magnetic resonance imaging (MRI) for diagnosis in patients with congenital heart disease.

The Echo Exam *Adult Congential Heart Disease*

Categories of Congenital Heart Disease

Congenital Stenotic Lesions

Subvalvular
Valvular
Supravalvular
Peripheral great vessels (aortic coarctation)

Congenital Regurgitant Lesions

Myomatous valve disease
Ebstein's anomaly

Abnormal Intracardiac Communications

Atrial septal defect
Ventricular septal defect
Patent ductus arteriosus

Abnormal Chamber and Great Vessel Connections

Transposition of the Great Arteries
Ventricular inversion (congenitally corrected
    transposition)
Tetralogy of Fallot
Tricuspid Atresia
Truncus Arteriosus

Approach to the Echocardiographic Examination in Adults with Congenital Heart Disease

Before the Examination

Review the clinical history
Obtain details of any prior surgical procedures
Review results of prior diagnostic tests
Formulate specific questions

Sequence of Examination

Identify cardiac chambers, great vessels, and their
    connections
Identify associated defects, and evaluate the physiology
    of each lesion
    Regurgitation and/or stenosis (quantitate as per
        Chapters 11 and 12)
    Shunts (calculate $Q_p{:}Q_s$)
    Pulmonary hypertension (calcuate pulmonary
        pressure)
    Ventricular dysfunction (measure ejection fraction if
        anatomy allows)

After the Examination

Integrate echo and Doppler findings with clinical data
Summarize findings
Identify which clinical questions remain unanswered, and
    suggest appropriate subsequent diagnostic tests

Clues to the Identification of Cardiac Structures in Adults with Congenital Heart Disease

Structure	Anatomic Feature	Echo Approach
Right atrium	Inferior vena cava enters right atrium	Start with subcostal approach to identify RA
Right ventricle	Prominent trabeculation Moderator band Infundibulum Tricuspid valve Apical location of annulus	Apical four-chamber view to compare annular insertions of two ventricles, parasternal for valve anatomy and infundibulum
Pulmonary artery	Bifurcates	Parasternal long-axis view or apical four-chamber view angulated very anteriorly
Left atrium	Pulmonary veins usually enter left atrium	Transesophageal imaging for pulmonary vein anatomy
Left ventricle	Mitral valve Basal location of annulus Fibrous continuity between anterior mitral leaflet and semilunar valve	Apical four-chamber view and parasternal long- and short-axis views
Aorta	Gives rise to aortic arch and arterial branches.	Start with parasternal long-axis view and move transducer superiorly to follow vessel to its branches

Examples

1. A 24-year-old with a history of a cardiac murmur has an echocardiogram which shows:

Right ventricular outflow velocity	1.6 m/s
Pulmonary artery velocity	3.1 m/s
Tricuspid regurgitant jet	3.4 m/s
Estimated right atrial pressure	5 mm Hg (small IVC with normal respiratory variation)

Because the right ventricular outflow velocity is elevated, the maximum pulmonic valve gradient should be calcuated using the proximal velocity in the Bernoulli equation:

$$\Delta P = 4(V^2_{jet} - V^2_{prox})$$
$$\Delta P = 4[(3.1)^2 - (1.6)^2] = 4[9.6 - 2.6] = 28 \text{ mm Hg}$$

If the proximal velocity is not included, the gradient would be overestimated at 38 mm Hg.

Estimated pulmonary systolic pressure is calculated by substracting the pulmonic valve gradient from the estimated right ventricular pressure because pulmonic stenosis is present:

$$PAP = (\Delta P_{RV-RA} + P_{RA}) - \Delta P_{RV-PA}$$
$$PAP = (4V^2_{TR} + P_{RA}) - \Delta P_{RV-PA} = [4(3.4)^2 + 5)] - 28 = 23 \text{ mm Hg}$$

Thus, pulmonary artery systolic pressure is normal even though the triscuspid regurgitant jet indicates a right ventricular systolic pressure of 51 mm Hg.

2. A 26-year-old woman undergoes echocardiography for symptoms of decreased exercise tolerance. She is found to have an enlarged right atrium and ventricle with paradoxic septal motion and the following Doppler data:

Right ventricular outflow	
Velocity	1.8 m/s
Velocity-time integral (VTI_{RVOT})	32 cm
Diameter	2.6 cm
Left ventricular outflow	
Velocity	1.1 m/s
Velocity-time integral (VTI_{LVOT})	16 cm
Diameter	2.4 cm

The right heart enlargement suggests an atrial septal defect may be present. The shunt ratio is calculated from the ratio of pulmonary flow (Q_p), measured in the right ventricular outflow tract and systemic flow (Q_s), measured in the left ventricular outflow tract. At each site, cross-sectional area is calcuated as the area of a circle:

$$CSA_{RVOT} = \pi(D/2)^2 = 3.14(2.6/2)^2 = 5.3 \text{ cm}^2$$
$$CSA_{LVOT} = \pi(D/2)^2 = 3.14(2.4/2)^2 = 4.5 \text{ cm}^2$$

Flow (stroke volume) at each site then is calculated:

$$Q_p = CSA_{RVOT} \times VTI_{RVOT} = 5.3 \text{ cm}^2 \times 32 \text{ cm} = 170 \text{ cm}^3$$
$$Q_s = CSA_{LVOT} \times VTI_{LVOT} = 4.5 \text{ cm}^2 \times 16 \text{ cm} = 72 \text{ cm}^3$$
$$\text{so that } Q_p{:}Q_s = 170/72 = 2.4$$

These calculations are consistent with a significant shunt that most likely will require closure to prevent progressive right heart dysfunction.

THE ECHO EXAM

Quick Reference Guide

The Echo Exam *Basic Principles*

Sound Waves

f = frequency
λ = wavelength
c = velocity of propagation
$c = \lambda f$

Ultrasound-Tissue Interaction

Reflection	Imaging
Scattering	Doppler
Refraction	Beam focusing
	Artifacts
Attenuation	Penetration

Resolution

Axial	Transducer frequency
	Bandwidth
	Pulse length
Lateral	Depth
Elevational	Depth

Frame Rate

Depth
Sector width

Imaging Instrument Settings

Transducer frequency
Power output
Gain
Time gain compensation (TCG)
Depth
Dynamic range
Sector width

Doppler Modalities

Pulsed	Spectral display
	Anatomic location
	Signal aliasing
CW	Spectral display
	High velocity flow
	Range ambiguity
Color	Visual 2D display
	Quantitation problematic

Doppler Equation

$$v = \frac{c(\Delta F)}{2F_T(\cos\theta)}$$

c = speed of sound in blood (1540 m/s)
θ is the intercept angle with flow
F_T = transducer frequency
ΔF = Doppler frequency shift

Spectral Doppler Instrument Settings

Power output
Receiver gain
Wall (high-pass) filters
Baseline shift
Velocity range
Post-processing
Sample volume depth (pulsed)
Sample volume length (pulsed)
Number of sample volumes (HPRF)

Ultrasound Safety

Bioeffects	Thermal
	Cavitation
	Other

Perform echos appropriately
Know power output and exposure intensities
Limit power output and exposure as possible

Optimization of Doppler Recordings

Modality	Data Optimization	Common Artifacts
Pulsed	2D guided with "frozen" image Parallel to flow Small sample volume Velocity scale at Nyquist limit Adjust baseline for aliasing Use low wall filters Adjust gain and dynamic range	Nonparallel angle with underestimation of velocity Signal aliasing. Nyquist limit = 1/2 pulse repetition frequency (PRF) Signal strength/noise
Continuous wave	Dedicated nonimaging transducer Parallel to flow Adjust velocity scale so flow fits and fills the displayed range Use high wall filters Adjust gain and dynamic range	Nonparallel angle with underestimation of velocity Range ambiguity Beam width Transit time effect
Color flow	Use minimal depth and sector width for flow of interest (best frame rate) Adjust gain just below random noise Color scale at Nyquist limit	Shadowing Ghosting Electronic interference

Principles of Doppler Quantitation

Method	Assumptions/Characteristics	Examples of Clinical Applications
Volume flow $SV = CSA \times VTI$	• Laminar flow • Flat flow profile • Cross-sectional area (CSA) and velocity time integral (VTI) measured at same site	• Cardiac output • Continuity equation for valve area • Regurgitant volume calculations • Intracardiac shunts, pulmonary-to-systemic flow ratio
Velocity-pressure relationship $\Delta P = 4v^2$	• Flow-limiting orifice • CW Doppler signal recorded parallel to flow	• Stenotic valve gradients • Calculation of pulmonary pressures • Left ventricular dP/dt
Spatial flow patterns	• Proximal flow convergence region • Narrow flow stream in orifice (vena contracta) • Downstream flow disturbance	• Detection of valve regurgitation and intracardiac shunts • Level of obstruction • Quantitation of regurgitant severity

The Echo Exam *Core Elements*

A complete Echo Exam consists of Core Elements plus Additional Components.

Modality	Window	View/Signal	Measurements
Clinical data		Indication for echo Key history and PE findings Previous cardiac imaging data Blood pressure at time of Echo Exam	
2D imaging	*Parasternal*	Long axis Short axis aortic valve Short axis mitral valve Short axis LV (papillary muscle level) Right ventricular inflow Right ventricular outflow	LV dimensions LV wall thickness Aortic root dimension LA dimension
	Apical	4-chamber Anteriorly angulated 4-chamber 2-chamber Long axis	Visual estimate of ejection fraction
	Subcostal	4-chamber IVC with respiration	
Pulsed Doppler	*Apical*	Left ventricular inflow at leaflet tips	E velocity A velocity
		Left ventricular outflow	LV outflow velocity

Color flow	*Parasternal*	Long axis
		Short axis of aortic and mitral valves
		RV inflow and outflow
			Color flow to identify
			  regurgitation of all 4 valves.
			  Measure vena contracta if
			  possible

	Apical	4-chamber Long-axis	Mitral, tricuspid and aortic valves
Continuous wave Doppler	*Parasternal*	Tricuspid valve Pulmonic valve	TR-jet velocity
	Apical	Aortic valve Mitral valve Tricuspid valve	Aortic regurgitation Mitral regurgitation TR-jet (PAP)

LV, left ventricle; IVC, inferior vena cava; TR, tricuspid regurgitation; PAP, pulmonary artery pressure.

The Echo Exam *Additional Components*

Abnormality on Core Elements	Additional Echo Exam Components (Chapter)
Reason for Echo	Additional components to address specific clinical question*
Left Ventricle	
Decreased ejection fraction	See Systolic Function and Dilated Cardiomyopathy (6, 9)
Abnormal LV filling velocities	See Diastolic Function (7)
Regional wall motion abnormality	See Ischemic Heart Disease (8)
Increased wall thickness	See Hypertrophic Cardiomyopathy, Restrictive Cardiomyopathy and Hypertensive Heart Disease (9)
Valves	
Imaging evidence for stenosis or an increased antegrade transvalvular velocity	See Valve Stenosis (11)
Regurgitation greater than mild on color flow imaging or CW Doppler	See Valve Regurgitation (12)
Prosthetic valve	See Prosthetic Valves (13)
Valve mass or suspected endocarditis	See Endocarditis and Masses (14, 15)
Right Heart	
Enlarged right ventricle	See Pulmonary Heart Disease and Congenital Heart Disease (9, 17)
Elevated TR-jet velocity	See Pulmonary Pressures (6)
Pericardium	
Pericardial Effusion	See Pericardial Effusion (10)
Pericardial thickening	See Constrictive Pericarditis (10)
Great Vessels	
Enlarged aorta	See Aortic Disease (16)

*The echo exam should always include additional components to address the clinical indication. For example, if the indication is "heart failure," additional components to evaluate systolic and diastolic function are needed even if the Core Elements do not show obvious abnormalities. If the indication is "cardiac source of embolus," the Additional Components for that diagnosis are needed.

The Echo Exam *Basic Transesophageal Exam*

Probe Position		View	Focus on
High Esophageal Set depth to include LV apex	0°	4-chamber	LV size and function (septum and lateral walls) RV size and systolic function LA and RA size Withdraw probe to see LA appendage Mitral and tricuspid valves Angulate anteriorly to see aortic valve
	~60°	2-chamber	LV size and function (inferior and anterior walls) LA and LA appendage Mitral valve
	~120°	Long-axis	LV size and function (anterior septum and posterior walls) LA size Mitral and aortic valves Withdraw probe to see ascending aorta
High Esophageal ↓ depth to optimize valves	~120°	Long-axis	Mitral valve anatomy and function Color Doppler for mitral regurgitation Antegrade mitral flow with pulsed Doppler Aortic valve anatomy and color flow
	~60°	2-chamber	Mitral valve anatomy and function Color Doppler for mitral regurgitation LA appendage imaging and Doppler flow
	0°	4-chamber	Mitral valve anatomy and function Color Doppler for mitral regurgitation Aortic valve (angulate anteriorly to "5-chamber" view) for anatomy and color flow Atrial septum
Transgastric	0°	Short-axis	LV wall motion, wall thickness, chamber dimensions RV size and function
	90°	Long-axis	LV and mitral valve Turn medially to image RV and tricuspid valve
Transgastric apical	0°	4-chamber	Useful for antegrade aortic flow but may still be non-parallel intercept angle
Transgastric to high esophageal	0°	Short axis descending aorta	Image aorta from the diaphragm to aortic arch

LV, left ventricular; RV, right ventricular; LA, left atrial; RA, right atrial.

The Echo Exam *Other Echocardiographic Modalities*

Modality	Instrumentation	Indications	Special Training
Intraoperative TEE	Transesophageal echo in the OR	Monitoring ventricular function Evaluation of valve repair and other complex procedures	Anesthesiologists with training in echocardiography
Stress echo	Digital cine loop image acquisition Exercise or pharmacologic stress	Suspected or known coronary diease Myocardial viability Valve and structural heart disease	Performance, risks and interpretation of stress studies
Contrast echo	Microbubbles for right or left heart contrast	Detection of patent foramen ovale LV endocardial definition	Intravenous administration of contrast agents
3D echo	Volumetric or 2D image acquisition Various display formats	Congenital heart disease, Rapid acquisition for LV regional function	Image acquisition and analysis
Intracardiac echo (ICE)	5–10 MHz catheter like intracardiac probe	Interventional procedures (ASD closure) EP procedures	Invasive cardiology training and experience
Intravascular ultrasound (IVUS)	30–50 MHz intracoronary catheter	Degree of coronary narrowing and plaque morphology training	Interventional cardiology
Hand-held ultrasound	Small, inexpensive ultrasound instruments	Beside evaluation by MD for pericardial effusion, LV global and regional function	At least level 1 echo training

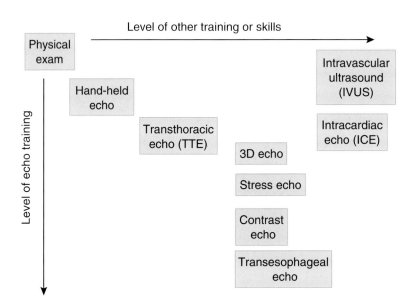

The Echo Exam *Indications for Transthoracic Echocardiography*

Clinical Diagnosis	Key Echo Findings	Limitations of Echo	Alternate Approaches
Valvular Heart Disease			
Valve stenosis	Etiology of stenosis, valve anatomy Transvalvular ΔP, valve area Chamber enlargement and hypertrophy LV and RV systolic function Associated valvular regurgitation	Possible underestimation of stenosis severity Possible coexisting coronary artery disease	Cardiac cath MRI
Valve regurgitation	Mechanism and etiology of regurgitation Severity of regurgitation Chamber enlargement LV and RV systolic function PA pressure estimate	TEE may be needed to evaluate mitral regurgitant severity and valve anatomy (esp. before MV repair)	Cardiac cath MRI
Prosthetic valve function	Evidence for stenosis Detection of regurgitation Chamber enlargement Ventricular function PA pressure estimate	Imaging prosthetic valves is limited by shadowing and reverberations TEE is needed for suspected prosthetic MR due to "masking" of the LA on TTE	Cardiac cath
Endocarditis	Detection of vegetations (TTE sensitivity 70–85%) Presence and degree of valve dysfunction Chamber enlargement and function Detection of abscess Possible prognostic implications	TEE more sensitive for detection of vegetations (>90%) A definite diagnosis of endocarditis also depends on bacteriologic criteria TEE more sensitive for abscess detection	Blood cultures and clinical findings also are diagnostic criteria for endocarditis
Coronary Artery Disease			
Acute myocardial infarction	Segmental wall motion abnormality reflects "myocardium at risk" Global LV function (EF) Complications: Acute MR vs. VSD Pericarditis LV thrombus, aneurysm RV infarct	Coronary artery anatomy itself not directly visualized	Coronary angio Radionuclide LV angio Cardiac cath
Angina	Global and segmental LV systolic function Exclude other causes of angina (e.g., AS, HOCM)	Resting wall motion may be normal despite significant CAD Stress echo needed to induce ischemia and wall motion abnormality	Coronary angio Stress thallium ETT
Pre-/post- revascularization	Assess wall thickening and endocardial motion at baseline Improvement in segmental function post-procedure	Dobutamine stress and/or contrast echo needed to detect viable but non-functioning myocardium	MRI PET Thallium ETT Contrast echocardiography
End-stage ischemic disease	Overall LV systolic function (EF) PA pressures Associated MR LV thrombus RV systolic function		Coronary angio Radionuclide EF

Continued

Clinical Diagnosis	Key Echo Findings	Limitations of Echo	Alternate Approaches
Cardiomyopathy			
Dilated	Chamber dilation (all four) LV and RV systolic function (qualitative and EF) Coexisting atrioventricular valve regurgitation PA systolic pressure LV thrombus	Indirect measures of LVEDP Accurate EF may be difficult if image quality poor.	Radionuclide EF LV and RV angiography
Restrictive	LV wall thickness LV systolic function LV diastolic function PA systolic pressure	Must be distinguished from constrictive pericarditis	Cardiac cath with direct, simultaneous RV and LV pressure measurement after volume loading
Hypertrophic	Pattern and extent of LV hypertrophy Dynamic LVOT obstruction (imaging and Doppler) Coexisting MR Diastolic LV dysfunction		
Hypertension	LV wall thickness and chamber dimensions LV mass LV systolic function Aortic root dilation, AR		
Pericardial Disease	Pericardial thickening Detection, size, and location of PE 2D signs of tamponade physiology Doppler signs of tamponade physiology	Diagnosis of tamponade is a hemodynamic and clinical diagnosis Constrictive pericarditis is a difficult diagnosis Not all patients with pericarditis have an effusion	Intracardiac pressure measurements for tamponade or constriction MRI or CT to detect pericardial thickening
Aortic Disease			
Aortic root dilation	Etiology of aortic dilation Aortic root diameter measurements Anatomy of sinuses of Valsalva (esp. Marfan's syndrome) Associated aortic regurgitation	May not visualize entire ascending aorta	CT, MRI Aortography, TEE
Aortic dissection	2D images of ascending aorta (PLAX, PSAX), aortic arch (SSN), descending thoracic (A2C), and proximal abdominal (SC) aorta Imaging of dissection "flap" Associated aortic regurgitation Ventricular function	TEE more sensitive (97%) and specific (100%) Cannot assess distal vascular beds	Aortography CT MRI TEE

Clinical Diagnosis	Key Echo Findings	Limitations of Echo	Alternate Approaches
Cardiac Masses			
LV thrombus	High sensitivity and specificity for diagnosis of LV thrombus Suspect with apical wall motion abnormality or diffuse LV systolic dysfunction	Technical artifacts can be misleading 5-MHz or higher frequency transducer and angulated apical views needed	LV thrombus may not be recognized on radionuclide or contrast angiography
LA thrombus	Low sensitivity for detection of LA thrombus, although specificity is high Suspect with LA enlargement, MV Disease	TEE is needed to detect LA thrombus reliability	TEE
Cardiac tumors	Size, location, and physiologic consequences of tumor mass	Extracardiac involvement not well seen Cannot distinguish benign from malignant, or tumor from thrombus	TEE CT MRI (with cardiac gating) Intracardiac echo
Pulmonary Hypertension			
	Estimate of PA pressure Evidence of left-sided heart disease to account for increased PA pressures RV size and systolic function (cor pulmonale) Associated TR	Indirect PA pressure measurement Unable to determine pulmonary vascular resistance accurately	Cardiac cath
Congenital Heart Disease			
	Detection and assessment of anatomic abnormalities Quantitation of physiologic abnormalities Chamber enlargement Ventricular function	No direct intracardiac pressure measurements Complicated anatomy may be difficult to evaluate if image quality is poor (TEE helpful)	MRI with 3D reconstruction Cardiac cath TEE 3D Echo

A2C, Apical two-chamber; Angio, angiography; AS, aortic stenosis; CAD, coronary artery disease; Cath, catheterization; CT, computed tomography; EF, ejection fraction; ETT, exercise treadmill test; HOCM, hypertrophic obstructive cardiomyopathy; LA, left atrial; LV, left ventricular; LVEDP, left ventricular end-diastolic pressure; LVOT, left ventricular outflow tract; MHz, megahertz; MR, mitral regurgitation; MRI, magnetic resonance imaging; MV, mitral valve; AP, pressure gradient; PA, pulmonary artery; PE, pericardial effusion; PET, position emission tomography; PLAX, parasternal long-axis; PSAX, parasternal short-axis; RV, right ventricular; SC, subcostal; SSN, suprasternal notch; 2D, two-dimensional; TEE, transesophageal echocardiography; TR, tricuspid regurgitation; TTE, transthoracic echocardiography; VSD, ventricular septal defect.

The Echo Exam *Systolic Function*

Global LV function	Wall thickness
	Internal dimensions/ volumes
	dP/dt
	Ejection Fraction
Regional LV function	Segmental wall motion
Global RV function	RV size
	RV systolic function
Pulmonary pressures	Pulmonary systolic pressure
Cardiac output	Stroke volume (SV) and Cardiac output (CO)

Example

A 57-year-old man with a recent inferior myocardial infarction now is hypotensive. Echocardiography shows:

LV wall thickness (diastole)	7 mm
LV end-diastolic dimension	57 mm
LV end-systolic dimension	38 mm
Apical biplane ejection fraction	52%
Time interval between 1 and 3 m/s on MR-Jet	30 msec
Segmental wall motion	Akinesis of basal and mid-LV segments of inferior and infero-lateral walls
RV size	Moderately increased
RV systolic function	Severely decreased
TR-jet velocity (V_{TR})	2.6 m/s
Inferior vena cava	Normal diameter with inspiratory change <50%
LV outflow tract diameter ($LVOT_D$)	2.4 cm
LVOT velocity time integral ($LV1_{LVOT}$)	10 cm
Heart rate (HR)	85 bpm

Discussion

The left ventricle is at the upper limits of normal in size with a mildly reduced ejection fraction and regional wall motion abnormalities consistent with a recent inferior myocardial infarction. Ejection fraction is evaluated qualitatively only when image quality is too poor for tracing endocardial borders for a biplane ejection fraction calculation.

Left ventricular dP/dt is calculated from the interval between 1 and 3 m/s on the MR jet signal (*dt*) as:

$$dP/dt = [4(V_2)^2 - 4(V_1)^2]/dt = [4(3)^2 - 4(1)^2]/dt$$
$$= [36 - 4 \, mmHg]/.030 \, s = 1067 \, mmHg/s$$

which is at the lower limits of normal (>1000 mmHg/s).

RV size and systolic function are graded qualitatively. The findings of a moderately dilated RV with severe systolic dysfunction in this patient are consistent with right ventricular infarction accompanying the inferior LV infarction, as the coronary artery that supplies the LV inferior wall also often supplies the RV free wall.

Right atrial pressure is mildly elevated (estimate 10–15 mm Hg) as shown by the <50% change in the diameter of a non-dilated inferior vena cava with respiration.

Pulmonary systolic pressure (PAP) is calculated from the tricuspid regurgitant jet velocity (V_{TR}) and estimate of right atrial pressure (RAP) as:

$$PAP = 4(V_{TR})^2 + RAP = 4(2.6)^2 + 10 = 27 + 10 = 37 \, mmHg$$

This is consistent with mild pulmonary hypertension.

Cardiac output (CO) is calculated using the LVOT diameter to calculate the circular cross sectional areas of flow:

$$CSA_{LVOT} = \pi(LVOT_D/2)^2 = 3.14(2.4/2)^2 = 4.5 \, cm^2$$

Stroke volume across the aortic valve ($cm^3 = mL$), then is:

$$SV_{LVOT} = (CSA_{LVOT} \times VTI_{LVOT}) = 4.5 \, cm^2 \times 10 \, cm = 45 \, cm^3$$

Cardiac output is:

$$CO = SV \times HR$$
$$= 45 \, mL \times 85 \, beats/min = 3830 \, mL/min \text{ or } 3.83 \, L/min$$

This low cardiac output is due to the right ventricular infarction and explains his hypotension.

Quantitation of Left and Right Ventricular Systolic Function

Parameter	Modality	View	Recording	Measurements
Ejection fraction	2D	Apical four-chamber and two-chamber	Adjust depth, optimize endocardial definition, harmonic imaging, contrast if needed	Careful tracing of endocardial borders at end-diastole and end-systole in both views
dP/dt	CW Doppler	MR jet, usually from apex	Pt positioning and transducer angulation to obtain highest velocity MR jet, decrease velocity scale, increased sweep speed	Time interval between 1 m/s and 3 m/s on Doppler MR velocity curve
PA pressures	CW Doppler	Parasternal and apical	Pt positioning and transducer angulation to obtain highest velocity TR jet	Estimate of RA pressure from size and appearance of IVC
Cardiac output	2D and pulsed Doppler	Parasternal LVOT diameter	Ultrasound beam perpendicular to LVOT with depth decreased and gain adjusted to see mid-systolic diameter.	LVOT diameter from inner edge to inner edge in mid-systole, adjacent and parallel to aortic valve.
		Apical LVOT velocity time integral	LVOT velocity from ant. angulated A4C view with sample volume just on LV side of aortic valve	Trace modal velocity of LVOT spectral Doppler envelope.

The Echo Exam *Diastolic Dysfunction*

Parameter	Physiologic Descriptor
Relaxation	$-dP/dt$ or tau
Compliance	dV/dt
Filling pressure	LV-EDP or LAP or PAW

EDP, end-diastolic pressure; LAP, left atrial pressure; PAWP, pulmonary artery wedge pressure.

Echo Exam

Left ventricular (LV) inflow at mitral leaflet tips
  E = Early diastolic filling velocity (m/s)
  A = Filling velocity after atrial contraction (m/s)
  DT = Deceleration time (msec)*

LV inflow at mitral annulus
  A_{dur} = duration of atrial filling velocity in msec

Myocardial tissue Doppler at base of septum
  E_m = Early diastolic filling velocity (m/s)
  A_m = Filling velocity after atrial contraction (m/s)

Isovolumic relaxation time
  IVRT = isovolumic relaxation time (msec)

Pulmonary venous inflow
  PV_S = peak systolic velocity
  PV_D = peak diastolic velocity
  PV_a = peak atrial reversal velocity
  a_{dur} = pulmonary vein atrial reversal duration

*DT, time interval from peak velocity to baseline, extrapolated from slope of diastolic deceleration curve.

Example

A 62-year-old man with amyloidosis has an echocardiogram that shows a symmetric increase in wall thickness with an ejection fraction of 52%. The following parameters of diastolic function are recorded.

E velocity	1.1 m/s
A velocity	0.6 m/s
Deceleration time (DT)	160 ms
A_{dur}	130 ms
E_m/A_m ratio	<1
IVRT	40 ms
PV_S/PV_D	<1
PV_a	0.4 m/s
a_{dur}	155

The E/A ratio is >1 but the E_m/A_m ratio is less than 1, indicating a pattern of pseudonormalization suggestive of moderate diastolic dysfunction with decreased compliance. Moderate diastolic dysfunction is confirmed by the short IVRT and relatively short deceleration time.

There also is evidence of elevated filling pressures with a $PV_a > 0.35$ m/s and with the duration of pulmonary vein atrial flow minus the duration of atrial flow at the mitral annulus >20 ms.

Quantitation of Diastolic Function

Parameter	Modality	View	Recording	Measurements
LV inflow at leaflet tips	Pulsed Doppler	A4C with 2–3 mm sample volume positioned at mitral leaflet tips	Parallel to flow Normal expiration Low wall filters	E and A peak velocities DT along outer edge of spectral envelope using linear slope from peak to baseline
LV inflow at annulus	Pulsed Doppler	A4C with 2 mm sample volume at mitral annulus	Parallel to flow, normal expiration, low wall filters	A_{dur}
Myocardial tissue Doppler	Pulsed Doppler	A4C with 2–3 mm sample volume placed within basal segment of septal wall	Very low gain settings Low wall filters	E_m and E_m/A_m
IVRT	Pulsed Doppler	Anteriorly angulated A4C with 3–5 mm sample volume midway between aortic and mitral valves	Clear aortic closing click and clear onset of transmitral flow, low wall filters	IVRT as time interval from middle of aortic closure click to onset of mitral flow
Pulmonary venous inflow	Pulsed Doppler (color to guide location)	Right superior pulmonary vein in A4C view using color flow to depict flow	2 mm sample volume 1–2 cm into pulmonary vein	PV_a, a_{dur}, and relative ratio of S/D

Classification of Diastolic Dysfunction

	Normal	Mild	Mild-Moderate	Moderate	Severe
Pathophysiology		↓ Relaxation	↓ Relaxation and ↑ LV-EDP	↓ Relaxation, ↓ Compliance, and ↑ LV-EDP	↓ Relaxation ↓↓ Compliance, and ↑↑ LV-EDP
E/A ratio	1–2	<1	<1	1.0–2.0	>2.0
E_m/A_m ratio	1–2	<1	<1	<1	>1
IVRT (ms)	50–100	>100	Normal	↓	↓
DT (ms)	150–200	>200	>200	150–200	<150
PV_S/PV_D	≥1	$PV_S > PV_D$	$PV_S > PV_D$	$PV_S < PV_D$	$PV_S \ll PV_D$
PV_a (m/s)	<0.35	<0.35	≥0.35	≥0.35	≥0.35
$a_{dur} - A_{dur}$ (ms)	<20	<20	≥20	≥20	≥20 ms

Based on the Canadian Consensus Guidelines (Rakowki et al: J Am Soc Echocadiogr 9:736–760, 1996; and Yamada et al: J Am Soc Echocardiogr 15:1238–1244, 2002), with modification to include tissue Doppler data; and Redfield: JAMA 289:194–202, 2003.

The Echo Exam *Ischemic Cardiac Disease*

Myocardial Ischemia

Stress echo modalities
   Treadmill exercise
   Supine bicycle
   Dobutamine
Digital cine-loop views
   Short axis mid-cavity
   Apical 4-chamber
   Apical 2-chamber
   Apical long-axis
Interpretation
   Exercise duration
   Heart rate and blood pressure
   Symptoms
   Wall motion at rest and with stress
   EF at rest and with stress
Utility
   Diagnosis of coronary artery disease
   Severity of disease
     Nnumber of vessels involved
     Extent of myocardium at risk
   Overall LV systolic function
   Diastolic LV function
   Clinical prognosis

Acute Myocardial Infarction

Detection of wall motion abnormalities
Evaluation of recurrent chest pain
Assessment of the response to reperfusion
Complications of acute myocardial infarction
   LV systolic dysfunction
   LV thrombus
   Aneurysm formation
   Acute mitral regurgitation
   Ventricular septal defect
   LV rupture (pseudoaneurysm)
   Pericardial effusion

LV Pseudoaneurysm

Abrupt transition from normal myocardium to aneurysm
Acute angle between myocardium and aneurysm
Narrow neck
Ratio of neck diameter to aneurysm diameter <0.5
May be lined with thrombus

End-Stage Ischemic Disease

LV systolic dysfunction
   Deceased ejection fraction
   Decreased dP/dt
   Regional pattern may be seen
RV systolic dysfunction
   May be present if RV infarction or if pulmonary
     pressures elevated
Mitral regurgitation (MR)
   Diverse mechanisms of ischemic MR
     LV dilation and systolic dysfunction
     Regional wall motion abnormality
     Papillary muscle dysfunction or rupture
   Quantitate severity (see Chapter 12)
LV aneurysm and thrombus formation

Stress Echocardiography

Parameter	Modality	View	Recording	Interpretation
Resting regional wall motion	2D	PSAX mid-cavity level Apical 4-chamber Apical 2-chamber Apical long-axis	Depth that includes only LV, optimize endocardial definition, use contrast if needed	Select optimal image from series of digital cine loops
Stress regional wall motion	2D	PSAX mid-cavity level Apical 4-chamber Apical 2-chamber Apical long-axis	Same depth as baseline, optimize endocardial definition, use contrast if needed	Compare optimal baseline and stress images in same views
Clinical and hemodynamic data		Symptoms Heart rate and rhythm Blood pressure	Continuous during exam, report values at each stage of stress	Maximal workload affects accuracy of echo results for detection of ischemia
LV systolic function	2D Doppler	Ejection fraction *dP/dt*	See section on systolic function for details	

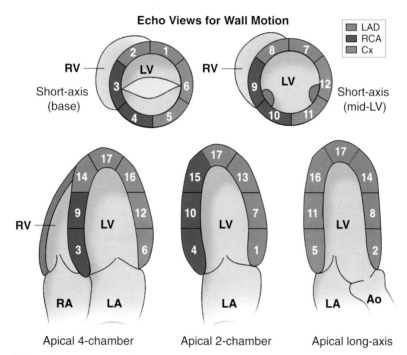

Echocardiographic views for wall motion evaluation. In the short-axis view, at the base and midventricular levels, the left ventricle is divided into the anterior (*1, 7*), anterior septal (*2, 8*), inferior septal (*3, 9*), inferior (*4, 10*), inferolateral (*5, 11*), and anterolateral (*6, 12*) segments. In the apical region, there are four segments: anterior (*13*), septal (*14*), inferior (*15*), and lateral (*16*) plus the tip of the apex (*17*). The territory of the left anterior descending artery is indicated in blue, the right coronary artery in red, and the left circumflex coronary artery in yellow.

The Echo Exam *Cardiomyopathies, Hypertensive and Pulmonary Heart Disease*

Echo Differential Diagnosis of Heart Failure

Ischemic disease
Valvular disease
Hypertensive heart disease
Cardiomyopathy
  Dilated
  Hypertrophic
  Restrictive

Pericardial disease
  Constriction
  Tamponade
Pulmonary heart disease

Cardiomyopathies: Typical Features

	Dilated	Hypertrophic	Restrictive
LV systolic function	Moderately-severely ↓	Normal	Normal
LV diastolic function	May be abnormal	Abnormal	Abnormal
LV hypertrophy	↑LV mass due to left ventricular dilation with normal wall thickness	Asymmetric LV hypertrophy	Concentric LV hypertrophy
Chamber dilation	All four chambers	Left and right atrial dilation if MR is present	Left and right atrial dilation
Outflow tract obstruction	Absent	Dynamic LV outflow tract obstruction may be present	Absent
Left ventricular end-diastolic pressure	Elevated	Elevated	Elevated
Pulmonary artery pressures	Elevated	Elevated	Elevated

Differentiation of Cause of Increased Wall Thickness

	Hypertensive Heart Disease	Hypertrophic Cardiomyopathy	Restrictive Cardiomyopathy
Left ventricular hypertrophy	+	+	+
Pattern of hypertrophy	Concentric	Asymmetric	Concentric
Clinical history of hypertension	+	Absent	Absent
Outflow obstruction	Midventricular cavity obliteration	Dynamic subaortic obstruction	Absent
RV hypertrophy	Absent	May be present	+
Pulmonary hypertension	Mild	Mild	Moderate
LV systolic function	Normal initially but may be reduced late in disease course	Normal	Normal initially but may be reduced late in disease course
LV diastolic function	Abnormal	Abnormal	Abnormal

+ = present.

Echo Approach to the Cardiomyopathies

Modality	Echo Views and Flows	Measurements
Imaging	LV size and systolic function	LV-EDV, LV-ESV Apical biplane EF
	Degree and pattern of LV hypertrophy	LV-mass
	Evidence for dynamic outflow tract obstruction	SAM of the mitral valve Aortic valve midsystolic closure
	RV size and systolic function	
	LA size	
Doppler Echo	Associated valvular regurgitation	Measure vena contracta, quantitate if more than mild
	LV diastolic function	Standard diastolic function evaluation with classification of severity and estimate of LV-EDP
	LV systolic function	dP/dt from MR jet Calculation of cardiac output
	Pulmonary pressures	TR-Jet and IVC for PA systolic pressure Evaluate PR jet for PA diastolic pressure Consider measures of pulmonary resistance
	Color, pulsed, and CW Doppler to quantitate outflow obstruction	Maximum outflow tract gradient

The Echo Exam *Pericardial Disease*

Pericardial Effusion

Views
Parasternal
Apical
Subcostal

Distinguish from pleural fluid

Size
Small (<0.5 cm)
Moderate (0.5–2.0 cm)
Large (>2.0 cm)

Diffuse vs loculated

Evaluate for tamponade physiology if moderate or large

Constrictive Pericarditis

M-mode/2D
Pericardial thickening
Normal LV size and systolic function
LA enlargement
Flattened diastolic wall motion
Abrupt posterior motion of the ventricular septum in early diastole
Dilated inferior vena cava and hepatic veins

Doppler
Prominent y descent on hepatic vein or superior vena cava flow pattern
LV inflow shows prominent E velocity with a rapid early diastolic deceleration slope and a small or absent A velocity
Increase in LV-IVRT by >20% on first beat after inspiration
Respiratory variations in RV/LV diastolic filling (difference >25%) with inspiratory ↑RV ↓LV filling with inspiration
Pulmonary venous flow shows prominent a wave and blunting of systolic phase

Pericardial Tamponade

Clinical Findings
Low cardiac output
Elevated venous pressures
Pulsus paradoxus
Hypotension

2D-Echo
Moderate-large pericardial effusion
Right atrial systolic collapse (duration greater than a third of systole)
Right ventricular diastolic collapse
Reciprocal respiratory changes in RV and LV volumes
Inferior vena cava plethora

Doppler
Respiratory variation in RV and LV diastolic filling
Increased RV filling on first beat after inspiration
Decreased LV filling on first beat after inspiration

LV Pseudoaneurysm

Abrupt transition from normal myocardium to aneurysm
Acute angle between myocardium and aneurysm
Narrow neck
Ratio of neck diameter to aneurysm diameter <0.5
May be lined with thrombus

The Echo Exam *Aortic Stenosis*

Valve anatomy	Calcific
	Bicuspid (2 leaflets in systole)
	Rheumatic
Stenosis severity	Jet velocity (V_{max})
	Mean pressure gradient (ΔP_{mean})
	LVOT:AS velocity ratio
	Aortic valve area (AVA)
Co-existing AR	Qualitative evaluation of severity
LV response	LV hypertrophy
	LV dimensions or volumes
	LV ejection fraction
Other findings	Pulmonary pressures
	Mitral regurgitation

LV, left ventricle; AR, aortic regurgitation.

Example

An 82-year-old woman presents with dyspnea on exertion and is noted to have a 3/6 systolic murmur at the base, radiating to the carotids with a single S2 and a diminished carotid upstrokes. Echocardiography shows a calcified aortic valve with:

Aortic jet velocity (V_{max})	4.2 m/s
Velocity time integral (VTI_{AS})	68 cm
Mean gradient	45 mm Hg
LV outflow tract diameter ($LVOT_D$)	2.1 cm
LVOT velocity (V_{LVOT})	0.9 m/s
Velocity time integral (VTI_{LVOT})	14 cm

The *maximum jet velocity* of 4.2 m/s indicates severe stenosis which is confirmed by calculation of maximum and mean pressure gradients.

Maximum pressure gradient is calculated from maximum aortic jet velocity (V_{max}) as:

$$\Delta P_{max} = 4(V_{max})^2 = 4(4.2)^2 = 71 \text{ mm Hg}$$

Mean pressure gradient is calculated by tracing the outer edge of the CW Doppler velocity curve, with the echo instrument calculating and then averaging instantaneous pressure gradients over the systolic ejection period. The simplified method for estimation of mean gradient is

$$\Delta P = 2.4(V_{max})^2 = 2.4 \ (4.2)^2 = 42 \text{ mm Hg}$$

In order to correct for transvalvular volume flow rate, the velocity ratio and valve area are calculated:

Velocity ratio is $V_{LVOT}/V_{max} = 0.9/4.2 = 0.21$
(dimensionless index)

Aortic valve area is

$$AVA = (CSA_{LVOT} \times VTI_{LVOT})/VTI_{AS\text{-}Jet}$$

Where cross-sectional area (CSA) of the LVOT is

$$CSA_{LVOT} = \pi(LVOT_D/2)^2 = 3.14(2.1/2)^2 = 3.46 \text{ cm}^2$$

Thus $AVA = (3.46 \text{ cm}^2 \times 14 \text{ cm})/68 \text{ cm} = 0.71 \text{ cm}^2$

Simplified formula for valve area is

$$AVA = (CSA_{LVOT} \times V_{LVOT})/V_{max}$$

Thus

$$AVA = (3.46 \text{ cm}^2 \times 0.9 \text{ cm/s})/4.2 \text{ cm/s} = 0.74 \text{ cm}^2$$

This mean gradient (>40 mm Hg), velocity ratio (<0.25) and valve area (<1.0 cm²) are all consistent with severe stenosis.

Quantitation of Aortic Stenosis Severity

Components	Modality	View	Recording	Measurements
LVOT diameter $LVOT_D$	2D	Parasternal long-axis	Adjust depth, optimize endocardial definition, zoom mode	Inner edge to inner edge of LVOT, parallel and adjacent to aortic valve, mid-systole
LVOT flow V_{LVOT} VTI_{LVOT}	Pulsed Doppler	Apical 4-chamber (anteriorly angulated)	Sample volume 2–3 mm, envelope of flow with defined peak, start with sample volume at valve and move apically	Trace modal velocity of spectral velocity curve
AS-Jet V_{max} $VTI_{AS\text{-}Jet}$	CW Doppler	Apical, SSN, other	Examination from multiple windows, careful positioning, and transducer angulation to obtain highest velocity signal	Measure maximum velocities at edge of intense velocity signal

The Echo Exam *Mitral Stenosis*

Valve anatomy	Valve thickness and mobility Calcification Commissural fusion Subvalvular involvement
Stenosis severity	2D valve area Mean pressure gradient Pressure half-time valve area
Left atrium	Size TEE for thrombus pre-valvuloplasty
Co-existing MR	Qualitative evaluation of severity
Pulmonary vasculature	Pulmonary systolic pressure Right ventricular size and function
Other findings	Aortic valve involvement Left ventricular size and systolic function

Example

A 26-year-old pregnant woman presents with dyspnea and is noted to have a diastolic murmur at the apex. Echocardiography shows rheumatic mitral stenosis with:

MVA_{2D} 0.8 cm^2
Mean ΔP 5 mm Hg
$T_{1/2}$ 260 ms

Mitral valve morphology score:
Leaflet thickness   2
Mobility   1
Calcification   1
Subvalvular   2
TOTAL   6

Tricuspid regurgitant jet velocity	3.1 m/s
Estimated RA pressure	10 mm Hg
Mitral regurgitation	Mild

Mean pressure gradient is calculated by tracing the outer edge of the CW Doppler velocity curve, with the echo instrument calculating and then averaging instantaneous pressure gradients over the systolic ejection period.

Doppler mitral valve area ($MVA_{Doppler}$) is calculated as

$$MVA_{Doppler} = 220/T_{1/2} = 220/260 = 0.85 \text{ cm}^2$$

The 2D mitral valve area and the pressure half-time valve area show reasonable agreement and both are consistent with severe mitral stenosis.

Pulmonary artery pressure (PAP) is

$$PAP = 4(V_{TR})^2 + RAP = 4(3.1)^2 + 10 \text{ mm Hg} = 48 \text{ mm Hg.}$$

Pulmonary pressure is moderately elevated consistent with a secondary response to severe mitral stenosis.

The mitral morphology score is low and only mild mitral regurgitation is present indicating a high likelihood of immediate and long-term success with balloon mitral valvuloplasty. A transesophageal echo is needed just before mitral valvuloplasty to evaluate for left atrial thrombus.

Quantitation of Mitral Stenosis Severity

Parameter	Modality	View	Recording	Measurements
2D valve area (MVA_{2D})	2D	Parasternal short-axis	Scan from apex to base to identify minimal valve area	Planimetry of inner edge of dark-light interface
Mean gradient (Mean ΔP)	HPRF Doppler	Apical 4-chamber or long-axis	Align Doppler beam parallel to MS jet. Adjust angle to obtain smooth envelope, clear peak and linear deceleration slope	Trace maximum velocity of spectral velocity curve
Pressure half-time ($T_{1/2}$)	HPRF Doppler	Apical 4-chamber or long-axis	Same as mean gradient. Adjust scale so velocity curve fills the screen. HPRF Doppler often has less noise than CW Doppler signal	Place line from maximum velocity along mid-diastolic linear slope

Classification of Aortic Stenosis Severity

	Mild	Severe
Jet velocity (m/s)	<3.0	>4.0
Mean gradient (mm Hg)	<20	>40
Velocity ratio	>0.50	<0.25
Valve area (cm²)	>1.5	<1.0

Classification of Mitral Stenosis Severity

	Mild	Severe
Mean gradient (mm Hg)	<5	>15
Pulmonary pressure (mmHg)	<30	>60
Valve area (cm²)	>1.5	<1.0

The Echo Exam *Aortic Regurgitation*

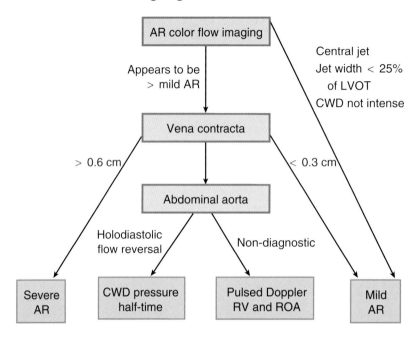

Quantitative Evaluation of Aortic Regurgitant Severity (ASE Guidelines)

Parameter	Mild	Severe
Jet width/LVOT	<25%	≥65%
Vena contracta (cm)	<0.3	>0.6
Pressure half-time (ms)	>500	<200
Regurgitant volume (mL/beat)	<30	≥60
Regurgitant fraction (%)	<30	≥50
Regurgitant orifice area (cm²)	<0.10	≥0.30

Quantitation of Aortic Regurgitation Severity

Parameter	Modality	View	Recording	Measurements
Vena contracta width	Color flow imaging	Parasternal long-axis	Angulate, decrease depth, narrow sector, zoom	Narrowest segment of regurgitant jet between proximal flow convergence and distal jet expansion
Descending aortic diastolic flow reversal	Pulsed Doppler	Subcostal and SSN	Sample volume 2–3 mm, decrease wall filters, adjust scale	Holodiastolic reversal of flow
CW Doppler signal (intensity, slope, VTI)	CW Doppler	Apical	Careful positioning, and transducer angulation to obtain clear signal	Compare signal intensity of retrograde to antegrade flow, measure half time from slope of signal edge
Volume flow at two sites (RV, RF,) ROA	2D and pulsed Doppler	Parasternal (2D) and apical	LVOT diameter and VTI Mitral annulus diameter and VTI	Calculations in example

Etiology	Valve abnormality
	Aortic root disease
Severity of regurgitation	Vena contracta width
	Descending aorta holosystolic flow reversal
	CW Doppler deceleration slope
	Calculation of RV, RF, and ROA
Coexisting aortic stenosis	Aortic jet velocity
Left ventricular response	LV dimensions or volumes
	LV ejection fraction
	dP/dt
Other findings	Aortic coarctation (with bicuspid valve)

Example

A 37-year-old man presents with an asymptomatic diastolic murmur. Echocardiography shows a bicuspid aortic valve with more than mild aortic regurgitation with:

Vena contracta width	5 mm
Descending aorta	Holodiastolic flow reversal in descending thoracic, but not proximal abdominal, aorta
CW Doppler	AR signal less dense than antegrade flow
	Pressure half-time = 400 ms
	VTI_{AR} = 204 cm
LVOT diameter ($LVOT_D$)	2.8 cm
VTI_{LVOT}	24 cm
Mitral annulus diameter	3.1 cm
VTI_{MA}	12 cm

The vena contracta width indicates more than mild aortic regurgitation, but this could be moderate or severe.

Holodiastolic flow reversal in the proximal abdominal aorta would be consistent with severe AR. Flow reversal in the descending thoracic aorta indicates at least moderate AR but is less specific for severe AR.

CW Doppler signal density indicates at least moderate AR and a pressure half-time >200 but <500 ms is also consistent with moderate or severe aortic regurgitation.

Next, regurgitant volume (RV), regurgitant fraction (RF) and regurgitant orifice area (ROA) are calculated.

Using the LVOT and mitral annulus diameters (MA_D), the circular cross-sectional areas of flow are calculated:

$$CSA_{LVOT} = \pi(LVOT_D/2)^2 = 3.14(2.8/2)^2 = 6.2\,cm^2$$

$$CSA_{MA} = \pi(MA_D/2)^2 = 3.14(3.1/2)^2 = 7.5\,cm^2$$

Stroke volume across each valve (cm^3 = ml), then is

$$SV_{LVOT} = (CSA_{LVOT} \times VTI_{LVOT}) = 6.2\,cm^2 \times 24\,cm$$
$$= 149\,cm^3$$

$$SV_{MA} = (CSA_{MA} \times VTI_{MA}) = 7.5\,cm^2 \times 12\,cm = 91\,cm^3$$

Regurgitant volume (RV) is calculated from transaortic flow (TSV, total stroke volume) and transmitral flow (FSV, forward stroke volume), as

$$RV = TSV - FSV = 149\,mL - 91\,mL = 58\,mL$$

Regurgitant fraction (RF) is

$$RF = RSV/TSV \times 100\% = 58\,mL/149\,mL \times 100\% = 39\%$$

Regurgitant orifice area (ROA) is

$$ROA = RSV/VTI_{AR} = 58\,cm^2/204\,cm \times 100\% = 0.28\,cm^2$$

The RV, RF, and ROA all are consistent with moderate (but nearly severe) aortic regurgitation.

The Echo Exam *Mitral Regurgitation*

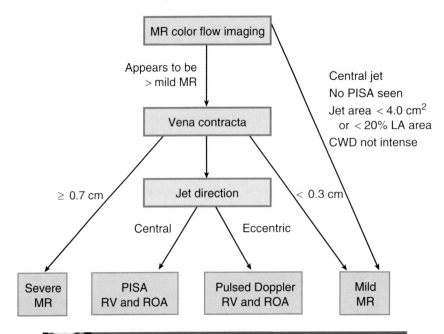

Quantitative Evaluation of Mitral Regurgitant Severity (ASE Guidelines)

Mitral Regurgitation	Mild	Severe
Jet area (cm²)	<4 cm² or <20% LA area	>40% LA area
Vena contracta (cm)	<0.3	≥0.7
Regurgitant volume (mL)	<30	≥60
Regurgitant fraction (%)	<30	≥50
Regurgitant orifice area (cm²)	<0.20	≥0.40

Quantitation of Mitral Regurgitation Severity

Parameter	Modality	View(s)	Recording	Measurements
Vena contracta width	Color flow imaging	Parasternal long-axis	Angulate, decrease depth, narrow sector, zoom	Narrowest segment of regurgitant jet between proximal flow convergence and distal jet expansion
Color flow imaging	Color flow imaging	Parasternal and apical	Narrow sector, decrease depth	Central vs. eccentric, anterior vs. posterior
CW Doppler signal	CW Doppler	Apical	Careful positioning, and transducer angulation to obtain clear signal	Compare signal intensity of retrograde to antegrade flow
Proximal isovelocity surface area	Color flow imaging	A4C or A-long axis	Decrease depth, narrow sector, zoom, adjust aliasing velocity	Adjust aliasing velocity so PISA is hemi-spherical, measure from aliasing boundary to orifice
Volume flow at two sites	2D and pulsed Doppler	Parasternal (2D) and apical	LVOT diameter and VTI Mitral annulus diameter and VTI	See calculations for aortic regurgitation example, with substitution of transmitral flow for TSV and transaortic flow for FSV
Pulmonary vein systolic flow reversal	Pulsed Doppler	A4C on TTE but TEE often needed	Pulmonary vein flow in all four veins	Qualitative; caution in patients in atrial fibrillation

Etiology	Primary valve disease
	Secondary (functional)
Severity of regurgitation	Vena contracta width
	Jet direction (central, eccentric)
	CW Doppler signal
	Calculation of RV, RF, and ROA
	Central jet: PISA method
	Eccentric jet: Volume flow at two sites
	Pulmonary vein flow reversal
Left ventricular response	LV dimensions or volumes
	LV ejection fraction
	dP/dt
Pulmonary vasculature	Pulmonary systolic pressure
	Right ventricular size and systolic function
Other findings	Left atrial size

Example

A 52-year-old man with a dilated cardiomyopathy presents with worsening heart failure symptoms. Echocardiography shows a dilated left ventricle with an ejection fraction of 32% and a central jet of mitral regurgitation with:

Vena contracta width	8 mm
CW Doppler	MR signal as dense as antegrade flow with no evidence for a v wave
	dP/dt =840 mm Hg/s
	Maximum MR velocity = 4.6 m/s
	VTI$_{MR}$ =150 cm
PISA radius	1.0 cm
Aliasing velocity	30 cm/s

Right superior pulmonary vein   Systolic flow reversal

The vena contracta width indicates severe mitral regurgitation.

CW Doppler signal density indicates moderate to severe MR and the absence of a v-wave suggests a chronic disease process. The *dP/dt* is <1000 mm Hg/s consistent with decreased left ventricular contractility.

Color flow indicates a central jet so the proximal isovelocity surface area (PISA) method can be used to quantitate regurgitant severity.

The *proximal isovelocity surface area (PISA)* is calculated from the radius measurement as

$$PISA = 2\pi r^2 = 2\pi(1.0\,cm)^2 = 6.3\,cm^2$$

The maximum *instantaneous regurgitant volume* (RV_{inst}) is calculated from PISA and the aliasing velocity ($V_{aliasing}$) as

$$RV_{inst} = PISA \times V_{aliasing} = 6.3\,cm^2 \times 30\,cm/s = 189\,cm^3/s$$

Maximum regurgitant orifice area (instantaneous) then is calculated from the RV and MR jet velocity (where 4.6 m/s = 460 cm/s)

$$ROA_{max} = RV_{max}/V_{MR} = (189\,cm^3/s)/460\,cm/s = 0.41\,cm^2$$

This ROA is consistent with severe mitral regurgitation.

Regurgitant volume over the systolic flow period can be estimated as

$$RV = ROA \times VTI_{MR} = 0.41\,cm^2 \times 150\,cm = 62\,cm^3 \text{ or ml}$$

This regurgitant volume also is consistent with severe mitral regurgitation.

If the jet is eccentric, quantitation should be performed using transaortic (forward) stroke volume and trans-mitral (total) stroke volume calculations, as illustrated for aortic regurgitation

The Echo Exam *Prosthetic Valves*

Transthoracic Examination

Imaging: Valve leaflet thickness and motion
LV size, wall thickness, and systolic function

Doppler: Antegrade prosthetic valve velocity
Evaluate for stenosis
Search carefully for regurgitation
Pulmonary artery pressures

Transthoracic Doppler Evaluation of Prosthetic Valves

Components	Modality	View	Recording	Measurements
Antegrade flow velocity	Pulsed or CW Doppler	Apical	Antegrade transmitral or transaortic velocity	Peak velocity (compare to normal values for valve type and size)
Measures of valve stenosis	Pulsed and CW Doppler	Apical	Careful positioning to obtain highest velocity signal	Mean gradient Aortic valves: ratio of LVOT to aortic velocity Mitral valve: pressure half-time
Valve regurgitation	Color imaging and CW Doppler	Parasternal apical, SSN	Jet origin, direction, and size on color	Vena contracta width
			CW Doppler of each valve	Intensity of CW Doppler signal
			Pulmonary vein flow	Pulmonary vein systolic flow reversal (MR)
			Descending aorta flow	Descending aorta flow reversal (AR)
Pulmonary pressures	CW Doppler	RV inflow and apical	TR-jet velocity IVC size and variation	Calculate PAP as $4v^2$ of TR jet plus estimated right atrial pressure

Transesophageal Examination

Imaging: Valve leaflet thickness and motion
Examine atrial side of mitral prostheses
LV size, wall thickness, and systolic function

Doppler: Antegrade prosthetic valve velocity
Evaluate for stenosis
Search carefully for regurgitation
Pulmonary artery pressures

Transesophageal Evaluation of Prosthetic Valves

Components	Modality	View	Recording	Limitations
Valve imaging	2D echo	High esophageal	Mitral valve in high esophageal four-chamber view Aortic valve in high esophageal long- and short-axis views	Aortic valve prosthesis may shadow anteior segments of the aortic valve With both aortic and mitral prostheses, the aortic shadow may obscure the mitral prosthesis
Antegrade flow velocity	Pulsed or CW Doppler	High esophageal or transgastric apical	Antegrade transmitral or transaortic velocity	Alignment of Doppler beam with transaortic valve flow may be problematic, compare with TTE data
Measures of valve stenosis	Pulsed and CW Doppler	High esophageal or transgastric apical	Careful positioning to obtain highest velocity signal	Mean gradient Aortic valves: ratio of LVOT to aortic velocity (alignment may be suboptimal) Mitral valve: pressure half-time
Valve regurgitation	Color imaging and CW Doppler	High esophageal with rotational scan	Document origin of jet and proximal flow acceleration, and jet size and direction	Measure vena contracta, record pulmonary venous flow pattern, search carefully for eccentric jets
Pulmonary pressures	CW Doppler	RV inflow and apical	TR-jet velocity IVC size and variation	Calculate PAP as $4v^2$ of TR jet plus estimated right atrial pressure. May be difficult to align Doppler beam parallel to TR jet, correlate with TTE data

Echocardiographic Signs of Prosthetic Valve Dysfunction

Increased antegrade velocity across the valve
Decreased valve area (continuity equation or $T_{1/2}$)
Increased regurgitation on color flow
Increased intensity of continuous-wave Doppler regurgitant signal
Progressive chamber dilation
Persistent left ventricular hypertrophy
Recurrent pulmonary hypertension

Example

A 62-year-old man with a mechanical mitral valve replacement 2 years ago for myxomatous mitral valve disease presents with increasing heart failure symptoms and a systolic murmur. He is in chronic atrial fibrillation.

Transthoracic echocardiography shows:

LA anterior-posterior dimension	5.7 cm
LV dimensions (systole/diastole)	6.2/3.8 cm
Ejection fraction	56%
Transmitral E-velocity	1.8 m/s
Mitral pressure half-time	100 ms
TR jet velocity	3.2 m/s
IVC size and variation	Normal

Color flow imaging shows ghosting and reverberations in the left atrial region but no definite regurgitant jet can be identified. Continuous-wave Doppler shows a mitral regurgitant signal that is incomplete in duration and not as dense as antegrade flow.

This transthoracic study is difficult to interpret without a previous study for comparison. The left atrial and left ventricular dilation and the borderline ejection fraction may be residual from before the valve surgery or could represent progressive changes after valve replacement. Pulmonary artery pressure (PAP) is moderately elevated at

$$PAP = 4(V_{TR})^2 + RAP = 4(3.2)^2 + 10 = 41 + 10$$
$$= 51 \text{ mm Hg}$$

Again, pulmonary hypertension may be residual or recurrent after valve surgery but the presence of pulmonary hypertension suggests the possibility of significant prosthetic mitral regurgitation. Although a clear regurgitant jet is not demonstrated due to shadowing and reverberations from the valve prosthesis, the high antegrade flow velocity with a short pressure half-time and detection of regurgitation with continuous wave Doppler indicate that further evaluation is needed.

Transesophageal echocardiography demonstrates a paravalvular mitral regurgitant jet with a proximal acceleration region seen at the lateral aspect of the annulus, a vena contracta width of 7 mm, and an eccentric jet directed along the posterior-lateral left atrial wall. The left pulmonary veins show definite systolic flow reversal, the right pulmonary veins show blunting of the normal systolic flow pattern. These findings are consistent with severe paraprosthetic regurgitation.

On transesophageal imaging the left ventricle was not well visualized due to shadowing and reverberations from the mitral prosthesis. Although transgastric short-axis views were obtained, ejection fraction could not be calculated. The maximum TR jet obtained on transesophageal echocardiography was 2.9 m/s. Because a higher jet was obtained on transthoracic imaging, the TEE jet most likely underestimates pulmonary pressures.

In summary, this patient has severe paraprosthetic mitral regurgitation with left atrial and left ventricular dilation, moderate pulmonary hypertension, and a borderline ejection fraction. As is typical with prosthetic valves, the combination of transthoracic and transesophageal echocardiography was needed for diagnosis.

The Echo Exam *Endocarditis*

Duke Criteria (Short Version)

Definite endocarditis = 2 major or

1 major + 3 minor or

5 minor criteria

Major criteria = Bacteremia with a typical organism

Echo evidence of endocarditis

Minor criteria = Predisposing condition

Fever

Vascular phenomenon

Immunologic phenomenon

Other microbiologic evidence

Echocardiographic Approach

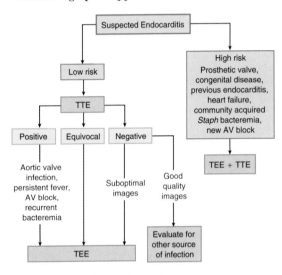

Detection of Valvular Vegetations

Start with standard views

Scan carefully between image planes

Use high-frequency transducer

Optimize image quality

Look for indirect signs (valve regurgitation, echolucent space, etc.)

TEE whenever risk is high or TTE is nondiagnostic

Difficult Issues in Echo Evalation for Endocarditis

Active versus healed vegetation

Nonbacterial thrombotic endocarditis (NBTE)

Abnormal underlying valve anatomy

Prosthetic valve

Detection of abscess

Need for clinical and microbiologic correlation

Example

A 28-year-old man with a bicuspid aortic valve presents with a 2-week history of fever and fatigue. Physical examination shows a blood pressure of 120/40 mm Hg and a harsh diastolic murmur at the left sternal border. Blood cultures (3 sets) are positive for *Streptococcus viridans*. With a predisposing factor, fevers, and positive blood culture results with a typical organism, the pretest likelihood of endocarditis is very high (>90%)

Transthoracic echocardiography shows a bicuspid aortic valve with a mass on the ventricular side of the leaflets with independent motion. LV size and systolic function are normal. Color flow Doppler shows aortic regurgitation with an eccentric jet and a vena contracta width of 7 mm, CW Doppler shows a dense signal with a pressure half time of 120 msec, and there is holodiastolic flow reversal in the proximal abdominal aorta.

The TTE findings are diagnostic for endocarditis so that this patient now has two major Duke critiera and a diagnosis of *definite endocarditis*. With his bicuspid valve, there may have been some degree of underlying regurgitation. However, the normal ventricular size and the short half time of the CW aortic regurgitant jet are consistent with superimposed *acute* aortic regurgitation. Aortic regurgitation is *severe* as evidenced by a wide vena contracta and holodiastolic flow reversal in the aorta.

The following day, a prolonged PR interval (first degree AV block) is noted on the ECG and transesphageal echocardiography is performed. The TEE shows an echolucent area in the aortic annulus region consistent with abscess and the patient is referred for prompt surgical intervention.

The Echo Exam *Cardiac Masses and Source of Embolus*

Structures That May Be Mistaken for an Abnormal Cardiac Mass

Left atrium	Dilated coronary sinus (persistent left superior vena cava)
	Raphe between left superior pulmonary vein and left atrial appendage
	Atrial suture line after cardiac transplant
	Beam-width artifact from calcified aortic valve, aortic valve prosthesis, or other echogenic target adjacent to the atrium
	Interatrial septal aneurysm
Right atrium	Crista terminalis
	Chiari network (Eustachian valve remnants)
	Lipomatous hypertrophy of the interatrial septum
	Trabeculation of right atrial appendage
	Atrial suture line after cardiac transplant
	Pacer wire, Swan-Ganz catheter, or central venous line
Left ventricle	Papillary muscles
	Left ventricular web (aberrant chordae)
	Prominent apical trabeculations
	Prominent mitral annular calcification
Right ventricle	Moderator band
	Papillary muscles
	Swan-Ganz catheter or pacer wire
Aortic valve	Nodules of Arantius
	Lambl's excrescences
	Base of valve leaflet seen *en face* in diastole
Mitral valve	Redundant chordae
	Myxomatous mitral valve tissue
Pulmonary artery	Left atrial appendage (just caudal to pulmonary artery)
Pericardium	Epicardial adipose tissue
	Fibrinous debris in a chronic organized pericardial effusion

Distinguishing Characteristics of Intracardiac Masses

Characteristic	Thrombus	Tumor	Vegetation
Location	LA (especially when enlarged or associated with MV disease)	LA (myxoma) Myocardium Pericardium Valves	Usually valvular Occasionally on ventricular wall or Chiari network
	LV (in setting of reduced systolic function or segmental wall abnormalities)		
Appearance	Usually discrete and somewhat spherical in shape *or* laminated against LV apex or LA wall	Various: may be circumscribed or may be irregular	Irregular shape, attached to the proximal (upstream) side of the valve with motion independent from the valve
Associated findings	Underlying etiology usually evident	Intracardiac obstruction depending on site of tumor	Valvular regurgitation usually present
	LV systolic dysfunction or segmental wall motion abnormalities (exception: eosinophilic heart disease)	Fevers, systemic signs of endocarditis, positive blood cultures	
	MV disease with LA enlargement		

LA, left atrium; MV, mitral valve; LV, left ventricle.

The Echo Exam *Diseases of the Great Vessels*

Examination of the Aorta

Aortic Segment	Modality	View	Recording	Limitations
Proximal aorta	TTE	Parasternal long axis	Images of sinuses of Valsalva, aortic annulus, and sinotubular junction	Shadowing of posterior aorta
	TEE	High esophageal long axis	Standard long-axis plane by rotating to about 120–130°	
Ascending	TTE	Parasternal long axis	Move transducer superiorly to image sinotubular junction and ascending aorta	Only limited segments visualized, variable between patients
	TTE Doppler	Apical	LVOT and ascending aorta flow recorded with pulsed or CW Doppler from an anteriorly angulated four-chamber view	Velocity underestimation if the angle between the Doppler beam and flow is not parallel
	TEE	High esophageal long axis	From long-axis view, move transducer superiorly to image ascending aorta	The distal ascending aorta may not be visualized
Arch	TTE	Suprasternal	Long- and short-axis views of aortic arch	Descending aorta appears to taper as it leaves the image plane
	TEE	High esophageal	From the short-axis view of the initial segment of the descending thoracic aorta, turn the probe toward the patient's right side and angulate inferiorly	View not obtained in all patients. The aortic segment at the junction of the ascending aorta and arch may not be visualized
Descending thoracic	TTE	Parastenal and modified apical views	Rotate from long-axis view to image thoracic aorta in long axis posterior to left ventricle From apical two-chamber view, use lateral angulation and clockwise rotation to image aorta	Depth of thoracic aorta on TTE limits image qualtiy. TEE usually needed for diagnosis
	TTE Doppler	Suprasternal	Descending aorta flow recorded with pulsed Doppler from SSN view	Low wall filters needed to evaluate for holodiastolic flow reversal
Proximal abdominal	TTE	Subcostal	Long axis of proximal abdominal aorta	Only the proximal segment is visualized
	TTE Doppler	Transgastric	Proximal abdominal aorta flow recorded with pulsed Doppler	Low wall filters needed to evaluate for holodiastolic flow reversal
	TEE	Transgastric	From the transgastric position, portions of the abdominal aorta may be seen posteriorly	Does not allow evaluation of entire abdominal aorta

Aortic Dissection

Dissection flap	In aortic lumen	
	Independent motion	
	True and false lumen	
	Entry sites	
	Thrombosis of false lumen	
Intramural hematoma		
Indirect findings	Aortic dilation	
	Aortic regugitation	
	Coronary ostial involvement	
	Pericardial effusion	

Sinus of Valsalva Aneurysm

Congenital	Complex shape
	Protrusion into RVOT
	Fenestrations
Acquired	Infection or inflammation
	Symetric shape
	Communication with aorta
	Potential for rupture

Aortic Atheroma

Complex (≥4 mm or mobile)
Associated with
   Coronary artery disease
   Cerebroembolic events

Complications of Thoracic Aortic Dissection

Aortic valve regurgitation
   Due to aortic dilation
   Due to leaflet flail
Coronary artery occlusion due to dissection at the orifice
   Ventricular fibrillation
   Acute myocardial infarction
Distal vessel obstruction or occlusion
   Carotid (stroke)
   Subclavian (upper limb ischemia)
Aortic rupture
   Into the pericardium
      Pericardial effusion
      Pericardial tamponade
   Into the mediastinum
   Into the pleural space
      Pleural effusion
      Exsanguination

The Echo Exam *Adult Congential Heart Disease*

Categories of Congenital Heart Disease

Congenital Stenotic Lesions

Subvalvular
Valvular
Supravalvular
Peripheral great vessels (aortic coarctation)

Congenital Regurgitant Lesions

Myomatous valve disease
Ebstein's anomaly

Abnormal Intracardiac Communications

Atrial septal defect
Ventricular septal defect
Patent ductus arteriosus

Abnormal Chamber and Great Vessel Connections

Transposition of the Great Arteries
Ventricular inversion (congenitally corrected
  transposition)
Tetralogy of Fallot
Tricuspid Atresia
Truncus Arteriosus

Approach to the Echocardiographic Examination in Adults with Congenital Heart Disease

Before the Examination

Review the clinical history
Obtain details of any prior surgical procedures
Review results of prior diagnostic tests
Formulate specific questions

Sequence of Examination

Identify cardiac chambers, great vessels, and their
  connections
Identify associated defects, and evaluate the physiology
of each lesion
  Regurgitation and/or stenosis (quantitate as per
    Chapters 11 and 12)
  Shunts (calculate Q_p:Q_s)
  Pulmonary hypertension (calcuate pulmonary
    pressure)
  Ventricular dysfunction (measure ejection fraction if
    anatomy allows)

After the Examination

Integrate echo and Doppler findings with clinical data
Summarize findings
Identify which clinical questions remain unanswered, and
suggest appropriate subsequent diagnostic tests

Clues to the Identification of Cardiac Structures in Adults with Congenital Heart Disease

Structure	Anatomic Feature	Echo Approach
Right atrium	Inferior vena cava enters right atrium	Start with subcostal approach to identify RA
Right ventricle	Prominent trabeculation Moderator band Infundibulum Tricuspid valve Apical location of annulus	Apical four-chamber view to compare annular insertions of two ventricles, parasternal for valve anatomy and infundibulum
Pulmonary artery	Bifurcates	Parasternal long-axis view or apical four-chamber view angulated very anteriorly
Left atrium	Pulmonary veins usually enter left atrium	Transesophageal imaging for pulmonary vein anatomy
Left ventricle	Mitral valve Basal location of annulus Fibrous continuity between anterior mitral leaflet and semilunar valve	Apical four-chamber view and parasternal long- and short-axis views
Aorta	Gives rise to aortic arch and arterial branches.	Start with parasternal long-axis view and move transducer superiorly to follow vessel to its branches

Examples

1. A 24-year-old with a history of a cardiac murmur has an echocardiogram which shows:

Right ventricular outflow velocity	1.6 m/s
Pulmonary artery velocity	3.1 m/s
Tricuspid regurgitant jet	3.4 m/s
Estimated right atrial pressure	5 mm Hg (small IVC with normal respiratory variation)

Because the right ventricular outflow velocity is elevated, the maximum pulmonic valve gradient should be calcuated using the proximal velocity in the Bernoulli equation:

$$\Delta P = 4(V^2_{jet} - V^2_{prox})$$
$$\Delta P = 4[(3.1)^2 - (1.6)^2] = 4[9.6 - 2.6] = 28 \text{ mm Hg}$$

If the proximal velocity is not included, the gradient would be overestimated at 38 mm Hg.

Estimated pulmonary systolic pressure is calculated by substracting the pulmonic valve gradient from the estimated right ventricular pressure because pulmonic stenosis is present:

$$PAP = (\Delta P_{RV-RA} + P_{RA}) - \Delta P_{RV-PA}$$
$$PAP = (4V^2_{TR} + P_{RA}) - \Delta P_{RV-PA} = [4(3.4)^2 + 5)] - 28 = 23 \text{ mm Hg}$$

Thus, pulmonary artery systolic pressure is normal even though the triscupid regurgitant jet indicates a right ventricular systolic pressure of 51 mm Hg.

2. A 26-year-old woman undergoes echocardiography for symptoms of decreased exercise tolerance. She is found to have an enlarged right atrium and ventricle with paradoxic septal motion and the following Doppler data:

Right ventricular outflow	
Velocity	1.8 m/s
Velocity-time integral (VTI$_{RVOT}$)	32 cm
Diameter	2.6 cm
Left ventricular outflow	
Velocity	1.1 m/s
Velocity-time integral (VTI$_{LVOT}$)	16 cm
Diameter	2.4 cm

The right heart enlargement suggests an atrial septal defect may be present. The shunt ratio is calculated from the ratio of pulmonary flow (Q_p), measured in the right ventricular outflow tract and systemic flow (Q_s), measured in the left ventricular outflow tract. At each site, cross-sectional area is calcuated as the area of a circle:

$$CSA_{RVOT} = \pi(D/2)^2 = 3.14(2.6/2)^2 = 5.3 \text{ cm}^2$$
$$CSA_{LVOT} = \pi(D/2)^2 = 3.14(2.4/2)^2 = 4.5 \text{ cm}^2$$

Flow (stroke volume) at each site then is calculated:

$$Q_p = CSA_{RVOT} \times VTI_{RVOT} = 5.3 \text{ cm}^2 \times 32 \text{ cm} = 170 \text{ cm}^3$$
$$Q_s = CSA_{LVOT} \times VTI_{LVOT} = 4.5 \text{ cm}^2 \times 16 \text{ cm} = 72 \text{ cm}^3$$
so that $Q_p:Q_s = 170/72 = 2.4$

These calculations are consistent with a significant shunt that most likely will require closure to prevent progressive right heart dysfunction.

INDEX

Note: Page numbers followed by f refer to figures; page numbers followed by t refer to tables.